BEST CHOICES
FROM
THE PEOPLE'S PHARMACY®

What You Need to Know *BEFORE* Your
Next Visit to the Doctor or Drugstore

BEST CHOICES
FROM
THE PEOPLE'S
PHARMACY

- Remedies That Will Surprise You
- Statistics That Will Shock You
- Ratings to Help Assess Your Treatment Options
- Drug Information That Could Save Your Life

JOE GRAEDON, MS, and TERESA GRAEDON, PhD

RODALE

Rodale books may be purchased for business or promotional use or for special sales. For information, please write to: Special Markets Department, Rodale Inc., 733 Third Avenue, New York, NY 10017

Printed in the United States of America

Rodale Inc. makes every effort to use acid-free ∞, recycled paper ♲.

Library of Congress Cataloging-in-Publication Data

Graedon, Joe.
    Best choices from the people's pharmacy : what you need to know before your next visit to the doctor or drugstore / Joe Graedon and Teresa Graedon.
        p.   cm.
    Includes index.
    ISBN-13 978–1–59486–407–0 hardcover
    ISBN-10 1–59486–407–1 hardcover
    1. Pharmacology—Popular works.   2. Drugs—Popular works.   3. Dietary supplements—Popular works.
    4. Consumer education—Popular works.   I. Graedon, Teresa, date   II. Title.
RM301.15.G69   2006
615'.1—dc22   2006028994

Distributed to the book trade by Holtzbrinck Publishers

4 6 8 10 9 7 5   hardcover

LIVE YOUR WHOLE LIFE™

We inspire and enable people to improve their lives and the world around them
For more of our products visit **rodalestore.com** or call 800-848-4735

TO THE MEMORY OF:

TOM FERGUSON, MD

A dear friend, colleague, and coauthor. He shared our goal of providing people with the tools they need to make informed health decisions. Tom had an unshakeable belief in asking people what health information they wanted to know instead of assuming that he knew what they needed. He had a vision of a new paradigm of health care where patients and professionals would collaborate as equals.

His curiosity was limitless and he generated ideas effortlessly. He was never condescending, always caring and compassionate. Tom had a brilliant mind and a gentle soul. We miss his passion, creativity, enthusiasm, and childlike delight in life.

CONTENTS

IMPORTANT NOTE
TO READERS

This book is not a substitute for the medical advice or care of a physician or other health-care professional. The reader must consult a physician in matters relating to his or her health, especially with regard to any signs or symptoms that may require diagnosis or medical attention. Any health problems that do not get better promptly or that get worse should be evaluated by an appropriate clinician and treated properly.

Home remedies are rarely tested in a scientific manner. They should never be used in lieu of suitable medical care. Information about adverse reactions or interactions with herbs, over-the-counter drugs, dietary supplements, or prescription medications is often lacking. The reader should not assume that the herbs, dietary supplements, home remedies, or drugs that are discussed in this book are safe. Every treatment has the potential to cause some side effects for some people.

The summary descriptions of adverse reactions, contraindications, and interactions that are provided with herbs, drugs, dietary supplements, and home remedies are abbreviated and do not represent the entire spectrum of potential problems that could occur. The reader should not assume that because a side effect or interaction is not mentioned in this book, the combination is therefore safe.

If you suspect that you or someone you care for is experiencing an adverse reaction from an herb, drug, dietary supplement, or home remedy, please consult a knowledgeable health professional immediately.

ACKNOWLEDGMENTS

Susan Berg, a patient editor who has helped introduce us to the powerful world of Rodale Books

Andy Eisan, a skilled library researcher who offered invaluable support during the deadline crunch

Alena Graedon, an amazing and creative daughter who helped us organize the sad statin letters for this book

Dave Graedon, a wonderful, kind son who offers steadfast support and comes through no matter what the challenge or the deadline pressure

Kit Gruelle, a loving friend who never fails to cheer us on with chocolate and hugs

Heather Jackson, a magnificent editor and innovator who came up with the idea for this book

Karen Moseley, a sparkling, supportive and superb assistant who has seen us through an interesting series of challenges and keeps us organized

Imogene Poplin, an optimistic assistant with a can-do attitude who has helped handle all our mail efficiently for more years than any of us can believe

Ralph Scallion, MD, a friend and colleague with a brilliant mind and a wonderful sense of humor who tries hard to keep us on the straight and narrow, even if we do like mood rings

Charlotte Sheedy, simply the best literary agent on the planet. We are forever grateful that Tom Ferguson brought us together and that we have worked on so many wonderful projects.

Lyn Siegel, an organized, caring, and creative producer, director, and office manager who successfully handles all the challenges we throw at her

Sybil Sternberg, a joyful and caring helper who has lit up our lives with her smile and her hugs

The listeners of The People's Pharmacy radio show and the readers of *The People's Pharmacy* books and newspaper columns. Your willingness to share your experiences and home remedies have made this book better.

The physicians and pharmacologists who were willing to play our desert island drug and dietary supplement game and share their wit and wisdom with our readers.

PREFACE

When Joe's father, Sid Graedon, said good-bye, he frequently added, "You're on your own." What he meant was that you had to rely on your own resources and common sense to get you through everyday life. Of course, if an emergency or a serious problem arose, he would be the first one there to help. But his sign-off was intended to encourage you to solve day-to-day challenges with creativity and optimism.

When you leave your doctor's office, you're on your own. If there's an emergency, you must act immediately to seek appropriate professional help. But the minor, day-to-day health challenges we all face require common sense, creativity, and some basic information about options. This book is an attempt to provide you with some tips and tools that may help you in that quest.

Our friend and colleague Tom Ferguson, MD, was a pioneer in the self-care movement. Tom firmly believed that well-informed people could be trusted to manage their own health. Tom coined the term *e-patients* to describe individuals who are equipped, enabled, empowered, and engaged in their health and health-care decisions. He envisioned health care as an equal partnership between e-patients and the health professionals and systems that support them. Our goal with this book is to strengthen that partnership by providing you with information that will enable you to work with your health-care professionals and make wise decisions about matters affecting your health.

In April 2006, the Government Accountability Office (GAO) released a devastating assessment of the FDA's drug safety oversight. The GAO—the investigative arm of Congress—studies how the federal government spends your tax dollars. In the case of the FDA, according to the GAO, you're not getting your money's worth. The report concluded that this federal watchdog agency was not doing a good enough job detecting drug safety problems and correcting them. That means you're on your own. Do not expect the FDA to protect you from a medication misadventure such as having a heart attack because you were taking the osteoarthritis drug Vioxx.

It may be comforting to think that someone else is looking out for you, but it is a mistake to delegate to someone else the responsibility for your own health. Too many errors are made in hospitals, pharmacies, and doctors' offices for patients to take health care for granted. According to the Institute of Medicine (IOM), a prestigious arm of the National Academy of Sciences, 1.5 million Americans are harmed each year as a result of medication mistakes. The report, "Preventing Medication Errors," was released in July 2006. It paints a bleak picture of hospital drug prescribing and dispensing: "When all types of errors are taken into account, a hospital patient can expect on average to be subjected to more than one medication error each day."

The IOM report makes several recommendations for reducing potentially deadly drug errors. One of these is for patients and their families to take on more responsibility for monitoring medications to make sure they are getting the appropriate treatment. That is our goal for this book. Your body is more complicated than your computer or your car, and it doesn't come with an owner's manual. You must be vigilant to protect yourself from dangerous drug reactions.

The People's Pharmacy has always sought to alert you to potential problems so you can be prepared. Forewarned is forearmed. For example, you may be shocked by the information in our chapter about generic drugs. Although we have been enthusiastic boosters of generic alternatives to pricey brand-name prescriptions for more than 30 years, we are now concerned about the FDA's ability to monitor their quality. We believe that you must be cautious when choosing generic drugs. Therefore, we give you some practical tips about how to safely save money on medicines. We also share some surprising insights about America's favorite drugs—acid suppressers to control heartburn and statins to lower cholesterol. While such medications do indeed save lives, they also have a darker side that you should be aware of.

You will find a range of options for treating a variety of common problems in this book. Some are simple and inexpensive. They may not always work, but then neither do pricey prescription drugs. In certain cases, well-controlled clinical trials support the use of alternative therapies. Other times, data are lacking. To make the right treatment choice, you will have to gauge how urgent the problem is, what level of risk you are willing to accept, and how much you are willing to pay. Then you will need to discuss all these concerns with your health-care professional.

Joe and Terry Graedon

HOW TO USE THIS BOOK

Our goal in writing this book is to give you a tool that will help you make informed choices about dealing with common health problems. By sharing this information with your physician and other health-care providers, you should be able to tailor your treatment to your special needs.

For more than 30 years, we have been evaluating prescription drugs, over-the-counter medications, dietary supplements, and home remedies. We have received tens of thousands of letters, e-mail messages, and other feedback from people who wanted to share their experiences and concerns with others. Many people prefer to try simple, affordable treatments first. They want the best choice for the money. That's what this book is all about.

You will find a continuum of options, from home remedies to the latest prescription breakthroughs. For underarm sweating, for example, a person might try simply applying milk of magnesia to his or her armpits. This unique approach is far cheaper than getting Botox injections, which do work amazingly well for heavy sweating. One mother wrote to us to say, "My daughter had skin reactions to all the deodorants she tried. The rash and itching were uncomfortable. She didn't like going without a deodorant because of the odor. The milk of magnesia solution you wrote about is both economical and effective."

Another reader shared this experience: "I used tart cherries to cure a gout attack and it worked. The real news is that the pain from osteoarthritis of the hip joint diminished also. I've been able to reduce my use of Celebrex from 400 milligrams per day to 200 milligrams per day and still have less pain." Celebrex (celecoxib) is not only expensive (400 milligrams costs more than $4 per pill), it also has potential side effects.

You will find this kind of story sprinkled throughout this book. We can think of no better way to share the wisdom of our readers than to let you read their stories. These anecdotes are not scientific, but they tell you about someone else's experience. Most of the stories you will read have no names or initials attached to protect people's privacy. Occasionally, we will identify a letter writer if the individual has specifically requested that we do so.

We have also surveyed the medical literature and tried, to the best of our ability, to identify therapies that are effective and the least likely to cause complications. But it is essential to understand that all treatments (both pharmaceutical and nondrug alternatives) have the potential to cause some undesirable effects for some people. That is why you must remain vigilant no matter what treatment you use. Some people develop liver enzyme elevations while taking acetaminophen (Tylenol) for headaches or back pain. Others may experience the same problem when using the Indian spice turmeric to ease their arthritis or psoriasis, or black cohosh to relieve menopausal hot flashes. Many people get diarrhea as a reaction to magnesium taken as a sleep aid. An excellent blood pressure drug like ramipril sometimes causes a life-threatening allergic reaction that makes it hard to breathe.

To use this book effectively, you need to pay attention to your body. Know how it reacts and note how it is responding to whatever treatment you are using. If your symptoms don't get better or they begin to worsen, contact your physician immediately. Use good, common sense. Whenever something doesn't seem quite right, don't ignore the signal. We hope the information you find in the following pages will facilitate your collaborations with your doctor, pharmacist, nurse, and other healthcare professionals.

At the beginning of each condition entry, a box highlights the main approaches used to treat that problem. Some treatments are marked with stars, which represent our evaluation of the particular therapy. To arrive at that rating, we factored in effectiveness, safety, and cost, plus an intangible People's Pharmacy perspective derived from our decades of experience. As with restaurants, five stars (★★★★★) represent our highest rating. Very few treatments merit such a commendation.

Within each condition entry, the approaches that have been awarded stars are summarized briefly in a "thumbnail" box. In it the use, benefits, and downsides of the treatment are described, as well as the approximate cost.

As you read each condition entry, you will find that we tend to start with lower-cost, simpler approaches and work our way up to the most powerful and priciest prescriptions. For example, we discuss the merits of drinking pomegranate juice for heart health before launching into an evaluation of statin-type cholesterol-lowering drugs like Lipitor. For some conditions, of course, the best and most cost-effective approach is a prescription medication.

Each condition entry concludes with a summary of our main recommendations. If you'd like a quick overview of treatments for a particular health concern, begin at the end of the section and browse through the summary. Once you know what the options are, you can select several that make sense for you. Read more about them in the chapter to see if they merit your consideration.

In addition to chapters about specific health conditions, you will find a special chapter called The People's Pharmacy Favorite Picks. This summarizes some of our favorite new home remedies and relates some amazing stories about individuals' experiences with them. We are the first to admit that many of these unique treatments are not backed up with scientific evidence, but over the years we have heard from so many grateful readers that these amusing approaches were helpful that we wanted to share them with you.

Another chapter discusses generic drugs. These less expensive versions of brand-name prescription medications have become a mainstay of cost control in medicine. For decades we promoted the use of generics instead of brand-name prescriptions as a way for patients to save money. You would expect that such drugs would feature prominently in any discussion of best choices. After all, generic drugs usually represent a substantial savings over brand names. Now, however, we are challenging the FDA and the medical establishment on the wisdom of trusting that all generics are of universally high quality. You may be shocked by what you read, but we have also told you how to utilize generic drugs selectively. You will also learn about other strategies for saving money on medicines. Incidentally, whenever you see a number at the end of a sentence in this book, it will lead you to the original research or review. These references to the medical literature can be found at the end of their respective sections. They should allow you and your health-care providers to look up the data for yourselves.

In the appendix is the story of a *People's Pharmacy* radio show listener who developed her own natural approach to control cholesterol. She lowered her "bad" LDL cholesterol by 44 points in 5 weeks and is a role model for what an informed and motivated person can accomplish. We hope you will be inspired by Laura Effel's story.

It should go without saying that this book is in no way intended to substitute for medical advice. But it may tip you off to some possibilities that your physician didn't think to mention. Be sure to discuss the treatment you are considering with him or her to make sure that it is safe for you and compatible with any other medications you may be taking. And never stop taking a prescription drug or change your dosage without medical consultation.

MAKING BEST CHOICES

This book is about choices. Our goal is to help you and your doctor select the most effective and affordable treatments for you and your family. In some cases, this may be a home remedy or a dietary supplement. But in many others, the best option could be a prescription medication.

We all make decisions about where to go for dinner, what movie to see, and which car to buy. Surprisingly, we have more information to help us make these choices wisely than we do about our health-care options.

We can check restaurant or movie reviews from trusted critics or consult *Consumer Reports* magazine for an impartial analysis of the best buys on toasters, mattresses, or automobiles. But where can you find objective information about the best way to treat arthritis, high cholesterol, or migraines?

Once upon a time most people relied primarily on physicians to make the decisions about treating these kinds of conditions. There were relatively few medicines, so doctors could know a lot about the handful they were prescribing. Doctors learned about these drugs in medical school or depended on research published in medical journals. People trusted their doctors to select the best medicine for them.

Now, there are thousands of medications to choose from, and there is no way a physician can master all the information about so many. In addition, the pharmaceutical industry has developed sophisticated strategies to influence doctors' prescribing patterns. Drug companies advertise their prescription drugs directly to you on television and the Web and in magazines and newspapers. They spend almost $5 billion a year trying to get you to "ask your doctor" about one of their products.

Physicians, nurses, pharmacists, and even medical office receptionists are also targets of a full-court press by drug companies. Sales reps routinely provide lunches, dinners, and doodads like pens and notepads in an effort to influence your doctor to prescribe their latest and most expensive medicine. They leave lots of free samples for the doctor to give away. This may seem like a great deal, but after the pills run out, you are stuck paying the bill for what is often a pricey prescription.

These tactics work amazingly well. Patients do ask their doctors for specific medicines that they see advertised, and physicians prescribe them quite often.[5] And physicians are also influenced by drug company marketing.[6] Even their conferences and continuing medical education are often supported by the pharmaceutical industry.[7] That, too, influences prescribing, but does not necessarily lead to the most cost-effective, safest choice for the patient.

PAYING FOR THE FREE LUNCH

- There are more than 100,000 drug sales reps in the United States[1]

- That's one sales rep for every four doctors

- Drug marketing costs $12 billion to $15 billion per year[2]

- That's $8,000 to $15,000 spent on marketing per year per doctor[3]

- 90 percent of continuing medical education materials for physicians are produced by drug companies[4]

DRUG PRICES

Whether or not prescription drug commercials on television actually increase the cost of the medicines, they certainly help these pricey pills sell. Americans are paying more than ever for their medications. We have been tracking prices for 30 years. As you look at the following table, you may be astonished to see that between 1975 and 1985 the cost of some popular prescriptions rose very little. But starting in the 1990s, prices took off. They've been climbing ever since.

PRICE INCREASES OF POPULAR DRUGS

DRUG*	1975	1985	1995	2005
Coumadin (10 mg)	$9.40	$13.85	$86.19	$133.49
Lanoxin (0.25 mg)	$1.00	$3.00	$8.59	$24.69
Lasix (40 mg)	$9.73	$8.95	$19.99	$39.49
Premarin (1.25 mg)	$6.90	$15.95	$46.89	$140.99
Valium (5 mg)	$8.99	$20.30	$62.29	$193.89
*Price is for 100 tablets from chain drugstores.				

Drug companies frequently justify the cost of their pills by citing the expenses of pharmaceutical research and development. All of these drugs were on the market before 1975, however, so their research costs were paid for decades ago. If cars or computers were priced like drugs, we would be paying tens of thousands for a laptop and no one could afford a Buick.

AARP conducted a survey of prescription drug manufacturers' prices and discovered that they have been accelerating for years, dramatically outpacing the overall rate of inflation.[8] Its analysis of 150 popular products shows that price tags on these brand-name drugs rose an average of 35 percent between 1999 and 2004. That's almost three times higher than overall inflation during that time, which amounted to 13.5 percent.[9]

The result of this trend is per-pill prices that take your breath away. The cost of the sleeping pill Ambien (zolpidem), which is advertised directly to consumers, jumped 11.9 percent in 1 year. A month's supply could cost about $100, more than $3 per pill. It's enough to keep you awake at night worrying about how to pay for your prescriptions. But if prescription drug prices give you a headache, beware. One of the most successful migraine medicines, Imitrex (sumatriptan), will cost you nearly $20 a tablet.

HEAD-TO-HEAD

People don't mind paying top dollar if they believe they are getting their money's worth. That's why so many consult *Consumer Reports* magazine when they are trying to decide what microwave oven, digital camera, or cell phone to purchase. Consumers Union makes an effort to test many of the brands buyers are likely to find in their local stores. All equipment is subjected to the same tests, and products are rated on how well they perform. Consumers can choose the product that is most appropriate based on the features that matter most to them. With cars, people can compare models based on cost, reliability, owner satisfaction, safety, and miles per gallon.

When it comes to drugs, however, such

head-to-head comparisons are rare. All a pharmaceutical company needs to do to get FDA approval for a new drug is show that the medicine is better than nothing (a placebo). If a sugar pill relieves headache symptoms for 38 percent of the test subjects and Drug X works for 50 percent, the FDA is likely to give the new compound the green light. That doesn't tell you beans about whether Drug X is better than Drug Y or Z or whether it is more or less likely to cause complications.

When a drug company does spend money for a clinical trial that compares its prized compound to a competing brand, it may be very cautious about how the experiment is conducted. Richard Smith, MD, former editor of the *British Medical Journal,* tells how pharmaceutical companies around the world stack the deck:

> • *Conduct a trial of your drug against a treatment known to be inferior*
> • *Trial your drugs against too low a dose of a competitor drug*
> • *Conduct a trial of your drug against too high a dose of a competitor drug (making your drug seem less toxic)*
> • *Present the results that are most likely to impress*[11]

What all this means is that doctors have a very hard time determining how one medicine stacks up against another, or even against alternative approaches. Is Nexium (esomeprazole) really better than Prilosec (omeprazole) or Prevacid (lansoprazole) for relieving heartburn? Does Zoloft (sertraline) alleviate depression better than Prozac (fluoxetine)? Which one has fewer side effects?

You might not mind paying a lot for the latest blood pressure medicine if it works better than everything else on the market and has the fewest side effects. Unfortunately, in one huge head-to-head trial, that's not how it worked.

Many physicians were shocked when a government-sponsored study (ALLHAT, the Antihypertensive and Lipid-Lowering Treatment to Prevent Heart Attack Trial) showed that an old-fashioned, dirt cheap diuretic outperformed newer and more expensive blood pressure–lowering drugs.[12] This was the largest hypertension study (more than 42,000 patients were enrolled) ever conducted. A 15¢ water pill called chlorthalidone did as well as or better than blood pressure drugs like Norvasc (amlodipine), Zestril (lisinopril), and Cardura (doxazosin) that can cost 10 times as much (Norvasc and Zestril can run more than $1.50 per pill). For the extra money, people got less protection from heart disease, heart failure, and stroke, as well as the possibility of experiencing more serious side effects.

Would you be amazed to learn that chlorthalidone is prescribed infrequently? It isn't even among the "top 300" prescription drugs. In contrast, Norvasc was the number three most-prescribed drug in the United States in 2004, with 30,929,000 prescriptions filled.[13]

Most physicians like to think they practice "evidence-based medicine." That's the catchword for rational medical care based on scientific research. But in this case, it's pretty clear that many doctors have ignored the data from this important head-to-head trial and bowed to the marketing muscle of Big Pharma. Our goal in this book is to let you know about this type of research so you can work with your doctor to get the best treatments for your money.

GETTING RESULTS

We all hope that whatever treatment we use will help us rather than harm us. That's why FDA approval seems so important. It surprises both physicians and patients to learn that many of the medications endorsed by the FDA fall far short of our expectations.

A few years ago, a podiatrist took us to task for suggesting home remedies for nail fungus. He wrote:

❝ *There are real, doctor-prescribed, FDA-approved, clinically tested medications to treat toenail fungus. These include topical Penlac or oral Lamisil or Sporanox. I have successfully treated hundreds of patients with these drugs.*

The unproven treatments you mentioned are little more than urban legends. In 23 years in practice, I have never seen even one patient who has responded favorably to Vicks VapoRub, dilute vinegar soaks, or vitamin E oil. Don't make me waste time dispelling these myths. ❞

Initially we felt chastised. What were we thinking by offering folk wisdom against FDA-approved "real" medicine? Then the mail started pouring in. Dozens of people responded to the podiatrist who had pooh-poohed home remedies. They reported having positive experiences with approaches such as Listerine or dilute vinegar soaks, with applications of Vicks VapoRub or tea tree oil. One pharmacist made the following arguments in our defense:

❝ *I would like to point out some facts about the FDA-approved drugs the podiatrist prefers (Lamisil, Penlac, Sporanox). Does this doctor know that Penlac's success rate for a complete cure, according to the manufacturer's prescribing information, is only 5.5 to 8.5 percent after 48 weeks? When using Sporanox, the percentage of overall success rises to a dizzying 35 percent.*

Also, does he know the costs of these medications? A bottle of Penlac costs $72.99. To reach 48 weeks of treatment once a day to a single affected nail, I conservatively estimate that the patient will need six bottles of the lacquer (one bottle approximately every other *month). So Penlac will cost the patient, without insurance, $437.94 to reach an outstanding 8.5 percent cure rate.*

For Sporanox, one pulse-pak costs $255.99. This is a 14-day supply. The manufacturer recommends 12 weeks of treatment, bringing the patient cost, without insurance, to $1,535.94! No wonder people are looking for alternatives to these medications. **"**

Most consumers have no idea what the actual success rate is for any prescription medication. One industry insider captured headlines when he told a scientific meeting: "The vast majority of drugs—more than 90 percent—only work in 30 or 50 percent of the people." This is a secret that drug companies would just as soon keep under wraps. Allen Roses, MD, worldwide vice president of genetics at GlaxoSmithKline, was discussing the value of genetically targeted therapy in overcoming the limitations of several classes of medicines.[14]

RESPONSE RATES[15]

THERAPEUTIC AREA	DRUG EFFICACY RATE
Alzheimer's disease	30%
Asthma	60%
Depression (SSRI)	62%
Diabetes	57%
Incontinence	40%
Migraine (acute)	52%
Oncology (cancer)	25%

As you can see, selective serotonin reuptake inhibitor (SSRI) antidepressants like Prozac, Paxil (paroxetine), and Zoloft are effective almost two-thirds of the time. When you compare that rate of efficacy to the effectiveness of inactive sugar pills, though, the benefits are surprisingly slim. Placebos generally produce improvement in 30 to 50 percent of depressed patients, so the drugs are just a bit better than the dummy pills. A review (called a meta-analysis) of many antidepressant studies in the *British Medical Journal* concluded that "selective serotonin reuptake inhibitors have no clinically meaningful advantage over placebo" and that "antidepressants have not been convincingly shown to affect the long-term outcome of depression or suicide rates."[16]

In any other business, people would demand better results, especially when they have to pay so much. But patients rarely question their doctors' prescriptions. They mostly assume their medicine has a much better track record than has actually been proven. They may be quite disappointed when they discover that their pricey medicine does not perform as well as they expected. Here's one reader's story:

" *Last year, I spent $1,200 on Lamisil to cure nail fungus. This 3-month program required a prescription, a blood test, and, of course, a visit to the doctor. Despite all this time and money, there was absolutely no improvement in my nails.*

I wrote to the company that makes Lamisil

and asked for some answers. Novartis replied with a form letter saying Lamisil did not necessarily cure nail fungus, and the company did not guarantee the efficacy of the product.

This flippant attitude made me mad. I could have used nothing and saved a great deal of money with the same result."

To add to the complexity, the medicine may cause a serious reaction. But if the doctor doesn't mention risks, a patient might not weigh the danger of side effects. We heard this tragic story from a reader:

"*My husband took Lamisil to treat toenail fungus. The drug worked, but was ultimately responsible for his death.*

The fine print for this prescription drug noted that it might cause neutropenia. For my husband, it did. This led to MDS (myelodysplastic syndrome), which was followed thereafter by AML (acute myeloid leukemia) and his subsequent death.

He had suffered with periodic flare-ups of toenail fungus and athlete's foot for most of his life. Neither of these conditions was life threatening. The Lamisil was!"

WHO'S GUARDING THE CHICKEN COOP?

How could a drug to cure toenail fungus cause a life-threatening blood disorder? Before any medication can be marketed, it has to be proven "safe and effective." We hope you now realize that effectiveness is only relative. Sadly, so is safety. The FDA routinely approves medications that can trigger dangerous, if not deadly, reactions.

The best-known example of this came to light in 2004 when Vioxx (rofecoxib) was taken off the market by the manufacturer. Renowned cardiologist Eric Topol, MD, was provost at the Cleveland Clinic Lerner College of Medicine. In an editorial in the *New England Journal of Medicine,* Dr. Topol estimated that as many as 160,000 people may have suffered heart attacks or strokes while taking Vioxx.[17] FDA safety officer David Graham, MD, estimated that 30,000 to 40,000 people may have died as a consequence.[18]

In Senate hearings, Dr. Graham declared, "I would argue that the FDA as currently configured is incapable of protecting America against another Vioxx. We are virtually defenseless. It is important that this committee and the American people understand that what has happened with Vioxx is really a symptom of something far more dangerous to the safety of the American people. Simply put, FDA and its Center for Drug Evaluation and Research are broken."[19]

More than 20 million people took Vioxx before it was yanked.[20] But tens of millions more have taken Celebrex (celecoxib), Bextra (valdecoxib), and other nonsteroidal anti-inflammatory drugs (NSAIDs) like diclofenac, ibuprofen, and naproxen. A disturbing analysis suggests that these medicines may also increase the risk of cardiovascular complications.[21]

What this means is that the FDA has let us all down. We asked Robert Temple, MD, one of the FDA's most senior scientists, why the agency hadn't detected the problem with Vioxx before Merck took the drug off the market. He admitted that MedWatch, the agency's surveillance system, can't detect common health problems. Instead, it catches unusual things like liver injury or strange blood disorders.[22]

If a drug causes an "ordinary" problem like heart attack, stroke, depression, or cancer, the FDA is unlikely to notice it. Perhaps that is why it took the National Institutes of Health's Women's Health Initiative study to discover that menopausal hormones such as Premarin and Prempro could cause heart attacks, strokes, or breast cancer. Consider that Premarin has been on the market since 1942. It took almost 60 years before physicians and patients were officially alerted to these potentially deadly complications.

The FDA was also slow to pick up on antidepressants' dangers. Prozac was launched in 1987 and within a few years became the most prescribed antidepressant on the market. Despite its popularity, questions began to arise about whether it might trigger suicidal thoughts. Most psychiatrists pooh-poohed this idea, maintaining that depressed people sometimes commit suicide regardless of treatment. The FDA and the manufacturer denied any link between Prozac and suicide. They discounted a 1990 article in the *American Journal of Psychiatry* describing cases of "intense violent suicidal preoccupation after 2 to 7 weeks of fluoxetine [Prozac] treatment."[23] Fifteen years later, on July 1, 2005, the FDA finally warned that "adults being treated with antidepressant medicines, particularly those being treated for depression, should be watched closely for worsening of depression and for increased suicidal thinking or behavior."[24]

The problems with Prozac and Vioxx have received lots of press coverage. One drug that has garnered far less attention is salmeterol. It is one of the most popular prescription asthma medications in the world, found in asthma inhalers such as Advair and Serevent. Although salmeterol has been on the market since 1994, it wasn't until May 2006 that the FDA required the manufacturer "to alert health-care professionals and patients that these medicines may increase the chance of severe asthma episodes, and death when those episodes occur." An analysis published in the *Annals of Internal Medicine* reported that "salmeterol may be responsible for approximately 4,000 of the 5,000 asthma-related deaths that occur in the United States each year."[25] People who use salmeterol for first-line asthma treatment should never stop this drug on their own, but they should check with their physicians to find out more about this controversial issue. Unfortunately, the lesson from these drug disasters is that you have to be extremely vigilant. Doctors rely on the FDA for crucial drug advice. But the feds count on drug companies to supply them with this information. This is like asking the fox to guard the chickens. What's more, once the FDA has approved a medication, the agency may feel a sense of responsibility for it. Admitting that a drug is causing problems, or even killing people, is tough.

BALANCING BENEFITS AGAINST RISKS

The whole point of this book is to help you and your physician weigh the benefits, risks, and costs of various treatments. Choosing the best approach to any given problem depends upon a variety of factors.

A life-threatening condition like cancer justifies drugs that are extremely expensive and highly toxic. But for less dangerous conditions, most people might prefer to start treatment with inexpensive, safer remedies. Just as a family on a tight budget may choose a car based on price and fuel efficiency, an individual without prescription drug insurance might want to consider inexpensive home remedies, over-the-counter treatments, or prescription drugs that are economical. Even folks with insurance may want to control their costs and minimize their risks.

" I assumed toenail fungus was a fact of life for me. It had spread to five or six toenails when I finally saw a dermatologist. The prescribed treatment was costly, and after it began, the dermatologist told me the odds of reinfection after treatment were around 50 percent.

I had a nightmare reaction to the pills a week later. I was in remote Finland, of all unlikely places, when I developed hives and severe itching. After 24 hours of nonstop nonsleep itching, I got through to my doctor and was told to stop taking the pills.

When I got home, I decided to try the vinegar treatment. I applied a drop of distilled white vinegar to my toenails with a cotton swab each time I got out of the shower. As the nails grew out, the fungus was completely gone, along with slight traces of athlete's foot.

Cost: Under $2 over 9 months
Side effects: None
Effectiveness: 100 percent (or 200 percent if you include the athlete's foot)"

How do you know what treatment is best for your condition? Most people assume that doctors have a sophisticated system for selecting the most appropriate medication for their patients. Someday that may be true, especially when genetic testing leads to targeted therapy. But as things currently stand, doctors frequently work by trial and error. They may prescribe a blood pressure medicine and ask you to come back in several weeks to see whether it is doing the job or whether you have experienced intolerable side effects.

In a sense, each prescription is an experiment. Some people may find that Zoloft is miraculous in its ability to relieve depression and allow them to function normally. Others may discover that Zoloft makes them anxious and dizzy, gives them diarrhea and insomnia, or ruins their love life. Because of this incredible variation in individual reactions, doctors cannot predict ahead of time how any given person will respond.

As a result, you'll do better if you are actively involved in this process. No one else can know how you are feeling. The most prescribed drug in the United States is one for pain. Nearly 100 million prescriptions are filled annually for the combination of hydrocodone and acetaminophen. But no one can assess your pain except you. Treatments to alleviate anxiety, depression, and insomnia are also best evaluated by the patient. But even conditions like high blood pressure, diabetes, elevated cholesterol, and thyroid imbalance require you to monitor your progress and give your doctor honest feedback.

If a certain medicine gives you a rash or makes you dizzy, don't just put up with it. Let your doctor know that it may be time to move on and try another option. Clear communication is essential for assessing whether the medicine is doing what it should and whether any side effects that crop up are too difficult to tolerate. According to one study, if patients tell their doctors about drug side effects and if the doctors are attentive and adjust the treatment, many harmful reactions can be avoided. The investigators concluded that nearly 8 million adverse events could be prevented "if patients and their physicians communicated better and if physicians acted more reliably to address medication symptoms."[26]

" *Some time ago, I saw my doctor because of generalized but constant muscle pain unrelated to physical activity. I hurt all over, especially in my calves. Pain remedies had no noticeable effect.*

I really felt I would be an invalid by age 60 if things continued as they were. My doctor did all sorts of tests, including blood work and x-rays, but found nothing definitive. I was in good health though I felt miserable!

He chalked it up to old age (56) and the beginnings of arthritis. I asked him specifically if it could be due to the Lipitor he had prescribed shortly before all this started. He said no, because my liver function tests were normal. It was easy for him to say, but I was finding it difficult to get through a normal day.

I then tried going off the Lipitor, and the pain went away! When I started it again, the pain came back, 2 days later. The doctor switched me to Zocor, but I had the same symptoms. "

We have heard from hundreds of people who have experienced severe, sometimes debilitating muscle pains associated with statin cholesterol-lowering drugs, such as Crestor (rosuvastatin), Lescol (fluvastatin), Lipitor (atorvastatin), Mevacor (lovastatin), Pravachol (pravastatin), and Zocor (simvastatin). Even when blood tests do not show any abnormalities, people can experience muscle or joint pain as well as weakness. Others have reported neuropathy (nerve damage), memory problems, and sexual difficulties. It would be easy for a physician to chalk up such symptoms to "aging." But you don't have to accept that explanation if it doesn't feel right. You need to listen to your body and pay attention when it complains. If lowering your cholesterol means that you can no longer exercise or enjoy an active social life because of pain, it's time to consider some other way to reduce the risk of heart disease.

As crucial as it is to keep track of your progress and report possible side effects to your doctor when you are taking prescription drugs, it is just as important, if not more so, to keep tabs on how you are doing if you are using over-the-counter medications, dietary supplements, or home remedies. Drugs such as Advil and Motrin IB (ibuprofen) and Aleve (naproxen) may carry risks similar to those of their prescription formulations, even though the dosage may be lower. Bleeding gastrointestinal ulcers are a potential complication that puts tens of thousands of people in the hospital each year.

Even natural products like turmeric, the yellow spice in curry powder and yellow mustard, may hold unexpected dangers. Many people have reported their success using turmeric or its active component, curcumin, to relieve arthritis pain or psoriasis. But we have also heard from some who have experienced severe rash and itching, elevated liver enzymes, and even a potentially life-threatening interaction with warfarin (Coumadin).

> *I started taking turmeric after reading that it could help my psoriasis, but I developed a severe rash. I stopped using it last week. The rash is still with me, but my biggest concern developed today.*
>
> *I went for a routine blood test, necessary because I use Coumadin due to a prior lung embolism. My doctor called me 3 hours later to tell me that the number, which should have been between 2 and 3, was at an extremely thin level of 13. I was told to come in immediately for a vitamin K shot. I think your readers should know about this type of reaction.*

Even though turmeric is a natural product commonly used in Indian food, its safety must not be taken for granted. When used as a botanical medicine, it should be treated with the same respect that other drugs get. That goes for any other herb, dietary supplement, or home remedy as well. Because there is always the potential for dangerous interactions between herbs, dietary supplements, and medications, it is essential that you consult a knowledgeable physician before considering any of these approaches.

SAVING MONEY, STAYING SAFE

Skyrocketing drug costs are wrecking everyone's budget. Ask any director of a hospital pharmacy and she will tell you that medicines are breaking the bank. Employers are complaining, state budgets are busted, and if you have to pay for your own prescriptions, you know firsthand how costly your pills are. Even the co-pays are getting outrageously expensive. Some insurance companies and HMOs are now charging a $40 or $50 co-pay for brand-name prescriptions.

Generic drugs are frequently promoted as the best solution to the high cost of prescription medicines. The savings can be dramatic. For example, at the beginning of this chapter, we listed the cost of 100 pills of Valium ($193.89). If you opted for the generic (diazepam) instead, you'd pay less than $20. Who wouldn't choose to take advantage of this kind of a deal? After all, generics are supposed to be identical to their brand-name counterparts.

But how good are they, really? The FDA maintains that generics are excellent. And the insurance companies that have embraced generics trust the FDA to guarantee equivalency. A generic is supposed to get into the bloodstream just like the original innovator drug and work exactly the same in the body.

For decades we agreed and recommended generics. After all, the FDA has stringent guidelines for approval. But we have become concerned that certain drugs may be harder to substitute. And we have heard from hundreds of readers who have astonishing stories to share.

Dilantin versus Phenytoin

My mother went on Dilantin in August 2003. In September she was admitted to a rehab hospital. Her neurologist told them to give her only Dilantin, not a generic substitute.

Later that month, she had four grand mal seizures and was taken to the emergency department at the hospital. When I got there she wasn't expected to make it. The ER doctor told me that he did not think my mom had even had her Dilantin the past few days because her level was so low. The next day I learned she had been given generic phenytoin instead of Dilantin for the last few days. I am convinced that is why she suffered seizures.

This is not the only report we have received about generic phenytoin. Other readers also have complained about having breakthrough seizures when they were switched from Dilantin to the generic. A study published in the journal *Neurology* revealed that several patients who were well controlled on Dilantin experienced seizures that required trips to the emergency room and even hospitalization after they began taking generic phenytoin.[27] After this study was published, the state of Minnesota reversed its rule to automatically switch patients to generic phenytoin.

Phenytoin is not the only drug that worries us. We have received many other complaints about generic drugs such as atenolol (Tenormin), fluoxetine (Prozac), omeprazole (Prilosec), and warfarin (Coumadin). Some drugs are tricky to use. Coumadin, for example, is an anticoagulant that requires careful dosage adjustment and monitoring.

Coumadin versus Warfarin

“I needed surgery for a torn rotator cuff in my shoulder. Before the operation, they found my heart was in atrial fibrillation, so the surgery was postponed until my blood could be thinned to prevent blood clots forming in the heart.

I got a prescription for Coumadin and the pharmacist gave me the generic, warfarin. I took it for a month, but we couldn't get my blood in order. My cardiologist finally checked on exactly what pill I was taking and was shocked to see that it was a generic. He said even though it is supposed to be the same, it is not. As soon as he switched me to real Coumadin, my blood responded and I was able to have the operation.”

Medications like Dilantin and Coumadin are known to have a "narrow therapeutic index." In doctor-speak, that means that there's not much room between too little drug—which undermines effectiveness—and too much drug—which puts people at risk of having a serious toxic reaction. We urge users of such medicines to consider carefully whether the potential savings they get with a generic drug is worth risking a significant health problem.

We have been investigating issues related to generic drugs and the potential dangers of counterfeiting for years. We have interviewed people at the FDA and the USP (United States Pharmacopeia), which sets standards for all prescription and over-the-counter medicines sold in the United States. For more details on this issue and suggestions for how to deal with some of the problems that may be associated with generic substitution, please turn to Generic Drug Quandary on page 15.

EXECUTIVE SUMMARY

By now, you should realize that FDA approval does not necessarily mean that a particular medicine will work for you or that it will be safe. Instead, you need to participate in the decision about what treatment to try and when to move on to something else. In How to Use This Book, on page xvii, there is a description of how you and your doctor can see at a glance what treatments might make sense.

REFERENCES

[1] Japsen, B. "Drug Sales Calls Wear on Doctors." *Chicago Tribune*, May 8, 2005.

[2] Blumenthal, D. "Doctors and Drug Companies." *N. Engl. J. Med.* 2004;351:1885–1890.

[3] Ibid.

[4] ACCME annual report data 2003. Chicago: Accreditation Council for Continuing Medical Education, 2003.

[5] Kravitz, R. L., et al. "Influence of Patients' Requests for Direct-to-Consumer Advertised Antidepressants: A Randomized Controlled Trial." *JAMA* 2005;293:1995–2002.

[6] Spurgeon, D. "Doctors Feel Pressurised by Direct to Consumer Advertising." *BMJ* 1999;391:1321.

[7] Relman, A. "Your Doctor's Drug Problem." *New York Times*, Nov. 18, 2003.

[8] Gross, D. J., et al. "Trends in Manufacturer Prices of Brand Name Prescription Drugs Used by Older Americans, 2000 through 2003." AARP #2004-06.

[9] Gross, D. J., et al. "Trends in Manufacturer Prices of Brand Name Prescription Drugs Used by Older Americans—2004 Year-End Update." AARP Public Policy Institute, April 2005.

[10] Avorn, J. Interview on *The People's Pharmacy* #536, March 26, 2005.

[11] Smith, R. op. cit.

[12] ALLHAT Officers and Coordinators for the ALLHAT Collaborative Research Group. "Major Outcomes in High-Risk Hypertensive Patients Randomized to Angiotensin-Converting Enzyme Inhibitor or Calcium Channel Blocker vs Diuretic: The Antihypertensive and Lipid-Lowering Treatment to Prevent Heart Attack Trial (ALLHAT)." *JAMA* 2002;288:2987–2997.

[13] "Top 200 Brand-Name Drugs by Units in 2004." *Drug Topics: The Online Newsmagazine for Pharmacists*, March 7, 2005.

[14] Connor, S. "Glaxo Chief: Our Drugs Do Not Work on Most Patients." *The Independent/UK*, Dec. 8, 2003.

[15] Ibid.

[16] Moncrieff, J., and Kirsch, I. "Efficacy of Antidepressants in Adults." *BMJ* 2005;331:155–159.

[17] Topol, E. J. "Failing the Public Health—Rofecoxib, Merck, and the FDA." *N. Engl. J. Med.* 2004;351:1707–1709.

[18] Goozner, M. "What Went Wrong? FDA Veteran David Graham Speaks Out on the Drug Safety Dilemma." *AARP Bulletin*, February 2005.

[19] Congressional Testimony of David J. Graham, MD, MPH, before Senate Finance Committee on Vioxx, November 18, 2004.

[20] Martinez, B. "Merck Doctor Likely to Testify in Vioxx Trial." *Wall Street Journal*, July 18, 2005:B1.

[21] Hipisley-Cox, J., and Coupland, C. "Risk of Myocardial Infarction in Patients Taking Cyclo-Oxygenase-2 Inhibitors or Conventional Non-Steroidal Anti-Inflammatory Drugs: Population Based Nested Case-Control Analysis." *BMJ* 2005;330:1366–1373.

[22] Temple, R. Personal Communication, November 18, 2004.

[23] Teicher, M. H., et al. "Emergence of Intense Suicidal Preoccupation During Fluoxetine Treatment." *Am. J. Psychiatry* 1990;147:207–210.

[24] "FDA Reviews Data for Antidepressant Use in Adults." FDA Talk Paper T05-25. July 1, 2005.

[25] Salpeter, S.R., et al. "Meta-Analysis: Effect of Long-Acting ß-Agonists on Severe Asthma Exacerbations and Asthma-Related Deaths." *Ann. Intern. Med.* 2006;144:904–912.

[26] Weingart, S. N., et al. "Patient-Reported Medication Symptoms in Primary Care." *Arch. Intern. Med.* 2005;165:234–240.

[27] Burkhardt, R. T., et al. "Lower Phenytoin Serum Levels in Persons Switched from Brand to Generic Phenytoin." *Neurology* 2004;63:1494–1496.

THE GENERIC DRUG QUANDARY: QUESTIONS ABOUT QUALITY

When most people think about getting the best bang for their prescription buck, generic drugs come immediately to mind. By substituting a generic drug for a brand-name product, it is possible to save hundreds or even thousands of dollars a year. For example, the antidepressant Prozac (fluoxetine) can cost more than $280 for a 1-month supply of 40-milligram pills. The same dose of generic fluoxetine could cost $40 to $60 a month, depending on the manufacturer and the pharmacy. Such savings are breathtaking. Imagine buying a car that was identical in all respects to a brand-new Mercedes-Benz, but at one-fifth the cost. Who wouldn't jump at that deal?

For decades we encouraged our readers and listeners to ask for generic prescriptions whenever possible. But now, we are having second thoughts because we worry about the FDA's ability to monitor the quality of the nation's drug supply. With prices skyrocketing, generic drugs may still represent the best choice in many situations, but you will need to be vigilant to save money without putting your health at risk.

When we started writing about pharmaceuticals back in the mid-1970s, medications were a steal. Americans spent about $11 billion to $12 billion on prescription drugs each year.[1,2] The average prescription in the drugstore cost $4.[3] Thirty years later, annual pharmaceutical sales have soared to roughly $180 billion and the average prescription costs $56.[4] Some of the most popular brand-name medicines, like Lipitor (atorvastatin), Nexium (esomeprazole), Plavix (clopidogrel), and Prevacid (lansoprazole), can easily cost more than $120 a month.

If you think that's a lot, hold on to your hat. People with cancer or rare medical conditions are at the mercy of an industry that has lost all sense of decency. At the time of this writing, Herceptin (trastuzumab), a drug for breast cancer patients, costs $3,200 per month. Avastin (bevacizumab) for colorectal cancer can cost $4,400 per month. Revlimid (lenalidomide), a treatment for multiple myeloma, could cost more than $70,000 per year. And Erbitux (cetuximab) for head and neck or colorectal cancer might exceed $110,000 annually.

Two decades ago we spoke with a drug company insider. This former executive related a top-level meeting in which this question was raised: "If you found a cure for cancer, what would you charge for it?" The executive who was being grilled admitted that they would almost have to give it away. At that time, pharmaceutical leaders feared they would be seen as unethical if they gouged patients for life-saving medicines.

“ How do drug companies decide what to charge? My husband is on chemotherapy and must have two medicines—Mitomycin for the cancer and Zofran to control the nausea. Together they come to over $900 every time he has treatment.

Between the doctor's bills and the medicine it won't be long before our life savings are gone. It is cheaper to lie down and die. ”

Those ethical restraints have disappeared. These days, cancer therapies have become the holy grail for profitability. Many new high-tech compounds don't cure people, but they do extend life. The drugs are more effective and often better tolerated than old-fashioned chemotherapy. A patient who survives an extra 10 years could run up a bill of $1 million.

If you suffer from a rare medical disorder it can be even worse. Cerezyme (imiglucerase) is a bioengineered enzyme for Gaucher disease. People who suffer with this uncommon condition accumulate fatty material in the brain, lungs, spleen, liver, and bone. Untreated, Gaucher's can cause a variety of severe bone and brain problems and even death. Cerezyme costs an average of $200,000 annually per patient. That includes babies and children who need lower doses. Some adults have to spend $600,000 a year to stay alive. That's more than $1,500 a day. No one can afford that kind of drug bill. Even with insurance, families struggle. Those without insurance have to impoverish themselves so they qualify for Medicaid and Medicare benefits.

Talk to a hospital administrator, an insurance company executive, a state treasurer, or an HMO bean counter and they will all tell you that prescription drug expenses are busting their budgets. Or just ask your Aunt Martha or the next-door neighbor about monthly medication bills. If she has diabetes, high blood pressure, elevated cholesterol, allergies, and acid reflux, her monthly bill could top $600.

NEXT-DOOR NEIGHBOR'S MONTHLY DRUG BILL*

Actos (pioglitazone) for diabetes	$188.99
Lipitor (atorvastatin) for high cholesterol	$121.99
Nexium (esomeprazole) for acid reflux	$158.99
Altace (ramipril) for hypertension	$ 55.99
Zyrtec (cetirizine) for allergies	$ 75.99
Total	$601.95
*A hypothetical patient who buys her medicine online from a major national pharmacy chain.	

Anyone without health insurance who is not eligible for Medicare is in deep doo-doo. Even someone with insurance is hardly home free. Co-payments for some prescription medicines are running $40 to $60 per month.

I am middle-aged and self-employed. My medication bills are astronomical. Because I own a modest home and have some retirement funds, I am not eligible for financial assistance.

What do people like me do when our monthly drug bills are in the hundreds of dollars? I empathize with the elderly and the very poor, but I wish you would recognize that those of us in the middle have financial problems too!

Sadly, Medicare Part D is not the stellar solution to pricey prescriptions that so many had hoped for. First, the participant has to pay a $250 deductible each year. Then you pay 25 percent of your prescription costs up to $2,250 (another $500). Don't forget the insurance company premium, which can run $40 or more per month. Once your drug expenses total $2,250, you hit the infamous "donut hole." That's when you will pay 100 percent of your prescription drug costs until you have kicked in an additional $2,850. Once your total yearly drug costs reach $5,100, the government steps in again and pays 95 percent of your bills. Then it starts all over again the following year.

The problem is that the donut hole is huge. Millions of Americans will discover that between their premiums and their monthly drug bills, they won't be able to make ends meet. Most won't make it through the donut hole each year and will be astonished to discover that they are spending up to $4,000 out of their own pocket on prescription medicine. For example, if you pay about $400 a month for your medicine, you will hit the hole sometime around May or June. For the rest of the year you will be responsible for all of your drug bills. By the end of December you will have spent almost, but not quite, the additional $2,850 necessary to emerge from the horrible hole.

GENERIC DRUGS TO THE RESCUE?

Once people sign up for Medicare Part D, many will be encouraged to switch from their physician-preferred brand-name products to less expensive generic alternatives. This will happen because insurance companies want to maximize profits and will create huge financial incentives for patients to buy generics. And once folks find themselves in the donut hole, they will often choose generics to save money themselves. Anyone without insurance will likely opt for generic drugs just to survive. We used to think that was a very good idea.

We have been scrutinizing drug prices carefully for 30 years. When we began this journey we were unabashedly pro-generics. We were swimming against the tide. The overwhelming majority of prescriptions filled in American pharmacies were for brand-name products. In those days, pharmacists and physicians frequently defended branded drugs as being superior in quality and worth every extra dime because they represented an investment in future pharmaceutical development. We were chastised for promoting generics, but we thought they represented a great deal for consumers.

We were highly critical of physicians who refused to write generics prescriptions. Joe even debated an industry spokesman about the generics controversy on *Good Morning America*.

For the next 2 decades we exhorted consumers to buy generics. This seemed like the best way to save money on expensive medications. A beta-blocker heart medicine like Tenormin could cost $50 to $55 for a month's supply, whereas the generic atenolol is only $7 to $8. The prescription heartburn drug Prilosec could cost as much as $155 for 30 pills. The

---

GENERICS RANT IN *THE PEOPLE'S PHARMACY*, 1976

The argument which your doctor will almost always resort to when defending his practice of prescribing expensive brands is that they are superior in quality to the el cheapo generic varieties. Since no one wants a prescription for lousy medicine, this approach usually shuts a patient up pretty fast. By the time the doctor is finished, you will probably apologize for mentioning the subject and end up meekly retreating with your tail between your legs. But does his argument hold water?

Now just so you know which side of the fence I [Joe] am on I am going to make the story crystal clear. If your doctor hands you this tired line, he is fooling you in the worst way. The inequality of drugs routine is usually just plain untrue.[5]

generic equivalent, omeprazole, could run as low as $25 to $35 for the same amount.

What's not to love about generic drugs? Since this book is all about the best choices for the money, you would think that we would once again be promoting generic options whenever possible.

The trouble is that every once in a while we get a letter from a reader of our newspaper column that suggests that all is not as idyllic in generics land as we had believed. At first we discounted such stories as unreliable. We assumed that people had a difficult time assessing the drug's true effectiveness. And frankly, we had invested so much intellectual energy in defending generics for so long that we just could not believe they weren't identical to their brand-name counterparts. The FDA told us repeatedly that generic drugs were held to exactly the same standards as brand-name products. We knew that the feds had very stringent rules for approving generic drugs and we just could not imagine that there could be a problem in Eden.

We began to have doubts about generic drugs several years ago, prompted by a mother who insisted that when she substituted generic methylphenidate for the brand-name Ritalin, it didn't work as well to control her son's attention-deficit/hyperactivity disorder (ADHD). She would send him off to school on the generic drug and he wouldn't perform as well. The teacher complained about his behavior and the mom could see for herself that the methylphenidate was not helping his attention span

or controlling his hyperactivity adequately. When she put him back on Ritalin, his behavior improved and he made it through the day at school with no problems.

When we asked pharmacists about this dilemma, some told us candidly that they too had heard such stories from their customers.

> *I was taking Hytrin to treat an enlarged prostate. When using Hytrin I had no problem urinating, but then the pharmacy substituted generic terazosin.*
>
> *Almost immediately I had trouble. I feel an urgent need to urinate, but the flow is almost nonexistent and does not relieve the pressure on my bladder. With Hytrin, I got up once at night to urinate. With terazosin, it is every hour throughout the night.*
>
> *I can easily understand why the generics are less costly. They aren't worth a tinker's darn.*

Once we took off our rose-colored glasses and began to ask questions, we heard some astonishing reports. One of the first involved thyroid medicine:

> *I have been treated for hypothyroidism for over 30 years, and have been on Synthroid 0.125 milligram for the past 10. This year my doctor wrote the prescription for a generic at the same dose. By the 4th day on the generic, I felt as though I was on the end of a tightly coiled spring. I couldn't sleep; I had a slight case of diarrhea; I was sweating more than usual; and my heart felt*

as though it would pound out of my chest. When I finally realized all this might be due to the change in medication, I had the pharmacist give me Synthroid instead. Almost immediately I calmed down, my heart stopped pounding so hard, and I was back to my normal self. Why should this drug have affected me so?"

The symptoms this person described are classic for an excessive dose of thyroid hormone. We began to wonder what was going on, but we still believed everything was pretty much hunky-dory. Then we heard from someone else: "My mother was switched from Lasix to a generic furosemide for heart failure. Her feet started to swell and she had trouble breathing. As soon as we got her back on Lasix she got better."

And this:

"*Several years ago I was diagnosed with persistent atrial fibrillation. My doctor prescribed Betapace, which controlled the irregular heartbeat beautifully.*

Recently, however, I ran out of my usual mail-in prescription. I got a new prescription from my cardiologist and had it filled at the local pharmacy (a 30-day supply to tide me over).

I did not request the brand name, so the prescription was filled with generic sotalol. Soon my heartbeat became so erratic that I went to see my cardiologist. She had me wear an event monitor for 30 days to see what was happening.

During that time my regular prescription for Betapace arrived, and I switched back from the generic to the brand-name drug. My erratic heartbeat went back to its usual nice steady rhythm almost immediately. When I returned to the doctor, she agreed the whole thing was probably due to the generic substitution."

We still could not believe anything was seriously wrong with generic drugs. We responded lamely to the son concerned about his mother's heart failure symptoms that "any change in medication requires close monitoring." As the stories began accumulating, though, we were gradually beginning to question our steadfast faith in generic drugs' invincibility.

"*I have taken Prozac for approximately 10 years with wonderful results. Approximately 1 to 2 weeks after a recent renewal I was aware that I was feeling withdrawn, depressed, and slightly anxious. My husband and co-workers also noted a change in me. While taking my morning dose, I happened to glance at the label and noticed that I was given the generic equivalent without my knowledge. It seems that my insurance coverage had changed and in order to keep my deductible lower, the generic switch was made.*

I immediately mentioned it to my doctor and pharmacist and had my prescription rewritten. Within several days I was my old self again. My co-payment went up for Prozac but my well-being is too important. I thought generics were acceptable, but now have a change of heart."

Ironically, just as we began to have doubts, everyone else seemed to embrace the lower-cost generics as the solution to high drug costs. The FDA was adamant that generic drugs were identical to their brand-name counterparts. Congress passed legislation to speed approval of generics in anticipation of a tidal wave of blockbuster brand-name drugs that were on the verge of losing patent protection, like the cholesterol-lowering drug Zocor (simvastatin) and the antidepressant Zoloft (sertraline).

Insurance companies and HMOs were doing everything in their power to switch people from pricey brands to generic alternatives. They created three- and four-tier co-payment schedules. If you and your doctor went along with a low-cost generic on the approved drug list, you might be charged only a $5 or $10 co-pay. If your physician selected a brand-name medicine on the formulary, it might cost $25. If she insisted that you needed a brand-name product not on the approved list, you might end up paying $40 to $60.

In some cases insurance companies were so eager for people to switch to low-cost medications that they waived co-payments entirely for 6 months to coax patients into using generics instead of brand-name drugs. It's hardly any wonder they were so excited about generics. In some cases the cost of the generic was less than the actual cost of the co-payment.

❝ *I'm an RN working full-time in a Coumadin clinic. We monitor and adjust the blood thinner Coumadin for over 3,000 patients and I can assure you generics make a difference.*

We had patients who had been in target range literally for years as long as they were on Coumadin. When they started taking generic warfarin we found they needed 20 to 30 percent more drug and were much harder to keep in range.

Those who went back to Coumadin went right back on their previous dose and stayed in target.

Generics may be "equivalent" but in a drug with a narrow therapeutic index they sure are not equal. ❞

THE GENERIC GOOSE CHASE

Eventually our concerns about the quality of generic drugs reached a tipping point. We had heard from so many people that they had experienced therapeutic failure or strange side effects while taking a generic drug that we decided it was time for an investigation. We asked Roger L. Williams, MD, executive vice president and chief executive officer of the United States Pharmacopeia (USP), what he thought about generic drugs. The USP is the organization that has been setting US pharmaceutical standards for more than 185 years, before there even was an FDA.[6] Before taking over the top job at USP, Dr. Williams worked at the FDA (from 1990 to 2000). There, he was deputy director for pharmaceutical science at the Center for Drug Evaluation and Research. He oversaw the division that reviews generic drug approval for the FDA.

Dr. Williams did not reassure us that everything was fine at the FDA. "My position as a clinician/scientist is that FDA could do a better job in controlling the quality of a generic," he said. "A specific flaw: the average criterion used to compare Test (generic) and Reference (pioneer) products doesn't assure switchability."[7]

Yikes! If Dr. Williams thinks the FDA could do a "better job in controlling quality of a generic," then we are in big trouble.

We heard the following from a reader with an insider's perspective:

> *My husband and I worked in the QC [quality control] lab of different drug companies. The FDA may require that drug X be between 90 percent to 110 percent of the stated dose. The companies that I worked for always had tighter limits on their name-brand drugs. The name-brand drug X may have 95 percent to 105 percent of the stated dose. Also the companies had many more tests (hardness and solubility) that the name-brand drugs had to pass.*
>
> *Saying that a generic and a brand name are equivalent is like saying that a teaspoon of granulated sugar and a sugar cube will dissolve the same way in a glass of iced tea. The biochemical use of the generic and brand name is not the same.*
>
> *Most doctors that I have been to do not have any idea that there are differences between the generic and brand name. They are not the same, even though both have passed the required FDA regulations.*

So, what does the FDA have to say about all this? We went straight to the Office of Generic Drugs at the FDA. We talked to Gary Buehler, RPh, director of the Office of Generic Drugs, along with Robert West, RPh, deputy director of the Office of Generic Drugs, and Cecelia Parise, RPh, regulatory policy advisor to the director of the Office of Generic Drugs.[8] These are the folks who oversee the FDA's approval process for generic drugs.

Because of all the reports we had seen from consumers, we asked these FDA staffers how the agency monitors generic drugs once they are approved and out on the market. They told us that they do about 50 to 100 "spot checks" a year. In addition, the FDA is supposed to inspect manufacturing plants every 2 years. They insisted that if there were a problem with a product, they would probably see it.

When we asked where consumers, pharmacists, and physicians could report a problem, their answer was vague: People could contact their local FDA office, something called MedWatch, or the FDA "Office of Compliance." It was clear that there was no consumer-friendly system in place to collect this kind of data.

> *I am a medical assistant for three orthopedic surgeons who do total joint replacements. One of my main duties is to call in refills for pain medication after surgery. Our surgeons specify brand-name medicines like Vicodin and Lortab because some generic substitutions don't relieve patients' pain.*

The next step in our quest for information was to talk to Nicholas Buhay, deputy director of the Division of Manufacturing and Product Quality in the Office of Compliance at the Center for Drug Evaluation and Research at the FDA.[9] We asked Nick about the monitoring process and he told us that the FDA has a program related to ensuring the quality, identity, purity, and strength of these products. He told us that there are about 50 inspectors devoted to the plants making all the generic drug products. He admitted that while the law calls for plants to be inspected every 2 years, there are not enough resources to accomplish that goal, so they have to "prioritize." Some small companies might be inspected only every 3 or 4 years. When we asked how people could report generic drug problems or submit samples for analysis, we once again felt that there was a lack of clarity and no formal process in place.

Finally, we were referred to Jay Schmid, team leader of the Postmarket Surveillance Team in the Division of Prescription Drug Compliance and Surveillance, part of the Office of Compliance at the Center for Drug Evaluation and Research for the FDA.[10] Jay has a total of six people working with him and "a lot of responsibility." We specifically wanted to know how Jay and his group check all the generic drugs that are on the market. He told us that they select about 50 or 60 different drugs (brand and generic) each year for analysis. They get them from a wholesaler in Virginia and send them to a lab in Detroit. Since they use four different lots for each test, that represents about 300 to 400 "finished dosage forms" per year.

> *My husband has been taking Prilosec for several years. Recently our local pharmacy substituted the generic form, omeprazole. He experienced itching on the palms of his hands and developed large raised red patches on his upper arms, thighs, groin, and trunk within a day of taking the generic drug. The reaction went away after he stopped the omeprazole and resumed the Prilosec.*

We came away from our conversations with the FDA frustrated and confused. We had talked to the people at the agency who are in charge of generic approvals and monitoring. They tried hard to convince us that everything is fine and dandy. We even went over their heads and shared some of our most compelling stories with Robert Temple, MD, one of the most senior and powerful FDA officials. He pretty much suggested that patients' perceptions that some generic drugs weren't working well were psychological and could not be related to any possible inferiority of the pills. He summed up the FDA perspective: "We do know these dramatic reports are often not reliable." Our repeated offers to visit the FDA and share these stories and discuss our concerns were met with indifference. We came away with the distinct impression that the FDA preferred to hear, see, and speak no evil about generic drugs.

> "The FD&C [Federal Food, Drug and Cosmetic] Act requires the FDA to inspect all medical manufacturers at least once every 2 years. However, it still appears that the FDA can't even find many of the companies it is supposed to visit."[11]
>
> —David Anast, *Biomedical Market Newsletter,* May 31, 2002

And yet we were left with a nagging suspicion that all was not right. The experiences that our readers were relating were incredibly moving. Then it struck us that the FDA pretty much trusts generic drug companies and the wholesalers who distribute these pills to be honest and play by the rules.

In other industries where safety is at stake and where there may be an incentive to cut corners or cheat, the government takes pains to carry out regular inspections. The Federal Aviation Administration regularly inspects aircraft for defects that might affect passenger safety. Customs inspectors check luggage for plant materials that might carry insect pests or diseases, not to mention checking for other illegal items. New buildings, old elevators, and all restaurants are inspected on a regular basis.

Let's be perfectly honest here. Although staffers have a hard time admitting it, the FDA really relies on the honor system. Inspectors are supposed to visit each drug manufacturing plant every 2 years, but the agency does not have the manpower or resources to accomplish this task. Consequently, several years may pass between visits. Shady operators may not be scrupulous about maintaining standards in the interim.

Most worrisome of all, the FDA's random testing system is a joke. Although a few bottles are selected for analysis each year, they amount to a relative handful. The FDA says it analyzes about 300 "finished dosage forms" annually, including both branded and generic medicines. That represents approximately 0.00001 percent of the 3 billion-plus prescriptions filled in community pharmacies each year. If you thought your chances of getting a speeding ticket were 1 in 10 million, you probably would not worry very much about obeying the speed limit. Compare that to your lifetime risk of being struck by lightning, which is estimated at just 1 in 3,000. If you were a less than honorable generic drug manufacturer or wholesaler, you would not have to worry much about getting caught by the FDA.

THE SMOKING GUN

Many of the letters and e-mail messages we had been reading were somewhat subjective. One person had her high blood pressure under good control for years while taking Zestril. When she was switched to the generic lisinopril, she said, her blood pressure shot up. Someone else who had successfully managed his severe chronic pain for 20 years with Vicodin complained that he got no pain relief and experienced withdrawal symptoms when he was switched to a generic "equivalent" (acetaminophen and hydrocodone). Compelling, yes, but not smoking-gun proof.

What really convinced us that the FDA was not fulfilling its promise to the American public was a seizure story. We received this poignant communication from a reader:

> " My mother went on Dilantin in August 2003. In September she was admitted to a rehab hospital. Her neurologist told them to give her only Dilantin, not a generic substitute.
>
> Later that month, she had four grand mal seizures and was taken to the emergency department at the hospital. When I got there she wasn't expected to make it. The ER doctor told me that he did not think my mom had even had her Dilantin the past few days because her level was so low. The next day I learned she had been given generic phenytoin instead of Dilantin for the last few days. I am convinced that is why she suffered seizures. "

We also were told this:

> " My husband has been taking Dilantin as a seizure preventive for some time with great success. A generic came out that would save him a lot of money, so he tried it and had a seizure. The neurologist made him promise not to do that again. "

We were pretty sure something strange was happening. A man who had been on Dilantin for decades switched to phenytoin and immediately started having seizure activity. It disappeared as soon as he went back on Dilantin. We had received so many similar reports of breakthrough seizures that we could not believe this was imaginary.

Then we found confirmation. Research published in the journal *Neurology* in October 2004 reported on a problem that was noticed in Minnesota soon after the state health plan mandated generic drug substitution.[12] Epileptic patients who had been controlled on Dilantin for years began to have seizures that required urgent clinic or emergency room visits or even hospitalization.

Health-care providers investigated eight patients who suffered serious seizures after being switched from the prescription antiepileptic medicine Dilantin to its generic equivalent, phenytoin. Blood levels dropped by roughly 30 percent when patients took a certain type of generic phenytoin. The researchers concluded that switching patients to generic phenytoin could be penny-wise but pound-foolish. The small cost savings could be wiped out with a single hospitalization.

Once again we contacted the FDA about the cases we had heard about regarding seizures associated with generic phenytoin. We inquired about the Minnesota research and requested a meeting to discuss this critical issue. We also wanted to follow up on many of our other generics concerns. Our request was ignored and we were told that the Dilantin issue was being investigated. We have never heard back about the outcome of the investigation.

Doctors Are Worried, Too

We're not the only ones worried about the quality of generic drugs. Many physicians also share our concerns. A 2006 survey carried out by Medco Health Solutions (a leader in managing prescription drug benefit programs) revealed a surprising lack of confidence in generics: "One quarter of the physicians surveyed stated that they do not believe generic medications to be chemically identical to their branded counterparts." The same survey found that "nearly one in five physicians believes generic drugs are less safe than brand-name medications, and more than one in four doctors (27 percent) believe generic medications will cause more side effects than brands."[13]

COUNTERFEIT DRUGS

Here's a dirty little secret that no one in government is talking about because it's too scary to share with the public: There is no organized system to verify that American drugs are genuine. Pharmaceuticals are now worth so much money that some criminals have discovered that it is easier, safer, and more lucrative to create and peddle counterfeits than to sell heroin or cocaine.

When most people think about counterfeit drugs, they picture some sleazy operator who sells bogus Viagra (sildenafil) from an offshore Web site to gullible victims in America. The FDA has bolstered this belief by warning people not to buy drugs over the Internet. No one imagines that counterfeit medications could be sitting on shelves in American pharmacies. And yet, according to investigative reporter Katherine Eban, "we have rings of counterfeiters who are operating in this country who are infiltrating our drug supply and selling their wares to corrupt wholesalers, who then sell to our retail pharmacies."[14] Eban documented her shocking revelations in the book *Dangerous Doses: How Counterfeiters Are Contaminating America's Drug Supply*.

Although the FDA has tried hard to scare the American public into thinking that Canada is a dangerous place to purchase pharmaceuticals, the truth is that Canadians have a far safer system for distributing drugs than we do in the United States. In Canada there are relatively few wholesalers. These are the middlemen who buy drugs from the drug manufacturers and distribute them to retail pharmacies. Canadian regulators do not allow widespread repackaging. When you get your bottle of pills from a pharmacist in Canada, it usually comes in the original sealed container from the drug company.

In the United States, there are hundreds, perhaps thousands, of wholesalers and repackagers. Huge batches of pills are taken out of big bottles and redistributed into lots of little bottles. Chances are good that most of your medications are in small pill bottles that came from a pharmacy. It is unusual in America to receive original, sealed drug company packaging, especially for generic medications.

Wholesalers in different parts of the country buy and sell from each other in ways that can be hard to track. Your medicine may have been manufactured by a small generics company in Florida, put into the drug distribution system there, shipped to New York, and sold to a hospital, a nursing home, or a repackager. From there the pills might be shipped to California or Louisiana, resold to another wholesaler, and eventually end up on the shelf at your local pharmacy. Rarely is the paper trail (a "pedigree") available, although it is required to assure the quality or origin of the medicine as it passes through this secondary supply chain.

What is astonishing to physicians, pharmacists, and patients is that the federal government has no system for verifying, testing, tracking, or monitoring this gray market. As you have already read, the FDA only analyzes about 1 bottle of pills out of every 10 million sold. Once medications get into the pipeline, they are pretty much home free. States are responsible for cracking down on counterfeit or subpotent pills, but few states have the resources or expertise to really monitor their drug supply. In many cases there may be only a couple of investigators to cover an entire state's drug distribution system.

One state that has taken a leadership role in counterfeit investigation is New York. The state's attorney general, Eliot Spitzer, has been digging into the secondary market to try to unearth how counterfeits get into the supply chain.

Most of the law enforcement attention that has been devoted to counterfeit drugs has focused on high-priced prescriptions. These are drugs like Lipitor (atorvastatin) for cholesterol control, Serostim (somatropin) for AIDS, and Epogen (epoetin alfa), Neupogen (filgrastim), and Procrit (erythropoietin) for blood disorders associated with cancer chemotherapy. What no one knows is whether the counterfeiters have penetrated the generics marketplace. As far as we can tell, investigators have not even bothered to look because they have figured that generic drugs are small potatoes. But this market has become huge, and it is cutthroat. Buyers decide which generics to purchase based almost exclusively on their cost. That creates incentives to cut corners. Raw materials purchased from India, China, or Indonesia may not be up to the same standards as those produced in Germany, France, or the United States.

You would think that drug companies would want to publicize the problems with counterfeits and encourage a crackdown. It turns out that many manufacturers would prefer to keep this problem under wraps.

CONVERSATION WITH JOSEPH BAKER ON *THE PEOPLE'S PHARMACY* **RADIO SHOW**[16]

Joseph Baker*: What we're doing is looking at what's called the secondary wholesale market. And basically that is a kind of gray area, really, in the market for drug distribution. You've got some large distributors that are national. Then you've got local distributors that get drugs from manufacturers or from other distributors and ship them to pharmacies. . . .

Part of the problem is that federal law contains a bit of a loophole that does not require all these distributors to keep a good record of where these drugs are coming from. But the other thing is that there are criminals at large here who are taking advantage of the system and would probably do so even if some of these controls were in place. So we've got to be really vigilant.

A few years ago there was a problem with counterfeit Lipitor entering the system. So it's not only very expensive drugs, but also drugs that many, many Americans now are taking on a daily basis in order to improve their quality of life or their health.

*Joseph Baker is the health-care bureau chief of the New York State Attorney General's office.

SAVING MONEY, STAYING SAFE

So what's a consumer to do? Although we are very concerned about counterfeit drugs and lax FDA monitoring, we do not think you need to give up on all generic drugs just yet. After all, they can represent a savings of 40 to 80 percent over the cost of some brand-name products. And the good news is that the FDA has announced that it has become very concerned about the counterfeit drug problem (though it still believes this is "quite rare within the US drug distribution system").[18] A task force for the agency has called for electronic "track and trace technology" that is supposed to ensure the keeping of a drug "pedigree" from manufacturer to pharmacy. This would provide an electronic chain of custody that could be checked as a medicine moves through the supply chain. In theory, such a system should reduce the risk of counterfeits. We applaud this effort and only hope that it can be implemented as smoothly and quickly as the FDA recommends.

Until we are certain that all generic drugs are identical, patients will have to be extra careful, especially with medications that have what is called a narrow therapeutic index (NTI). That generally means that there is not much difference between a safe dose and a toxic dose. These medications require special vigilance when dosing.

> "It has been very difficult to obtain citable factual information about the extent of the problem of counterfeit drugs. Drug companies keep the information they have strictly confidential. The reason given for this secrecy is that companies are afraid that if it becomes known that one of their products has been counterfeited, people will stop buying it and purchase a competitor's product even after the counterfeit product has been destroyed."[17]
>
> —M. M. Reidenberg and B. A. Conner, *Clinical Pharmacology and Experimental Therapeutics*, 2001

THE GRAEDONS' GUIDE TO NTI DRUGS

GENERIC NAME	BRAND NAME
Amiodarone	Cordarone
Carbamazepine	Tegretol
Clindamycin	Cleocin
Clonidine	Catapres
Cyclosporine	Sandimmune
Digoxin	Lanoxin
Divalproex	Depakote
Ethosuximide	Zarontin
Isoproterenol	Isuprel
Levothyroxine	Synthroid
Lithium	Eskalith, Lithobid
Phenytoin	Dilantin
Prazosin	Minipress
Primidone	Mysoline
Procainamide	Pronestyl
Quinidine gluconate	Quinaglute
Quinidine sulfate	Quinidex
Theophylline	Theo-24, Theolair, Uniphyl
Valproic acid	Depakene
Warfarin	Coumadin

Our standards for classifying NTI drugs are significantly higher than those of many other institutions, but we could easily add dozens more to this list. The guidelines we used are certainly different from those used by many insurance companies, the FDA, and HMOs, none of which believe there is a problem when NTI drugs are dispensed generically. We always believe in erring on the side of caution, however. In our opinion, these medications are safest when they come from a single manufacturer. If you can afford the brand-name drugs or your insurance company will spring for them, we think that is the way to go. If you are forced to select a generic drug because of budgetary constraints or insurance company rules, find out who the generic manufacturer is and try to stick with that one company to avoid possible variation between products.

> *I took 10 milligrams of lisinopril from generics company X for about a year with satisfactory results. Then my local pharmacy closed and I was switched to Eckerd. They filled my prescription with lisinopril from company Y. Within days my blood pressure increased markedly.*
>
> *After a couple of weeks I became suspicious and had Eckerd order and fill my prescription with company X's lisinopril. (I gave the Eckerd pharmacist detailed records of my blood pressure readings immediately proceeding and during the generic switch so he was cooperative.)*
>
> *Shortly after returning to lisinopril from company X, my blood pressure decreased to earlier, acceptable readings.*

Just because your medicine is not on our list of NTI drugs does not necessarily mean a generic is fine for you. We have received way too many letters and e-mail messages relating therapeutic failures or side effects that occurred when someone was switched from a branded product to a generic or from a generic made by one company to another company's knockoff.

GUIDELINES FOR USING GENERIC DRUGS

We have no way to prove that there is anything wrong with the generic drugs that people have written us about. But their stories are so compelling that we cannot ignore them. We do not want you to end up in trouble, the way some folks have, so we have developed some guidelines to help you monitor your progress.

1. **Keep track of your numbers.** If you are taking a medication that involves any kind of quantitative measurement, detail your progress. People with hypertension need to monitor their blood pressure daily. Someone with diabetes should be tracking blood sugar levels just as rigorously. Any changes that are associated with medication switching should alert you to a problem. Consult both your physician and your pharmacist about appropriate solutions.

> *I am a type 2 diabetic on Glucophage and Glucotrol. My fasting blood sugar was hovering*

between 84 to 94 mg/dl every day when I was taking the brand-name medicines.

My health insurance provider decided to save money and switched me to generic drugs. The result was an overnight increase in glucose level to over 140 mg/dl with no change in eating behavior. 99

2. **Keep lab records.** Make sure your physician always provides you with a record of your laboratory results. Track these numbers in a diary or on a computer. Anyone with lipid problems should track cholesterol and triglyceride levels. People taking Coumadin (warfarin) must be scrupulous about monitoring lab values like INR or PT. Those who are hypothyroid should be notified about TSH, T_3, and T_4 readings. Anyone on diuretics should stay on top of potassium and magnesium levels.

3. **Monitor subjective responses.** Some medications affect your body in subtle or not so subtle ways. People who are hypothyroid can monitor their TSH level from a lab test, but they can also tell if their metabolism gets out of whack. Parents can pay attention to children with symptoms of ADHD. Insomniacs can tell how well they are sleeping and people with depression can assess their mood.

4. **Experiment on yourself.** Pay attention to your body! If you suspect that a generic is not performing for you, do an experiment. Keep a detailed diary of your subjective feelings and reactions. If you are taking a medi-

cine for an enlarged prostate, count the number of times you get up to go to the bathroom each night. Then switch back to the brand-name drug. Do this several times and try to determine if there really is a difference. Report your results to your doctor— and never stop taking any medicine without first checking with your doctor.

66 *Ten years ago my doctor put me on a combination of hydrochlorothiazide and Zestril to control my blood pressure. Last year my prescription drug plan switched me to the generic, lisinopril. After taking it for 3 weeks, I started to experience increasingly severe dizziness and finally loss of balance.*

I stopped taking all medication to see if that had caused the problem, and gradually the dizziness subsided and disappeared. I started the Zestril again with good blood pressure readings and no side effects. 99

5. **Monitor side effects.** Keep a careful record of things like dizziness, rash, heartburn, nausea, and diarrhea. If you suspect that a drug switch is responsible for a new adverse reaction, let your physician know promptly.

Generic substitution is not the only problem you have to face. Many insurance companies have restricted drug lists. That means they only pay for one or two medications in a particular class. Contrary to popular belief, not all drugs in a class are created equal. Some people do far better on one medicine than another, even when they are supposedly interchangeable.

Several years ago we heard from a mail carrier about his experience with drug substitution. He had taken Zantac (ranitidine) for years to treat severe heartburn brought on by a hiatal hernia. It kept the condition under control with no side effects. Then his managed care company decided to save money on his prescription by having his doctor switch the prescription to cimetidine (generic Tagamet). In theory, the two drugs work in a similar fashion.

In less than 2 weeks, though, the mailman had developed pancreatic inflammation and was in the intensive care unit of the hospital. He nearly died and needed months to recover. After he was discharged from the hospital, his insurance company still refused to cover Zantac. That is despite the fact that his doctors confirmed that cimetidine had caused the life-threatening complication that had cost the managed care company tens of thousands of dollars. He paid for his next Zantac prescription out of his own pocket.

If you find that you cannot tolerate a generic medication or even an alternative brand, make sure your doctor stands up to the insurance company for you. There should be an appeals process so your doctor can prescribe the best choice for your condition, whether or not it is on the formulary.

6. Report problems to the FDA. Our experience with the FDA has been frustrating to say the least, but that does not mean we should give up. Whenever you suspect that you have experienced a therapeutic failure or any other problem with a generic, report it to MedWatch. Contact the FDA on the Web at www.fda.gov/medwatch or call 888-463-6332.

Gary Buehler, RPh, is director of the Office of Generic Drugs. He has told us that if a generic drug is not performing adequately, it can be analyzed. "We can send the samples to our lab (St. Louis or White Oak) for analysis," he said. "They can perform an analysis for content of active ingredient. If we have enough samples, we can perform other testing (dissolution), but the usual interest is in content of active."

Ask your pharmacist for the name of the manufacturer of your generic product, the lot number, and when it was dispensed. The FDA needs this information for its investigation. Include a short description of what happened (or didn't happen) while you were taking the generic medicine. Send samples to:

Gary Buehler, RPh, Director
Office of Generic Drugs
US Food and Drug Administration
5600 Fishers Lane
Rockville, MD 20857-0001

BUYING MEDICINES ONLINE FROM CANADA

It is illegal to import drugs from Canada or any other country if they are available in the

United States. That said, neither the FDA nor Customs has been enthusiastic about prosecuting grannies for purchasing blood pressure pills or breast cancer medication from outlets in other countries. Many state governments have set up Web sites to facilitate purchasing from north of the border to save their citizens money.

Despite the FDA's disapproval, we believe that the Canadian system is less susceptible to being infiltrated with counterfeit drugs. If you travel north of the border you can verify that you are purchasing from a bona fide pharmacy. If you buy your drugs online, you might get fooled by a pharmacy that claims to be in Canada but is really somewhere else, such as Vanuatu. Keep in mind that generic drugs are generally cheaper in the United States than in Canada, but the quality control may be better north of the border. Brand-name products are usually significantly less expensive in Canada.

To make sure you are dealing with a legitimate Canadian online pharmacy you may wish to follow these guidelines:

- All Canadian pharmacies must be licensed in their province and must post their provincial pharmacy license number on their Web site. Make sure it is there.
- Look for a physical address on the Web site. It should be somewhere in Canada.
- Telephone the Provincial Regulatory Authority to confirm that the license is genuine. You can find the regulators listed online at www.napra.org and www.pharmacists.ca.

- Look for a toll-free number for calls from the United States.
- Use the toll-free number to speak to a customer service representative or pharmacist.
- The pharmacy must require a prescription written by a licensed physician to fill it.
- Make sure the pharmacy requires you to fill out a medical history, including any drug allergies you have and a list of other medicines you are taking.
- The pharmacy must require a signed patient agreement before the order is processed.
- Look for the certification seal of the Canadian International Pharmacy Association (CIPA) on the Web site.
- Don't buy any drugs from e-mail spam or pop-up ads that offer super-low prices or narcotics. There's no telling where they come from.

Here are some Canadian pharmacy Web sites that are legitimate:

www.canadapharmacy.com   800-891-0844
www.canadawaydrugs.com   877-507-3061
www.doctorsolve.com   866-732-0305
www.medicationscanada.com   866-481-5817
www.oneworldrx.com   888-533-9900
www.rxnorth.com   888-700-1119

CONCLUSIONS

Choosing generic drugs can save you a great deal of money, and in some cases the generic prescription may be the best choice for the money. If you can monitor your response by measuring something like blood sugar, cholesterol, blood pressure, or anticoagulant effect, you will be able to tell whether a generic is working as well as the brand-name drug.

Paying attention to your subjective response is also important, particularly when it comes to side effects. If your generic antidepressant doesn't ease your depression, tell your doctor it's not working well for you. If your pain level has increased on a generic analgesic, let your doctor know. Although the honchos at the FDA discount such experiences, we believe that your ability to assess your body's reaction is a valuable tool in helping you and your doctor choose the best treatment for your condition.

If you worry about generic drug quality in the United States or you want to save money on a brand-name product, Canadian pharmacies may be an alternative. In our opinion, quality control there is better than it is in the United States. Buying prescription medicine from Canada makes particular sense for people who do not have insurance to cover drug costs and for Medicare recipients who expect their drug bills to total more than $2,250 but less than $5,100 on medications during the year. Follow the guidelines on the previous pages to avoid taking unnecessary risks when buying online.

10 Tips for Saving Money on Medicine

1. Seek lifestyle remedies whenever possible. Exercise, weight loss, and relaxation techniques may help control blood pressure, cholesterol, anxiety, depression, and insomnia.

2. Consider nondrug alternatives. Home remedies and dietary supplements like the ones we discuss throughout this book may be helpful and far less expensive. Vinegar soaks for nail fungus and athlete's foot or turmeric for joint pain may be surprisingly effective.

3. Ask your pharmacist about nonprescription products. In many cases an over-the-counter drug is less expensive than prescribed medications. The allergy medicine NasalCrom (cromolyn) and the heartburn medicine Prilosec OTC (omeprazole) might help you avoid pricey prescriptions.

4. Ask your MD for the most cost-effective prescription. There may be several medicines for your condition. Your physician may be able to select one that gets the job done affordably. Ask your doctor and pharmacist if it is safe for you to split your pills. In the crazy world of pharmaceuticals, the prices for 5-milligram, 10-milligram, and 20-milligram pills are often similar. Not all tablets can be split safely, however.

5. Find out if you are eligible for free medicine. The pharmaceutical industry maintains a program to help people who are in serious financial need obtain their prescription drugs. To find out if you qualify, you can visit www.helpingpatients.org or call 888-477-2669.

6. Take advantage of the Medicare Part D benefit. If you are eligible, this program makes sense despite the donut hole. As we write this, you pay $750 plus your insurance premiums while Uncle Sam kicks in $1,500 for your first $2,250 in medication bills.

7. Dodge the dastardly donut hole. Once your total medication bill reaches $2,250 for the year, you enter the "donut hole," where you are responsible for 100 percent of your medication costs. If you will probably spend less than $2,850 more for the rest of the year, consider buying from Canada.

8. Be vigilant when considering choosing a generic version of your prescription. As long as your medicine does not have a narrow therapeutic index (see the NTI list on page 29) and you follow our Guidelines for Using Generic Drugs (on page 30), you can save a significant amount.

9. Control your quantity. When starting a new prescription, ask for a free sample to see if the medicine agrees with you and will work. If that is not possible, have the pharmacist dispense a trial dose. Once you know the medicine is right for you, you can save money by buying in bulk. Check big-box pharmacies like Costco for deals.

10. Shop around. Comparison shopping still makes sense. You will discover that prices vary enormously between pharmacies and even among online or mail-order services. One way to compare prices is by going online at www.pharmacychecker.com. When you visit this site and enter your medication, you will see the prices charged by a variety of online drugstores from the United States and other countries. Exercise good judgment about where you buy your prescription medicine.

REFERENCES

[1] Rucker, D. T. "Drug Use Data, Sources, and Limitations." *JAMA* 1971;230:888–890.

[2] "PM's Consumer Expenditure Study Shows HBA Sales $23.2 Billion." *Product Marketing* 31st Annual Edition, July 1978. pp. A–V.

[3] "For the 1st Time 7 Generic Drugs Climb to the Top 50." *Pharmacy Times* 1972;38(4):30–35.

[4] Gebhart, F. "2005 Rx Market: The Highs and Lows." *Drug Topics* 2006;March 20.

[5] Graedon, J. *The People's Pharmacy: A Guide to Prescription Drugs, Home Remedies, and Over-the-Counter Medications.* New York: St. Martin's Press, 1976. p. 293.

[6] "About USP—An Overview: Who We Are." USP Web site, 2006.

[7] Williams, R. L. Personal Communication, August, 6, 2002.

[8] Buehler, G., West, R., and Parise, C. Personal Communication, August 1, 2002.

[9] Buhay, N. Personal Communication, September 13, 2002.

[10] Schmid, J. Personal Communication, November 25, 2002.

[11] Anast, D. "The FDA Doesn't Even Know Who to Regulate." *Biomedical Market Newsletter* May 31, 2002.

[12] Burkhardt, R. T., et al. "Lower Phenytoin Serum Levels in Persons Switched from Brand to Generic Phenytoin." *Neurology* 2004;63:1494–1496.

[13] "Survey Reveals Seven out of 10 Doctors Concerned about Safety of Prescription Medicines: Risk/ Benefit Thinking Supports Generics." Medco Health Solutions, Inc., May 18, 2006.

[14] *The People's Pharmacy* Radio Show, # 557. "Dangerous Doses," broadcast September 24, 2005, with Katherine Eban, Joe Baker, and Cesar Arias.

[15] *The People's Pharmacy* radio show, # 557, broadcast September 24, 2005, with Katherine Eban.

[16] *The People's Pharmacy* radio show, # 557, broadcast September 24, 2005, with Joseph Baker, health-care bureau chief of the New York State Attorney General's Office.

[17] Reidenberg, M. M., and Conner, B. A. "Counterfeit and Substandard Drugs." *Clin. Pharmacol. Exp. Ther.* 2001;69:189–193.

[18] FDA Counterfeit Drug Task Force Report 2006 Update, June 8, 2006.

BEST CHOICES

ACNE

• Avoid sugar and refined carbs and cut back on milk	
• Try an over-the-counter product with benzoyl peroxide	★★★
• Ask your MD about a prescription for clindamycin gel	★★★★
• Apply prescription-strength tretinoin gel	★★★
• Discuss Nicomide-T gel with your doctor	★★★
• Ask your doctor about isotretinoin	★★
• Ask your doctor about photodynamic therapy	★★★

Acne is usually thought of as an adolescent problem, but dermatologists have been treating adults with blemishes for years. The technical term for such outbreaks of pimples is *acne vulgaris*. Common skin bacteria (mostly *Propionibacterium acnes*), the production of oils by the skin, and even the impact of hormones all seem to play a role in determining who gets acne and how severe it will be. When an oil-producing hair follicle becomes plugged up and the bacteria go to work feasting on the fatty acids trapped inside it, the body often reacts with inflammation. That's what makes the pimple so sore and red.

Based on this scenario, there are four ways to tackle the problem of acne: discourage the bacteria, reduce the production of oil, control the hormones, or lower the level of inflammation. In practice, dermatologists mostly focus on bacteria and oil production. But perhaps trying to lower the level of inflammation is more practical than they think.

The Anti-Acne Diet

Dietary recommendations for acne sufferers have a checkered history. Way back when, teen-agers were told to lay off the cheeseburgers and french fries. If they stayed away from high-fat foods like milk shakes and chocolate, they were told, they'd have lovely, clear skin.

We don't know how many kids with acne in the 1960s and 1970s followed that advice, but eventually dermatologists changed their minds. They did some studies and discovered that the amount of fat in the diet didn't seem to correlate very well with the severity of blemishes. So they told their adolescent patients, "Never mind." Diet was not considered a significant risk factor for acne.

Then a few dermatologists began to wonder if that advice was correct. An international team of investigators reported that clinical examination of 1,200 residents of Papua New Guinea (Kitavan Island) and of 115 hunter-gatherers from Paraguay did not turn up a single case of acne.[1] Since 70 to 95 percent of adolescents and approximately half of people more than 26 years of age have facial acne in Westernized societies, the difference was striking. The researchers proposed that diet might play an important role. Specifically, they noted that the native peoples consume a diet composed of low-glycemic-index foods, with a minimum of refined foods, especially refined carbohydrates such as sugar and flour. (Presumably, their diets are also low in the unnatural trans fatty acids as well, since these are equally linked to processed foods.[2]) Perhaps, the scientists hypothesized, this diet that minimizes insulin spikes might also benefit the skin.

● ● ●

Q. My 14-year-old daughter has had moderate acne for nearly 2 years. There are always 5 to 10 small pimples on her forehead, and now she has 10 to 20 pimples on her cheeks as well.

Clearasil left bleach stains on her clothes. Antibiotics the doctor prescribed didn't help and even seemed to make matters worse. The doctor suggested birth control pills, but that is not an option we'd entertain. Are there any natural remedies that might work? What about diet?

A. The purported link between acne and diet is controversial. Teens once were told to avoid chocolate and high-fat foods. That turned out to be unhelpful.

Research published in the *Archives of Dermatology* suggests, however, that diet actually may make a differ-

ence. Populations on low-carb diets that don't make blood sugar rise quickly may be less prone to blemishes. Your daughter might try avoiding foods like candy, cookies, french fries, potato chips, sugar, and white flour to see if it helps her complexion.

● ● ●

Not all dermatologists have welcomed this new look at the possible role of diet. The epidemiological comparison suggesting that diet might be relevant in the development of acne triggered a series of comments under titles such as "Diet and Acne Revisited" and "The Unwelcome Return of the Acne Diet."[3,4,5]

It isn't altogether clear why this development should be so unwelcome. Nutrition science is gradually reaching a consensus that a low-glycemic diet, one with the least amount of trans fats as well as saturated fat, is probably preferable for long-term health in many respects. Such a dietary pattern seems to lower the risk of diabetes and heart disease. Encouraging young people to adopt healthy dietary habits at a time when they would be motivated by the short-term benefit of clearer skin might be a good public health strategy. Most patients seem to think that diet is important in treating acne, and they expect dietary recommendations from their doctors.[6] In the meantime, dermatologists should be conducting research to determine if this dietary hypothesis is solid or if it is as far-out as many doctors think.

Refined carbohydrates and trans fats like margarine might not be the only dietary culprits. A different study reviewed the dietary and dermatological histories of 47,355 female nurses and concluded that the more milk these women drank in adolescence, the more likely they were to have had severe acne as teenagers.[7] The Harvard scientists who conducted this research suggest that hormones and growth factors found in milk might contribute to this problem.

It appears that a good deal more research is needed before there will be a clear answer to the question of whether diet affects acne. In the meantime, motivated acne sufferers can do their own experimentation to find out if including less processed food and less milk in their diet might result in fewer blemishes.

> *My son recently returned from a 5-day camping trip where he didn't have milk or any of his acne medicine. To my surprise, his face looked beautiful. Maybe there's a connection between clear skin and no milk. The dermatologist suggested eliminating milk to see what happens.*

Home Remedies

People have devised a number of potions to put on their faces as home treatments for blemishes. There's really no good evidence that any of them work, but they might be worth a try. We heard from a man who had tried washing his face with milk every day as a teenager and found it helpful. He wasn't able to convince his daughter to try the same approach, though. We haven't seen any evidence that a milk face wash is effective, but it seems like a low-risk adventure. In India, milk is mixed with ground nutmeg and applied to blemishes as a treatment.

Another approach is the clay mask. Versions of this are sold in drugstores and at cosmetics counters. We don't know why it would work, but it has been popular for a long time.

• • •

Q. *I taught pottery at a vocational program in the Dominican Republic some years ago. My teenage students often smeared liquid local clay from our workshop on their faces as a cure for acne. The treatment worked.*

A. We've never seen a scientifically solid study of clay for treating acne. But clearly, clay masks have been used as a complexion aid for centuries. We don't know if American teenagers would be willing to embrace such a treatment, but stranger things have become popular.

• • •

Clay is not the only traditional "poultice" that has been applied to blemishes. We've heard of one home remedy that calls for mixing a teaspoon of powdered nutmeg with a teaspoon of honey and putting it on the zit for 20 minutes.[8] Then it is rinsed off, just as the nutmeg-milk mixture or milk alone would be. Still another variant is to apply a paste of ground cinnamon and honey to the blemishes and leave it on overnight. Whether any of these will actually clear up pimples is a mystery to us. They have not been put to the rigors of scientific study.

One natural product that has been studied is tea tree oil in a 5 percent gel. An Australian study compared a gel composed of an extract of the Australian tree *Melaleuca alternifolia* to a standard over-the-counter (OTC) acne treatment, benzoyl peroxide.[9] The scientists who conducted the 124-patient study wanted to see if the antimicrobial activity of the tea tree product would be useful. They found that although the initial response was slower, the benefits were comparable for noninflamed lesions after 3 months of treatment. Benzoyl peroxide was significantly better at reducing inflamed lesions, but it also produced significantly more undesirable side effects, such as skin dryness, stinging, itching, burning, and redness. If you can't find a water-based tea tree oil gel, look for a cleanser with tea tree oil, which should be readily available. Some people are allergic to tea tree oil, so try a bit on the inside of your forearm first to make sure you don't have a reaction. Watch for redness, itching, or irritation.

Speaking of cleansers, it is a myth that acne is caused by dirt that needs to be scoured off with a harsh or gritty cleanser. Simply washing the face gently each morning and evening with a nondrying cleanser such as Dove, Cetaphil, or CeraVe is recommended. Cosmetics and sunscreens should be noncomedogenic, which means they don't contribute to blackheads. This information should be on the label.

● ● ●

Q. *I am 39 years old and plagued with acne on my chin and neck. The dermatologist has given me topical prescription creams that haven't done much good, and has said my only other choice would be oral antibiotics.*

Recently I started applying Neosporin ointment to the affected areas of my face. The difference is miraculous! I am practically blemish free after only 2 weeks of this treatment. Any blemishes I do get are very small and disappear within a few days of applying the Neosporin. Have you heard of this? My teenager tells me that some of her friends do the same.

A. Neosporin contains the antibacterial ingredients polymyxin B, bacitracin, and neomycin. It is used for first aid to keep minor cuts from becoming infected. Your use of Neosporin is new to us. If you stop getting good results, check back with your doctor. There are a number of other prescription treatments for acne that should help. Some people develop serious skin reactions to neomycin.

• • •

Over-the-Counter Treatment: Benzoyl Peroxide

Benzoyl peroxide is the primary ingredient in most OTC acne treatments. This compound has antimicrobial activity and is usually quite effective for mild acne.

• • •

Q. *My teenage son has a mild case of acne, but to him it is* huge. *He washes with strong cleansers and uses a variety of acne medicines. Can you recommend something that will clear up his skin so he doesn't scrub so much? His face is bright red after all the washing, and I don't think that is good.*

A. You're right! Acne is not caused by dirt, so vigorous washing won't help. It may even make things worse.

OTC benzoyl peroxide (Benzac, Clearasil Acne Treatment, Oxy 5, etc.) should do the job. If not, your son should see a dermatologist. Retin-A (tretinoin) and/or antibiotics can work wonders.

• • •

Benzoyl peroxide is found in a number of different products, from cleansing bars and liquid cleansers to lotions and even shaving creams. Read the instructions on the label and follow them; the procedure varies a little for the different forms. Benzoyl peroxide can dry the skin and cause irritation. If that happens, use it a little less frequently or look for a product with a lower concentration of the ingredient. Some individuals are allergic to benzoyl peroxide and break out in hives or swelling, so try it out on your forearm first to make sure you will not react badly. If you do, you will have to forgo benzoyl peroxide treatment and look for another way to manage your acne.

A few nonprescription acne products contain active ingredients other than benzoyl

★★★ Benzoyl Peroxide

Benzoyl peroxide unplugs pores and discourages the growth of skin bacteria. It is not, however, an antibiotic, and skin bacteria don't seem to develop resistance to it. Follow the instructions on the product label for application and use.

Side effects: Skin irritation, dryness, redness, scaling, and rash

Downside: Acne may worsen initially before improving. Use the product for 6 weeks to 2 months to evaluate its effectiveness.

Cost: Varies, depending on the product; approximately $20 to $30 for a month's worth of gel

peroxide. Resorcinol is generally used in combination with sulfur (Clearasil Adult Care contains them both). Salicylic acid is also found in some OTC acne products. None of these should be used in combination with benzoyl peroxide. All may irritate and dry the skin, and they should not be combined with other products that might irritate the skin.

Prescription Lotions and Gels

If treatment with benzoyl peroxide doesn't get your pimples under control within a couple of months, check with a physician. Dermatologists often prescribe topical antibiotic gels or lotions in addition to or instead of benzoyl peroxide. Erythromycin and clindamycin are old standbys. Because they have been so widely used, however, bacteria have begun to develop resistance to them.[10] As a result, dermatologists have been restricting their use and instead turning to other approaches.

One other medication that is being prescribed is azelaic acid (Azelex, Finevin). Like benzoyl peroxide, this topical treatment seems to keep pores from clogging and to discourage the multiplication and spread of bacteria. It too may result in burning, stinging, redness, or dryness of the skin. In rare instances, dark skin exposed to azelaic acid may develop lighter patches. If you have a cold sore or fever blister that gets worse while you are using an azelaic acid product, notify the prescribing physician immediately.

★★★★ Clindamycin Gel (Cleocin T, Clinda-Derm, Evoclin Topical Foam)

Clindamycin is an antibiotic that can be applied to the skin to fight acne-causing bacteria. It may take 2 months to see significant improvement, but generally this treatment is effective. Other topical antibiotics such as erythromycin gel are also effective.

Some prescription products combine an antibiotic with benzoyl peroxide for greater effectiveness. These include BenzaClin and Duac Gel (clindamycin plus benzoyl peroxide) and Benzamycin (erythromycin plus benzoyl peroxide). These are effective but expensive because no generic equivalents are available.

Side effects: Itching, burning, dryness, and peeling. A rare but very serious and dangerous side effect of clindamycin that is extremely unlikely to occur but still possible with the topical form is pseudomembranous colitis. Notify your doctor *immediately* if you develop persistent or bloody diarrhea.

Downside: Skin bacteria (*P. acnes*) are beginning to develop resistance to topical clindamycin.

Cost: Approximately $50 for a 60-gram tube

★★★ Tretinoin Gel (Retin-A)

Retin-A speeds up cell turnover and normalizes the lower levels of the skin. With 6 weeks or more of treatment, it is frequently very helpful against acne.

Side effects: Stinging, dryness, redness, flaking, and irritation

Downside: Retin-A makes skin more sensitive to sunburn and sun damage, so stay out of the sun and use effective protection against ultraviolet rays.

Cost: $35 to $50 for 15 grams

Tretinoin or a similar compound in the vitamin A family can be very effective in treating acne and reducing the inflammation associated with severe acne. Using topical vitamin A–like compounds (retinoids) early in the course of acne lessens the likelihood of scarring, a complication of the condition. Some doctors prescribe tretinoin together with benzoyl peroxide or with an oral antibiotic such as doxycycline to clear the skin faster. Because it works on the deeper cellular layers of the skin and speeds up cell turnover, it can also bring pimples to the surface more quickly. This means that acne may seem to be getting worse at first rather than better, but with patience the condition should clear up. Tretinoin is also used to smooth out wrinkles due to sun damage.

There is another prescription gel or cream that is based on a vitamin. Nicomide-T gel or cream contains nicotinamide, a form of niacin. Like Retin-A, it is topical but not an antibiotic, so theoretically bacteria should not develop resistance to it. A preliminary study showed that Nicomide-T gel is as effective as clindamycin gel in reducing blemishes.[11] Other research confirmed that it can protect the skin and is less likely to dry it than a number of other acne treatments.[12, 13] It is not clear whether Nicomide-T is as effective as Retin-A, though some studies conducted by the manufacturer, Sirius Laboratories, suggest that adding it to other treatments boosts the effectiveness of both.

Prescription Pills for Acne

When topical antibiotics don't do the job, dermatologists may prescribe oral medication to get the antibiotic into the bloodstream rather

★★★ Nicomide-T

This topical treatment has been flying under the radar for years. Some dermatologists tell us that it should have anti-inflammatory action and may be better tolerated than benzoyl peroxide.

Side effects: Redness, dryness, and burning

Downside: Hard to find, although it is available from many online pharmacies. May take several weeks to work. Physicians and pharmacists seem unaware of its effectiveness, and studies are few.

Cost: Approximately $30 for a 30-gram tube

than just on the surface of the skin. Tetracycline and clindamycin have been widely prescribed, but some acne-causing bacteria have developed resistance to them. Now, dermatologists may be more likely to prescribe minocycline. Although this antibiotic works against acne, it is not clear that it is either more effective than other oral antibiotics or less likely to cause undesirable reactions.[14]

Anyone who is prescribed oral antibiotics needs to know when to take them and whether they should delay taking other treatments, such as supplements or antacids. Patients should discuss all the pros and cons of oral (*systemic*) antibiotic therapy with the doctor prescribing it. Certain drugs may cause rare but potentially serious side effects, such as the pseudomembranous colitis that is sometimes seen with clindamycin.

One study found that people using antibiotics (oral or topical) to treat their acne were about twice as likely to come down with an upper respiratory tract infection.[15] Colds, flus, and similar upper respiratory tract infections are usually self-limited and rarely a serious threat to health, but it makes sense to evaluate whether the acne is in fact affecting your life so much that you'd be willing to trade it for a cold. It might not make sense to take an antibiotic for mild acne that is not too bothersome.

After completing a course of antibiotic treatment, acne patients may be able to keep their skin clear by using tretinoin gel or a similar product.[16] Adapalene or tazarotene gel may also be useful.[17] Using such a topical medicine as follow-up therapy can reduce the amount of antibiotic exposure.

Hormone Treatment

Because hormones, especially androgens like testosterone, play a role in acne, changing the balance of these natural compounds in the body can be helpful in some cases. Many young women benefit from taking birth control pills for their acne. This treatment stops the hormone surges and also probably reduces the amount of testosterone that is available to stimulate oil-producing hair follicles and make mischief. Keep in mind, though, that young women who take oral contraceptives for an extended period may have a lowered libido for quite a long time after discontinuing the treatment.[18] (Parents of teenagers may not consider this a negative factor, but it can be very troublesome for a woman in her twenties or thirties.)

• • •

Q. *You had a question about a teenage girl with acne. Nothing the dermatologist prescribed had worked, and her mother refused to consider birth control pills for her.*

My heart goes out to her. I too have suffered with acne my whole life, starting when I was 10 years old. I am now 35.

My parents took me to dermatologists who prescribed pills and creams;

we changed my diet; we tried sun expo-sure and no sun exposure. They kept trying because they knew my self-esteem was suffering. Acne makes you feel ugly.

At the age of 16 I saw a gynecologist who suggested birth control pills. I was raised a strict Irish-Catholic, but Mom was open to anything that might help me. Within 2 months of starting birth control pills, my skin was considerably better!

I am one of those people whose body loves the pills. As soon as I stop taking them, my skin starts to break out. I hope my experience will help convince that mother that birth control pills could be the magic she wants for her daughter.

A. When all else fails, birth control pills can be helpful. The hormones counter-act testosterone. Yes, young women make this male hormone too. Not every woman tolerates oral contraceptives as well as you do, but doctors frequently prescribe them for hard-to-treat acne.

● ● ●

A dermatologist may also prescribe a very old-fashioned blood pressure drug called spironolactone by itself or in combination with birth control pills. This is an "off label" use of spironolactone, but one with quite a long history. Spironolactone seems to help reduce the action of testosterone or other androgen hormones. That may explain why it is also used to treat women who have excessive facial hair (hirsutism). The dose that dermatologists use for acne is usually one-fourth that used for hirsutism.

Spironolactone is a potassium-preserving diuretic and must not be combined with potassium supplements or other potassium-preserving medications. In addition, spironolactone carries a black-box warning in its prescribing information that tells doctors in the strongest way possible that this drug causes cancer in animal studies. Generally, therefore, physicians prescribe it only for a limited time. Women are urged not to become pregnant while on this medicine. When it is used in combination with oral contraceptives, that shouldn't be as much of a concern.

Isotretinoin

Dermatologists have one last big gun, a powerful medicine to use in desperate cases when nothing else has worked. Isotretinoin has stirred a lot of emotions—from excitement to fear—because it is so effective but also has some extremely serious side effects. This drug is approved for severe cystic acne, and it really should be reserved for acne that is not responding to other treatments.

From the time of its introduction, the maker of Accutane strove to get across the point that this drug can cause birth defects. Women who take this medication must not get pregnant while they are on the drug or for sev-

★★ Isotretinoin (Accutane, Amnesteem, Claravis, Sotret)

Isotretinoin is chemically related to vitamin A, so it controls cell division. Four to 5 months of treatment usually results in significant clearing of acne, sometimes lasting years.

Common side effects: Dry lips and mouth; dry, crusty skin; upset stomach; hair loss; nosebleed; sun sensitivity; elevated cholesterol; and reduced night vision

Serious side effects: Birth defects; depression, potentially leading to suicidal thoughts or behaviors; inflammation of the pancreas; pressure on the brain (pseudotumor cerebri) causing severe headache

Downside: Despite efforts to keep this drug away from pregnant women, each year some babies are exposed in utero and born with birth defects. Women *must* use two different and effective means of contraception throughout the time they are taking isotretinoin.

Cost: Varies widely from about $100 to $400 for 1 month of treatment

eral months after stopping it. (The compound stays in the body for a while.) Nonetheless, the manufacturer's warnings have not been enough. Every year some women on isotretinoin do conceive, despite all the precautions. As a result, the FDA and the manufacturer have limited the access to this medicine. To prescribe it, a dermatologist must have enrolled in the iPLEDGE program, which educates physicians about the drug. Patients are also required to enroll in the iPLEDGE program and view the educational DVD before taking the first dose. The program uses telephone- and computer-based tracking to verify that female patients are getting regular pregnancy tests to ensure that they do not take this medication during pregnancy. Patients who do not enroll in the program cannot get their prescriptions filled. More information is available online at www.ipledgeprogram.com.

• • •

Q. *I have been on Accutane to treat bad acne for almost a month. I have taken 26 tablets, but stopped taking it when I thought I might be pregnant.*

I found out yesterday that I am indeed pregnant, and I am scared. I want to have this baby, but after reading about the drug causing birth defects, I am not sure. What should I do?

A. We were shocked to learn that you have become pregnant while taking Accutane. This acne medicine can cause very serious birth defects in a fetus.

That is why the manufacturer recommends every woman have a pregnancy test before she starts on this drug and use effective contraception throughout therapy. Every time a pill is removed from its packaging, a symbol reminds the patient not to take this drug during pregnancy.

Please discuss this serious matter with your physician and your partner. The drug company can provide further information about your odds of having a baby with severe health problems.

• • •

Blue Light Photodynamic Therapy

The latest thing in acne treatment is the Dusa Blue Light. The FDA initially approved this therapy for treating precancerous skin lesions called *actinic keratoses*. The approach utilizes a special photosensitizing chemical, aminolevulinic acid (Levulan Kerastick), that is applied to the skin for 30 to 40 minutes. It is then rinsed off and the patient sits in front of the Dusa Blue Light for 8 to 12 minutes. This special fluorescent tube emits a narrow band of blue light (417-nanometer wavelength). It is not a laser. It looks like an ordinary fluorescent light.

This photodynamic therapy reverses precancerous damage to the skin and also seems to undo some of the effects of long-term sun exposure. In addition, this treatment appears to change the hair follicle and make the environment inhospitable for acne-causing bacteria. Dermatologists who adopted the Blue Light early on seem quite enthusiastic about its use for hard-to-treat acne. There is also a hint that it may help "rejuvenate" skin by reducing wrinkles and improving skin texture.

★★★ Dusa Blue Light

For people with precancerous skin lesions or severe acne, the Blue Light may be a valuable tool. The skin may look worse for a few days, but within a week or two the acne should clear up significantly. Results may last several months.

This photodynamic therapy requires a two-step process: First a photosensitizing chemical (Levulan Kerastick) is applied to the skin and then removed. Then the skin is exposed to the special light.

Side effects: Crusting, stinging, and redness

Downside: Cannot be used if you have active cold sores (herpes simplex) or warts, if you've recently had chemotherapy, or if you are pregnant. People who have used isotretinoin within the last year may not be able to undergo Blue Light therapy. Stay out of the sun and avoid fluorescent light exposure for a couple of days after treatment.

Cost: Varies according to the practitioner. Some plastic surgeons charge $500 to $1,000 for a series of treatments.

Conclusions

Blemishes are a common part of adolescence, but they also trouble many people well into adulthood. Changes in hormone levels seem to aggravate acne. Most treatments are aimed at killing or slowing down bacteria that are commonly present on and in the skin, and this usually works well until or unless the bacteria develop resistance. Stress seems to make acne worse (which is why college students have more zits during the week of final exams), but given the fact that stress is so hard to avoid, almost no treatments focus on controlling it. There are many approaches to acne treatment; if self-care does not prove effective, a dermatologist should be able to prescribe a therapy that will help.

• Change your diet. A low-glycemic-index diet with very little sugar and other refined carbohydrates might improve skin significantly, and it will have other health benefits as well. Other things to avoid: milk and trans fatty acids, which are found in margarine and shortening. A study of dairy products and acne is currently under way.

• Facial masks of clay may remove excess oil and help clear the skin. Other topical treatments include nutmeg mixed with milk or honey to make a paste for pimples. A tea tree oil gel (5 percent) is worth trying.

• Wash morning and evening with a gentle nonsoap cleanser. Using a harsh or abrasive product may aggravate acne.

• Ask your doctor about applying a topical antibiotic such as clindamycin or erythromy-cin. They can be helpful, but skin bacteria are developing resistance to these drugs.

• Check with your doctor regarding a prescription for Retin-A. Be vigilant about protecting your skin from the sun or any other source of ultraviolet radiation while you are using this medicine.

• Ask about Nicomide-T gel or cream. This vitamin-based topical medicine can reduce inflammation and may be almost as effective as some topical antibiotics.

• Oral antibiotics may work even when topical antibiotics do not. Be sure to ask your doctor about side effects and interactions, and follow the dosing instructions carefully.

• Women may benefit from birth control pills. Sometimes the diuretic spironolactone provides additional anti-acne power.

• For severe acne that has not responded to other treatments, isotretinoin (Accutane, Sotret, etc.) is an option. Discuss the risks and benefits thoroughly with your dermatologist before starting on a 5-month course of these pills. Because isotretinoin causes birth defects, women are required by the manufacturer to verify before taking any of this medication that they are not pregnant, and to confirm it again each month during treatment. They must also use two effective forms of contraception during the course of treatment.

• Ask your dermatologist if Dusa Blue Light (photodynamic therapy) is appropriate for you. It should be administered by a dermatologist or plastic surgeon experienced with its use.

ALLERGIES

• Install an Aprilaire HEPA-type air filter	★★★★
• Use a high-quality vacuum cleaner (Miele)	★★★★
• Rinse your nasal passages with saltwater	
• Try vitamin C	
• Experiment with the herbs stinging nettle and butterbur	★★★
• Take quercetin and bromelain	
• Try NasalCrom (cromolyn) spray to prevent allergy symptoms	★★★★
• Look for loratadine, an over-the-counter antihistamine	★★★★
• Ask your doctor about a steroid nasal spray	★★★★★
• Consider pseudoephedrine for symptomatic relief	

Breathing is basic. Most of the time we take it for granted. But if your nose is congested and your sinuses are stopped up, you are miserable. For one thing, your head feels as if it's full of cotton. Studies have found that people suffering from allergies frequently experience sleep difficulties, fatigue, poor concentration, drowsiness, irritability, delayed reaction times, memory problems, and cognitive impairment.[19] When you are in the middle of an allergy attack it is hard to drive safely even if you are not sneezing. Making decisions or operating other kinds of machinery can also be problematic.

Paradoxically, although antihistamines are the mainstay of allergy treatment, they can also cause drowsiness, delayed reaction times, sedation, and cognitive impairment. Even the so-called second-generation nonsedating antihistamines that are so heavily advertised to consumers may not be as benign as drug companies would have you believe.[20] When given in doses that are adequate to relieve symptoms, some of these nonsedating antihistamines may also make people drowsy and impair performance.[21]

Research has shown that driving skills are affected with both the older and the newer antihistamines.[22] A massive study conducted for the National Highway Traffic Safety Administration discovered that driving while drowsy—no matter what the cause—increased the risk of a crash or near crash by four to six times.[23]

Physicians often think of allergies as more of a nuisance than a life-threatening condition. But we now realize that impairment poses huge risks if people are driving. And allergy symptoms don't just occur in the spring and fall, when pollen is in the air. Nowadays many folks are congested all year long. At last count, 50 million people are sensitive to things like dust mites, cat dander, cockroaches, mold spores, and pollens from oak, elm, and maple trees as well as ragweed and rye, blue, and Bermuda grasses.[24] Symptoms include nasal stuffiness, runny nose, itching, sneezing, and coughing. Chronic sinusitis, which may develop as a consequence of allergies, affects more than 30 million people. And asthma, which can be life threatening, often has an allergic and inflammatory component.

What is so scary about these statistics is that they keep going up. No one knows why, but it appears that more people are suffering than ever before.

Your Home Environment

People are now exposed to a chemical soup at home and in the workplace. Buildings are tightly sealed for energy efficiency and may trap chemical gasses and dust from a variety of sources. Cleaning agents left on floors and other surfaces dry and can eventually circulate on dust particles throughout the house or workplace and be inhaled with each breath. Fire retardants and other chemicals used in fabrics and foams in furniture, mattresses, and electrical insulation can be irritating to the airway. Mold can flourish wherever there is humidity—in basements, crawl spaces, bathrooms, air conditioners, and automobile air ducts.

It is crazy to treat the symptoms of allergies if you don't examine your environment and try to eliminate what's causing the problem in the first place. If you lived in a house with faulty wiring that kept blowing fuses or tripping the circuit breakers every day, it would be foolish to ignore the underlying problem. Continually throwing the circuit breaker to the on position or replacing fuses might leave you vulnerable to a fire. In the old days, people sometimes stuck a penny in the fuse box to bypass the warning system completely. No doubt some homes burned down as a result.

We know of one family that moved into a charming old house. Within a few months, the dad starting sniffling and sneezing. Then he developed asthma for the first time in his life. Not long after, both children also became congested and had periodic bouts of asthma. They were all treated with various medications to relieve their symptoms. It wasn't until they moved that their symptoms eventually went away and their need for allergy and asthma drugs disappeared.

No dermatologist in his right mind would keep prescribing prednisone to someone who showed up with a poison ivy outbreak every other week. At some point the dermatologist would tell this patient to stay away from poison ivy to avoid the itchy, red rash in the first place. We wish allergists and lung experts would do more than prescribe antihistamines, bronchodilators, and corticosteroids for their patients. If they actually visited their patients' homes or workplaces they might discover the cause of the symptoms.

Of course, that is not going to happen. Instead, you will have to become your own Sherlock Holmes, sniffing out the culprits if you can. In some cases it might even be worthwhile to employ a certified environmental engineer to look for sources of allergens in a house or apartment. Watch out for charlatans, though. There are lots of quacks out there who would love nothing more than to sell you a pricey home inspection and cleanup. Make sure that whoever analyzes your living space isn't selling a service or recommending an organization they have a financial relationship with.

Air Filters and Dehumidification

It is impossible to eliminate all the airborne allergens that trigger symptoms, but you can reduce the amount of dust floating around your rooms. Forget the old-fashioned fiberglass filters that only capture large particles. That is like trying to catch mosquitoes with a fishnet. We are not big fans of ozone-type air "purifiers" either. The fine folks at *Consumer Reports* warn that many small room-size ionizing air cleaners (or "electrostatic precipitators") can generate ozone.[25] As far as we're concerned, ozone is the last thing someone with allergies or asthma needs, since it can be irritating and decrease lung function.

Our first choice in air-cleaning technology is the HEPA (high-efficiency particulate air) filter. These devices are made of densely packed fibers that look like thick paper. The filters are pleated or folded and look like a mini-accordion. That way they maximize the air's contact with the filter. Industrial-strength HEPA filters are used in computer clean rooms, pharmaceutical manufacturing plants, and hospitals, where it is essential to trap very small dust particles.

To install a whole-house HEPA filter you will need professional help. Ask a heating and air-conditioning (HVAC) expert whether they can retrofit such a system for your home. We

---

★★★★ Aprilaire Whole-House Air Cleaner

This high-efficiency particulate air (HEPA)-type filter is highly efficient, uses no electricity, lasts 1 to 2 years, and captures most pollen, mold spores, and large dust particles. The box that holds the filter needs to be installed next to your furnace by a heating, ventilating, and air-conditioning (HVAC) professional.

An alternative to the HEPA-type air filter is the Aprilaire Model 5000 Electronic Air Cleaner. *Consumer Reports* consistently gives this system its highest score.[26]

Downside: The Aprilaire HEPA-type filter needs to be changed every year or two. Initial installation requires a professional. The electronic alternative is pricey.

Cost: Initial installation of the HEPA filter box is done by your HVAC expert. Should cost less than $200. A packet of two filters is $50 to $60. The Aprilaire Model 5000 Electronic Air Cleaner is roughly $600. Installation can run an additional $200.

think the Aprilaire Media Air Cleaner (formerly Space-Gard) is the place to start (800-334-6011 or on the Web at www.aprilaire.com). This HEPA-type filter achieves 99 percent efficiency for particles bigger than five microns and 95 percent efficiency for the smallest one-micron-sized particles. (Pollen and mold spores usually range from 10 to 100 microns.) The longer you use the filter, the more efficient it becomes, at least to a point. It should be changed every one to two years.

If you cannot afford either a HEPA filter or an electronic air cleaner, consider the less efficient, do-it-yourself 4-inch American Air Filter for around $40 or the 1-inch 3M Filtrete for about $25. These should fit into your existing air return system in place of the old-fashioned filter you may be using.

We find it astonishing that there hasn't been more clinical research on home air filtration. Pharmaceutical companies have spent hundreds of millions, if not billions, of dollars testing drugs to relieve symptoms. Only a pittance has been devoted to air quality in the home and its relationship to symptom relief.

One review of the available research concluded that "Among patients with allergies and asthma, use of air filters is associated with fewer symptoms."[27] A small study showed that a HEPA air cleaner could reduce the amount of cat allergen levels in the house, but it did not demonstrate improvement in nasal symptom scores.[28] Another tiny study showed that a HEPA filter could reduce dog allergens in the air.[29]

A pilot study in two daycare centers demonstrated that when a HEPA filter was combined with a dehumidification system, airborne fungal spores were substantially diminished.[30] Most people do not realize how serious dampness and humidity are for the home environment. Wherever there is moisture, mold has a marvelous opportunity to multiply. Mold spores can be highly allergenic.

The solution is to get rid of the source of the moisture and keep dampness under control by dehumidifying. The drier your home castle, the less likely it is that there will be mold, mildew, and dust mites. These latter nasty little critters live in mattresses, bedding, carpets, and furniture. Mite poop is also highly allergenic and is responsible for many people's discomfort. Dry air makes it harder for mites to flourish.

By the way, we used to encourage folks with allergies or asthma to encase their mattresses and pillows with allergen-impermeable bed covers. The goal was to separate the allergy sufferer from the mite poop. Sadly, well-conducted clinical trials have established conclusively that this effort is ineffective.[31, 32, 33]

Vacuum Cleaners

You can reduce dust and pollen with good air filtration, but you can never eliminate it. A decent vacuum cleaner can go a long way toward reducing the dirt and dust that can cause allergies. But many machines suck up dust and allergens at one end and spew them out with the exhaust at the other end. These vacuum cleaners may actually cause more problems for the allergy sufferer.

According to *Consumer Reports*, vacuum cleaner models "with a HEPA filter have been very effective at reducing emissions. However, some models that don't have HEPA filters have performed just as well in our tests, and such vacuums may cost less than HEPA models."[34]

The Sears Kenmore canister models generally scored high in the *Consumer Reports* testing. The Progressive 25512 model, at $300, was a "*Consumer Reports* Best Buy." Miele vacuums come with HEPA filters and range from $500 to $800. We have been very pleased with ours. The Bosch Premium, at around $800, and the Aerus Lux Guardian, at roughly $1,200, also come with HEPA filters and score well.

★★★★ Miele Solaris Electro Plus

Choosing a vacuum cleaner is a highly personal decision. We like this Miele machine because it comes with a HEPA filter, is highly rated by *Consumer Reports*, and has served us successfully for years. You may find the Sears canister vacuum just as effective at a substantially lower cost.

Downside: A little on the pricey side. Filter needs to be changed regularly.

Cost: Approximately $800

Nondrug Approaches for Allergies

Even if you created a perfect living environment by eliminating carpets and rugs, minimizing stuffed furniture, banning your pets to the outdoors, and filtering your air, you could never truly eliminate allergens from your personal space. And every time you go outside, you are vulnerable to whatever is in the air. So, what can you do to minimize your reaction to pollen and all the other nasties flowing through your nose every time you breathe?

Nose Cleaning with Neti

Americans have a hard time imagining that you can clean your internal environment. But the Ayurvedic tradition of India encourages nasal washing with what's known as a neti pot. This porcelain container looks a little like Aladdin's lamp. It allows saltwater to be poured into one nostril and exit out the other. This washing process is supposed to clear the nasal passages of dust, pollen, and other allergens.

You can find neti pots at some health-food stores or by calling the Himalayan Institute at 800-822-4547. Visit their Web site at www.netipot.org to get an idea of what we are talking about. A ceramic pot costs $18 to $20.

"*For years I was troubled with allergies. But I have discovered the following natural approach. I use a neti pot to wash my sinuses with salt water. Sinus and ear infections are now a thing of the distant past. Many people are grossed out at even the suggestion of pouring something into their noses, but the sensation is really very pleasant, if done properly (with lukewarm filtered water and mild saline solution).*

I also vacuum my bedding daily to get rid of dust mites. "

Vitamin C

We are the first to acknowledge that vitamin C studies are squishy. There just have not been large, well-conducted clinical trials to test the effectiveness of ascorbic acid (vitamin C) against allergic disorders. The allergists will rightfully say that without decent data they cannot recommend this vitamin.

Nevertheless, some research suggests that this nutrient might help reduce allergy symptoms through a kind of antihistamine action.[35,36] There is also the possibility that vitamin C modulates immune-system reactivity and has anti-inflammatory effects.[37] The benefits, if they exist, appear fairly short-lived.

That's why the general recommendation is to take 500 milligrams of ascorbic acid three or four times a day.[38]

Stinging Nettle (Urtica dioica)

The very name of this herb is enough to scare many folks away. If you were to come into contact with stinging nettle, which grows widely throughout Europe and North America, you would have even more misgivings. Touching the tiny hairs on this plant can cause an impressive rash that can itch and sting for up to 12 hours.

It is ironic that these hairs contain a witches' brew of irritating chemicals, including histamine and formic acid (also found in ant stings), yet the herb may be helpful in controlling allergy symptoms. When the leaves and other parts of the aboveground plant are extracted and swallowed, they may offer some fascinating pharmacological benefits.[39]

In Europe, where *Urtica dioica* is quite popu-

★★★ Stinging Nettle (*Urtica dioica*)

This herb is well known in Europe, where it is used primarily to relieve allergy symptoms and improve urinary flow in cases of benign prostate enlargement. The dose that has been used for treating nasal symptoms is 300 milligrams of freeze-dried *Urtica dioica* per day.

Side effects: This herb is usually well tolerated. Mild digestive upset has been reported, especially if it is taken on an empty stomach. Some people may experience an allergic rash and should discontinue use immediately if this occurs.

Downside: Large, well-controlled trials are lacking. Better research is needed before we can give this herb a ringing endorsement.

Cost: Approximately $5 to $10 for a month's supply

---

lar, physicians have been prescribing it to treat allergies for a long time. One double-blind trial noted that 58 percent of the study participants had good relief of symptoms.[40] Almost half of the patients said that stinging nettle was just as effective, if not more so, than their standard allergy medicine. Why something that contains histamine might actually help to relieve allergic symptoms is somewhat mysterious. Investigators suspect that it may help to modulate the immune response.[41]

● ● ●

Q. *I feel like I am caught between a rock and a hard place. My allergies are awful, but most antihistamines and decongestants warn that they're not to be used by men like me. I have an enlarged prostate, so Benadryl and Sudafed are off limits. Is there anything natural that would help my allergies and not aggravate my prostate problem?*

A. Most over-the-counter (OTC) allergy medicines contain either an antihistamine or a decongestant that can make urination more difficult for a man with an enlarged prostate. An herbal remedy that might substitute is stinging nettle (*Urtica dioica*).

According to European research, extracts of this herb can do double duty to relieve allergy symptoms and help improve urine flow in men with benign prostate enlargement. Side effects are uncommon.

● ● ●

Now that the value of saw palmetto has been called into question for treating benign prostate enlargement (BPH),[42] some men may want to consider stinging nettle instead. *Urtica dioica* has been used to treat BPH in Europe for decades. There are good reasons why this herb might be effective. For one thing, stinging nettle root affects sex hormone–binding globulin and its ability to interact with hormones like testosterone. Another key player in prostate problems, epidermal growth factor, is inhibited by 53 percent by stinging nettle lectins. In addition, this herbal extract has anti-inflammatory activity that interferes with an enzyme (Na/K-ATPase) that is necessary for prostate cell growth.

Most important, human studies have shown that nettle root extract improves urine flow and decreases the amount of urine left in the bladder after voiding. Many men with an enlarged prostate report that the herb reduces the number of times they have to get up at night to go to the bathroom.

❝ *I read a letter in your column about a man with allergies. Because of an enlarged prostate, he couldn't take the usual over-the-counter antihistamines.*

You suggested the herb "stinging nettle" as a substitute that might relieve allergy symptoms and improve the flow of urine. My husband looked these stinging nettles up and began taking them. He has improved 100 percent in both his allergy condition and his prostate symptom of frequent urination. In addition, his PSA number has come down!

The urologist said, "Yes, I've heard of it, and it helps some but not others." We are so glad you mentioned this herbal medicine, and we have shared the information with others. **"**

Butterbur (Petasites hybridus)

Another interesting allergy treatment involves the herb butterbur. This botanical medicine has been used to treat symptoms of migraine headaches, asthma, and allergy. It has anti-inflammatory activity and blocks the formation of compounds called leukotrienes (pronounced lew-co-TRY-eens). These rascals cause all sorts of mischief in the nose, including itching, sneezing, swelling, and congestion. In some respects, leukotrienes may be even more of a problem than histamine. Leukotrienes contribute to the inflammatory cascade that underlies both allergy and asthma. The prescription asthma and allergy drug Singulair (montelukast) also works by inhibiting leukotriene formation.

Swiss researchers compared butterbur with the antihistamine cetirizine (Zyrtec) in a randomized, double-blind study. They found that both products were equally effective at controlling symptoms, but butterbur was significantly less sedating than Zyrtec.[43]

• • •

Q. *I have suffered from chronic sinusitis, which in turn led to bronchitis and frequently into pneumonia. My physician put me on Allegra and then switched me to Clarinex.*

I continued to have sinusitis and pneumonia annually for 5 years, so my doctor sent me to an allergist. He diagnosed several allergies and added a prescription for Nasacort to the Clarinex.

Two years ago, having suffered through another bout of sinusitis and pneumonia, I saw an integrative alternative medicine physician. He took me off Clarinex and prescribed butterbur, stinging nettles, and quercitin instead. I've taken this combination for 2 years and it has reduced the frequency of the sinusitis.

I read that I should take butterbur only 6 weeks a year. Now I am concerned about the danger of liver damage.

A. Pharmacologist David Kroll, PhD, offered this clarification on butterbur. "I wanted to follow up on a reader who wrote to your newspaper column regarding the potential liver toxicity of butterbur (*Petasites hybridus*), an herb that's become popular due to positive efficacy trials in migraine prevention and allergic rhinitis. While the herb is

potentially toxic to the liver, it shouldn't be a problem with high-quality products like Petadolex. I do fear that some less honorable companies may latch onto this herb and not take such care with the high-tech extraction process that is necessary to reduce the risk. That might lead to some major liver injury cases."

• • •

There is one fly in the ointment, however. Concerns have been raised about potential liver toxicity associated with compounds in butterbur. If the herbal preparation is not manufactured under very stringent quality-control conditions, there could be problems. As a result, we suggest that people use butterbur only temporarily (say, for 6 weeks during hay fever season) and that they monitor their liver enzyme activity with medical supervision. One product that should be safe is Petadolex. The German manufacturer is Weber and Weber, and it is available in the United States.

Quercetin and Bromelain

Two other natural products that may be worth consideration against allergies are quercetin and bromelain. Quercetin is an antioxidant flavonoid that is found in many fruits, vegetables, and herbs. The anti-inflammatory effect of quercetin helps stabilize mast cells. These are the cells in your eyes, nose, and lungs (and other places in your body) that are highly sensitive to allergens.

Think of mast cells as floating mines. When they come into contact with allergens like ragweed pollen or dust mite poop, a switch gets thrown on these cellular "mines" and all hell breaks loose. Mast cells start releasing histamine and other chemicals called *kinins* (pronounced KYE-nins), which then turn on a cascade of other nasty things like leukotrienes and prostaglandins. The end result is sneezing, itching, inflammation, and congestion.

Quercetin, especially when combined with bromelain (an enzyme derived from pineapple), seems to stabilize mast cells and make them less likely to trigger the release of such chemicals.[44,45,46]

We think such an approach may be more logical than trying to block the effect of histamine with antihistamines.

Think of it this way. If your mast cells are like a barn holding in a bunch of wild horses (histamine molecules), then what would be more efficient—reinforcing the door and walls of the barn to keep those wild histamines inside or trying to protect all the grass in your pasture from having those histamine "horses" nibbling away at it? Antihistamines are like a chemical barrier that tries to protect your grass once the horses are out of the barn. But they are not 100 percent efficient, and some histamine will always find a target and wreak havoc. Keeping the barn closed tightly (or the mast cells stabilized) seems to us to be a more effective approach.

Allergy Medications

NASALCROM (CROMOLYN)

Speaking of stabilizing mast cells, another way to do this is with a nasal spray. Cromolyn (Nasal-Crom) was first introduced as a prescription product in 1983. NasalCrom went over the counter in 1997. Cromolyn, the active ingredient in NasalCrom, was originally derived from an herb, the fruit of bishop's weed (*Ammi visnaga*), which was traditionally used to treat asthma.

The compound cromolyn stabilizes highly sensitive mast cells in the lining of the nose and lungs so they can better resist the onslaught of pollen. It won't cause drowsiness or cognitive impairment and, if used regularly, it is quite effective. Unlike decongestant nose sprays, there is no need to fear developing dependency.

Cromolyn is available in eyedrops (Crolom) for itchy, red eyes due to allergies. There is also an aerosol inhaler (Intal) for treating asthma. Both products require a prescription, whereas NasalCrom does not require your physician's assistance.

• • •

Q. *I'm going to visit my daughter in a few weeks and she has two cats that have the run of the house. When I'm there, I suffer runny nose, watery eyes, and sneezing from the cat hairs that are all over the house and furniture.*

Can you recommend something over-the-counter for me to take during the visit?

A. NasalCrom is a nasal spray that can be quite effective if taken preventively. You will need to start spritzing several days before arriving so you can stabilize the cells in your nose and protect them against cat allergens.

If you also took the oral antihistamine Claritin (loratadine), you might be able to minimize the sneezing and allergic reactions.

• • •

★★★★ NasalCrom (cromolyn sodium)

This nonprescription nasal spray is often ignored by doctors, but it is a valuable tool in the fight against nasal allergies. By stabilizing mast cells in the nose, NasalCrom makes it harder for histamine and other inflammatory chemicals to be released and do their dirty work.

Side effects: Cromolyn is very safe and does not cause drowsiness or rebound nasal congestion the way OTC nasal decongestants can. Some people may experience temporary sneezing, nasal burning, or a bad taste in their mouth.

Downside: You must use NasalCrom at least four times a day to really benefit. Some experts believe it is much less effective than intranasal corticosteroids.

Cost: Approximately $17 to $20 for a 1- to 2-month supply

ANTIHISTAMINES

Antihistamines have been the mainstay of allergy treatment for decades. The so-called first-generation drugs like diphenhydramine (Benadryl), brompheniramine (Dimetane, Dimetapp), and chlorpheniramine (Chlor-Trimeton) are linked to drowsiness and cognitive impairment.[47] Second-generation antihistamines such as cetirizine (Zyrtec), desloratadine (Clarinex), fexofenadine (Allegra), and loratadine (Claritin) have been promoted as nonsedating. Because they were supposed to be so much safer and better tolerated than the old-fashioned drugs, many came with a very steep price tag ($2 to $3 per pill). But there is growing concern that when given in doses that are adequate to relieve allergy symptoms, even these newer compounds may cause some sedation in some patients and produce mild impairment.[48] Researchers now believe that "a clear and consistent distinction between sedating and nonsedating antihistamines does not exist."[49]

What this means is that the allergy victim is truly caught on the horns of a dilemma. Suffering with allergies makes you spacey, sleepy, and irritable and can impair your ability to function. Antihistamines can also cause sedation and impair performance. If such drugs only partially control symptoms (a fairly common situation), then you may end up with the worst situation of all—sedation from the medicine *and* from the allergic condition.[50]

In such a confusing situation, we would normally suggest that the allergy sufferer experiment with a variety of antihistamines to try and determine which one works best and is least troublesome in terms of side effects. The

---

★★★★ Loratadine (Claritin, Alavert)

Claritin used to be the most widely prescribed antihistamine on the market. When it lost patent protection, the company took it OTC. Compared to many of the older nonprescription antihistamines, loratadine is probably less likely to cause drowsiness at recommended doses. We have seen no data to suggest that it is less effective than pricier prescription antihistamines.

Side effects: Headache, sleepiness, dry mouth, fatigue, jitteriness, and stomach upset. Liver problems may be a rare adverse reaction.

Downside: More expensive than old-fashioned antihistamines. Insurance companies may deny you affordable access to drugs like Allegra now that loratadine is available OTC. Loratadine may cause sedation and impair driving in susceptible people. Do not assume you are safe behind the wheel.

Cost: Approximately $5 to $10 for a month's supply when purchased generically in bulk. The brand-name Claritin can cost two to four times that much.

---

difficulty is that people are notoriously bad at assessing their level of impairment. There is a warning on the label of Benadryl and many other OTC allergy medicines reminding users that "marked drowsiness may occur" and urging them to "be careful when driving a motor vehicle or operating machinery." Such cautions are as meaningless as telling a drunk to be careful behind the wheel. In fact, researchers have reported that diphenhydramine "had a greater impact on driving than alcohol did."[51] These scientists discovered that "drowsiness ratings were not a good predictor of impairment, suggesting that drivers cannot use drowsiness to indicate when they should not drive."

By the way, did you know that you could be arrested for driving while impaired after taking an OTC allergy pill? If your driving skills are not up to par, an officer can give you a ticket even though you have no alcohol in your system.

So, dear reader, we have no easy answers. We would like to say, if you have allergies, do not drive, especially if you are taking antihistamines. That would be the only prudent thing. We know that some people will disobey such a suggestion, however. Some experts believe that fexofenadine (Allegra) may be one of the least sedating and safer antihistamines to take if you must drive.[52,53] Others point out that even this nonsedating antihistamine may pose problems at higher doses.[54] If driving or operating machinery is essential or if you must make important decisions, we encourage you to look for other options besides oral antihistamines.

There is now a prescription antihistamine nasal spray called azelastine (Astelin). It is fairly fast acting but has the disadvantage of requiring twice-daily nasal spritzing. Some data suggest it may be as effective as oral antihistamines. Side effects may include a bitter taste in the mouth (20 percent of patients), headache, drowsiness (11 percent of patients), nasal burning or inflammation, sore throat, dry mouth, sneezing, fatigue, and dizziness. A 1-ounce bottle can cost $75 to $85. Not exactly a perfect solution to the problem, eh?

CORTICOSTEROID NASAL SPRAYS

The big revolution in allergy treatment involves the use of steroid nasal sprays. Allergists have known for decades that cortisone-like drugs (prednisone, for example) can dampen the reactions of an overactive immune system and calm allergy symptoms amazingly well. The trouble is that relief comes at a stiff price. So many side effects are associated with oral corticosteroids that few physicians would ever consider prescribing such medications for nasal allergy symptoms except as a last resort. Even then, cautious doctors prescribe medications like prednisone for the shortest period of time necessary. Adverse reactions can include irritability, insomnia, anxiety, high blood pressure, potassium depletion, headache, nausea, and dizziness.

INTRANASAL CORTICOSTEROIDS

GENERIC	BRAND NAME
Beclomethasone	Beconase AQ
Budesonide	Rhinocort Aqua
Flunisolide	Nasarel
Fluticasone	Flonase
Mometasone	Nasonex
Triamcinolone	Nasacort AQ

Not surprisingly, people wanted the benefits of steroids without the risks. That's where nasal sprays come in. There are about a half-dozen different intranasal corticosteroids available by prescription. Most experts would say that these formulations are the most effective allergy treatment available. Although it may take a week for the benefits to reach peak effect, these sprays should relieve allergy symptoms such as itching, sneezing, and congestion quite well. They are pricey, however. A small bottle can run $85 to $95. At the time of this writing, generic flunisolide costs around $40. We cannot say whether one spray is better or safer than another.

The general consensus is that there are few, if any, systemic side effects associated with topical steroids. In other words, the experts do not believe people absorb enough of the drugs into the system to cause much, if any, concern.[55] One study did report growth suppression in children, but other research has not confirmed this complication. There have been rare reports of nasal perforation (creating a hole between the nostrils) and increased pressure within the eyes. More common are local reactions such as irritation and burning in the nose, sore throat, nasal dryness, nosebleed, and headache.

LEUKOTRIENE MODIFIER MONTELUKAST (SINGULAIR)

We used to think Singulair was a very cool drug. It is an oral prescription medicine that blocks the effects of those inflammatory chemicals called leukotrienes. So, it only made

★★★★★ Corticosteroid Nasal Sprays

Most allergy experts believe that these steroid sprays are the most effective treatments available and should be the first-line therapy. They are not likely to cause drowsiness or sedation and should be safe for people who must drive or operate machinery.

Side effects: Nasal irritation, stinging, burning, and bleeding. Other adverse reactions may include sore throat (and, rarely, yeast infections), headache, nausea, and cough. Rare adverse reactions may include perforation of the septum, nasal ulcers, reduced growth rate in children, glaucoma, cataracts, and asthma symptoms.

Downside: These drugs are pricey and may alter the senses of taste and smell.

Cost: Approximately $85 to $95 for brand-name nasal sprays. Generic flunisolide is $35 to $40 per bottle.

sense to us that a drug like Singulair would relieve symptoms. This medication is widely prescribed to ease the breathing problems associated with asthma.

Research suggests, however, that Singulair is only modestly effective for alleviating itching, sneezing, congestion, and runny nose. It is roughly comparable to antihistamines such as loratadine (Claritin). One study reported that Singulair, which costs more than $3 per pill, was no more effective than the oral decongestant pseudoephedrine (Sudafed) for relieving typical allergy symptoms.[56] Generic pseudoephedrine is far less expensive than Singulair. It is harder to purchase these days because pharmacists can only dispense it from behind the counter. You don't need a prescription, but you will have to sign for it. Too many people used pseudoephedrine to make the illegal drug methamphetamine, so states and the federal government cracked down on easy access.

The research demonstrating that pseudoephedrine is quite effective in relieving allergy symptoms has forced us to reevaluate this old and inexpensive vasoconstrictor. It works by shrinking blood vessels in the nose. Perhaps that's why so many drug companies now add this OTC ingredient to their antihistamines. Whenever you see a *D* appended to the name of an allergy medicine, you can pretty much assume that there is a decongestant on board, and frequently it is pseudoephedrine. It is found in Allegra-D, Claritin-D, Clarinex-D, Zyrtec-D, and other similar formulations.

● ● ●

Q. *I would like to point out a side effect of allergy medications that contain pseudoephedrine for nasal decongestion. Taking Claritin-D left me completely unable to fall asleep. I was literally up all night with a racing heartbeat.*

I have had insomnia problems before, so I did not immediately associate this with the medication and continued to take it for 5 days. I was so sleep deprived that I couldn't work.

I finally read the warning about nervousness, dizziness, or sleeplessness. I called my doctor, who said I should switch to Claritin (non-D). On this drug I sleep like a baby.

I found that some OTC allergy medicines I had taken for years also contain pseudoephedrine. I suspect this contributed to my earlier insomnia problems.

I urge anyone with insomnia to check all medications for pseudoephedrine. It does not affect everyone, but some of us just can't handle even a small amount.

A. Millions of people struggle with insomnia and many don't realize that the medicines they take may be contributing to their problem.

Decongestants aren't the only culprits. Antihistamines, antidepressants, asthma medicines, blood pressure pills,

and pain relievers are some of the drugs that can cause insomnia.

● ● ●

As popular as pseudoephedrine may be, there are some side effects to be alert for. Many people complain of insomnia, anxiety, agitation, headache, nausea, dizziness, and tremor. The most serious adverse reactions are elevated blood pressure and irregular heart rhythms. Men with prostate enlargement must avoid this decongestant because it can make urination much more difficult.

Conclusions

Allergies don't get the respect they deserve. When you complain about your congestion, most friends and family members will barely sympathize. But allergies can slow you down and make you dangerous behind the wheel. Finding the right treatment to ease your symptoms without causing worse problems is a challenge. Combining several options, including environmental control, may be the most effective solution for solving this common problem.

- Use a HEPA-type air filter and a dehumidifier to remove allergens from the air you breathe and make the environment inhospitable for the three Ms of allergy—mold, mildew, and mites.
- Get a high-quality vacuum cleaner that won't spew dust and dirt back into the air. Miele models rank high on our list.
- Wash your nasal passages with saline. A neti pot will help.
- Consider an herbal approach such as stinging nettle (*Urtica dioica*) or butterbur (*Petasites hybridus*). Men with prostate enlargement may find nettles especially helpful since some OTC allergy medicines may make this condition worse.
- The natural products quercetin and bromelain may help stabilize mast cells and prevent histamine release.
- Cromolyn (NasalCrom) is an OTC remedy that also stabilizes mast cells. It should be used preventively before exposure to allergens occurs. Cromolyn does not cause drowsiness.
- Oral antihistamines can control symptoms, but they may also make you dangerous on the highways. Even nonsedating products may interfere with driving ability. Generic loratadine (Claritin) is now available without a prescription.
- Among prescription allergy medicines, steroid nasal sprays offer the most effective symptom relief with a minimum of side effects. The cost is significant, since they are available only by prescription. One generic variety (flunisolide) is less expensive than brand-name products like Flonase and Rhinocort AQ.
- Pseudoephedrine can be surprisingly effective at controlling allergy symptoms. Beware of side effects such as insomnia, nervousness, high blood pressure, and irregular heart rhythms.

ARTHRITIS

• Eat a diet rich in selenium	
• Get 1,000 IU of vitamin D daily	★★★★★
• Follow a Mediterranean diet	
• Take aspirin to relieve pain and control inflammation	★★★★
• Try naproxen for pain relief	★★
• Ask your doctor about a prescription for Pennsaid (diclofenic)	★★★★
• Experiment with fish oil and green-lipped mussels	★★
• Try gin-drenched raisins	
• Consider Certo and grape juice	★★★★★
• Drink pomegranate juice	★★★★
• Sip vinegar with apple and grape juices	
• Drink cherry juice	
• Take turmeric	★★★★
• Try boswellia	
• Consider acupuncture	★★★

No one really knows how many people suffer from arthritis and related inflammatory conditions. The folks at the CDC (Centers for Disease Control and Prevention), who are in charge of tracking such things, put the number at close to 70 million. That includes more than 43 million adults diagnosed by doctors and another 23 million who have symptoms but have not been officially diagnosed.[57,58] That means one in three adults is afflicted with some form of arthritis.

If you think that's a lot of folks, you ain't seen nothin' yet. Aging baby boomers are about to discover up close and personal what it's like to suffer from chronic inflammation. The CDC estimates that by 2030 we will add another 22 million to the list of people in pain.[59] Arthritis will become the biggest obstacle to enjoyable retirement for the boomer generation.

With so many suffering, it's hardly any wonder we're all desperate for relief. Shaking hands, buttoning a shirt, or typing on a computer keyboard can be difficult if your fingers hurt. But who can give up e-mail? We communicate with the world through our fingers.

Everyone tells us that exercise is the most important thing we can do for our overall health. Yet it's hard to walk, jog, or play tennis or golf if your knees, hips, and shoulders are sore.

No wonder we turn to drugs to relieve our inflammation and ease the pain. A friend who hiked the Appalachian Trail dubbed ibuprofen "vitamin I." Weekend warriors frequently rely on Advil (ibuprofen) or Aleve (naproxen) before, during, and after tennis matches, basketball games, or karate competitions. We now know that most of the medications used for arthritis can have potentially serious side effects.

We're caught in a classic double bind. Without something to control inflammation, pain limits our activities, which is not good for our health. Take the medicine, however, and we risk all sorts of complications, from high blood pressure and kidney problems to heart attacks and strokes. Some popular anti-inflammatory drugs may even make our arthritis worse.

Corticosteroids

When cortisone was first introduced in the 1950s it was heralded as a wonder drug. Doctors became overnight heroes because they helped patients who had been crippled by rheumatoid arthritis get out of bed and begin functioning again. Even people with milder conditions like osteoarthritis, allergies,

COMMON CORTICOSTEROIDS

- Cortisone
- Dexamethasone
- Hydrocortisone
- Methylprednisolone
- Prednisolone
- Prednisone
- Triamcinolone

SIDE EFFECTS OF CORTICOSTEROIDS

- Cataracts
- Osteoporosis
- Diabetes
- Spontaneous fractures
- Bone deterioration
- Insomnia
- Irritability
- Glaucoma
- Fluid retention
- Weight gain
- Moon face
- Infections
- High blood pressure
- Blood clots
- Potassium loss
- Stomach ulcers
- Muscle weakness
- Blood clots
- Menstrual disturbances
- Impaired wound healing
- Fatigue
- Steroid "psychosis"

asthma, and eczema were thrilled because corticosteroids relieved their symptoms amazingly well. But the very reason these medications were so successful was also their Achilles heel. As great as they are at easing inflammation, they profoundly affect cells throughout the body. Taking high doses for long periods of time is a little like dancing with the devil.

Once people woke up to the downside of steroids, the drugs lost their luster and fell into disfavor. Don't get us wrong, though. These medications are incredibly valuable, especially for short-term use. People experiencing an arthritis flare-up, a bad sunburn, or a terrible case of poison ivy will benefit immensely from a pulsed dose of corticosteroids. When Joe went deaf in one ear, a course of prednisone restored his hearing. If used cautiously and with respect for their risks, these drugs can be extremely valuable. But using corticosteroids regularly to treat arthritis is a slippery slope.

NSAIDs

After the roller-coaster ride with cortisone, you would think that the medical establishment would have been more careful about the next big thing. Maybe doctors were so anxious to find something safer for arthritis that they didn't appreciate that they might be jumping from the frying pan into the fire.

Aspirin was the first nonsteroidal anti-inflammatory drug (NSAID). It was introduced in 1899 and was a mainstay of arthritis treatment for most of a century. Aspirin works a little differently from other drugs in this class and has advantages that make it unique. For almost 100 years aspirin was the Rodney Dangerfield of the drugstore. It got relatively little respect. Because aspirin was available over the counter, it took physicians a long time

---

NON-ASPIRIN NSAIDS

- Celecoxib (Celebrex)
- Diclofenac (Cataflam, Voltaren)
- Etodolac (Lodine)
- Fenoprofen (Nalfon)
- Flurbiprofen (Ansaid)
- Ibuprofen (Advil, Motrin, etc.)
- Indomethacin (Indocin)
- Ketoprofen (Orudis, Oruvail)
- Ketorolac (Toradol)
- Meloxicam (Mobic)
- Nabumetone (Relafen)
- Naproxen (Aleve, Anaprox, Naprosyn)
- Oxaprozin (Daypro)
- Piroxicam (Feldene)
- Sulindac (Clinoril)
- Tolmetin (Tolectin)

---

to appreciate how valuable it could be against heart attacks, strokes, and even cancer. Because it has been around for so many years, doctors have often assumed that newer medicines would provide better pain relief. And they (and their patients) have often been disappointed.

The launch of prescription indomethacin (Indocin) in 1965 really put NSAIDs on the map. These drugs became some of the most successful pharmaceuticals of their time. Whenever a new anti-inflammatory drug came along, it generated tremendous excitement.

Drugs like sulindac (Clinoril), piroxicam (Feldene), ibuprofen (Motrin), and naproxen (Naprosyn) had their time in the limelight. Then along would come something newer and doctors would switch their allegiance.

Those of us who have observed this game of medicinal musical chairs for more than 40 years have become somewhat cynical about this class of pain relievers. The fickle switching from one drug to another suggests to us that no particular NSAID really stands out. There have not been really great head-to-head clinical trials that prove one drug is superior to another or significantly safer than others in the class.

If truth be told, these drugs really don't work all that well when it comes to relieving the pain and inflammation of arthritis, especially of the knee. Despite the fact that tens of millions of people have spent countless billions of dollars on these medications, there are surprisingly few data demonstrating long-term benefit with their use. A scientific analysis of 23 different studies was published in the *British Medical Journal* in 2004. This meta-analysis involved more than 10,000 patients and revealed a shocking discovery: "NSAIDs can reduce short-term pain in osteoarthritis of the knee slightly better than placebo, but the current analysis does not support prolonged use of NSAIDs for this condition. As serious adverse effects are associated with oral NSAIDs, only limited use can be recommended."[60]

What a bombshell! This review of the world's medical literature on NSAIDs con-cluded that such drugs are reasonable only for short-term use. But arthritis is a long-term affair. The only conclusion we can draw: Regular use of such drugs is inappropriate for a chronic condition like arthritis.

Even more alarming, some evidence suggests that these medications may actually be harmful to arthritic joints.[61,62,63] Researchers in the Netherlands followed more than 1,600 patients for several years. Patients who had been taking the NSAID diclofenac (Arthrotec, Cataflam, Voltaren) experienced greater joint deterioration as determined by x-ray evidence. The authors concluded, "Our data suggest that diclofenac may not be harmless and may induce accelerated progression of hip and knee OA [osteoarthritis]."[64]

OTC Mistake?

When NSAIDs like ibuprofen (Advil, Cap-Profen, Excedrin IB, Genpril, Haltran, Ibuprin, Ibuprohm, Ibu-Tab, Medipren, Midol IB, Motrin IB, Nuprin, Pamprin IB, Profen, etc.) and naproxen (Aleve) were approved for over-the-counter (OTC) sale, millions of people were delighted to have access to these powerful anti-inflammatory drugs. An Rx-to-OTC switch was a radical concept back in 1984. Even though the FDA assured consumers that such drugs were so safe that they did not require medical supervision, many physicians opposed the plan. They feared that side effects such as rash, fluid retention, high blood pressure, gastritis, and ulcers might make these drugs too dangerous for casual use. The FDA ignored the worriers.

Dear reader, we cannot tell you whether the decision to make NSAIDs available OTC was a blessing or a curse. The FDA has been incredibly inept at keeping track of adverse reactions to prescription medications. The agency's track record on nonprescription pills is even worse. So, we really do not know how many ulcers, heart attacks, or other serious complications have occurred because of easy access to NSAIDs.

What we do know is that people are gobbling down these drugs almost like candy. Based on scientific surveys (Roper and the National Consumers League), it is estimated that 23 million Americans use a nonprescription NSAID (ibuprofen or naproxen) every day.[65] Only about one in five consumers bothers to read the directions on the label and fewer than one in three checks out dosing instructions. Perhaps that's why one-fourth of them take more than the recommended dose. Scarier still, roughly half of the people surveyed were unaware of the potential for NSAID toxicity or just plain didn't care.[66]

NSAID Nastiness

The biggest recognized drawback to NSAIDs has always been their tendency to cause digestive tract distress. That's because of how they work in the body. These drugs block the manufacture of a class of chemicals called prostaglandins. These hormonelike compounds have

> "OTC analgesics including NSAIDs are widely used, are frequently taken inappropriately and potentially dangerously, and users are generally unaware of the potential for adverse side effects."[67]
>
> —C. Mel Wilcox et al., *Journal of Rheumatology*, 2005

a profound impact on cells throughout the body.

If you sprain your ankle, have a tooth extracted, or develop arthritis, you will experience pain, redness, warmth, and inflammation. This is in large measure due to prostaglandins made by a protein called cyclo-oxygenase-2 (COX-2). Blocking their formation with NSAIDs like ibuprofen or naproxen means there is less inflammation and pain.

But some prostaglandins made by another protein, COX-1, are beneficial. They protect the stomach lining from damage. If you disrupt their production by blocking COX-1 with NSAIDs, many people complain of symptoms such as nausea, indigestion, abdominal pain, constipation, and diarrhea. It is estimated that more than half of the people taking NSAIDs experience unpleasant gastrointestinal (GI) symptoms.[68]

Far more worrisome are ulcers, which can bleed or, in the worst case, perforate. A bleeding ulcer or a hole in the stomach wall can very quickly turn into a life-threatening crisis. All too often there are no early warning symptoms that someone is on the verge of disaster.

Although it is hard to know exactly how many people are affected each year, experts estimate that more than 100,000 are hospitalized because of complications caused by

"If deaths from gastrointestinal toxic effects of NSAIDs were tabulated separately in the National Vital Statistics reports, these effects would constitute the 15th most common cause of death in the United States. Yet these toxic effects remain largely a 'silent epidemic,' with many physicians and most patients unaware of the magnitude of the problem.[69] Furthermore, the mortality statistics do not include deaths ascribed to the use of over-the-counter NSAIDs."[70]

—Michael M. Wolfe et al., *The New England Journal of Medicine,* 1999

NSAIDs and more than 16,000 die.[71] The researchers admit these numbers are probably conservative.

Although most physicians have known for a long time that NSAIDs can be hard on the stomach, they didn't realize that the same drugs can be disastrous for the small intestine. That's because until recently the small intestine could not be examined directly. Now a small video camera the size of a capsule can be swallowed and the image it transmits can be monitored on a television as the capsule passes into the small intestine. Investigators discovered in a preliminary study that 71 percent of the patients taking NSAIDs had erosions or ulcers in their small intestine, compared to only 10 percent of those not taking these drugs.[72] This unexpected finding suggests that NSAID damage to the intestinal tract is even more common and serious than previously suspected.

Frequently, aspirin is sold with an enteric coating that protects the stomach from harm. The coating is designed to dissolve in the small intestine instead, releasing the aspirin there. When we asked gastroenterologist Waqar Qureshi, MD, chief of endoscopy at Baylor University and the Michael E. DeBakey Veterans Affairs Medical Center in Houston, about such formulations, he said, "Enteric-coated drugs might, in fact, cause more damage than regular medications."[73] This is because the damage occurs in the small intestine, where the tissue is less resistant to irritating chemicals than the stomach is and where the damage may go undetected.

The COX-2 Catastrophe

With such GI toxicity associated with NSAIDs, it's hardly any wonder that doctors and patients were excited to learn about COX-2 inhibitors. Vioxx, Bextra, and Celebrex were introduced with the idea that they would be gentler on the stomach than other NSAIDs. That's because these newfangled members of the class were supposed to be "selective." They would block only the COX-2 enzyme, relieving inflammation as well as aspirin or other NSAIDs do. By sparing the COX-1 enzyme, prostaglandins would be created to protect the stomach from irritation. The promise: pain relief with much less risk of digestive upset or stomach ulcers.

As soon as COX-2 inhibitors were introduced in 1999, they took off like rocket ships. Aggressive advertising directed at consumers and enthusiastic prescribing by physicians turned Celebrex and Vioxx into overnight sensations. Tens of millions of people started popping these pills in the hope that they would relieve pain without the usual problems.

There was just one big *oops*. By selectively blocking the COX-2 enzyme to relieve inflammation, a crucial prostaglandin called *prostacyclin* was also reduced. This compound is our friend. It dilates blood vessels and keeps the sticky part of blood, called platelets, from clumping together to form clots. Without adequate amounts of prostacyclin circulating throughout the body, there is an increased risk of blood clots that can trigger heart attacks and strokes.

Early in the development of COX-2 inhibitors some researchers worried that there could be cardiovascular dangers. In 2000, a large Vioxx study suggested that the pain reliever could cause an increased risk of heart attacks and other vascular complications.[74]

Neither the FDA nor the manufacturer acted on those early warning flags. In one of the darkest hours in the history of American medicine, millions were allowed to continue taking COX-2 inhibitors until the fall of 2004. By then the handwriting was on the wall. First Vioxx and then Bextra were pulled off the market. In the interim, it is estimated that more than 100,000 people who had been taking COX-2 inhibitors suffered heart attacks and strokes.[75] According to FDA safety officer David Graham, MD, as many as 40,000 people may have died.[76]

The Broken Promise

If COX-2 inhibitors like Vioxx, Bextra, and Celebrex had truly protected the digestive tract from damage, it might have been easier to justify their approval, aggressive marketing tactics, and high prices. But an editorial in the *Journal of the American Medical Association* described the science behind COX-2 inhibitors as a "house of cards" based on wishful thinking. They were marketed "with unrealistic expectations about pain relief, marked gastrointestinal protection, and safety."[77]

Canadian researchers tracked hospital admissions caused by gastrointestinal bleeding before and after the introduction of COX-2 inhibitors (Vioxx, Celebrex, and Mobic). Instead of dropping when the new drugs became available, as investigators had expected, the rate of hemorrhage and hospitalization for older people paradoxically rose by 10 percent.[78] British researchers asked a similar question: Would COX-2 inhibitors be easier on the stomach than traditional NSAIDs? The answer: There was no evidence to suggest that the newer drugs were less harmful to the digestive tract.[79] In hindsight, it looks as if we were all sold an expensive bill of goods.

FDA NSAID WARNING

"NSAIDs may cause an increased risk of serious cardiovascular thrombotic events, myocardial infarction [heart attack], and stroke, which can be fatal."[80]
—FDA Public Health Advisory, April 7, 2005

Other NSAID Troubles

No sooner did the FDA wake up to the risk of heart attacks and strokes associated with COX-2 inhibitors than the agency had to deal with the possibility that other NSAIDs might pose a similar problem. Decades after these drugs began to be marketed, the FDA reviewed the data and decided that all such prescription pain relievers should carry a stronger black-box warning.

The FDA goes on to warn that people with risk factors for cardiovascular disease are especially vulnerable to these life-threatening problems. That includes almost everyone with arthritis. If you accumulate enough birthdays to develop osteoarthritis, you are bound to have some hardening of the arteries. But that's not all. The FDA has gone on to emphasize other problems with NSAIDs as well.

It is easy for your eyes to glaze over when looking at such a list. You may also assume that some of these potential side effects are rare events, but that could be a dangerous assumption. A study of older and potentially sicker patients revealed a startling incidence of kidney damage associated with Celebrex. More than 20 percent of the people taking this COX-2 inhibitor experienced kidney toxicity (fluid retention, high blood pressure, and kidney failure).[81] If patients had some kidney impairment before the study started (a common situation in older people), the likelihood of kidney toxicity jumped to more than 50 percent! We assume other NSAIDs are likely to have a similar effect on kidney function.

OTHER NSAID ADVERSE EFFECTS

- High blood pressure
- Fluid retention, edema
- Congestive heart failure
- Stomach ulcer (bleeding)
- Perforation of the stomach
- Perforation of the small intestine
- Perforation of the large intestine
- Kidney damage
- Severe allergic reaction
- Skin rash (toxic)
- Itching
- Stevens-Johnson syndrome
- Liver damage
- Blood disorders (anemia)
- Asthma worsening

NSAID Survival Strategy

By now it should be clear that nonsteroidal anti-inflammatory drugs, including the COX-2 inhibitors, can be trouble with a capital T! They aren't all that effective for arthritis, especially of the knee. Some NSAIDs may actually contribute to joint deterioration if they are taken for years. Then there's the risk of serious side effects like bleeding ulcers, hypertension, heart attacks, strokes, and kidney or liver damage. Why would anyone in his or her right mind take such medicine?

★★★★ Aspirin

Aspirin prevents blood clots and lowers the risk of heart attacks and strokes. Unlike other NSAIDs, it does not raise blood pressure.

Aspirin remains the best buy for pain relief. At pennies a day, it reduces the inflammation that is at the root of so many chronic ailments, including arthritis, diabetes, and Alzheimer's disease. Regular aspirin users seem to develop fewer cancers of the colon, rectum, prostate, pancreas, ovary, skin, lung, and breast.

Downside: Damage to the stomach lining. The potential for indigestion, gastritis, and ulcers makes this drug inappropriate for many. Bleeding or perforated ulcers can be life threatening. Anyone on long-term aspirin therapy must be under medical supervision.

Cost: Approximately $2 to 5 per month

The most obvious answer is that there aren't very many pharmaceutical alternatives. Doctors have relatively little to offer beyond NSAIDs when it comes to pain and inflammation. And sometimes you hurt so much that you need something to help you move your bones around. When used in the short-term and with appropriate safeguards, it may be possible to take an NSAID. But which one should you consider?

Aspirin remains our first choice by far. No other NSAID or OTC pain reliever has ever been proven more effective. In addition, aspirin reduces the risk of heart attacks and thrombotic (clotting) strokes. As a bonus, there is growing evidence that aspirin may diminish the likelihood of developing many common cancers. We discourage the use of enteric-coated aspirin because this merely moves the aspirin to the small intestine, where it can do serious damage.

Our preferred method for taking aspirin is as a liquid. In Europe, Australia, Canada, New Zealand, and dozens of other countries you can find several soluble, effervescent aspirin products. Brands like Aspro and Disprin are very popular because all you do is drop the aspirin tablets into a glass of water, where they fizzle and dissolve within seconds. This makes them a little faster acting and possibly a little less irritating to the stomach (though there is no guarantee of protection).

Soluble aspirin never really caught on in the United States, except in the form of Alka-Seltzer. It is a combination of aspirin, sodium bicarbonate, and citric acid advertised for

---

ASPIRIN AND BAKING SODA

Although it will not be identical to Alka-Seltzer, you can create your own buffered, soluble aspirin. In a glass, combine:

- 2 uncoated aspirins
- 8 ounces club soda or sparkling water
- ½ teaspoon baking soda
- Juice from ¼ wedge lemon

Wait till the aspirins dissolve and then drink. This formula is not appropriate for people on a sodium-restricted diet.

relief of "acid indigestion, sour stomach, heartburn with headache, body aches and pains." The trouble with Alka-Seltzer is that it's way more expensive than plain aspirin and there's too much sodium for folks who have congestive heart failure or salt-sensitive hypertension.

If you would prefer not to pay an arm and a leg for fizzy aspirin, you could make your own soluble aspirin for a fraction of the cost. All you have to do is buy some club soda or sparkling water. Drop two regular-strength aspirin tablets in the fizzy water and let them dissolve. It will take a couple of minutes.

Aspirin-Like Drugs

One of the best arthritis buys in the pharmacy is a frequently overlooked prescription drug called salsalate. It has been around for so long that many physicians have forgotten about it. Because salsalate is available generically, the cost should only be the amount of your co-pay. Even without insurance, the cost shouldn't be much more than $1 a day.

Salsalate is a kissing cousin to aspirin (it is salicylsalicylic acid instead of acetylsalicylic acid). Because it lacks the acetyl group, salsalate behaves differently in the body. Studies done 20 to 30 years ago suggest that it may be a little less irritating to the stomach than aspirin because it is absorbed only from the small intestine. (There are no data on whether it irritates the small intestine the way enteric-coated aspirin does.)

Salsalate is just as effective as aspirin at relieving joint pain or morning stiffness. Unfortunately, it probably won't prevent blood clots or heart attacks the way aspirin does. Salsalate may also be a little more likely to cause dizziness or ringing in the ears. It does require medical supervision, just as any NSAID does, and probably has similar side effects.

Another aspirin-like arthritis medicine that is often overlooked is choline magnesium trisalicylate (Tricosal, Trilasate, Trisalicylate). It too requires a prescription and should cost a lot less than $1 a day. Like salsalate, it may be a little less irritating to the stomach than aspirin. Again, it provides no extra protection against heart attacks or strokes.

Ibuprofen and Naproxen

For those who cannot tolerate aspirin or who want a traditional NSAID to get them over a hump, which drugs would we consider using? This is an incredibly difficult call because of the new and alarming data linking these drugs to heart attacks. If forced to recommend something, we would probably fall back on naproxen. For one thing, it is a good deal. When prescribed generically the co-pay should

BRANDS OF SALSALATE

- Amigesic
- Artha-G
- Disalcid
- Mono-Gesic
- Salflex
- Salsitab

be $10 or less a month. Even when purchased over the counter the cost should be no more than 15 cents per day. That compares to as much as $4 to $7 a day for Celebrex.

One study found that ibuprofen and naproxen are not associated with accelerated progression of hip and knee arthritis the way some other NSAIDs are.[83] Another possible plus with these two drugs may be a somewhat safer cardiovascular profile. One epidemiological study demonstrated no increased risk of heart attacks or other cardiovascular complications with these two pain relievers when they were used for short periods of time.[84] Another study, unfortunately, found that NSAIDs like ibuprofen increase the risk of a second heart attack.[85] A Danish study of nearly 60,000 heart attack survivors showed that NSAIDs such as Celebrex, ibuprofen, and diclofenac were linked to an increased risk of heart attack death. This complication showed up within several weeks of starting on the pain reliever. The researchers concluded that heart attack survivors need to be very cautious about the kind of pain reliever they use.

Even people who have not had a heart attack need to be wary about NSAIDs. Anyone with high blood pressure, high cholesterol, blockage in a coronary artery, or kidney problems is likely to be at increased risk of a heart attack when taking such pain relievers.[86]

Finnish investigators studied more than 33,000 heart attack patients hospitalized between 2000 and 2003. By comparing them to 139,000 control subjects, the researchers found that taking any NSAID increased the

SIGNS OF TROUBLE!*

- Chest pain
- Shortness of breath or sudden weakness
- Slurred speech or paralysis
- Severe stomach pain or indigestion
- Black, tarry stools
- Sudden weight gain
- Trouble removing a ring
- Skin rash, itching, blisters, fever
- Nausea, fatigue, yellow eyes, flu symptoms

*If any of these symptoms occur, contact your physician immediately or visit urgent care.

chance of a heart attack by approximately 40 percent.[87]

For those who think taking aspirin together with a drug like Advil or Aleve might diminish any risk of a blood clot, think again. There are no clear-cut data to support that notion. There is even some worry that drugs like ibuprofen and naproxen might undo the cardiovascular protective benefits of aspirin.[88,89] Be wary of interactions with other medications, especially blood pressure drugs (ACE inhibitors), furosemide (Lasix), lithium (Eskalith, Cibalith, Lithane, Lithobid, Lithotabs), methotrexate (Rheumatrex, Trexal), and blood thinners like warfarin (Coumadin).

Of course anyone who opts to use an NSAID must treat these drugs with the respect they deserve. Treatment for more than 10 days requires medical supervision and great vigilance. Remember, there may be an increased risk for heart attack, hypertension, heart failure, kidney problems, and ulcers.

To counteract the risk of serious GI toxicity, many gastroenterologists now routinely recommend acid-suppressing drugs called PPIs (proton pump inhibitors) in combination with NSAIDs. Medications such as esomeprazole (Nexium), lansoprazole (Prevacid), omeprazole (Prilosec), pantoprazole (Protonix), and rabeprazole (Aciphex) are supposed to diminish the likelihood of NSAID-induced stomach upset and ulcers.[92] Despite this belief, there is no guarantee that such drugs can prevent all ulcers or perforations. A review of the use of low-dose aspirin in the *New England Journal of Medicine* cautions against any sense of complacency. This should apply to all NSAIDs.

Topical NSAIDs

Americans have been deprived of an arthritis treatment that is widely available all over the world. Topical NSAIDs (gels, creams, and sprays) are very popular with patients and physicians in Europe, Australia, Canada, Italy, New Zealand, and dozens of other countries, but they are virtually ignored in the United States. The very same drugs (diclofenac, ibuprofen, ketoprofen, ketorolac, piroxicam, etc.) that cause so much mischief when taken orally can be applied to the skin with little, if any, risk of stomach ulcers, kidney problems, heart attacks, strokes, or other systemic complications. Except for aspirin-like compounds (salicylates) found in OTC products like Aspercreme, BenGay, Myoflex crème, and Sportscreme, you will not find topical NSAIDs on pharmacy shelves in the United States. That's because the FDA has never approved these formulations for topical use.

PPI CAUTION

"Although there seems to be a general agreement among gastroenterologists that proton pump inhibitors should be prescribed to high-risk patients taking low-dose aspirin,[90] such a strategy has not been widely adopted because of a lack of definitive evidence to support it."[91]

—Carlo Patrono et al., *The New England Journal of Medicine*, 2005

How effective are topical NSAIDs for relieving the pain and inflammation of arthritis? Over the years there have been dozens of clinical trials of such products for both temporary (acute) discomfort and longer-term (chronic) treatment.[93] One review of 26 double-blind, placebo-controlled trials involving 2,853 patients concluded that "topical NSAIDs were effective and safe in treating acute painful conditions for 1 week."[94]

Okay, okay! We hear you: "One week, big deal." Another review examined 14 double-blind, placebo-controlled trials including almost 1,500 patients. The conclusion: "Topical NSAIDs were effective and safe in treating chronic musculoskeletal conditions for 2 weeks."[95] That's a little better, but still not a long-term solution. One sour note comes from the thorough and objective Cochrane Library. The reviewers for this organization analyze all available evidence, published and unpublished, and provide their assessment of various treatments. This 2004 review looked at studies of use of topical NSAIDs for longer than 2 weeks and determined that "after 2 weeks there was no evidence of efficacy superior to placebo. No trial data support the long-term use of topical NSAIDs in osteoarthritis."[96]

Based on this summary we would be inclined to suggest that topical NSAIDs be used for 2 weeks or less to relieve an acute arthritis flare-up. On the brighter side, there are now four newer clinical trials of use for 3 to 12 weeks.[97, 98] Investigators specifically looked at osteoarthritis of the knee. In each

study, diclofenac (Pennsaid or Voltaren Emugel) was superior to placebo in providing relief, with only "minor local irritation and no significant systemic adverse events."[99, 100] In a 12-week head-to-head comparison of oral diclofenac with topical diclofenac (Pennsaid Lotion), their effectiveness was comparable. But side effects like nausea, indigestion, stomach pain, and liver damage were much more likely to occur with the oral NSAID.[101]

Pennsaid Lotion is interesting because the formulation relies on DMSO (dimethyl sulfoxide) to help get the drug through the skin and into the area of the joint where pain relief is desired. DMSO is a solvent that is uniquely able to penetrate the skin and carry medications with it. We have long wondered why drug companies were not using DMSO to facilitate absorption. Now the makers of Pennsaid have done just that.

So, how can you get topical NSAIDs? If you were in Australia you could purchase products like piroxicam (Feldene Gel), ibuprofen (Nurofen Gel), ketoprofen (Orudis Gel), and diclofenac (Voltaren Emulgel) over the counter without a prescription. At this time that is impossible in the United States. Nevertheless, it is possible to purchase oral ibuprofen and ketoprofen over the counter. That means a compounding pharmacist (one who mixes raw ingredients into finished products) can legally purchase ibuprofen or ketoprofen powder, make a cream or a gel, and sell it to you without a prescription.

An alternative would be to shop online for one of the brands mentioned above. Since they

This topical NSAID has been shown to provide lasting relief from the pain and inflammation of osteoarthritis. It may produce some skin irritation, but does not appear to cause significant systemic toxicity, as oral diclofenac does.

Side effects: Skin dryness, flakiness, and rash

Downside: Not available in the United States. Available by prescription in Canada, Finland, Iceland, Italy, Greece, Portugal, the United Kingdom, and elsewhere.

Cost: Approximately $60 to $120 per month

are nonprescription in many countries, you may be able to purchase them and not have US Customs give you any problems. One final option, and our number one recommendation, is to have a US physician write a prescription for Pennsaid. This topical form of diclofenac has been tested in several clinical trials and found to produce long-lasting relief from osteoarthritis. You would then need to contact a Canadian pharmacy online or by phone to have the prescription filled. Since this drug is not available in the United States, you should be able to import it legally without incurring the wrath of the FDA.

Alternatives for Arthritis

Many physicians complain about alternative therapies on the grounds that they are not sci-

entifically valid or FDA approved. But we have just established that FDA-sanctioned drugs like corticosteroids, NSAIDs, and COX-2 inhibitors have caused untold misery and countless deaths. Many of the treatments you will now read about have not been tested in double-blind, randomized, placebo-controlled trials the way Vioxx and Bextra were. Nevertheless, we doubt that any could trigger the kind of public health catastrophe these "well tested" pharmaceuticals have caused.

Some of the approaches you will read about will seem illogical. Others will have a surprising amount of research behind them. One thing we do not know is whether combining some of these alternative approaches will enhance their effectiveness. All we can suggest is trial and error. Some folks tell us that gin-soaked raisins have provided almost miraculous relief from arthritis pain. Others tell us this remedy is worthless. We cannot explain why one person would get such a dramatic benefit while another would find it ineffective. Then again, we cannot explain why one person's headache will quickly disappear after taking two aspirin tablets and someone else will get zero relief. Each of us is a complex biological system that responds differently to drugs, herbs, dietary supplements, and home remedies. The best we can do is to pay careful attention to how our body responds to whatever treatments we try.

You Are What You Eat

No one really understands why some people develop osteoarthritis at a relatively early age while others seem fairly immune to aches and pains well into their eighties. We used to think this kind of arthritis was due to wear and tear. If you accumulated enough birthdays, the theory went, you were bound to damage joints. But that's not always true. There are people in their nineties who get around amazingly well without a lot of pain or stiffness while a lot of fiftysomethings can barely go up and down stairs. Athletes are not necessarily more likely to develop osteoarthritis than couch potatoes, though football players and those who damage their joints are at greater risk.

In some respects the couch potato may be in greater danger of developing joint problems than many athletes. If you are overweight, you put more strain on your knees and hips and increase your risk for later problems. We are also beginning to learn that what you eat may influence your risk of arthritis.

Good Foods versus Bad Foods

Q. *I was eating a piece of chocolate when a friend said, "That's not good for your arthritis." Since then, another friend told me to avoid tomatoes.*

All this advice is confusing me. Are there really foods I should avoid and are there any foods that might help arthritis?

A BENEFIT OF LOSING WEIGHT

"It actually doesn't take that much weight loss to make a difference. You can lose as little as 10 to 12 pounds and cut your risk of developing symptomatic knee osteoarthritis in half."[102]

—Joanne Jordan, MD, MPH, Associate Director of the University of North Carolina Thurston Arthritis Research Center

---

A. Researchers at Tufts University reported that small changes in diet may make a difference in arthritis control.[103] Omega-3 fatty acids, found primarily in fish but also in flaxseeds, pecans, walnuts, tofu, and green leafy vegetables, help fight inflammation. Common oils such as corn, sunflower, and safflower are full of omega-6 fatty acids that may actually promote inflammation and joint pain.

• • •

The researchers suggest having at least six servings a day of produce (three vegetables and three fruits) to get adequate vitamin C and beta-carotene. They also recommend substituting fish (a 3-ounce serving every other day), beans (½ cup), and nuts (1 ounce) for meat. Vitamin D and fish oil supplements (for those who cannot stomach fish) may also be helpful. These foods seem to provide anti-inflammatory nutrients that may help relieve joint pain.

Chocolate and tomatoes may trigger pain for some sensitive individuals. Most folks, however, don't have to avoid these treats. You'll have to be your own judge on whether specific foods trigger your discomfort.

SELENIUM

A growing body of data suggests that there are anti-inflammatory foods that may promote joint health, and that a lack of certain nutrients may be risky for joints. Epidemiologists have known for some time that low levels of selenium in the diet of persons living in parts of China, North Korea, and Siberia increased the risk of a kind of early onset osteoarthritis (Kashin-Beck osteoarthropathy).[105] Researchers have discovered that low selenium may also pose a risk for US citizens. They carefully measured the amount of selenium in the toenails of 940 rural and suburban North Carolinians. This technique allows for a scientific estimate of selenium exposure over a prolonged period. Scientists then compared knee x-rays to the level of selenium in each person's system. They found that people with a high selenium level were 40 to 50 percent less likely to experience knee osteoarthritis than were individuals who were low in selenium.[106]

Should you be taking a selenium supplement to ward off arthritis? So far, there are no data to suggest that that would work. We always encourage people to try to get their nutrients from the most natural source possible—food! Neverthe-less, there are data to suggest that selenium is essential for good health. It appears to be involved in regulating inflammation and immune function, helping to ward off infection and maybe even prevent cancers of the prostate, esophagus, stomach, and lungs.[107, 108] Eating a couple of Brazil nuts three or four times a week could be one of the safest and tastiest ways to get extra selenium in the diet. Don't pig out, however. Joanne Jordan, MD, MPH, advises against consuming much more than 400 micrograms of selenium daily. Excess selenium (prolonged intake of more than 1 mg daily) may be toxic. Symptoms of toxicity include brittle hair and nails, skin rash, fatigue, nausea, and vomiting.

HIGH SELENIUM FOODS

FOOD	SELENIUM CONTENT
Brazil nuts	544 mcg per 1 oz serving
Chicken liver	71 mcg per 3 oz serving
Tuna (canned)	63 mcg per 3 oz serving
Mackerel	53 mcg per 3 oz serving
Spaghetti with meat sauce	34 mcg per serving
Sunflower seeds	26 mcg per 1 oz serving
Wheat germ	22 mcg per 1 oz serving
Chicken breast	20 mcg per 3.5 oz serving
Oatmeal (prepared)	12 mcg per cup
Egg	14 mcg per medium egg

BETA-CRYPTOXANTHIN AND ZEAXANTHIN SOURCES

- Carrots
- Cilantro
- Corn
- Oranges
- Papayas
- Peaches
- Pumpkins
- Red bell peppers
- Tangerines
- Watermelon

ORANGE JUICE

A glass of fresh orange juice may seem like an indulgence, but if it could help prevent inflammation and arthritis it would be well worth the time and expense. A study published in the *American Journal of Clinical Nutrition* (August 2005) suggests that you might want to think of OJ as preventive medicine.

The investigators followed more than 25,000 people between 1993 and 2001. The subjects who consumed the most antioxidant carotenoids (specifically, beta-cryptoxanthin and zeaxanthin) were the least likely to develop inflammatory arthritis.[109] These compounds are found in yellow and orange fruits and vegetables. The researchers determined that the amount of beta-cryptoxanthin in just one glass of freshly squeezed orange juice daily is enough

to reduce the risk of inflammatory conditions such as rheumatoid arthritis.

The Sunshine Vitamin

We are often asked what we would take with us to a desert island. If we could take only one drug it would be aspirin, the cheapest and most versatile medicine in the pharmacy. If we could take only one vitamin it would be vitamin D. The really good news is that we wouldn't have to take it along. It's already there. Vitamin D is the cheapest nutrient in the world because you don't have to pay a penny for it. All you need is a few minutes of sun exposure every day and your body will make all the vitamin D you need.

This compound is essential for overall good health and yet millions of people are deficient in vitamin D. That's because they are totally

★★★★★ Vitamin D

The sunshine vitamin is the best deal in town because it is free. This nutrient is associated with a lower risk of osteoporosis, fractures, depression, cancer, and arthritis. Five to 10 minutes of sun exposure (without sunscreen) on the hands, arms, and face every 2 or 3 days is enough to do the job for most people.[110]

If oral supplements are necessary because sun exposure is not practical, we recommend anywhere from 800 IU to 1,200 IU per day. Do not overdose, though. Keep your total intake under 2,000 IU daily.

confused about sun exposure. Dermatologists have been issuing dire warnings for decades. They tell us that the sun causes wrinkles, age spots, and skin cancer. If we go out in the sun without slathering on the sunscreen, we've been led to believe we're living dangerously.

If we spend a lot of time soaking up the rays this is indisputably true. On the other hand, research has been mounting that sunshine prevents cancer. Numerous studies have demonstrated that cancers of the colon, breast, prostate, and lung are less common among people who get some regular sun exposure.

Sunshine is important because it stimulates the production of vitamin D in the skin. It is possible to overdose with oral supplementation, but the skin only makes as much as the body can use. Unfortunately, many Americans do not get enough vitamin D. They spend most of their time inside. Even in the summer they may prefer to spend their time in air-conditioned comfort. If they do engage in outside activities, they put on a high SPF sunscreen before they even go out the door. This dramatically reduces the amount of vitamin D the skin can make.

Vitamin D that is made in the skin circulates throughout the body. Tissues that need to use vitamin D as a hormone are capable of transforming it into the activated compound that seems to be responsible for its cancer-preventing properties. The form of vitamin D produced by sun-exposed skin may be more efficient for this use than that in oral supplements.

Don't get us wrong, though. Supplements can be helpful, especially for those who do not get enough sunlight. Research published in the *American Journal of Public Health* (February 2006) reports that when people take 1,000 IU of vitamin D daily the risk of getting colorectal cancer is cut in half and the chance of coming down with either breast or ovarian cancer is reduced by one-third.

In addition to the anticancer benefits of vitamin D, research shows that this nutrient is crucial for strong bones. When people take at least 800 IU daily they reduce their risk of hip fracture by 26 percent.[111] The potential power of vitamin D to help prevent the progression of osteoarthritis (OA) is equally astonishing. The Framingham Heart Study has been following people in that Massachusetts community for more than 50 years. Researchers have been especially interested in lifestyle, diet, and heart disease data. But they have also considered other health issues, including arthritis.

In 1996 a landmark study was published in the *Annals of Internal Medicine* that went almost unnoticed. Investigators reported that Framingham participants with low intake and low serum levels of vitamin D had "an increased risk for progression of osteoarthritis of the knee."[112] In fact, these citizens were three times more likely to have their OA progress than were those with high levels of vitamin D. Although the study did not demonstrate that vitamin D could prevent the development of arthritis, the researchers were bold enough to suggest that people who have OA and modest vitamin D intake "may benefit from increased vitamin D intake or exposure to sunlight."[113] We don't know yet whether regular vitamin D intake (or sun exposure) will prevent osteoporosis, but we wouldn't be at all surprised if that were the case.

The Mediterranean Diet

There is growing recognition that certain foods may increase inflammation while others dampen the body's inflammatory responses. Numerous epidemiological studies suggest that both the prevalence and severity of rheumatoid arthritis may be lower in regions where people consume more fish, olive oil, fruits, vegetables, and legumes.[114, 115]

Normally you think of Greece, Crete, or Italy when you think about this sort of Mediterranean diet. That's why it comes as such a delightful surprise to learn that researchers tested this diet at a rheumatology center in southeastern Sweden. To enhance compliance with the diet, investigators supplied the human guinea pigs

---

THE MEDITERRANEAN DIET

There is no one exact "Mediterranean" diet, but common elements include:

• Olive oil

• Fish and poultry

• Lots of vegetables and fruits

• Legumes, nuts, and seeds

• Eggs

• Wine

---

with free olive oil, canola oil, margarine made from canola oil, frozen vegetables, and tea. Subjects who were randomly assigned to the Mediterranean diet achieved "a reduction in inflammatory activity, an increase in physical function and improved vitality."[116]

Additional research suggests that when people increase their intake of omega-3 and monounsaturated fats and reduce their consumption of omega-6 fatty acids, inflammation is decreased and there is a better clinical outcome.[117]

OMEGA-3 VS. OMEGA-6 FATS

OMEGA-3 AND MONOUNSATURATED FATS	OMEGA-6 FATS
Almond oil	Corn oil
Avocado oil	Cottonseed oil
Canola oil	Peanut oil
Olive oil	Safflower oil
Walnut oil	Sesame oil
	Sunflower oil

FISH OIL

No matter how careful you are about your diet, it may be hard to dramatically alter your ratio of omega-6 fats (which are pro-inflammatory) to omega-3 fats (anti-inflammatory). That's because vegetable oils that are high in omega-6 fatty acids (corn, safflower, sunflower) are ubiquitous in everything from cookies and crackers to soups and sauces.

Our great-grandparents had a healthier

★★ Fish Oil

There is little clinical evidence to support the value of fish oil against osteoarthritis. Nevertheless, the preliminary data look encouraging, and fish oil is one of the more effective anti-inflammatory compounds we know of.

Downside: A word of caution: High doses of fish oil may increase the risk of bleeding when combined with aspirin or other anticoagulants such as warfarin (Coumadin). Check with a physician before taking fish oil on a regular basis. Physicians we have consulted often recommend 1 to 3 grams daily.

Cost: Varies widely

ratio of omega-6 to omega-3 fats, probably in the realm of two or three to one. They ate meat from animals that were grass fed and therefore much higher in omega-3 fats. And they didn't have vending machines loaded with snacks. Today, various estimates are that we have a ratio of omega-6 fats to omega-3 fats of 10 or even 25 to 1.[118]

Our grandparents had another tradition that kept their omega-6 to omega-3 ratio under control: cod liver oil! As awful as it tasted, this old-fashioned remedy was loaded with omega-3 fatty acids. In the 18th century cod liver oil was considered a useful arthritis remedy. The trouble with this dietary supplement is that it contains way too much vitamin A, which may be bad for bones. Scientists have reported that high intake of vitamin A from cod liver oil in Sweden and Norway is associated with weaker bones, osteoporosis, and an increased risk of hip fracture.[119]

To get around this problem, pharmaceutical-grade fish oil might be very helpful. Barry Sears, PhD (of Zone Diet fame), recommends between 3 and 8 grams total of EPA (eicosapentaenoic acid) and DHA (docosahexaenoic acid) daily to calm inflammation.[120] According to Dr. Sears, that's roughly 1 to 3 teaspoons of fish oil or 4 to 12 capsules (depending on the brand).

How effective is fish oil in calming the pain and inflammation of osteoarthritis? Unfortunately, we don't have great randomized, double-blind, placebo-controlled trials to prove its benefit. An astonishing amount of

FISH OIL BREAKFAST SMOOTHIE

To enhance absorption and minimize taste, combine these ingredients in a blender:

- 1 to 3 teaspoons pharmaceutical-grade fish oil
- 1 tablespoon whey protein powder
- 1 teaspoon powdered egg white
- ½ frozen banana (peel before freezing)
- 1 cup frozen fruit
- 1 cup low-fat yogurt
- ½ cup grape, cherry, orange, or pomegranate juice

Blend at high speed until completely pureed, with no pieces of powder, fruit, or yogurt visible.

data suggests that fish oil is good against heart disease, though, and some tantalizing research indicates that omega-3 dietary supplements are "of benefit to human patients suffering from joint disease."[121] A man who listens to our syndicated public radio show offered his own experience with fish oil:

> **I had quite a bit of pain in my joints, particularly my knees. Then I started taking fish oil with omega-3 fatty acids. It has completely eliminated all the pain in the joints. I've been taking them for about 2 months and all the pain is gone. I take one capsule in the morning and that's it. Not only that, but it has virtually eliminated the clicking in my knees. When I would stand they would click. That's almost gone, and the pain is definitely gone.**
>
> **To find out if it was just a temporary thing that wouldn't work, I laid off of the fish oil for 3 or 4 days and there was the pain again.**
>
> **—Rex in Little Rock, Arkansas**

GREEN-LIPPED MUSSELS

The green-lipped mussels (GLMs) of New Zealand are getting a lot of buzz these days as another excellent source of anti-inflammatory omega-3 fatty acids.[122] They are definitely more exotic than plain old fish oil. A small, double-blind study of GLMs in arthritic dogs showed significant improvement of arthritis symptoms.[123] Veterinary studies are intriguing because we doubt that pets are particularly susceptible to a placebo effect.

We don't know if a lipid oil extract of green-lipped mussels will work as well for humans. We would love to see large, double-blind, placebo-controlled trials testing it. Several studies are now under way. In the meantime, if you would like to consider the GLM approach, you should be able to find the oil extract in your health-food store or on the Web. Not all brands of GLM are created equal. You may want to look for Lyprinol, which seems, according to our research, to be a quality product. It may take at least a month or two for results to start to show up.[124] If there is no improvement after 3 months, give up on those green-lipped mussels.

The Raisin Remedy

Until 1994 we never gave much thought to home remedies for arthritis. We assumed that the only effective treatments for inflammation were to be found in the drugstore. But in May of that year a letter arrived that changed the way we think about a lot of things. A reader of our newspaper column inquired about the value of soaking golden raisins in gin and then eating nine a day. We laughed at such a pre-

---

RAISIN RECIPE

- 1 box (15 ounces) golden raisins
- 1 pint good gin

Pour the gin over the raisins in a bowl. Cover with a towel and allow the gin to evaporate (it takes up to a week). Transfer the moist raisins to a covered jar and place it in refrigerator. Eat nine daily.

---

posterous idea but decided to share it anyway just for fun. That was the beginning of an extraordinary journey into the amazing world of arthritis home remedies.

Since we published the original recipe for gin-soaked golden raisins, we have received hundreds and hundreds of letters and e-mail messages from people all around the world. Many are astonished at the power of this remedy. Others say it isn't worth a damn. Of course, we also heard from folks who told us that the FDA-approved drug Vioxx was worthless for their arthritis while others insisted it was like a miracle.

Many physicians believe that the raisin remedy is placebo power at work. They maintain that any perceived benefit is merely mental. All we can say in response is that many folks do their own "challenge" testing. We have heard many stories like this:

> *Gin and golden raisins have kept me pain free for over a year. I ran out of gin, and went 1 week without this treatment. At the end of the week, the pain and stiffness in my knees came back, and it was very uncomfortable to sit down or get up from a chair. Needless to say, I went out that day and bought more gin.*

Cashiers in liquor stores periodically tell us about senior citizens who surreptitiously buy a bottle of gin for their arthritis. They don't want their friends or neighbors to know their little secret. Some say the nine daily raisins help their knees. Others insist the remedy relieves the pain and inflammation in their neck or elbows.

> *My mother has arthritis in the joint of one of her little fingers. The joint was frozen and she was in constant pain. Since she started eating gin-soaked golden raisins, the pain is gone and she is able to play tennis twice a week without discomfort. My mother just turned 81!*
>
> *We also suggested the raisins to a friend who was visiting from Norway. She has suffered years of pain from rheumatoid arthritis. After only a week of gin-soaked golden raisins, her pain was already starting to subside. I don't know what it is, but it seems to be very effective.*

We have heard all sorts of explanations for why the raisin remedy might work. Some think it's the juniper berry extract used to make gin. Others insist that the sulfite preservative used to bleach golden raisins provides the magic. (It also makes this remedy off-limits for anyone with a sulfite allergy.) And then there are all sorts of variations on the raisin remedy theme. One woman offered this: "I've been amused by your discussions of gin-soaked raisins for arthritis. My Dutch mother soaked diced dried apricots in gin for 2 weeks before consuming them. She said this relieved her aches and pains!"

We have even heard that instead of using regular gin, people should be using sloe gin:

> *People who don't get relief from golden raisins and gin should try the original remedy, passed down in my family for generations. It is nine dark raisins soaked in sloe gin. It could be the sloe*

berry that does the trick. This remedy is dark purple and delicious."

Sloe gin is made from the berries of the blackthorn shrub. In Europe, a syrup of sloe berries has been used traditionally for digestive disorders.

Although we cannot explain the power of gin and raisins, we can only say that it started us on a great adventure. Read on for some more amazing arthritis tales.

Grape Juice and Certo

In March 1998 we received word of another astonishing home remedy. It opened our eyes to all sorts of other possibilities.

> *My wife and I tried your golden raisins and gin for arthritis and we were unimpressed. We have discovered something else, though. Take 2 teaspoons of Certo [fruit pectin] dissolved in 3 ounces of grape juice. Do this three times a day. We have been told to cut back to 1 teaspoon Certo in grape juice twice a day after the joints quit aching.*
>
> *We buy Certo in the grocery store near the canning jars. It's simple and cheap and seems to be helping. I am on Coumadin so I can't take anti-inflammatory drugs like Advil or Aleve."*

The moment we shared this alternative approach to arthritis, the response was over-

> "The berries of juniper ('Wacholder') were a favorite remedy prescribed for a variety of ailments by the 19th-century priest and healer Sebastian Kneipp, who was revered as a saint by his patients and dismissed as a quack by the medical profession.
>
> According to a German chart in our house that describes herbal remedies, juniper cures rheumatism, gout, skin disorders, and the common cold, presumably in that order of effectiveness."
>
> —H.H. Stadelmaier, PhD, Professor Emeritus, Materials Science and Engineering, North Carolina State University

whelming. It was as if the floodgates had opened. We heard from people who had been using this remedy for decades. One woman reported that her grandmother had been relying on Certo and grape juice since the 1940s.

★★★★★ Grape Juice and Certo

We offer three different recipes for this remedy:

• 2 teaspoons Certo in 3 ounces grape juice (three times daily)

• 1 tablespoon Certo in 8 ounces grape juice (once daily)

• 1 packet Certo in 64 ounces of grape juice (drink 6 to 8 ounces daily)

We personally opt for the third recipe because it is the most convenient. Home remedies are, by their nature, not scientific. Go with what works best for you.

This is one of our few five-star remedies because it is inexpensive and may do triple duty by relieving inflammation, increasing the flexibility of blood vessels, and lowering cholesterol. Do not take statin drugs at the same time; they may not be absorbed well.

When Grandma went to Florida for a 2-week vacation she skipped the remedy. By the time she got home she was in major pain and cried as she crawled into bed. Two weeks after resuming the Certo and grape juice, Grandma was fine again.

For those who have never done any home canning, Certo is a mystery. This product was introduced in Canada in 1919 for jam and jelly manufacturers. It was first sold to home canners as Certo in 1923 as a thickening agent. Without plant pectin, jam would be runny and not very appetizing. Today, liquid Certo is sold by Kraft and is still used to thicken jams and jellies. It can be found in most supermarkets in the home canning section.

Aging athletes have been especially delighted with this home remedy. Bill Weinacht is an octogenarian who was a world-class sprinter (the 100 meters) in his age category. To his disappointment, osteoarthritis of the knees had reduced him to racewalking. But after trying the grape juice and Certo recipe, he reported, *"voilà,"* back to sprinting. Bill wasn't the only athlete to report success. We have heard from other runners as well:

" *I want to describe a home remedy that has made dramatic improvements in my osteoarthritis. I am now 60 years old and have had no cartilage in my right knee since 1967.*

I have led an active lifestyle: running (quit 15 years ago after running 34,582 miles, lifetime), basketball (half-court basketball, twice weekly, for 40 years), and walking (1 to 3 miles daily). In the last several years my arthritis symptoms had worsened. The pain was continuous, and the swelling of the knee was significant. I was forced to use a leg brace and then a cane. I had trouble sleeping, and was considering a total knee replacement.

Then a business associate mentioned that some friends had found relief from their osteoarthritis by using a home remedy: Each morning swallow 2 teaspoons of liquid pectin in 4 to 6 ounces of grape juice. The pectin I use is for making fruit jams at home and carries the tradename Certo.

Within 8 hours my pain diminished to almost zero, the swelling was reduced significantly, and I slept all night without interruption for the first time in years. I no longer need my brace or my cane.

These positive results have continued every single day since starting the regimen. I made no other changes in medications, supplements, diet, or activities and have continued the regimen faithfully every day.

Come to the Maverick Athletic Club most Saturday mornings and watch me play half-court basketball with men half my age. My right knee is still "arthritic bone on arthritic bone," but I have surprising mobility and only very moderate discomfort. "
—Kent Hedman, Arlington, Texas

We cannot promise that drinking purple grape juice with Certo will eliminate the need for knee replacement surgery, but we no longer think of this as just a quirky home remedy. There is growing scientific evidence that grape juice has powerful anti-inflammatory activity. Polyphenols are natural antioxidant compounds found in many foods such as blueberries, cherries, grapes, chocolate, parsley, and tea. One particular subset of polyphenols called *proanthocyanidins* (PAs) is of particular interest. These antioxidant flavonoids give fruits their tart or astringent flavor. They are of great interest because PAs have many health benefits. They appear to reduce the risk of blood clots by making platelets less sticky while also making blood vessels more flexible.[125]

The USDA reports that serving for serving, grape juice has more PAs than any other beverage including apple juice, cranberry juice, red wine, or tea.[126] Researchers have shown that grape juice can raise good HDL cholesterol, reduce the oxidation of bad LDL cholesterol, diminish platelet stickiness, and reduce inflammation that can lead to atherosclerosis.[127, 128] If grape juice can have such a profound impact on the inflammatory reactions that contribute to coronary artery disease, we can imagine that this simple beverage might also be affecting inflammation in joint tissue.

66 *Last year my cholesterol was 284. I read your column about ½ cup apple cider vinegar mixed with 4 cups apple and 3 cups grape juice, and began taking 6 ounces of this tonic every morning before breakfast.*

Slowly but surely my cholesterol has dropped. Now it is down to 212. In addition, the arthritis pain in my knee is gone. 99

Juice and Vinegar

D.C. Jarvis, MD, wrote about the value of vinegar and honey in 1958 in his classic book, *A Vermont Country Doctor's Guide to Good Health*. Over the years readers have shared their success with a variety of juice and vinegar recipes. Sometimes people come up with their own imaginative combinations, which is how home remedies get started in the first place. Because there is no clinical research behind these recipes, we cannot tell you which, if any, would work best for you. Here are several worth consideration:

66 *My husband and I are interested in arthritis remedies. We've been taking cider vinegar and honey in a cup of hot water to ease the pain in our finger joints. Even so, my husband's thumbs hurt so much he could hardly grasp anything, and I recently developed a hard painful lump on my right ring finger.*

We read in your column about a solution of five parts grape juice, three parts apple juice, and one part cider vinegar. Then we also read about Certo and grape juice. We decided to combine these remedies and added two parts of Certo to the apple-grape-cider mixture. Within a couple of weeks the lump on my finger went away and the finger became less painful and stiff. 99

This last remedy came from Bud of Dallas, Texas, who shared the following story:

66 *The man that once owned the Dallas Cowboys gave me his arthritis remedy and it's been a god-*

VINEGAR AND JUICE #1

- 1 cup vinegar
- ⅓ cup honey
- 16 ounces grape juice
- 32 ounces apple juice

  Drink a couple of ounces daily.

VINEGAR AND JUICE #2

- 1 part cider vinegar
- 3 parts apple juice
- 5 parts grape juice

  Drink ½ cup daily.

VINEGAR AND JUICE #3

- 1 teaspoon orange gelatin powder
- ½ teaspoon apple cider vinegar
- ½ teaspoon honey
- 6 ounces water

  Stir ingredients together and drink daily.

send. It's 1 teaspoon of a mixture of 50 percent apple cider vinegar and 50 percent honey (I mix a quart for a month or so supply) added to a 6-ounce glass of water with a teaspoon of Knox orange-flavored gelatin powder stirred in and dissolved. Within a few weeks I regained virtually 100 percent use of my knuckles which had really become stiff, sore, and painful to use! Exact measure of the three does not seem to be critical. I just eyeball them, stir, and drink. Hope it works as well for others as it does for me."

Pomegranate Juice

If you've ever eaten a pomegranate you know that it is powerful. The bright red color and unique flavor make pomegranates really special. They played an important role in Greek mythology in the story of Persephone, daughter of the harvest goddess, Demeter. Hades, the lord of the underworld, kidnapped the beautiful maiden. Because she ate a few pomegranate seeds before being rescued, she had to spend several months every year in the underworld with him. According to the myth, that's when the earth was forced to endure winter.

Thousands of years later, pomegranates are still getting attention, especially in the scientific community. Researchers report that they are rich in antioxidants that can keep bad LDL cholesterol from oxidizing.[129] This degra-

---

★★★★ Pomegranates

What's not to love about pomegranates? The fruit is delicious and rich in antioxidants. Scientific studies have demonstrated that the juice may reduce the risk of heart disease, erectile dysfunction, and prostate and breast cancer. Pomegranate juice extract may also calm inflammation around joints and slow cartilage destruction.

Downside: Pomegranates might interact with some drugs in a manner similar to grapefruit. Anyone taking prescription medicine should check for possible interactions.

dation of LDL seems to be a key step in the development of atherosclerosis. In addition, pomegranate juice, like grape juice and aspirin, can help keep blood platelets from clumping together to form unwanted clots. Data also suggest that pomegranate juice may enhance oxygen flow to the heart in patients who have coronary artery disease and might even help combat erectile dysfunction.[130] Preliminary research in animals suggests that pomegranate juice may help prevent prostate cancer.

Most important to this discussion, pomegranates may be valuable in combating arthritis. Scientists at Case Western Reserve University have reported in the *Journal of Nutrition* that tissue cultures of human cartilage cells respond to pomegranate extract.[131] Inflammation is reduced and the enzymes that break down cartilage become less active.

Tariq Haqqi, PhD, is professor of medicine at Case Western Reserve University and the lead investigator in this research. He told us that pomegranate juice extract is very, very effective at inhibiting the production of mediators of cartilage degradation that are found in osteoarthritic joints. He admitted that both he and his wife are now big believers in pomegranate juice extract and are drinking it regularly in the hope of inhibiting the induction or progression of osteoarthritis.[132]

Cherry Juice

We have been writing about the value of cherries (fresh, dried, or frozen cherries; cherry juice; and even cherry extract capsules) against gout for many years. This is another one of those remedies about which the old wives were way out in front of the scientists. In 2003, investigators at the University of California at Davis conducted a little study on 10 healthy women between 22 and 40 years of age. They measured the urate level and other inflammatory markers in blood samples before and after a dose of bing cherries (280 grams). High levels of urate (uric acid) in the blood can cause gout attacks. The crystals precipitate around joints (especially in the big toe) and cause severe inflammation and excruciating pain.

The investigators reported in the *Journal of Nutrition*: "The decrease in plasma urate after cherry consumption supports the anti-gout reputation of cherries. The trend toward decreased plasma concentrations of the inflammatory markers CRP [C-reactive protein] and NO [nitric oxide] adds to the in vitro evidence that compounds in cherries may inhibit inflammatory pathways."[133]

> **My sister has had two recent episodes of gout. Because she has no health insurance, she could not afford to go to the doctor.**
>
> **I gave her some samples of an anti-inflammatory medicine I had on hand. She took them, but got relief only when she started eating sour cherries. Someone told her it was an old remedy to eat six sour cherries a day.**

There has been less evidence regarding cherries or cherry juice and arthritis. A small study published in an obscure Texas medical journal in 1950 suggested that they have some benefit against both gout and arthritis, but it has been ignored for decades.[134] We did hear from one senior citizen, though: "I was on Celebrex but had side effects. A friend recommended that I try Brownwood Acres tart cherry juice. It took 4 weeks to kick in, but at the ripe old age of 79 I'm tap-dancing again. It worked for me."

> *I recommend CherryFlex, a low-carb pill that works well for arthritis and is much more convenient than drinking cherry juice.*
>
> *As a nurse I was skeptical when someone mentioned CherryFlex. Nevertheless, I tried it after the Vioxx disaster and have gotten good relief from arthritis.*

Herbs

Long before aspirin was a gleam in Bayer's eye, herbs were used to soothe inflammation and relieve pain. Willow bark, the precursor to modern-day aspirin, was recommended by Chinese healers in 500 BC. The Greek physician Dioscorides prescribed willow bark during the 1st century to ease inflammation. And in India, herbs such as turmeric, ginger, and boswellia have been used for thousands of years. This doesn't mean they are perfectly safe, but it does give us some comfort to realize that many of these natural plant products have been used in food as well as for medicinal purposes.

TURMERIC (CURCUMA LONGA)

Turmeric has been used in India for millennia. This spice gives curry its distinctive color. You will also find it in yellow mustard. Ayurvedic and Chinese healers have known about the medicinal properties of turmeric for a very long time. They have relied on turmeric to treat a wide variety of inflammatory conditions as well as disorders of the digestive tract, liver, and skin. Now, Western scientists are catching up. The amount of research going on with curcumin, the active ingredient in turmeric, is nothing short of astonishing. If you search online with PubMed, a service of the National Library of Medicine, you will discover more than 1,400 journal articles citing curcumin.

Researchers from all over the world are now

★★★★ Turmeric (curcumin)

This yellow spice has been used for thousands of years in Ayurvedic medicine. Its diverse anticancer, anti-inflammatory, and immune-modulating activities make it one of the most exciting compounds in the food pharmacy. Preliminary research and reports from readers suggest that turmeric may help ease joint pain, psoriasis, and other inflammatory conditions.

Side effects: Skin rash, liver enzyme elevation, and increased risk of bleeding when used in combination with warfarin (Coumadin)

looking into the amazingly diverse physiological activity of curcumin. Scientists are exploring the possibility that this natural product may help prevent or assist in the treatment of a variety of cancers (breast, colon, rectum, pancreas, prostate, lung, melanoma, multiple myeloma, leukemias). The cardiovascular protective effects of curcumin may reduce the risk of atherosclerosis and diminish the damage done to heart muscle during a heart attack. Preliminary animal research suggests that curcumin may be beneficial in helping to control blood sugar in diabetic rats and in diminishing the consequences of oxidative stress brought on by diabetes. And curcumin's immune-modulating and anti-inflammatory properties are being explored in the treatment of irritable bowel syndrome, multiple sclerosis, Alzheimer's disease, and psoriasis.

After reading about turmeric in your column, I started using 1 teaspoon in my scrambled eggs each morning. My arthritis has greatly improved, and I have far less pain when I walk.

I work in my yard every few weeks, weeding, hoeing, mowing, and pruning. Usually I am sore for days after this work. But this last time, since I started taking turmeric, I had no soreness the next day.

Because turmeric is used traditionally in India as an anti-inflammatory agent, it is not surprising that researchers would begin investigating curcumin's action against arthritis.

Preliminary results suggest that the spice may have unique cellular activity that protects cartilage.[135] Several human clinical trials suggest that curcumin is an anti-inflammatory and appears to be reasonably safe.[136]

Readers have shared their experiences with turmeric. Putting this spice on cereal (as one reader did) or in scrambled eggs strikes us as somewhat bizarre. One woman told us that she takes turmeric pills instead and they relieved her arthritis pain. When she stopped temporarily, the pain returned. She resumed taking the turmeric pills and the pain disappeared. Another reader reported that she got relief from her aching knees and her desire to gamble.

All my life my knees have ached at night. I would use Aleve, arthritis-strength aspirin, or Tylenol and usually woke up and had to take more about 3 a.m. I was worried that I was going to burn a hole in my stomach with the amount of aspirin and other pain relievers I was taking.

I read in your column about using turmeric for arthritis pain and I bought some turmeric capsules. I took one with milk and a cookie at bedtime and slept pain-free all night and every night since then. It is almost miraculous.

There is another interesting effect. I used to enjoy playing the slot machines. With video slot machines in bars and restaurants here in Oregon, I was playing the slots once or twice a week. I felt I was a little too interested in the slots but I'd still find myself spending more on them than I intended. Since that first capsule of turmeric, I have had no interest whatsoever in gambling. It was like flipping off a switch.

I'd think this was simply an odd coincidence, but I recall reading about a prescription drug with the opposite effect. It triggered a gambling compulsion that went away when the drug was discontinued. Gambling is hard to kick, so I thought you might be interested in my experience. Turmeric has been a godsend to me on two fronts."

BOSWELLIA (BOSWELLIA SERRATA)

Ayurvedic Indian healers have been using boswellia (Indian frankincense) to treat rheumatism for a very long time. More recently, Swiss veterinarians tested a dietary supplement containing an extract of boswellia. They found that it provided "symptomatic support in canine osteoarthritic disease."[137] After several weeks of treatment the dogs had less lameness and stiffness.

"*I suffer from fibromyalgia, which is extremely painful. Lately I have found that the herb boswellia is very helpful for morning stiffness. There are no side effects, and the results are very quick. It doesn't eliminate pain, but reducing my stiffness makes the morning less difficult. Others with fibromyalgia might want to know about this.*"

A small human study (randomized, double-blind, and placebo-controlled) conducted at the Indira Gandhi Medical College in Nagpur, India, also confirmed an anti-inflammatory and anti-arthritic benefit with boswellia. The researchers reported: "All patients receiving drug [boswellia] treatment reported decrease in knee pain, increased knee flexion, and increased walking distance."[138]

Side effects seem uncommon (digestive tract upset is one possibility), but there have been relatively few long-term studies of any of these anti-inflammatory herbs or spices. It is hard to predict the consequences of regular dosing at levels that are significantly higher than those found in food. It is also unclear whether compounds like curcumin or boswellia will interact with prescription medicines. We have heard from readers that curcumin can make anticoagulants like warfarin (Coumadin) more dangerous and this may be true with other herbs and spices (like ginger).

Some herb manufacturers combine both boswellia and curcumin in their products. A small study suggests that such a mixture could be helpful in relieving knee tenderness and increasing pain-free walking time.[139] We cannot tell you which products are of a high quality. You will have to experiment on your own to determine whether this is an approach that will be helpful.

OTHER ANTI-INFLAMMATORY HERBS

There are several other herbal preparations that may be helpful against arthritis. Ginger (*Zingiber officinale*) is often thought of as a digestive aid to settle the stomach or relieve the nausea associated with motion sickness. It can help block the manufacture of some prostaglandins, though, and might be helpful against joint inflammation.

One well-conducted clinical trial published in the journal *Arthritis and Rheumatism* reported that a standardized, highly purified ginger extract reduced knee pain.[140] The product is made by the Danish company Eurovita and sold under the name Zinaxin. Because this is such a concentrated ginger formula, side effects and drug interactions (especially with anticoagulants) are possible. Some subjects reported belching, indigestion, and nausea related to this formulation.

Another herb for rheumatism is stinging nettle (*Urtica dioica*). An extract or tea made of leaves and stems can be taken for joint pain. According to herb expert James Duke, PhD, some people with access to fresh leaves "sting" themselves on the sore joints to achieve symptomatic relief. To our surprise we found that British physicians had actually tested this approach for thumb and finger arthritis. A controlled trial of such "nettle sting" therapy published in the *Journal of the Royal Society of Medicine* confirmed that it produced a statistically significant improvement over the placebo deadnettle leaf (*Lamium album*).[141] Less hardy souls may prefer a liniment with a spirit extract of the leaves.

Speaking of liniments, folks have been rubbing concoctions on sore joints for centuries. The essence of hot chili peppers is capsaicin. It gives the kick to salsa and hot sauce. When applied to the skin, capsaicin stimulates nerve

fibers to release a chemical called *substance P.* With repeated exposure, substance P is thought to be depleted from the nerve cells, which in turn results in diminished discomfort. Creams containing capsaicin are used to treat diabetic neuropathy, postherpetic neuralgia (residual pain from a shingles attack), and osteoarthritis. Not terrifically effective for arthritis, such creams also have a fairly high incidence of side effects. Roughly one-third of subjects in clinical trials experienced local adverse events, including burning, stinging, and redness.

Dietary Supplements

With all the bad news about prescription arthritis drugs it is hardly any wonder that dietary supplements have become hugely successful in the health-food stores. In fact, they have jumped from the fruit-and-nut locales to the pharmacy and even big-box discount stores like Wal-Mart and Costco. Sales of glucosamine and chondroitin have been spectacular, exceeding $700 million annually. Can it last?

GLUCOSAMINE AND CHONDROITIN

Ever since Jason Theodosakis, MD, wrote his giant bestseller, *The Arthritis Cure*, glucosamine and chondroitin (G&C) have been the most popular alternative treatments for osteoarthritis. The promise was that these dietary supplements would relieve pain and inflammation and repair damaged cartilage. How good is the evidence that G&C live up to this reputation?

Over the years there have been numerous studies published in medical journals. A review in the *Journal of the American Medical Association* of all the studies published between 1966 and 1999 concluded: "Trials of glucosamine and chondroitin preparations for OA [osteoarthritis] symptoms demonstrate moderate to large effects, but quality issues and likely publication bias suggest that these effects are exaggerated. Nevertheless, some degree of efficacy appears probable for these preparations."[143]

Another analysis of 15 well-conducted trials of G&C for knee arthritis concluded that there was "structural efficacy" but called for further research.[144] So far, so good. People with arthritis had reason to believe that their investment in G&C products would pay off in terms of symptomatic relief and joint protection.

Then came the big disappointment. The National Institutes of Health funded the largest, most expensive ($14 million), and most definitive clinical trial ever undertaken to determine the effectiveness of G&C. Nearly 1,600 patients were recruited from 16 academic rheumatology centers around the United States. GAIT—Glucosamine/Chondroitin Arthritis Intervention Trial—was the Big Kahuna of clinical studies. These dietary supplements were going to be tested as if they were standard drugs. Subjects were randomly assigned to receive glucosamine, chondroitin, G&C together, Celebrex, or placebo. Investigators were looking for a relatively modest 20 percent improvement in knee pain by the end of 6 months.

The envelope was opened at the 2005 Annual Meeting of the American College of Rheumatology. Daniel Clegg, MD, chief of the Division of Rheumatology at the University of Utah School of Medicine, announced the findings: "As expected, celecoxib [Celebrex] improved knee pain in patients with osteoarthritis. For the study as a whole, the supple-

---

THE GRAEDONS' G&C GUIDELINES

If you have mild knee arthritis, glucosamine and chondroitin probably won't do you much good. If you're really hurting, these dietary supplements might help somewhat. They're worth a try for a few months to see whether you get relief.

Adverse events appear to be "generally mild." Please have your cholesterol levels measured before starting on G&C and periodically thereafter to make sure they don't go up while on these supplements. Although not proven scientifically, we have heard from people who have experienced just such a complication.

ments [glucosamine and chondroitin] were not shown to be effective."[145]

Wow! This multimillion-dollar, comprehensive trial had laid a giant goose egg. But no sooner were the results out than the spinmeisters for the nutraceutical industry tried to turn lemons into lemonade. Press releases were issued stating that GAIT was "Good News for Osteoarthritis Sufferers. If you're one of the 21 million consumers coping with osteoarthritis (OA) . . . the GAIT study demonstrates that there may be a safe and affordable way to help manage your pain."[146]

Here's the straight and skinny on GAIT. Patients with mild knee pain saw no statistical improvement while taking G&C compared with placebo; 62.9 percent responded to glucosamine and chondroitin given together, whereas 61.7 percent got benefit from placebo and 70.3 percent responded to Celebrex.

The investigators did report that "an exploratory analysis suggested that the combination of glucosamine and chondroitin might be effective in osteoarthritis patients who had moderate to severe knee pain." This subset of patients with worse pain did appear to get statistically significant benefit: 79.2 percent on G&C experienced pain relief compared to 69.4 percent on Celebrex and 54.3 percent on placebo. These results were not overwhelming, though, since the researchers were careful to qualify the data as "exploratory" and the result as "might be effective." When the patients with "moderate to severe" osteoarthritis were lumped together with those with "mild" arthritis, there was no statistically significant improvement compared to placebo. All in all, we would have to say that the outcome of this gigantic study was disappointing.

> "I am a runner and have had problems with my knees. Last year I started taking glucosamine and chondroitin and was very pleased with the pain relief.
>
> I read in your column that some people have higher cholesterol when they take these supplements. Sure enough, when I had my physical, my total cholesterol had gone from 190 to over 250. My blood pressure was also up and my doctor is talking about medication.
>
> I stopped the glucosamine and chondroitin and am hoping my readings will come back down. But now my knees ache again."

MSM and SAMe

Methylsulfonylmethane (MSM) is a naturally occurring compound found in many fruits and vegetables. It has been widely promoted as an arthritis remedy, but there is very little research to support the testimonials. One preliminary study reported some relief from pain but not stiffness.[147] Despite the lack of scientific proof, some readers do report success with this dietary supplement. We heard from one postmenopausal woman who reported that MSM not only eased her arthritis pain but also had some unexpected benefits.

> "I went to my local natural pharmacy and said I was taking glucosamine and chondroitin

because when I hit menopause I developed arthritis pain in my hands. The folks there suggested I take MSM as well. They said to increase the dose gradually because it gives you diarrhea if you bump it suddenly. I'm taking a great deal of it and I have no unpleasant side effects. It controls the pain beautifully.

I did discover one fantastic side effect. I was also having another issue with menopause. My hair was thinning, falling out in clumps. But as soon as I started taking all this MSM my hair became gorgeous, my skin soft, and my nails fantastic. I look beautiful! I'm going to be 55 soon and my husband says I look at least 10 years younger."

S-adenosyl-L-methionine (SAMe) is a natural compound found in the body. It is crucial to many biochemical reactions because it is a methyl group "donor." This means it plays a role in the manufacture of proteins, DNA, RNA, and many other essential molecules.

SAMe has been used in Europe as an antidepressant as well as an anti-inflammatory in the treatment of arthritis. There have been relatively few good clinical trials for its effect in osteoarthritis. A meta-analysis of existing research concluded that SAMe "appears to be as effective as NSAIDs in reducing pain and improving functional limitation in patients with OA without the adverse effects often associated with NSAID therapies."[148] Despite this optimistic assessment, the authors pointed out that there have been no well-conducted long-term studies of SAMe against arthritis. Although this dietary supplement may be helpful, we will await additional data before giving it an endorsement.

Acupuncture

Let's face it, acupuncture is still mysterious to most Western physicians. American medical education has a very hard time grappling with things outside the dominant paradigm. Talk about chi or energy flow and most traditionally trained physicians will look at you as if you are from a distant planet. And yet Chinese healers have been practicing acupuncture for thousands of years. How effective is it for relieving symptoms of arthritis?

Well-conducted clinical trials published in such reputable journals as the *Lancet*, the *Annals of Internal Medicine*, and the *British Medical Journal* confirm that acupuncture can be a useful adjunct to osteoarthritis therapy. So how do researchers do randomized, controlled acupuncture studies? In drug studies subjects never know whether they are receiving real medicine or look-alike sham pills. It's possible to do the

---

★★★ Acupuncture

Several well-controlled trials of acupuncture suggest that it provides statistically significant relief of pain and stiffness and restores physical function. We may not understand exactly how it works, but as an adjunct to other treatments, acupuncture appears worthwhile.

If the practitioner is skilled in the art and science of acupuncture, side effects appear to be minimal.

---

same thing with acupuncture. Investigators fool their volunteers by inserting needles into sham acupuncture locations or by using mock plastic needles that give the sensation of acupuncture without actually penetrating the skin.

One large, long-term (26-week) study supervised by researchers at the University of Maryland carried out just such a controlled protocol. Acupuncture relieved pain and improved function without side effects.[150] Another research group found that when true acupuncture was added to NSAID (diclofenac) therapy, it was more effective than drug treatment alone.[151]

How long do the effects of acupuncture last? One fascinating study compared 8 weeks of standard acupuncture (average of 17 needles) to minimal acupuncture (average of 12 needles) or nothing. The researchers reported that at the end of the 8-week session, "acupuncture treatment had significant and clinically relevant short-term effects when compared to minimal acupuncture or no acupuncture in patients with osteoarthritis of the knee."[152] Although the benefits persisted for weeks after the treatment was discontinued, they were not statistically significant after 26 weeks and had virtually disappeared 1 year later.

Magnet Therapy

If you think physicians get upset when you talk about acupuncture, just wait till you mention magnets. This concept is guaranteed to drive most traditionally trained doctors up the wall because it does not fit with anything they have learned in medical school. To most, the idea is preposterous. They believe it is sheer quackery and wouldn't believe magnets could relieve arthritis pain regardless of the scientific evidence. Truthfully, we have a hard time swallowing this approach ourselves because we cannot imagine how magnets would work.

On the other side of the equation is the popularity of magnets. Several years ago sales were reported at $5 billion annually. An individual magnetic bracelet is relatively cheap and without side effects. Of course just because they are affordable and popular does not mean they are worth a damn.

So, are there any valid data to support magnet therapy? Unfortunately, there has not been a lot of great research done. A small, double-blind, placebo-controlled trial conducted by Harvard researchers did demonstrate effectiveness.

Magnetic Bracelets

Investigators used a bracelet containing standard neodymium magnets set in a steel backing cup, with the open side facing the ventral wrist. The field strength of the magnet at the wrist contact surface was 170 to 200 mTesla (a measure of magnetic strength). That is the equivalent of 1,700 to 2,000 gauss (another measure of magnetic strength).

Caution: Magnets are *not* appropriate for pregnant women, people with pacemakers or metal implants, or those using electromagnetic equipment such as insulin pumps or sleep apnea machines. Also, keep magnets away from credit card strips, computer disks, and watches.

To locate companies that sell magnetic bracelets, use a search engine like Google to search for "neodymium magnetic bracelet." We found several companies that can be reached without a computer. We make no recommendations or warrantees, so please exercise appropriate caution if you decide to order. They include:

Magnetic Therapy Sales Specialists   888-883-0813

Ace Magnetics   800-599-9098

Synergy for Life   888-311-2963

The cost of a magnetic bracelet is approximately $60 to $100.

A much more impressive study concluded that: "Pain from osteoarthritis of the hip and knee decreases when wearing magnetic bracelets."[153] These investigators came up with a thoughtful game plan. They gave some subjects standard-strength (170 to 200 mTesla) neodymium magnetic bracelets (which can be purchased on the Web or in specialty stores). Others received weak magnetic bracelets (12 to 30 mTesla) or nonmagnetic bracelets. The investigators employed weak magnets so that subjects would not be able to test their bracelet against iron and scope out the "real" from the subtherapeutic bracelet. They found that after 12 weeks the real magnetic bracelets were as effective as oral NSAIDs, topical NSAID creams, and exercise therapy. Not only were pain and stiffness diminished, but physical function improved.

Of course the skeptics come out of the woodwork when we write about magnetic bracelets. Some say this is pure snake oil. Others maintain that discussing magnet therapy will open the floodgates to other "fringe treatments, such

HARVARD MAGNET STUDY

"Despite our small sample size, magnets showed statistically significant efficacy compared to placebo after 4 hours under rigorously controlled conditions."[154]

—P.M. Wolsko et al., *Alternative Therapies in Health and Medicine*, 2004

as laetrile and coffee enemas for cancer." We disagree. We think most folks will use common sense when it comes to magnet therapy. Although we need to see better research before we can endorse this approach for arthritis, a magnetic bracelet seems relatively inexpensive, safe, and intriguing as an adjunct treatment.

A Skeptic Speaks Out

Q. *I cannot believe you would write about magnetic bracelets for arthritis. This is just a bunch of hooey designed to loosen the purse strings of gullible readers.*

I am surprised you would give credence to any "study" of this nonsense. This bunk should be consigned to the trashcan.

A. We agree that magnet therapy seems far-fetched, but just because we don't understand how something works doesn't mean we should ignore it.

The well-designed study you refer to was reported in the *British Medical Journal* (December 16, 2004). The researchers randomly assigned patients to wear a bracelet containing a strong magnet, a weak magnet, or nonmagnetic washers.

After 3 months the patients wearing the strong magnets had measurable relief from hip and knee pain. The placebo effect is hard to eliminate in such studies, but these scientists did

their best to control for it. Even though they could not explain how magnet therapy works, they summarized, "Whatever the mechanism, the benefit from magnetic bracelets seems clinically useful."

● ● ●

Conclusions

We hope we have not overwhelmed you with arthritis options. We have offered lots of ideas because there is no way to predict what will work the best for any given individual. There is no test to determine if someone will benefit from gin-soaked raisins or Certo in grape juice. Of course, the same thing applies to drugs like Advil or Celebrex.

Selecting the best approaches for you requires trial and error. There may be synergy between some of these remedies. One person may find that combining acupuncture and a magnetic bracelet with curcumin and pomegranate juice is the magic formula. Another person might discover that applying Pennsaid Lotion to sore joints, taking the herb boswellia, and drinking grape juice and Certo does the trick.

None of these approaches is a substitute for good medical management. Blending home remedies with medications such as Pennsaid or Voltaren Emulgel may offer the maximum benefit. A short course of ibuprofen or naproxen may also be called for when arthritis pain flares up. On the next page, you will find an overview of our recommendations in this chapter.

• Preventing arthritis beats trying to treat it. Keep weight under control, drink fresh-squeezed orange juice, and follow a Mediterranean diet. Get 10 to 15 minutes of sunshine on your face and hands several days a week or take 800 to 1,200 IU of vitamin D daily.

• Aspirin is the best buy in the pharmacy. It relieves pain and inflammation while reducing the risk of heart attack, stroke, and many cancers. Beware of its potential to cause ulcers. Medical supervision is essential for long-term use.

• Topical NSAIDs reduce the risk of stomach irritation and ulceration. Pennsaid and other prescription NSAID creams and gels are available online from abroad. A compounding pharmacist in the United States can make a ketoprofen gel or cream without a prescription.

• Fish oil or green-lipped mussel oil extract can supply valuable omega-3 fatty acids.

These anti-inflammatory compounds are helpful against heart disease, arthritis, and other chronic conditions.

• Home remedies such as gin-soaked raisins, Certo and grape juice, or vinegar and juice may be effective. Other juices that may have anti-inflammatory benefits include pomegranate and cherry.

• Turmeric is a spice that does triple duty. It comes from the ancient Ayurvedic healing tradition and may relieve inflammation. In addition to joint pain, some people find that it helps psoriasis. It's also being studied for its effects against a wide variety of cancers.

• Glucosamine and chondroitin remain controversial. People with moderate to severe pain may benefit from their use even though those with mild arthritis probably won't.

• Acupuncture may offer significant pain relief. Seek a qualified acupuncturist for such treatment.

CONSTIPATION

• Get enough fluid and fiber	
• Eat prunes, apples, or apricots	
• Sprinkle ground flaxseed on cereal	★★★★★
• Chew sugarless gum	★★★★
• Use psyllium powder	★★★★
• Try docusate for less straining	★★
• Use milk of magnesia for quick relief (occasional use)	★★★
• Ask your doctor about a prescription for MiraLax	★★

Many people feel that regularity is the key to good health. Is this true or is it a myth? Grandmothers around the world have promoted daily bowel movements for generations, but there is no evidence that a trip to the bathroom each morning is necessary. People vary in the frequency that suits them best. Some do well on a schedule of no more than three times a week. Others feel good on a schedule as frequent as a few times a day.

Constipation is defined as unsatisfactory defecation[155], but doctors and patients don't always agree on what is most important. Physicians may prefer objective measures like the number of days between bowel movements. But people may be as concerned about consistency as frequency. They complain about the effort of passing hard "golf balls" or "bricks."

Sometimes physicians dismiss constipation as a minor complaint. While it is not usually life threatening, constipation can be serious. Almost 100,000 people are hospitalized each year for constipation-related problems. Many more suffer considerable distress and reduced quality of life as a result of this common condition.

Fluids and fiber are the cornerstones of constipation prevention. Those who are constipated are often urged to drink more water. Adequate fluid (at least 6 glasses of water a day) is essential, but unless someone is actually dehydrated, drinking extra water does not solve the problem of hard stools. Together with fiber, though, the fluids may help. The first step, of course, is to make sure that the diet contains at least 25 grams of fiber a day. That may take some doing, but it can be accomplished with 5 to 10 servings of vegetables and fruits a day, along with whole grains rather than refined bread, pasta, crackers, and the like. For some people, though, even that may not be enough to conquer constipation completely.

If constipation arises suddenly or if it starts to interfere with everyday activities, it makes sense to check in with your doctor. There are some conditions, such as an underactive thyroid gland or Parkinson's disease, that can lead to constipation. In those cases the underlying disease needs to be treated.

Warning signs that should trigger a doctor's visit include blood in the stool or bleeding from the rectum; dark, tarry stool; weight loss of 10 pounds or more; a family history of colon cancer; or a positive Hemoccult test, a way of identifying invisible blood in the stool.[156] Be sure to tell the doctor about any of these issues, so the proper work-up can be done.

People taking medications or even supplements should also check with their doctor to see whether one of these might be responsible. A surprising number of prescription drugs can trigger constipation as a side effect. Because of the impact that constipation can have on their sense of well-being, patients sometimes become upset if doctors don't warn them that a prescribed medication may interfere with bowel function. Narcotics are among the most notorious offenders, but there are many others. Sometimes, switching to a differ-

SOME DRUGS THAT MAY LEAD TO CONSTIPATION

- Abilify (aripiprazole)
- Actonel (risedronate)
- Anaprox (naproxen)
- Arimidex (anastrozole)
- Asacol (mesalamine)
- Casodex (bicalutamide)
- Cataflam (diclofenac)
- Catapres (clonidine)
- Cenestin (synthetic conjugated estrogens)
- Clinoril (sulindac)
- Clorpres (clonidine and chlorthalidone)
- Clozaril (clozapine)
- Cognex (tacrine)
- Cordarone (amiodarone)
- Covera-HS (verapamil)
- Creon (pancreatin)
- Cymbalta (duloxetine)
- Detrol (tolterodine)
- Ditropan XL (oxybutynin)
- Duragesic (fentanyl)
- EC-Naprosyn (naproxen)
- Effexor (venlafaxine)
- Femara (letrozole)
- Geodon (ziprasidone)
- Gleevec (imatinib)
- Imdur (isosorbide mononitrate)
- Kadian (morphine sulfate)
- Kytril (granisetron)
- Lexapro (escitalopram)
- Lotronex (alosetron)
- Lyrica (pregabalin)
- Meridia (sibutramine)
- Mirapex (pramipexole)
- Myfortic (mycophenolic acid)
- Nalfon (fenoprofen)
- Naprosyn (naproxen)
- Orap (pimozide)
- OxyContin (oxycodone)
- Pacerone (amiodarone)
- Pancrease MT (pancrelipase)
- Paxil (paroxetine)
- Permax (pergolide)
- Rapamune (sirolimus)
- Relafen (nabumetone)
- Remeron (mirtazapine)
- Requip (ropinirole)
- Retrovir (zidovudine)
- Risperdal (risperidone)
- Rythmol (propafenone)
- Thalomid (thalidomide)
- Topamax (topiramate)
- Vicodin (hydrocodone and acetaminophen)
- Zofran (ondansetron)
- Zoloft (sertraline)
- Zyprexa (olanzapine)

ent medicine can ease the problem. The physician should always be involved in such a decision, because some of these drugs may be essential treatment for a serious condition such as cancer or AIDS.

Dietary Approaches

For uncomplicated constipation, focus on increasing the high-fiber foods in the diet. Sometimes, people buy a loaf of soft-and-squishy "wheat" bread and figure that's all they need to do to get extra fiber. Wrong! Unfortunately, the "wheat" label may just be a marketing ploy. Consumers need to read the ingredient list to see if the first ingredient is whole-wheat flour. That's a good start.

Even better is to actually consume the whole grains in pilafs or porridges, which is one rea-

son we are so fond of steel-cut oats. (Also, they taste wonderful.) One of our favorite high-fiber breakfasts is steel-cut oats with extras: blackberries or pieces of apple, together with walnuts or almonds, topped with a sprinkling of freshly ground flaxseed. To boost the protein content of this breakfast, we stir in some egg white while the oats are cooking.

• • •

Q. *My wife is bedridden with emphysema and osteoporosis. Her fractured vertebrae are due to the steroids she takes for emphysema.*

The doctor suggested calcium to strengthen her brittle bones. Then she had a problem with bowel movements

---

FOODS THAT ARE HIGH IN FIBER

- Apples
- Barley
- Beans
- Blackberries
- Bran
- Bran cereal
- Broccoli
- Bulgur wheat
- Chickpeas
- Fiber One cereal
- Figs
- Lentils

- Lima beans
- Oat bran
- Oats (steel-cut)
- Pears
- Popcorn
- Prunes
- Raisins
- Split peas
- Uncle Sam Cereal
- Wheat berries
- Winter squash

because of not getting any exercise.

This caused her great distress until she tried eating a quarter of an apple every evening. The apple has made her regular again.

A. Thanks so much for reminding us all of the importance of fiber in the diet. This may help explain the wisdom behind Grandmother's recommendation of an apple a day.

• • •

Prunes

Why are the marketers changing the name of prunes to "dried plums"? While it is an accurate designation, it's not particularly catchy. Instead, it is an attempt to get away from the image of self-treatment for constipation that "prune" or "prune juice" conjures up.

• • •

Q. *A year ago I had a serious problem with constipation (over 2 weeks!). I tried everything I could, including Metamucil, Ex-Lax, milk of magnesia, and a Fleet enema with no results. A visit to the doctor resulted in a prescription but still no relief.*

Then I remembered: Prunes are laxatives. I bought some prune juice with pulp and drank 4 ounces a day with

plenty of water. Within a few days I was back to normal.

For a few months I drank some every other morning to keep me regular. Now I only need it once a week. Prune juice with pulp is my salvation.

A. Prunes are a time-honored home remedy for constipation. Researchers have confirmed what grandmothers always knew: Prunes stimulate the digestive tract.

In 1951 scientists discovered an ingredient in prunes that is closely related to the chemical laxative oxyphenisatin. This product was taken off the market when it was linked to liver damage.

Experts for the *Harvard Health Letter* suggest, "It is unlikely that moderate consumption [of prune juice] would cause any problems, but prune use, like everything else, should be prudent."

• • •

Prunes are said to be loaded with antioxidant phytonutrients, so they are a healthy choice if consumed in moderation. They are not the only dried fruit that can be helpful in an attempt to overcome constipation. Dried figs and even apricots provide a little variety. They may not have any specifically laxative components, but they certainly are good sources of fiber, and some people find them quite helpful.

> **"Dried apricots (two a day) and plenty of water can relieve constipation. It helps me and has helped my friends."**

FLAXSEED

Another source of fiber is not nearly as well known as prunes. Flaxseed has long been used as a source of soluble fiber. It is one of the ingredients in an old-fashioned cold cereal, Uncle Sam Cereal. Once marketed as a "natural laxative," it is now being touted as a low-glycemic-index or low-carb food. The primary ingredients are wheat berries and flaxseed. Both should help to keep things moving in the right direction.

> **"Constipation has been my problem for more years than I want to count. Psyllium seed barely works.**
>
> **My solution is flaxseeds ground in my coffee grinder. I keep it in small batches in the refrigerator and take ½ teaspoon with a glass of juice or water daily. Sometimes I sprinkle it on my cereal or put it in a fruit smoothie. I like the nutty taste and it has been like a miracle for me."**

Besides combating constipation, flaxseed is an excellent source of omega-3 fatty acids and has the added advantage of lowering cholesterol at least modestly. The seeds keep well, but once they are ground (a blender or a coffee grinder works well), they go rancid quickly. Ground flaxseed meal should be kept in the refrigerator or even in the freezer. Someone with a tendency to constipation might well want to get in the habit of

---

★ ★ ★ ★ ★ Flaxseed

Ground flaxseed is a good source of soluble fiber. Not only is it helpful against constipation, it can aid in lowering cholesterol and may help reduce the hot flashes of menopause. Flaxseed is an excellent plant source of omega-3 fatty acids.

Downside: Keeps well until ground, then is susceptible to going rancid. Keep ground flaxseed in the refrigerator for no more than 10 days to 2 weeks.

Cost: Approximately $4 to $5 per month (around 13¢ a dose)

---

incorporating ground flaxseed into meals.

Another way to get the benefits of flax is to make a solution. Simmer 2 tablespoons of flaxseed in 3 quarts of water for 15 minutes. Cool the liquid and strain it. It should be kept in the refrigerator. Add 2 ounces a day to fruit juice.

SUGARLESS GUM

It might be surprising to learn that something as simple and inexpensive as sugarless gum could counter constipation quite effectively. By the way, the converse is also true. People sometimes have problems with chronic diarrhea because of their gum-chewing habits. Sugarless candy has the same impact.

● ● ●

Q. *I read with interest and sympathy a letter about problems with constipa-*

tion. I wanted to share something that has helped me.

After hearing some people complain that sugar-free jelly beans gave them diarrhea if eaten in quantity, I decided to see if they would help my frequent constipation. I have found that if I eat 30 sugar-free jelly beans with a glass of water half an hour before bedtime, I stay regular. I hope this idea might help others with the same problem.

A. Thanks for the tip. Many people find that the sweeteners in sugar-free candy can cause diarrhea. How clever of you to turn that side effect to your advantage! Each person will have to experiment to find the right "dose."

● ● ●

★★★★ Sugarless Gum

Pick a flavor that you like and experiment to find the right dose. The "sugar alcohols" used to sweeten sugarless gum—maltitol, sorbitol, mannitol, and xylitol—are not absorbed from the digestive tract. They act as "osmotic laxatives." Chewing sugarless gum does not contribute to tooth decay. A gum containing xylitol might even help fight ear infections.

Side effect: Diarrhea
Downside: Many sugarless gums contain aspartame, which some people prefer to avoid.
Cost: Approximately 7¢ to 15¢ a dose

Over-the-Counter Remedies

Laxatives are among the most popular products in the pharmacy. Hundreds of millions of dollars are spent each year on these over-the-counter remedies. But overuse of such products can be a serious problem.

● ● ●

Q. *My 19-year-old daughter and her girlfriend have been taking laxatives for weight control for several months. They also take over-the-counter diet pills.*

My main concern is about the abuse of laxatives. Would you please print the harmful effects laxatives can cause? She won't listen to me!

A. Chronic laxative abuse can undermine the body's ability to eliminate waste on its own. We have heard from many elderly people who started using laxatives in their youth and became dependent upon them.

We are more concerned, however, about the potential interactions these young women might experience. Strong laxatives can deplete the body of potassium.

Laxatives are not an effective tool for lasting weight loss. Dietary counseling and exercise may be more helpful in the long run.

● ● ●

We generally suggest that people avoid stimulant chemicals like aloe, cascara sagrada, senna, and castor oil. These can be irritating to the digestive tract. Some of these compounds can interfere with proper nutrition, and chronic use might make a person more susceptible to weakened bones.

Bulk-Forming Laxatives

The first step in treating constipation is to increase your intake of fiber. Since dietary fiber may not be enough, there are several possible sources of fiber sold as "bulking agents" in the pharmacy. Psyllium is a naturally derived fiber from blond ispaghula seed (*Plantago ovata*). It can usually be bought quite inexpensively. There are also some alternative types of fiber.

Adequate fluid intake is crucial when taking fiber. Swallowing fiber such as psyllium without enough water could lead to choking as a result of the product clumping and swelling in the esophagus. Other digestive tract blockage is also possible if fluid intake is inadequate.[157]

If psyllium is not satisfactory, other possible fiber sources are available. Polycarbophil (Equalactin, FiberCon, Fiber-Lax, Konsyl Fiber) may be the next step. Other options include methylcellulose (Citrucel) and powdered cellulose (UniFiber). There's no good evidence to suggest that any one of these is superior to the others overall, but people do have their favorites.

No bulk-forming laxative should be taken if the person is nauseated, vomiting, running a fever, or suffering abdominal pain. Such symptoms deserve prompt medical attention.

" *I've had such frustration with constipation over the years. I've tried a lot of remedies, but the ones that worked were too harsh. Then a friend*

★★★★ Psyllium

Sold under a number of brand names, including Metamucil, Fiberall, Konsyl, Perdiem Fiber Therapy, Reguloid, and Serutan. Store brands, available in most drugstore chains, are more economical. Psyllium (1 tablespoon in 8 ounces of water three times a day) is approved both for constipation and for lowering cholesterol. It may take a few days to observe the effects. Psyllium is considered safe for daily use. Sugar-free brands may be more economical, but most contain aspartame, which some people would rather avoid.

Side effects: Flatulence, bloating, or diarrhea; severe allergic reactions
Downside: May interfere with the absorption of other drugs taken at the same time. Many people object to the gloppy or gritty texture of dissolved psyllium fiber.
Cost: Approximately 8¢ to 30¢ per dose

told me about UniFiber. It is a very fine powder, and I combine it with canned peaches or home-made oat bran muffins. It really regulates my system with no diarrhea or cramping. "

Stool Softeners

When the main problem is that the stool is hard, the best remedy may be a stool softener. These are also recommended for people who have had abdominal or colorectal surgery or an episiotomy during labor and delivery and must avoid straining.

Old-fashioned mineral oil is the best-known product in this category. It should be used for only a short time, though. Mineral oil is petroleum-based and is not absorbed into the body. But it can interfere with the absorption of important fat-soluble nutrients, such as vitamin A, vitamin D, vitamin E, and vitamin K. Over weeks or months, this could be detrimental to health.

The doctors' choice in stool softeners is usually docusate sodium or docusate calcium. Although the evidence of their effectiveness is

★★ Docusate Sodium

Available as Colace and Ex-Lax Stool Softener, and generically under various store brand names. Acts a wetting agent to help stool absorb more water and thus become softer. Expect this product to take up to 3 or 4 days to work.

Side effects: Rash, throat irritation, nausea
Cost: Approximately 25¢ to 50¢ per dose

★★★ Milk of Magnesia

This usually works fairly rapidly, within several hours. Each dose should be taken with 8 ounces of water. It is intended for occasional use *only*.

Side effects: Diarrhea, nausea, weakness
Downside: This laxative contains magnesium, so it should not be used by people with kidney disease. It may disrupt the balance of minerals and fluid in the body.
Cost: Approximately 50¢ to 75¢ per dose

not strong,[158] they are widely used. They might work better in a postsurgical situation than they do for chronic constipation.

Osmotic Laxatives

Compounds that attract water into the digestive tract add moisture to the stool. This softens it and may even help hurry it along. Such agents are called osmotic laxatives. We've already discussed sugarless gum, which works in this manner. It also exemplifies the downside of these laxatives: Getting the balance just right can be difficult. It's not rare for a person to experience diarrhea as a side effect if the dose is too high. Some old familiar remedies fall into this category. Both Epsom salts and milk of magnesia are osmotic laxatives.

Prescription Laxatives

Chronic constipation can be extremely frustrating. If lifestyle changes and over-the-counter approaches are unsuccessful, people turn to their doctors hoping for a miracle. In this situation, miracles are few and far between. Physicians do have a few drugs they can prescribe that may be helpful. One is a type of osmotic laxative called lactulose (Chronulac, Duphalac, Kristalose) that has been around quite a long time. This is a type of sugar that is not absorbed well, so it pulls water into the intestines. It may take a day or 2 to produce results, and it can result in cramping, gas, or diarrhea.

Doctors have another option as well. A prescription laxative containing polyethylene glycol, an ingredient quite similar to those used for cleansing the colon prior to a colonoscopy, can be used for desperate cases. MiraLax is not supposed to be used for more than 2 weeks at a time, however. MiraLax is an osmotic laxative.

★★ MiraLax

Contains polyethylene glycol, or PEG. It comes as a powder to be dissolved in juice, water, coffee, or tea. Expect results in 2 to 4 days. Do not use for more than 2 weeks.

Side effects: Diarrhea, abdominal cramping, nausea, gas

Downside: Prolonged or excessive use may upset the balance of fluids and minerals in the body or result in laxative dependence.

Cost: Approximately $1.40 to $2 per dose; one dose per day

The doctors' big gun in prescription products is Zelnorm (tegaserod). It was developed for people who have irritable bowel syndrome with constipation as the predominant symptom. It has also been approved for chronic constipation in adults under the age of 65. Your doctor will be able to evaluate if this last resort is appropriate for you. There have been instances of serious, dehydrating diarrhea that required hospitalization. Another dangerous side effect that worries us is ischemic colitis, a condition in which blood supply to part of the intestine shuts down. It has not been established whether Zelnorm was responsible for this frightening complication. Nevertheless, this drug is probably appropriate only when everything else has failed.

10 Tips for Combating Constipation

1. Pay attention to your diet. Getting plenty of fiber and fluid is essential. In addition, though, some foods tend to be constipating. Cheese has a reputation in this regard, but coconut, which can help ease diarrhea, may be constipating if too much is eaten. Other people have warned of the effects of pomegranate, mango, or peanut butter. The tannins in tea may also contribute to constipation.

2. Sip warm water with a tablespoon of blackstrap molasses. This sweetener contains a number of minerals. Some people find it a tasty way to cope with constipation. Another old-fashioned home remedy for

constipation is drinking lemon juice in a cup of hot water first thing in the morning. Afterward, rinse your mouth with plain water, to protect your teeth.

3. Simmer 2 tablespoons of flaxseed in 3 quarts of water for 15 minutes. Cool, strain, and add 2 ounces of the liquid to orange juice every day. An alternative is to use freshly ground flaxseed on cereal or other foods.

4. Chew sugar-free gum. Experiment to find the appropriate dose. Or, if you prefer, eat sugar-free candy. Either may ease constipation; don't overdo it.

5. Take psyllium powder in 8 ounces of water. For when you're traveling, Metamucil makes psyllium cookies that are easier to carry, but they're also more expensive and higher in calories.

6. Stay away from traditional laxative herbs such as aloe, cascara sagrada, and senna. They are harsh and overstimulate the digestive tract. Very occasional use may be acceptable, but overuse can lead to dependence. Instead, try dong quai, ginger, or milk thistle.

7. Load up on vitamin C. Some people find that about 2,000 milligrams a day is enough to trigger diarrhea. Finding the dose that works for you and backing off just slightly is one approach that may work. Do not try this if you have ever had kidney stones, because excess vitamin C raises oxalate excretion and might increase the risk of a recurrence.[159]

8. Stir a couple teaspoons of Swedish bitters into a cup of water. Hot water or herb tea may work best. It also comes in capsules that are convenient for when traveling.

9. Experiment with a bulk-forming laxative. Some people find that UniFiber or Citrucel works better for them than psyllium.

10. Make sure you get enough magnesium, especially if you are taking calcium supplements. Calcium carbonate can be constipating, but magnesium can help offset this tendency. We generally advise people that a dose above 300 milligrams of magnesium per day may cause diarrhea. The maximum short-term dose of magnesium advised on the label of Phillips' Milk of Magnesia is 2,000 milligrams for adults. Do not take magnesium or milk of magnesia if you have kidney disease.

Conclusions

Constipation accompanied by pain, nausea, vomiting, or fever should not be ignored. It deserves medical attention. Even without such symptoms, persistent constipation should also be brought to a physician's attention. Uncomplicated constipation may respond to home treatment.

• Begin with diet. Make sure you get six to eight 8-ounce glasses of water or other fluids daily. Concentrate on increasing fiber, and make sure you get 25 to 35 grams daily.

• Ask your doctor to check whether a medical condition or medication may be causing your constipation.

- Eat fruit. Apples, dried apricots, and (in moderation) dried plums, aka prunes, are a wonderful way to establish regularity when needed.
- Sprinkle ground flaxseed on your food, or take a solution of simmered flaxseed in juice.
- Chew sugarless gum or enjoy sugar-free candy for its laxative effect.
- Take psyllium as directed, with an 8-ounce glass of water.
- Docusate may soften stools and ease straining.
- Milk of magnesia may give relatively quick relief, but should not be overused. It's off-limits for anyone with kidney trouble.
- Prescription drugs such as MiraLax are intended for short-term use of less than 2 weeks.

COUGH

Get a prescription for codeine cough syrup	★★★★
Smear Vicks VapoRub on the soles of the feet	★★★★
Add thyme to chicken broth	★★★
Enjoy a bit of dark chocolate	★★
Sip a glass of Concord grape juice	★

Trying to ease a cough can be a frustrating experience. If it arrived with a cold or another upper respiratory tract infection, it's likely to go away eventually, but those 2 or 3 weeks of suffering until it does can be miserable. Way back before the end of the last century, Americans could buy cough medicines that worked. Codeine-containing antitussive syrups were widely available without prescription. Physicians also recommended terpin hydrate, an expectorant, from the late 1800s until the early 1990s. In theory, an expectorant simply loosens up the stuff in the lungs and makes it easier to cough up. But many people found that terpin hydrate offered more benefit.

● ● ●

Q. *For years I used terpin hydrate as an expectorant when I had a cough. It worked.*

It was sold over the counter and one small bottle would last me the entire cold season.

Over-the-counter cough remedies on the market today are no better than water. They just do NOT work.

Is terpin hydrate still available? I've never found another cough syrup that works so well, but I can't find it in my local drugstores.

A. Terpin hydrate was a popular cough medicine from the late 1800s until the early 1990s. Then the FDA banned it on the grounds that it had not been proven effective.

As an expectorant, terpin hydrate was supposed to loosen mucus and relieve coughs. It was derived from natural sources such as oil of turpentine or compounds found in oregano, thyme, and eucalyptus.

Terpin hydrate is no longer available in the United States. Instead, you may want to try a different old-fashioned remedy. Vicks VapoRub contains similar ingredients: oil of turpentine, thymol, and eucalyptol. Don't take it internally. Just rub it on the chest or the soles of the feet to ease a cough.

Another approach is thyme tea. Use ½ teaspoon of dried thyme leaves from the kitchen spice shelf per cup of tea. Some people like to add lemon and honey. Others prefer chicken bouillon for flavor.

● ● ●

Terpin hydrate was removed from the market because the FDA did not receive enough data to support its use when they were reviewing over-the-counter (OTC) drugs for effectiveness. (A high-ranking FDA official admitted to us off the record that he had used it and found it helpful. But the agency needed real data, not testimonials.) Perhaps the fact that it had been around for so long and no one company had a strong vested interest in it meant that no one wanted to invest in research on terpin hydrate. Or maybe it really doesn't work quite as well as people believed. But in any event, after it was banned, Americans needed to look for other cough remedies.

Codeine Cough Medicine

Codeine at prescription doses is generally considered an effective cough suppressant, but even the lower-dose OTC forms are becoming much harder to find. If you have a cough, your doctor might write you a prescription. It is legal in some states for people to buy low-dose codeine cough syrups if they sign for them. Presumably, that step offers extra security against abuse. But even where OTC codeine is legal, many chain drugstores won't sell it without a prescription. They simply don't want to be bothered. If you live in a state where codeine may be sold without a prescription, check with an independent pharmacy. Otherwise, ask your physician about a prescription. Codeine can be constipating, and long-term use can lead to dependence. But for a short-term annoying hack, this is a very helpful medication.

Dextromethorphan

By far the most readily available cough medicine is dextromethorphan. It is the primary ingredient in most OTC cough syrups, including Robitussin DM (the DM stands for dextromethorphan) and many other popular brands. Dextromethorphan has been almost the only choice for nonprescription cough relief for years. It is considered fairly safe because (unlike codeine) it is not classified as a narcotic.

The effectiveness of dextromethorphan has been questioned, however. The American College of Chest Physicians issued guidelines in 2006 on the diagnosis and management of cough that discourage the use of dextromethorphan or any other OTC cough medicine. According to Richard Irwin, MD, the head of the committee that developed the guidelines, "There is no clinical evidence that over-the-counter cough expectorants or suppressants actually relieve cough." That's a pretty discouraging view, since very few coughs actually warrant a doctor's attention. If the cough has lasted for more than a couple of weeks, or if you are otherwise sick, then you should by all means see your doctor. But a regular cough from a cold probably won't benefit from anything your doctor can do.

Home Remedies

There's no good evidence for most of the home remedies that we are going to suggest. No one has done studies to see if thyme tea or horehound drops will really help. On the other hand, these approaches are inexpensive, so you can try them and judge for yourself if they work.

Vicks VapoRub

Vicks VapoRub shouldn't really be classified as a home remedy. It is, after all, a perfectly respectable OTC product that has been a popular way to treat colds for more than a hundred years. According to the history, North Carolina pharmacist Lunsford Richardson set out to formulate a vaporizing cold salve for his own family. His children had come down with bad chest colds and the standard treatments of the day were messy and unsatisfactory.

The result of his effort was Vicks VapoRub. With its distinctive blue jar and unforgettable aroma, Vicks became known around the world as a remedy for congestion and other cold symptoms. It still contains the original formula: menthol, camphor, eucalyptus oil,

★★★★ Vicks VapoRub

Many of the herbal oils in this old-fashioned salve seem to help ease a cough. Menthol is found in many cough drops, and thymol has a reputation for fighting cough. VapoRub is even approved by the FDA for relieving congestion and cough.

You could apply it to the throat and chest, as the instructions suggest, but go ahead and try it on the soles of the feet for a nighttime cough.

Downside: Not for internal use. Keep away from broken skin. Do not apply inside nostrils. No studies confirm that applying Vicks to the soles of the feet will work to calm cough.

Cost: Approximately $6 to $10 for a jar, which will last quite a while

cedarleaf oil, nutmeg oil, thymol, and turpentine oil in a petrolatum base. Parents everywhere rub Vicks VapoRub on their children's chests to ease their coughs.

> *My son continues to have problems with ear infections, although he had tubes put in them at 8 months old. He is now 30 months old and has an ear infection with nasal and chest congestion.*
>
> *I was looking for home remedies for coughs when I found your Web site. I read the idea of putting Vicks VapoRub on the soles of the feet. Within 10 minutes he was asleep without a cough.*

We heard from a nurse who had learned from someone in her church that Vicks could be smeared on the soles of the feet to ease a nighttime cough. As she admitted, this sounded a little crazy, but she was desperate enough to try it on her 4-year-old daughter. When she did, they both finally were able to sleep through the night. We don't know why Vicks on the soles of the feet would work any

better than Vicks on the chest. Perhaps it doesn't. But we do know that we have heard from hundreds of people who have tried this trick and had success. We have used it ourselves and been pleased. Be sure to put on socks to protect the bed sheets.

Thyme

Coughs frequently are a consequence of colds, and chicken soup is a time-honored cold remedy. Beyond its long history of use for this purpose (the Jewish philosopher Maimonides is said to have recommended it), there is even research to demonstrate its value for relieving congestion from colds.[160] So it is little wonder that chicken soup flavored with thyme can be helpful.

> *My husband recently had a spell of heavy, non-productive coughing and couldn't reach his doctor. Robitussin DM didn't do a thing. He went 2 nights with very little sleep and was miserable.*
>
> *I made him some chicken soup for supper, and after he ate a bowl of it he stopped cough-*

ing. During the night he started up again. With more chicken soup, the coughing stopped immediately and he finished the night sleeping well.

I recalled what I'd put into the soup, and zeroed in on two herbs from my garden—three fresh sage leaves and some dried thyme. On the Internet I found that sage can calm a cough and thyme has been widely used as cough medicine.

I made him 2 cups of thyme tea before he went to bed the next evening and he slept the whole night through. I think our experience shows that thyme is a good remedy to keep around until the doctor calls back."

★★★ Thyme

Thyme contains compounds such as thymol and carvacrol. This herb is listed in the *PDR for Herbal Medicines* as indicated for cough and bronchitis. One to 2 grams of dried thyme leaves ($\frac{1}{2}$ to 1 teaspoon) are used to make a cup of tea. The recommended daily dosage is 10 grams spaced over the course of the day.

Side effects: None known
Cost: Inexpensive

Chicken soup with thyme is one way to get the essence of thyme. Another is to make a cup of thyme tea. Ordinary thyme leaves from the kitchen spice cupboard will work just fine—$\frac{1}{2}$ teaspoon to a cup of hot water, steeped for about 5 minutes.

One reader reported getting a cough remedy over the counter when traveling in Germany. She found it very useful, much better than Robitussin DM, and wondered what it was. The medicine, called Makatussin, came as drops to be put on a sugar cube or in tea and contained *Thymianfluidextrakt* and *Sternanisol*. These are extract of thyme and star anise oil. The German government has approved both herbs for colds and coughs, confirming what our readers have found for themselves.

Other Herbs

A number of other herbs have traditionally been used for uncomplicated coughs. Lico-rice is classic for sore throat and cough. It can raise blood pressure, so we don't recommend it for people with hypertension, but for short-term use, it could be helpful. Menthol seems to have been approved by the FDA, since it is found in most OTC cough drops (as well as Vicks VapoRub). Linden flower tea is a European favorite for cough, but may be difficult to find in this country. Elderberry flowers can also be collected and dried for use in tea as a "homegrown" cough remedy. You'd have a hard time finding elderberry flowers in a store, although there are some elderberry products that use the berries themselves, rather than the flowers.

● ● ●

Q. *With my high blood pressure, it's hard to find cold or cough medicine that is safe. My sister recommended*

black elderberry extract and zinc. It did the trick.

A. Elderberry-flower tea is a traditional remedy for colds and coughs. Many herbalists believe elderberry is more effective than echinacea.

Studies of zinc used against colds have produced mixed results, some positive but others negative. Neither remedy should increase blood pressure, though.

● ● ●

Ginger tea is one of our favorite cold remedies, and it also may help to ease a cough. One animal study found that a component of ginger called *shogaol* worked at least as well as dextromethorphan against cough. That may mean simply that shogaol is just as good as placebo, now that the effectiveness of dextromethorphan is in question. Nevertheless, ginger tea is tasty and not very expensive.

Another old-fashioned approach to calming a cough is horehound. Candies flavored with this herb are still available in some stores and catalogs (such as the Vermont Country Store) that pride themselves on carrying old-time products. There's no good research for any of these herbal products, but also no indication that they would cause any serious reactions, either.

Some people find that sucking on a piece of hard candy works quite well to ease a daytime cough, whether or not the candy has any active ingredients such as licorice or menthol in it. One scientist has suggested that part of the reason most cough syrup is sweet is not only to mask the nasty flavor of dextromethorphan, but also to recruit the brain's own opioids, endorphins, in calming the cough.[161] Since opioids are very effective against cough, this is an appealing hypothesis.

Chocolate

Another possible remedy for a simple cough may surprise you. Chocolate lovers though we are, we never suspected that theobromine, one of the essential components of chocolate and cocoa, would have any benefit against cough. But that is exactly what British researchers found in experiments with guinea pigs.[162] They gave the guinea pigs citric acid to make them cough, then gave them theobromine purified from cocoa. The theobromine overcame the induced cough. An experiment in humans confirmed that theobromine is also effective against coughs in people.

The question is, how much chocolate does it take, and in what form? Unfortunately, we do not have an answer to that extremely practical issue. The researchers used theobromine alone, which is not available to the rest of us. But all of us have access to chocolate. You could do some experiments of your own to find the most palatable and effective cough-suppressing chocolate.

Here's what pediatrician Alan Greene, MD, says about using chocolate against cough:

How much chocolate would this be? Chocolate preparations vary widely, depending on their cocoa content, but dark chocolate often has up to about 450 milligrams of theobromine per ounce. Milk chocolate has far, far less. Two ounces of dark chocolate was about the amount of theobromine used for the adults in the study. Half that may be plenty for kids (but of course there is still a lot to learn about this marvelous food). Will that much chocolate keep them awake? Even though theobromine is structurally related to caffeine, studies have shown it doesn't interfere with sleep at those amounts. I used some fine dark chocolate for my own family during our latest viral cough illness, and our coughs disappeared nicely. What a pleasant way to get through a cold!

One other odd cough remedy may be worth a try. This one has not been tested in guinea pigs, but some people find that drinking Concord grape juice helps to ward off colds and ease coughs. There is research demonstrating that Concord grape juice has measurable anti-inflammatory activity.[163] But we don't know what component of grape juice, if any, might be contributing to its cough-calming effect.

• • •

Q. *My wife used to get sore throats every winter. They'd hang on for weeks and develop into a loud, hacking cough. Until she recovered, neither of us would get much sleep.*

Then I remembered that my sister had a similar problem with her four growing boys. In desperation, she tried a remedy she read about: drinking "red" grape juice regularly.

My wife and I started drinking a glass of Concord grape juice every day fall through spring, and the problem vanished. Since then, we've almost never had a bad cough.

We drink half a glass of grape juice and add a half glass of water. Do you know why this works?

A. Purple grape juice has a surprising number of potential health benefits. Research has shown that it can reduce bad cholesterol, lower blood pressure, and help keep blood vessels flexible. There are even some data to suggest

★★ Chocolate

Theobromine has been tested and shown to be effective in suppressing a cough. We don't know of any way to get theobromine except to eat some chocolate, preferably dark chocolate. Savor it, and remember that it has other health benefits if consumed in moderation.

Side effects: Allergy is possible.
Downside: Dose unknown. Excess chocolate consumption may lead to weight gain.
Cost: Highly variable; no prescription dispensing fees

that certain ingredients in grapes may support the immune system. Whether this effect would help ward off sore throats and coughs we do not know.

• • •

Treating Cough in Children

It is hard on parents to listen to a child coughing away. It may even be hard on the youngster. Sometimes coughs keep them awake at night. And because children are so susceptible to colds and other respiratory tract viruses, they seem to get a lot of coughs. But parents should refrain from rushing to the drugstore for cough remedies. A study published in *Pediatrics* found that the two main ingredients in OTC cough medicine, dextromethorphan and diphenhydramine, were no better at easing children's coughs than a placebo syrup was.[164]

According to the lead author, Ian Paul, MD, assistant professor of pediatrics at Penn State Hershey Medical Center, "One of the conclu-

---

★ Grape Juice

Concord grape juice has anti-inflammatory properties, but we don't know of any studies that confirm it has cough suppressant activity.

Side effects: None known

Cost: About $4 to $5 for a 64-ounce bottle

---

sions you could come to from the results of our study is that these medicines don't work [for kids]. And in fact this is what evidence-based reviews of the medical literature have found before, that the existing evidence doesn't support the use of these medicines for acute cough due to a cold."[165] In addition, these medicines are not without risk. According to Dr. Paul, the children who received the standard ingredient in most cough medicines, dextromethorphan (DM), had a harder time falling asleep. That's the last thing an anxious parent wants for a sick kid.

What to do? For a nighttime cough, we are partial to Vicks on the soles of the feet. Grape juice is certainly popular with most youngsters and would be worth a try. And during the day, a lunch of chicken soup with thyme in it would not be amiss. We don't know for sure that any of these remedies will work for kids, though. We have received many testimonials on vanquishing kids' coughs with Vicks, however, so we suspect it is likely to help.

Conclusions

These suggestions are not intended for a cough that has lasted longer than a few weeks, or one that is accompanied by fever, pain, or other symptoms of serious illness. They are aimed primarily at the annoying but not dangerous cough that often crops up at the tail end of a cold or the "flu" and hangs in there even though the patient is feeling much better otherwise.

When it comes to coughs and colds, be very cautious about medicating children. Although there are lots of products on the market aimed at kids, very few have been tested on children. And often, when they are tested on children, they don't seem to work very well. For youngsters, less is definitely better.

- Codeine-containing cough syrup is one of the most effective remedies for cough. It may be difficult to purchase without a prescription. But if your cough is troubling you, ask your doctor to write one. Don't overuse it, because it can be constipating.
- Vicks VapoRub, with its familiar aroma of menthol, camphor, and eucalyptus, is worth trying. If you don't want to put it on your chest, try it on the soles of your feet (under your socks) for a cough-free night.
- Chicken soup with thyme is a comfort food that could help control a cough.
- Several herbal teas may be helpful. Try ginger, mint (menthol), elderflower, or linden flower tea. Sweetening the tea slightly with honey may help the brain's own opioids kick in to help with that cough.
- Suck on hard candy flavored with licorice or horehound.
- The theobromine found in chocolate is active against cough. Perhaps the best way to get it is to melt a square or two of dark chocolate in your mouth.
- Concord grape juice has its enthusiasts, and very little risk.

DANDRUFF

• Soak the scalp with Listerine original-formula (amber) mouthwash	★★★★
• Smear some Vicks VapoRub on itchy spots	
• Make an herbal rinse with sage or rosemary	★★★
• Slather yogurt on the scalp	
• Use a dilute vinegar rinse after washing the hair	★★★★
• Rotate dandruff shampoos to maintain effectiveness	
• Shampoo with Nizoral A-D	★★★★

Dandruff may be dastardly, but in general, it is not a serious medical condition. Though people who have it may by frustrated by it, or even desperate for relief, doctors don't get too excited when they see it. The flakes are not life threatening. They never require surgery. They are not contagious and, unlike flatulence, they don't drive others away. But a bad case of dandruff makes people self-conscious, and thanks to decades of advertising, may even carry a social stigma.

Skin cells die and are sloughed off every day, all over the body. But on the scalp, they may clump together and form flakes that stick in the hair or fall to the shoulders, and are unpleasantly visible on a black polo shirt. If the flakes are especially large and numerous and the scalp is particularly itchy and red, a dermatologist might identify the problem as seborrheic dermatitis. This condition may also affect the face. In some people, patches of skin on the forehead (including the eyebrows), the sides of the nose, and the chin seem to be especially susceptible to developing reddish, itchy scales.

> " *I fought dandruff for 30 years. Even my eyebrows itched. I only bought light-colored clothing that wouldn't show flakes.*
>
> *My dermatologist recommended various shampoos that didn't work. When I changed doctors, my new doctor said my "dandruff" was a yeast infection. She recommended Nizoral shampoo. I only have to use it about once a month and I have no more flakes or itching.*
>
> *I know this story isn't as dramatic as finding a cure for cancer, but solving an annoyance like this is truly liberating.* "

Dermatologists usually distinguish between dandruff and seborrheic dermatitis, but researchers now believe that both conditions can be traced to the skin's reaction to yeast that lives on its surface. This fungus, *Malassezia globo* and related species, sets up housekeeping, especially where the skin is secreting oils.[166] The fungus then produces oils of its own, which irritate the skin.[167] The resulting reaction is the excessive flaking typical of dandruff or the redness and itching on the scalp and face that characterize seborrheic dermatitis. Presumably, the big difference between dandruff and seborrheic dermatitis is the amount of irritation that results.

Malassezia yeast normally inhabit the skin; nobody seems to know exactly why some people are more irritated by *Malassezia* by-products than others. It might have something to do with hormones, or diet, or the activity of the immune system. Because dermatologists don't know how to change individual susceptibility, the basic approach has been just to kill off as many of the yeastie beasties as is practical without hurting the scalp. This not only makes sense, it actually works most of the time. And it also explains why some dandruff shampoos seem to lose effectiveness over time. Presumably, the yeast can develop resistance.

Once in a while, people taking an oral antifungal drug for another problem report that it gets rid of their dandruff. But even for superdandruff (aka seborrheic dermatitis of the scalp), an oral antifungal is too big a cannon to consider seriously. Why risk potentially serious side effects over dandruff?

• • •

Q. *I had dandruff for more than 20 years and tried all sorts of medicated sham-*

poos with no success. About 2 years ago I got a fungus under the nail of my big toe. My podiatrist put me on Lamisil, a pill a day for 3 months.

While I was taking it, my dandruff cleared up and quit itching. The Lamisil did not get rid of my nail fungus, but it seems to have cured the dandruff.

A. We're not surprised to learn that the antifungal medicine you took for your nail infection cleared up your dandruff. Dermatologists think that dandruff is caused, in part, by yeast. Antifungal medicines could eliminate the yeast.

• • •

Home Remedies for Dandruff

Anyone who has had dandruff knows that ordinary shampooing, while it may help for a little while, just doesn't make much difference. But a lot of people have discovered some rather interesting home remedies that can be helpful. We've collected a few that are low cost and low risk, even though there is not much evidence that they work more than occasionally. Use your own common sense in selecting those that seem worth a try.

Herbal Products

What would you think of putting mouthwash in your hair? It may not be the first thing that comes to mind, but quite a few people assure us that Listerine (the amber-colored original formula) can banish dandruff. We first heard this idea from a man who said his veterinarian recommended a mixture of Listerine and baby oil to treat itchy "hot spots" that caused his dog to keep licking its coat. It worked well for the dog, so he experimented on himself! We caution animal lovers to check with your own vet before trying this at home. And we would be especially wary about trying anything of this sort on cats, since they groom themselves so assiduously.

• • •

Q. *Have you ever heard of using Listerine for dandruff? Someone told me he heard it on the radio.*

A. A gentleman called in to our public radio show with an amazing story about Listerine mixed with baby oil. His veterinarian had recommended this combination for relieving itchy spots on his Dobermans and horses. He found that it worked and tried it for his own dandruff. He told us that it gets rid of dandruff in 2 to 3 days.

• • •

In the early 20th century and throughout the World War II era, Listerine was actually promoted as a dandruff treatment. Presumably the company dropped that claim when the FDA demanded proof. It's not too far-fetched to believe, though. Listerine contains a number of herbal oils that have antifungal action, such as thymol, eucalyptol, and menthol. These ingredients might work together to knock down *Malassezia* and thus control flaking. The alcohol in Listerine might also have some antifungal action.

> 66 *I have suffered from severe dandruff all of my life, and nothing helped. I tried washing my hair with Listerine, and have been dandruff free since. It's nothing short of a miracle cure.* 99

The ingredient list for Listerine overlaps quite a bit with the list for another familiar old-fashioned product, Vicks VapoRub. Vicks contains camphor, thymol, menthol, eucalyptus oil, turpentine oil, cedarleaf oil, and nutmeg oil. Although Vicks is not promoted as working against fungus, many people find it helpful in fighting nail fungus, which is notoriously difficult to treat. Others report that it can be effective for the red, itchy flakes of seborrheic dermatitis on the face or behind the ears.

The drawback to using Vicks against dandruff is that the base is petroleum jelly. Washing this goo out of hair could be a real challenge!

People have tried a lot of different techniques to get petrolatum out of hair. The one technique that appears to be most reliable, and easiest, is to work mineral oil into the glop to "cut" it and then wash that out with shampoo or with Dawn dish detergent. It may take several latherings. Some folks are willing to try this treatment repeatedly, but many find that once is enough to convince them to try another method.

● ● ●

★★★★ Listerine

Original Listerine contains a mixture of herbal oils with antifungal action. Currently, it is not promoted as a dandruff cure, but it was once marketed for this purpose. Wet the scalp well with Listerine and leave it on for 5 minutes before shampooing.

Downside: May sting on application. Mouthwash aroma might linger after shampooing.

Cost: Approximately $8 to $10 for a 1½-liter bottle (around 15¢ per treatment)

Q. *I've been suffering with scaly dandruff for 3 years. I've spent an enormous amount of money on medicines prescribed by the dermatologist, but none is a cure.*

Last year I read in your column about people treating fungus-infected toenails with Vicks VapoRub. I thought I would try it for my problem. A bottle of Vicks cost me just over $5.

The Vicks softened those itchy scales and in just 2 weeks I have no more nasty flakes. Thank you for helping people like me on a low income.

A. We've never heard of using Vicks VapoRub against dandruff. This condition has been linked to yeast on the scalp, however, and is treated with antifungal shampoo.

The essential oils in Vicks are reported to have some activity against fungus. We're glad to hear it worked for you, but we wonder: How did you wash the Vicks out?

● ● ●

We heard from one individual who was experimenting with coloring her hair naturally. She made an herbal tea out of sage (but did not tell us how she made it). Then she used the sage tea as a rinse after each shampoo. To her astonishment, she realized that her dandruff had disappeared. Being of a scientific turn of mind, she stopped using the sage tea rinse. Sure enough, her dandruff came right back. She was very pleased to have found an inexpensive way to treat dandruff.

● ● ●

Q. *I used to rinse my hair with a decoction I made from rosemary plants that I grew in my herb garden.*

My hair tends to be the "fly-away" sort, but rosemary made it manageable and also eliminated dandruff. It made my hair smell nice, too. Growing the rosemary myself made my hair rinse a

renewable resource that came from my own yard and saved me money.

A. Rosemary has a reputation as being good for hair, so we are not surprised that your home remedy is helpful. Some people are sensitive to rosemary oil, however, and may develop a rash.

● ● ●

One of the important components of rosemary oil is camphor (along with cineole, alpha-pinene, and limonene). It also contains rosmarinic acid and carnosol. Sage, on the other hand, contains thujone, cineole, and rosmarinic acid.[168] If you plan to try one of these herbal teas as a scalp rinse, use a teaspoon of dried herb for a generous cup (8 or 9 ounces) of hot water. Steep sage tea for 5 minutes before straining; let rosemary tea steep for 15 minutes. If you have fresh herbs from

★★★ Herbal Rinse

After washing the hair, rinse with a tea made of sage or rosemary leaves.[169]

Downside: Some people may have an allergic skin reaction. To be safe, test a spot on your inner arm the day before you plan to use it on your scalp.

Cost: Varies. Using rosemary or sage from the garden is free. Buying herbs in bulk results in a cost of about 5¢ per dose.

the garden, use a tablespoon of fresh leaves for your cup of tea. Let it cool before pouring it over your scalp so you won't scald your scalp by accident.

Kitchen Magic

People can be quite ingenious when they are faced with a problem like dandruff, so it's little wonder that some folks have tried putting common foods on the scalp. One herbal author recommends smearing yogurt onto the scalp after shampooing, allowing it to sit for 15 minutes, and then washing it out.[170] Don't use just any yogurt, though. It should be a type with active cultures (read the label). Yogurt is fairly acidic, and that may make the skin less appealing to fungus. Then again, perhaps those live cultures do their own bit to discourage yeast. We have not tried this remedy and don't know how well it would work.

> **All my life I have used dilute vinegar to rinse my hair after shampooing. It works well against dandruff and you can also use it on your feet to stop odor. Best of all, it's cheap!**

We have heard from a number of people who use vinegar as a rinse after shampooing. Some insist upon apple cider vinegar, while others go with inexpensive white vinegar. Like yogurt, vinegar is acidic. Acid disrupts the environment for many fungi that live on human skin. It stands to reason that it would also work against *Malassezia*.

In fact, when the problem is a fungal infec-

★★★★ Vinegar

It may take a little experimentation to find the right dilution. One part vinegar to five parts water would be safe, but might not be strong enough. One part vinegar to one part water would probably be strong enough to fight the fungus, but it might also sting the scalp. Apply the rinse after shampooing, let it stay on the scalp for 5 minutes, then rinse it with clear water to get rid of the vinegar aroma.

Side effect: Possible skin irritation
Downside: Without the final water rinse, you might smell like a pickle.
Cost: About $1 per quart

---

tion of the ear that makes it itch, one ear-nose-and-throat specialist recommends a solution made of one part white vinegar to five parts tepid water. The ear is flushed gently three times a day, and the fungus usually responds. Such a dilution might work as a scalp rinse. Then again, it is possible that a solution as strong as one part vinegar to two or three parts water would not be too harsh for the scalp.

One other food that could be used against dandruff could make you very popular with Pooh and other fictional bears. Honey, it turns out, is active against *Malassezia* yeast.[171] This might be a lot more convenient to use against seborrheic dermatitis on the face than on the scalp to treat dandruff. But if one were feeling brave, or extra-sweet, it would be possible to mix honey with water, apply it to the scalp for 10 or 15 minutes, and then wash it off. Honey probably wouldn't be much messier than yogurt, though it certainly would be more expensive than vinegar.

Over-the-Counter Remedies

Dandruff shampoos are readily available, and most are backed up by research showing that they affect yeast on the scalp and reduce flaking and itching. Keep in mind, though, that *Malassezia* may develop resistance to shampoos they are exposed to on a regular basis. As a result, it makes sense to rotate the type of medicated shampoo you use every month or two.

You might start, for example, with a shampoo such as Head & Shoulders, Pert Plus for dandruff, or Suave Dandruff 2 in 1 that contains zinc pyrithione. Research has shown that zinc pyrithione kills *Malassezia* and other fungi,[172] which is why these shampoos are usually effective for dandruff. After 6 weeks or so, though, you should switch to an entirely different category of dandruff shampoo.

A medicated shampoo like Nizoral A-D, which contains ketoconazole, would be one option. This antifungal drug also kills *Malassezia* and has some anti-inflammatory action as well.[173] This shampoo is to be used twice a week at first, then only as often as necessary once the flakes are under control. Keep the suds away from the eyes, of course, but you can use Nizoral to wash any skin affected by fungus (patches of seborrheic dermatitis, jock itch, athlete's foot, and the like).

★★★★ Nizoral A-D

This shampoo contains the antifungal drug ketoconazole. (Make sure you buy the medicated shampoo. Nonmedicated Nizoral A-D is also available, but it won't fight dandruff.) Nizoral shampoo is also available by prescription at twice the strength (2 percent).

Side effects: Rash, allergic reaction. To be safe, test a spot on your inner arm before you use it on your scalp.

Downside: Relatively expensive

Cost: Approximately 80¢ to $1.30 per wash

Selenium sulfide is yet another antifungal ingredient. It is found in Selsun Blue, Glo-Sel, and Exsel shampoos.

There are two other categories of dandruff shampoo. One contains coal tar (a category that includes Denorex, Ionil T Plus, Neutrogena T/Sal, and Zetar). This ingredient acts against flaking and helps quell itching as well. The other contains salicylate acid and sulfur, which loosen the flakes and help them break into smaller (and thus less visible) pieces. These are shampoos such as Meted, Pernox, and Sebulex.

It surely doesn't make sense to try all of these medicated shampoos, or even all of the various categories. Switching back and forth among three different categories would probably be just fine. The idea is simply not to let *Malassezia* get too accustomed to whatever it is you are using.

Give any dandruff shampoo enough time to

fight the fungus. That is, after first washing off the surface dirt with any shampoo you please, lather up the medicated shampoo and leave it on for at least 5 minutes. This is harder than it sounds. After all, you may not want to waste water in the shower, but standing around wet and shivering for 5 minutes is also not appealing. You'll have to use your ingenuity to solve this problem, but if you can, you'll find the dandruff shampoo is far more effective. Here's a hint: Shampoo first, then wash the rest of your body while you let the suds sink in.

When you are done washing your hair, resist the urge to blow it dry, at least once in a while. Hair dryers are hard on the scalp and seem to make flaking worse.

Prescription Shampoos

A stronger formulation of Nizoral shampoo is available by prescription. Doctors have a couple of other prescription possibilities as well, in case the other options aren't effective enough. One of these is Loprox shampoo (ciclopirox). This antifungal agent also has some anti-inflammatory activity, which is useful when skin is itchy and red.[174] Needless to say, a prescription shampoo is more expensive than the nonprescription approaches. No head-to-head studies have been done to compare it and find out if it is also more effective.

Conclusions

Dandruff and seborrheic dermatitis both seem to result from a reaction to yeast that normally live on the skin. Scientists don't know why some people react while others do not, nor are they sure why *Malassezia* yeast seems to grow more vigorously on some people's skin than on others'. But research has shown that making life hard for the yeast usually controls the flaking and itching that are so bothersome. If any of these remedies make matters worse, stop the treatment right away and give your skin time to recover before you try anything else. When in doubt, check with a dermatologist!

- Drench the scalp with Listerine original (amber) mouthwash before shampooing. The herbal oils and alcohol in Listerine discourage the growth of yeast on the scalp.
- Smear some Vicks VapoRub on itchy, red, scaly spots. It contains many of the same antifungal herbal oils as Listerine. It can be very difficult to remove Vicks from hair, though.
- Brew some herbal tea with sage or rosemary. Use it as a rinse after shampooing your hair.
- Slather yogurt containing live cultures on the scalp. Leave it for 15 minutes before shampooing it out. Unlike the petrolatum in Vicks VapoRub, yogurt should be fairly easy to wash out.
- Make a rinse with vinegar diluted at least two to one in water. Some people prefer apple cider vinegar, while others use the cheapest white vinegar.
- Switch from one type of dandruff shampoo to another every 6 to 8 weeks. Don't give *Malassezia* a chance to adapt.

• Try using Nizoral A-D shampoo twice a week, then cut back and use it only as often as needed to keep flaking under control.

• If none of this helps, check with your doctor. Perhaps your condition is not ordinary dandruff.

• A prescription shampoo such as Loprox may help when other measures have failed.

DEPRESSION

• Report suicidal thoughts to a health professional	
• Ask your doctor if fluoxetine (generic) is appropriate for you	★★★
• Discuss bupropion if sexual side effects from fluoxetine become a problem	★★★
• Consider cognitive behavioral therapy	★★★★
• Try vigorous exercise 5 days a week	
• Spend time outside in the sun or get a bright light	
• Add fish oil to your dietary regimen	
• Ask your doctor if St. John's wort would be safe	★★★
• Inquire about Emsam when other treatments fail	

Almost everyone knows what it's like to feel sad. Losing a pet, a friend, or a loved one is devastating. Being fired or getting a divorce can send you into a tailspin. An accident or a serious disease affects not only the physical body but also the psyche. For a while there is little pleasure to be had in life. It can be as if darkness has settled into your bones and sucked the joy right out of the marrow.

Most of us eventually recover from the boulders that are dropped on us. But some people never manage to dig themselves out of a hole. According to the National Institute of Mental Health, major depression affects about 15 million people each year. One in five of us will experience some form of depression sometime during our lifetime.[175]

When the fog descends, people may forget what it's like to feel happy. Sleep becomes next to impossible—or all you want to do. Food loses its appeal and its flavor. Those with major depression often have a low energy level; they find it hard to mobilize themselves to finish projects or visit friends or family. They feel gloomy and down in the dumps for weeks or even months. They doubt their abilities and feel pessimistic much of the time. Just remembering simple things becomes an overwhelming challenge. They may experience thoughts of suicide—a hallmark of major depression.

SIGNS OF DEPRESSION

- Feeling sad, gloomy, or "empty" for more than a few weeks
- Feeling hopeless
- Feeling helpless or worthless
- Insomnia, early-morning wakening, or persistently sleeping too much
- Feeling worn-down, fatigued, or like you're moving in slow motion
- Loss of appetite: eating because it's necessary rather than because the food tastes good and satisfies hunger
- Loss of interest in sex
- Restlessness or agitation, pacing the floor
- Difficulty with concentration and with remembering simple things; indecisiveness
- Physical complaints such as headache or pain that don't get better when treated
- Thoughts of death or suicide

Such a mood disorder requires professional help immediately. Let us repeat that. If any of the symptoms above apply to you or someone you care about, seek highly qualified assistance right now! Digging out from a depression should never be a do-it-yourself project. You cannot pull yourself up by the bootstraps or tough it out on your own. Chronic depression increases the risk for heart disease, stroke, diabetes, and other serious conditions and must not be ignored. The suggestions we will discuss in this chapter are meant to supplement whatever your health professional may offer you in the way of help.

The Good Old Days

As remarkable as this may sound, some people actually coped surprisingly well with depression 50 to 100 years ago. They intuitively knew that there were some strategies that worked. For one thing, they looked around for someone to talk to. It might have been a pastor, a friend, a neighbor, or a relative. If they could afford it, they went to a psychologist or psychiatrist for counseling. Just talking things out sometimes seemed to help.

People also exercised. It might have been a physically exhausting task like chopping wood, hoeing a field or hiking through the woods. In those days, people spent more time outdoors working hard and walking from here to there. Nowadays we go from the air-conditioned comfort of our house or apartment to the air-conditioned comfort of a car, bus, or train to the air-conditioned comfort of an office or mall. We rarely spend time outside in the sun, and the only "workout" we get is at the gym or health club.

Oh yes, there was one more thing. In the good old days, especially during the winter, mothers made their kids swallow a spoonful of cod liver oil. It was never clear exactly what cod liver oil was good for, but mothers seemed to know that fish oil had beneficial properties. It was just "good for you," no matter how bad it tasted.

Well, it turns out that virtually all of those quaint old strategies have now been proven helpful against depression. As you will learn shortly, research has shown that fish oil, exercise, light exposure, and cognitive behavioral therapy are surprisingly effective in dealing with depression.

Drug Therapy

Fifty years ago "talking therapy" was considered essential in the treatment of depression. Psychologists and psychiatrists saw lots of patients who suffered from mild to moderate depression. But during the 1970s *biological psychiatry* took off. The medical profession embraced the theory that depression was primarily caused by an imbalance of chemicals in the brain. Many health professionals adopted the belief that a depressed person only needed antidepressant medication to normalize brain biochemistry. All you had to do was "feed your head" the *right* chemicals and the depression would disappear.

During those heady days many patients were given tricyclic antidepressants to soothe their troubled psyches. Medications like amitriptyline (Elavil), desipramine (Norpramin, Pertofrane), doxepin (Adapin, Sinequan), imipramine (Janimine, Tofranil), and nortriptyline (Aventyl, Pamelor) were prescribed in huge numbers. Never mind that such drugs caused drowsiness, fatigue, constipation, dry mouth, dental problems, weight gain, blurred vision, urinary difficulties, dizziness, disturbed concentration, impaired memory, mental confusion, sexual dysfunction, and impotence.

Although these medications did help many people get out of the depths of despair, the side effects were sometimes as depressing as the depression itself. Imagine what it would be like to put on 30 or 40 pounds, feel mentally cloudy and constipated most of the time, and have no sex life. But insurance companies liked these medications. It seemed far more cost-effective to have an internist or a family practice doctor prescribe an antidepressant than to approve a lengthy series of counseling sessions with a psychologist or psychiatrist.

Then along came Prozac (fluoxetine). In 1987 when it was introduced, this antidepressant hardly made a splash. First-year sales were just barely respectable, but more than doubled in the second year. By the third year, Americans spent more on Prozac than on all other antidepressants combined. Everyone seemed to fall in love with Prozac—physicians, pharmacists, patients, and, most of all, the big payers (insurance companies and HMOs).

Prozac—a selective serotonin reuptake inhibitor, or SSRI—was so successful because it got great PR, and because it seemed to have fewer side effects than traditional tricyclic antidepressants. At least it was less likely to cause sedation, dizziness, constipation, or dry mouth. It also was more effective—or at least that was the impression among physicians and patients. There were never any data to support that belief, but that didn't stop the media blitz. Prozac even made the cover of *Newsweek* and *Time* magazines. Once people decided it was the new wonder drug, other pharmaceutical manufacturers were desperate to get in the game. The race was on.

It wasn't long before the wannabes started showing up, trying to claim a piece of the Prozac pie. Today the competitors include bupropion (Wellbutrin), citalopram (Celexa), duloxetine (Cymbalta), escitalopram (Lexapro), nefazodone (Serzone), paroxetine (Paxil), sertraline (Zoloft), and venlafaxine (Effexor). Almost 190 million prescriptions are written for these antidepressants each year, with sales exceeding $12 billion.[176]

Such meds are being prescribed enthusiastically for a wide range of other health problems, too. The pharmaceutical industry has promoted some of these antidepressants for conditions such as obsessive-compulsive disorder, panic attacks, hot flashes, premenstrual distress, nervousness, and shyness ("social anxiety disorder").

Almost from the beginning, though, these drugs have been controversial. In the original clinical trial for Prozac, 15 percent of patients in the study dropped out because they felt worse instead of better—a statistic that was not widely publicized. Anxiety, insomnia, restlessness, nausea, and tremors caused distress for some people. There also was a high incidence of sexual dysfunction with the SSRIs. But the real controversy has always swirled around whether Prozac and similar compounds could trigger thoughts of suicide or homicide in some people.

Antidepressants and Suicide

In 1988, we received a letter from a grieving physician. His daughter had been prescribed Prozac for an eating disorder; a month later she took her life by hanging herself. This ophthalmologist was convinced that Prozac had contributed to her tragic death. At the time, we discounted this story—which we now regret—and told him that depressed people sometimes take desperate action and may try to harm themselves when they start treatment. Later, he responded that his daughter had never been depressed, nor had she been acting like a person who planned to take her life.

In 1990 an article appeared in the *American Journal of Psychiatry* describing a half-dozen patients who developed "intense violent suicidal preoccupation after 2 to 7 weeks of fluoxetine treatment."[177] This report stirred up quite a lot of concern, but many psychiatrists downplayed the connection. When we asked the drug company and the FDA about this report, we were told that depressed people sometimes commit suicide and that the drug was not to blame.

Over the last 18 years we have heard of many other instances in which people became preoccupied with harming themselves or others after starting on an antidepressant. A man taking Zoloft awoke in the middle of the night with a strong urge to kill himself. A woman reported wild thoughts on Prozac about ramming her car into other cars and getting a gun to kill an irritating co-worker. Another woman told us that she experienced an overwhelming urge to open her car door and jump out of the vehicle while it was going at 50 miles an hour down the highway.

> *My son Mike was prescribed Paxil for depression while he was a graduate teaching assistant at New Mexico State University. Around day 13 he slipped into a mood that I had never seen before. He never came out of it. Four days later he shot himself in the temple with a .22 rifle. He had taken Paxil for 17 days.*
>
> *I hold the FDA and GlaxoSmithKline (maker of Paxil) responsible for my son's suicide. No one should ever have to look at a son or daughter's tombstone!*

Whenever we discussed our concerns with psychiatrists, drug companies, or FDA officials, we were told that such events were purely coincidental. Our federal watchdog insisted that the medicines could not have been responsible for such tragic outcomes. But when British drug regulators began warning physicians that SSRI-type medications might trigger suicidal thoughts, agitation, and self-injury in young patients, the whole ball of yarn began to come unraveled.

Eventually, an FDA staffer, Andrew Mosholder, MD, MPH, was given the task of analyzing 22 studies. His conclusion: "Short-term pediatric trials of antidepressant drugs demonstrate an increased rate of suicidal events with active drug compared to placebo." He also said that there is not adequate information to tell if antidepressants other than Prozac are effective for children.

The idea that drugs designed to fight depression and prevent suicide could potentially make things worse for some kids seemed to shock FDA officials to the core. Initially, Dr. Mosholder was muzzled. Eventually, though,

FDA JULY 1, 2005, PUBLIC HEALTH ADVISORY

• Adults being treated with antidepressant medicines, particularly those being treated for depression, should be watched closely for worsening of depression and for increased suicidal thinking or behavior.

• Close observation of adults may be especially important when antidepressant medications are started for the first time or when doses for the specific drugs prescribed have been changed.

• Adults whose symptoms worsen while being treated with antidepressants, including an increase in suicidal thinking or behavior, should be evaluated by their health-care professional.

the data convinced even the FDA hardliners. Belatedly, the agency issued warnings about suicidal thinking and antidepressants.

These cautions came far too late to prevent many terrible tragedies over nearly 2 decades. As difficult as it has been for psychiatrists and FDA officials to contemplate, people taking SSRI-type antidepressants are sometimes preoccupied with thoughts of suicide or homicide. Harvard psychiatrist Joseph Glenmullen, MD, has criticized the makers of SSRI-type antidepressants for delaying adequate warnings.[178] The maker of Effexor XR added "homicidal ideation" to its label years after the drug was introduced. The company considers this a very rare adverse event and does not believe the drug can be causally linked to actual homicides. But there have been a number of high-profile violent events associated with antidepressants. Causal or not, this controversy continues to simmer.

The entire SSRI-suicide story strikes us as mishandled. Just as with the Vioxx (rofecoxib) scandal, it has seemed to us that FDA officials have been more intent on protecting the pharmaceutical companies' profits than the public health.

STAR*D Disappointment

To add even more confusion to this already sordid affair, the reputation these drugs have enjoyed as being highly effective against depression is now suspect. Remember that placebo-controlled trials are the gold standard that everyone is supposed to adhere to. Drug companies are required to show that their expensive antidepressants are significantly superior to a placebo. But an "analysis of 96 antidepressant trials between 1979 and 1996 showed that in 52 percent of them, the effect of the antidepressant could not be distinguished from that of placebo."[179] In other words, "more than half of all recent clinical trials of commonly used antidepressants failed to show statistical superiority for the drug over placebo."[180]

That, dear reader, is almost beyond belief. It suggests that either placebos—sugar pills—are amazingly effective in relieving depression or that current antidepressants are not all that impressive.

Another overview of many clinical trials concludes that the latter is the case. It goes even further and suggests that "recent meta-analyses show selective serotonin reuptake inhibitors have no clinically meaningful advantage over placebo. . . . Antidepressants have not been convincingly shown to affect the long-term outcome of depression or suicide rates."[181] Of course, this kind of analysis relies on the statistical manipulation and combining of many smaller studies. As compelling as the conclusions may be, they do not substitute for really big, well-conducted trials.

The largest and most definitive study of depression and antidepressant medications was a $35 million project, funded by the National Institutes of Health, called the STAR*D (Sequenced Treatment Alternatives to Relieve Depression) trial. This was no drug company whitewash. This was your tax money at work. What made this research so valuable was that the investigators looked at actual recovery from depression ("remission"), not just some symptom improvement. Recovery is, after all, what depressed patients really care about.

The antidepressants used in the STAR*D trial were bupropion SR (Wellbutrin SR), citalopram (Celexa), sertraline (Zoloft), and venlafaxine XR (Effexor XR). When the long-awaited results were published in the *New England Journal of Medicine* (March 2006), they were surprisingly disappointing. About one-fourth of the patients achieved real remission, regardless of the type of antidepressant that was taken.[182] What makes this so discouraging is that these patients got optimal treatment. They received intense evaluation and a level of care not usually available to the average patient. If the depressed folks in this study had been treated in a more typical manner, "the remission rate probably would have been significantly lower—perhaps even in the single digits."[183] That's abysmal.

If there is any good news that came out of the STAR*D research, it is that when a different antidepressant medication was substituted after initial treatment failure, about one in three patients finally did achieve remission.[184, 185] What this means is that antidepressants actually do what they are supposed to do (cure depression) about half the time. Depending upon your perspective, that means the glass is either half full or half empty.

We are happy to learn that 50 percent of the patients in this trial got better. But even under these ideal conditions, half did not, regardless of the type of medicine used. That means that an awful lot of people are suffering drug side effects without benefit. And since there were no placebo controls in STAR*D, we have no idea how many folks might have improved if they had received sugar pills instead of drugs.

So how can you determine which antidepressant is best for you? In truth, it is extremely difficult for physicians and patients to make clear decisions about safety and effectiveness when it comes to these medications. Despite all the hype from the drug companies, it is hard to prove that one type of antidepressant is better than another one.[186]

Newer drugs like Cymbalta affect both serotonin and another neurotransmitter called *norepinephrine* (hence their name serotonin/norepinephrine reuptake inhibitors, or SNRIs). This dual action is supposed to make such drugs more effective. It has certainly driven up the cost. A single Cymbalta pill can cost between $3 and $4. A *Wall Street Journal* review reported that when Cymbalta was compared head-to-head with venlafaxine (Effexor), an older drug in this class, "Cymbalta wasn't significantly different from Effexor in treating depression."[187]

The bottom line is that there are no "best choices" when it comes to these kinds of antidepressants. All these drugs are roughly similar in effectiveness, and all have the potential to cause serious adverse reactions for some people. Anyone who experiences anxiety, agitation, irritability, and especially thoughts of violence toward himself or others should contact a health professional immediately!

Watch Out for Withdrawal!

There is one other complication associated with these antidepressants that is rarely discussed. Sudden discontinuation of drugs like Effexor, Paxil, Serzone, and Zoloft may cause unexpected symptoms. We have heard from many patients that they experienced dizziness, nausea, insomnia, headaches, nervousness, sweating, shakiness (like a bad hangover), weakness, visual disturbances, and an inability to concentrate. One reader called the problem "Paxil Head," like having your head stuck in a blender.

" *I take Zoloft, and have tried to stop taking it several times. Each time I stop I experience a very strange thing. Doctors, nurses, and pharmacists dismiss me like I'm a nut case, but I swear this is true. I get electrical shocklike sensations in my head and become extremely dizzy. I absolutely know this is associated with not taking Zoloft. Not 2 hours after I resume taking it again the symptoms, which are overwhelming, disappear completely. I would like to get off of this drug but have no idea how to do so, especially*

★★★ Fluoxetine (Prozac)

Fluoxetine is a stand-in for all SSRI-type drugs. Although there are subtle variations between medications in this class, there are more similarities than differences.

Side effects: Headache, nausea, dizziness, diarrhea, nervousness, anxiety, and insomnia are relatively common and may affect up to one-fourth of the patients who take SSRI-type medications. Some people may experience drowsiness or dizziness. Delayed ejaculation, inability to achieve orgasm, and decreased sexual desire are common complications of this entire class of drugs. Less frequent problems may include decreased appetite, indigestion, sweating, mania, dry mouth, heart palpitations, tremor, chills, constipation, blurred vision, memory problems, confusion, rash, and joint pains. Blood sugar control or thyroid function may be altered. Seizures, while uncommon, have been reported in roughly 0.1 to 0.2 percent of patients, an incidence comparable to that seen with older antidepressants. Any thoughts of suicide or violence must be reported to a physician immediately!

Downside: SSRI-type medications like Prozac can interact with many other drugs. Make sure your physician and pharmacist double-check to verify that any other medicine, herb, or dietary supplement you take is safe with your antidepressant.

Cost: Approximately $130 to $140 for a month's supply of Prozac. Generic fluoxetine costs $16 to $20 for the same amount.

when I cannot function without it and no one recognizes I'm having any trouble. They just think I'm crazy."

What is so sad about this particular problem is that no one really knows how common withdrawal symptoms are. There are, as far as we can tell, few good guidelines for helping people overcome this complication. So we do not know how long people will experience dizziness, shocklike sensations, or nausea after they stop a drug like Zoloft. Drug companies are not particularly interested in developing protocols for discontinuing SSRI/SNRI-type medications, since they would then need to admit they have a problem on their hands. That means that patients and physicians are on their own.

Gradual tapering over several weeks may be necessary. We have heard from some doctors that they switch patients over to fluoxetine and then taper it very slowly. That's because Prozac lingers in the body and may be less likely to trigger withdrawal symptoms

Despite all the controversy, we still think Prozac is worthy of consideration, especially since it is less likely to precipitate withdrawal symptoms when discontinued. And we are not convinced that other SSRI/SNRIs are more effective. Many people benefit dramatically from this or another SSRI or SNRI. Prozac is now available generically as fluoxetine, so the cost factor is less problematic. We're not convinced, though, that all generic fluoxetine is created equal. Some patients report therapeutic failures on this generic (see Generic Drug Quandary for details).

Since there is no way to predict whether someone will benefit more from one antidepressant than another, this is mostly a process of trial and error. It may take 4 to 6 weeks to begin to see improvement, so it is important to

★★★ Bupropion (Wellbutrin)

This antidepressant is less likely to interfere with sexuality and may even be helpful for people who have experienced diminished libido. It is also available generically, so there is a cost savings. People tend to feel energized rather than sluggish when taking bupropion.

Side effects: Common complaints include insomnia, dry mouth, anxiety or agitation, headache, nausea, and dizziness. Less common adverse reactions that we are aware of include mania, seizures, irregular heart rhythms, skin rash, hallucinations, paranoia, high blood pressure, and migraine.

Downside: Bupropion can interact with many other medications. Make sure your physician and pharmacist double-check to verify that any other medicine, herb, or dietary supplement you take is safe with your antidepressant. Any thoughts of suicide or violence must be reported to a physician immediately!

Cost: Approximately $130 to $150 for a month's supply of brand-name Wellbutrin SR; generic bupropion SR runs roughly $60 to $70 for a similar amount.

give each medication a fair trial. If no success is achieved after a few drugs in the same class are tried, then it may be time to move on to another category.

Bupropion (Wellbutrin) may offer certain advantages over other SSRI-type drugs. For one thing, it is far less likely to interfere with sexuality. Some have even reported that it restores libido.

Some people do benefit from old-fashioned tricyclic-type antidepressants such as desipramine, imipramine, and nortriptyline. For people who become agitated or anxious on an SSRI/SNRI or find that bupropion keeps them wide awake, tricyclics may offer an acceptable alternative.

There is also a completely different kind of antidepressant that comes as a skin patch (Emsam). We will discuss it at the end of this chapter.

Nondrug Therapy: Back to the Future

At the beginning of this chapter we suggested some old-fashioned approaches to treating depression that might be worth reconsidering. We were referring to seemingly archaic practices such as counseling, exercise, and fish oil. Surprisingly, there is some scientific support for these quaint concepts.

Talking Therapy

In our rush-rush world, people rarely take time to talk anymore. The idea that someone could actually sit down for an hour or so and discuss the issues that are causing distress seems outdated. Insurance companies and "mangled care organizations" may not be thrilled at the prospect of paying a psychologist or psychiatrist $100 to $200 a week to do counseling for several months. The bean counters seem to prefer paying for prescription drugs indefinitely. What is so bizarre about this ass-backwards approach is that psychotherapy can enhance the effectiveness of medications and can be stopped once it has been successful. That seems cost-effective to us.

For those in the know, *cognitive behavioral therapy*, *interpersonal therapy*, and *problem-solving therapy* are surprisingly effective for mild to moderate depression.[188] Cognitive behavioral therapy (CBT) got traction in the 1970s. In a

★★★★ Cognitive Behavioral Therapy

The results of well-conducted research suggest that cognitive behavioral therapy (CBT) is as effective as antidepressants in treating depression. The benefits are long lasting and we don't know of any serious side effects to talking therapy.

Downside: Such treatment can be expensive and it requires an experienced psychotherapist. Identifying someone who has the requisite expertise may not be that easy.

Cost: Approximately $100 to $200 per session. This is highly variable depending upon the practitioner's skill level and location. Several sessions may be required.

nutshell, this therapy works on the premise that depression arises from dysfunctional thoughts and beliefs. We are all influenced by our early learning experiences. When those thought processes are dysfunctional, they can be triggered by situations later in life and produce depression and other psychiatric symptoms. The trick here is to have skilled therapists help patients identify and challenge negative automatic thoughts so that behavior can be changed.[189]

One study found that "cognitive therapy can be as effective as medications for the initial treatment of moderate to severe major depression but this degree of effectiveness may depend on a high level of therapist experience or expertise."[190] Another study found that "cognitive therapy has an enduring effect that extends beyond the end of treatment. It seems to be as effective as keeping patients on medication."[191]

Exercise

As effective as talking therapy may be for depression, exercise may also be beneficial. Investigators have known for decades that aerobic exercise can improve mood and outlook. Recent research backs this up. A review confirms that exercise can benefit mental health, helping to alleviate depression as well as improve physical health.[192] According to Canadian reviewers, there is "irrefutable evidence" that physical activity can be effective against depression.[193]

One study was dubbed DOSE, for Depression Outcomes Study of Exercise. Men and women between 20 and 45 years of age with mild to moderate depression were asked to exercise for various amounts of time ranging up to 30 minutes of moderate-intensity movement almost every day of the week. That allowed the investigators to compare the "dose response" from exercise. They found that low-intensity exercise was no better than placebo, but high-intensity exercise was an effective treatment.[194]

Bright Light

To give your exercise a jump start, go outside and get a little sun on your face. There is growing evidence that light therapy can be beneficial against depression. One eminent psychiatrist reviewed the literature, expecting to find that the research was awful and the therapy didn't work. Instead, after reviewing the data objectively, he came to the conclusion that phototherapy was "comparable to what has been described in the clinical literature for conventional medications to treat depression. The findings are as strong or as striking."[195, 196]

Bright light therapy is helpful not only for seasonal affective disorder (SAD), which frequently occurs during the winter, but also for depression that occurs at any time of the year. There is evidence that light can enhance the effects of exercise as well as the antidepressant action of medications like citalopram (Celexa).[197, 198]

Fish Oil

Grandma might have been right that cod liver oil is good for your mind as well as your body.

She may not have had the benefit of randomized, placebo-controlled trials, but we do. Most of them show that fish oil can be helpful against depression.[199] We're hoping that there will be more studies in the future to determine the best dose of DHA and EPA, the main fatty acids in fish oil. We're not thrilled with cod liver oil, per se. These days you can obtain pharmaceutical-grade fish oil that does not have the excessive levels of vitamin A you often find in cod liver oil. Too much vitamin A is bad for your bones.

St. John's Wort

The medical community has had a very hard time grappling with research suggesting that an herb might be as good as an antidepressant like fluoxetine (Prozac) for relieving depression. Nevertheless, there have been dozens of clinical trials demonstrating that St. John's wort can be effective in treating mild to moderate depression.[200] In some studies, St. John's wort works as well as prescription antidepressants, and it usually has fewer troublesome side effects.

St. John's wort has long been prescribed in Europe for treating depression and other mood disorders. Although there are studies showing that the extract is not better than placebo, there are several showing that it works at least as well as prescription antidepressants. Most trials indicate that St. John's wort appears to be safe and well tolerated, perhaps better tolerated than a pharmaceutical antidepressant.

The way St. John's wort acts to relieve depression is not known. Scientists don't even know which of its many constituents might be responsible for the activity. This makes it hard to select an extract appropriately. Only standardized extracts, preferably ones that have been tested

---

★★★ St. John's Wort (*Hypericum perforatum*)

Some people may find that St. John's wort is an effective antidepressant. As long as it is taken under medical supervision and caution is exercised regarding drug interactions, we think it is worth consideration.

Side effects: Side effects are uncommon and usually mild. Unlike many prescription antidepressants, St. John's wort does not cause sexual dysfunction. Digestive upset has been reported. Allergic reactions are possible.

Downside: St. John's wort can cause photosensitization, making the skin and the eyes vulnerable to damage from sunlight. St. John's wort interacts dangerously with a wide range of prescription medications. Ask your pharmacist or your doctor to check on this possibility if you contemplate taking St. John's wort together with any other medicine.

Cost: Approximately $15 to $20 a month for Kira brand

---

and found effective, should be used. Three standardized products that have been tested in Germany are available here. The brand names are Kira, Movana, and Perika.

The Selegiline (Emsam) Patch

The latest and most interesting chapter in antidepressant therapy involves a prescription skin patch containing the drug selegiline (Emsam). This transdermal medication works in a completely different manner from most current antidepressants. It is called a monoamine oxidase inhibitor (MAOI). Such drugs were among the first antidepressants ever developed. But they lost their luster because of a potentially deadly interaction with many foods, beverages, and drugs. The "cheese effect," as it came to be known, could cause extremely high blood pressure when a person taking a medication like Marplan or Parnate ate an aged cheese such as cheddar. This could result in a stroke.

• • •

Q. *What can you tell me about selegiline? The vet prescribed it for my elderly dog. She had been very agitated, pacing for hours at a time (sometimes 12 or 15 hours straight!). She would pace until she dropped from exhaustion, sleep for half a day, then get up and start pacing again. She was also drooling excessively, digging compulsively, deliberately knocking things over, and urinating in the house whenever I left.*

My vet said these are all symptoms of senile dementia in dogs. I think it was precipitated by the death of my other dog. They had been together for more than 12 years and she just couldn't handle being alone.

Several days after she started on selegiline all those behaviors stopped completely. It was amazing. She started acting like herself again. After seeing how much it helped my dog, I would definitely take it myself. Do they ever prescribe it for people with memory problems?

A. Our veterinary consultant, Andrea Frost, DVM, says that selegiline can be helpful for dogs with the canine equivalent of senile dementia. When an old dog gets lost in his own house or becomes incontinent because he can't remember to ask to go out, quality of life for the owner, if not for the dog, has really declined.

Not every dog has as dramatic a response as yours, but selegiline can help buy some old dogs a little more quality time with their human families.

Selegiline is used in human medicine to treat people with Parkinson's disease and depression. It has been studied against Alzheimer's disease with mixed results.

• • •

The good news is that this new-generation MAOI is far less likely to cause such problems. In the lowest-dose skin patch, there is no food prohibition. When people take higher doses (9 or 12 milligrams), however, they do have to be careful about foods containing tyramine (beef liver, blue cheese, bologna, Brie, broad beans, Camembert, cheddar, Chianti, chicken liver, draft beer, miso soup, Parmesan cheese, pepperoni, salami, sauerkraut, and yeast extract) because their blood pressure could rise dangerously high.

Emsam should not be combined with other antidepressants or St. John's wort. It is crucial to check with your pharmacist and your physician before combining any other medication when you are using Emsam.

In double-blind trials, scientists determined that Emsam is significantly more effective than placebo. The most common side effects include irritation where the patch is applied to the skin, rash, indigestion, headache, insomnia, diarrhea, dry mouth, and dizziness when standing up suddenly. Sexual side effects appear to be uncommon. Anyone who experiences thoughts of suicide while using this patch should contact the prescribing physician immediately.

Conclusions

If there is one lesson you should learn from this book it is that everyone responds differently to various treatments. That is as true for relieving depression as for lowering cholesterol or controlling diabetes. Some people find that Prozac is an absolute miracle, lifting them from the despair of lifelong depression. Others find it makes them irritable, jittery, and incredibly uncomfortable. There is no good way to predict how any individual will react, so the best advice we can give is to stay vigilant.

If you start to feel better on an antidepressant, that's great. If you experience no improvement or get worse, contact your health-care professional immediately and seek alternatives. In some cases, combining several approaches such as vigorous exercise, fish oil, and light therapy may be as effective as prescription medicine.

• Depression can take the wind out of your sails. Do not expect that you will be able to pull yourself together on your own. Seek help from friends, family, and qualified professionals.

• Antidepressants can be very helpful for some people. There is no clear evidence that one is superior to another. Trial and error may be the only way to tell which one will produce the best results for you.

• Suicidal thoughts are now recognized as a potential complication of virtually all antidepressant therapy. Family and friends should be especially vigilant during the first few weeks of treatment and whenever your dosage is changed.

• Stopping some antidepressants suddenly can be difficult. Switching to a longer-acting medication like fluoxetine and then gradually tapering the dose may overcome the withdrawal symptoms. This should be carefully supervised by a knowledgeable physician.

•Alternative therapies such as exercise, light therapy, fish oil, and St. John's wort may be helpful.

•Emsam (selegiline) is a new antidepressant skin patch that may offer an alternative to the usual SSRI-type medications.

DIABETES

• Control weight	
• Eat a low-carbohydrate diet	
• Enjoy a little dark chocolate	★★
• Drink coffee	★★★
• Exercise regularly	★★★★★
• Sweeten foods with stevia	★★★
• Add cinnamon to meals	★★★★
• Monitor blood sugar regularly	
• Get adequate vitamin D	★★★★★
• Control stress	
• Ask your doctor about metformin (Glucophage)	★★★
• Discuss pioglitazone (Actos) with your doctor	★★★★
• Ask your doctor about repaglinide (Prandin)	★★

Diabetes is one of the major health problems affecting Americans. In this condition, cells of the body can't get energy from the sugar (glucose) circulating in the blood. They may literally starve to death in the midst of plenty. Imagine yourself in a lifeboat in the middle of the ocean. You are desperately thirsty, surrounded by water, but there's not a drop to drink. A diabetic's bloodstream has too much glucose, but because insulin is lacking or not effective, it cannot transport this sugar into the cells that need it.

This metabolic disruption creates conditions ripe for heart disease and stroke. Other potential complications include nerve damage (known as *neuropathy*), sexual dysfunction, kidney disease, and even blindness. But if diabetes is successfully treated so that blood sugar is kept within or close to the normal range, the complication rate can be minimized.

Experts estimate that 20 million Americans have diabetes. That's nearly 7 percent of the population. Unfortunately, nearly one-third of these diabetics have not been diagnosed and consequently are not being treated. One of the best ways to prevent complications from diabetes is to control blood sugar carefully. The good news is that keeping blood sugar within normal limits can cut the risk of life-threatening consequences such as heart attack and stroke nearly in half.[201]

Doctors classify the disease into two categories. In type 1 diabetes, the immune system attacks the pancreas and destroys the cells that make insulin. Since insulin is crucial for glucose to get into the cells from the bloodstream, the type 1 diabetic must get insulin from somewhere else. Usually, this means injections, often several times a day. (Inhaled insulin may offer another option.) This disease has also been termed *insulin-dependent diabetes*, which is descriptive, or *juvenile diabetes*, which is not very helpful. Not all people newly diagnosed with type 1 diabetes are children, and not all children diagnosed with out-of-control blood sugar have type 1 diabetes. Because this disease is so complicated and requires such careful medical supervision, it will not be covered in this chapter.

In type 2 diabetes, by contrast, there is insulin in the bloodstream, sometimes too much of it, but the cells become resistant to its action. Many people with type 2 diabetes are able to control their blood sugar level with diet, exercise, and oral medication. As a result, type 2 diabetes is also referred to as *non-insulin-dependent diabetes*, or *adult-onset diabetes*. The latter term is left over from a simpler time. With the increase in childhood obesity, more and more children are being diagnosed with type 2 diabetes all the time. Type 2 diabetes is the most common kind, and it is increasing at an alarming rate. The Centers for Disease Control and Prevention projects that one in three children under the age of 5 will develop this kind of diabetes during their lifetime. If they are Latino, the odds are that one in two will become diabetic.[202]

Everyone agrees that diabetes has reached epidemic levels. What is unclear is why. Most experts blame the problem on obesity and inactivity. But there are voices in the wilderness suggesting that there may be other factors that are also contributing to this public health nightmare. Some suggest that high-fructose corn syrup, which is widely used as an inexpensive sweetener in juice, soft drinks, and processed foods, might predispose people to diabetes. In animal research this sugar leads to insulin resistance and poor glucose tolerance.[203] Until this controversy is sorted out, we discourage the consumption of foods and beverages containing high-fructose corn syrup.

Another even scarier scenario involves the compound bisphenol A (BPA). You've probably never heard of this chemical, but the chances are very good that you have it circulating in your body. BPA shows up in the bloodstream of 95 percent of Americans. BPA is a common compound found in plastic. There may be some in your water bottle or jug. It is also in the plastic lining of cans of soft drinks and beer. Canned foods, food storage containers, pacifiers, baby teethers, and dental sealants may contain BPA.

The plastic industry will tell you that small amounts of BPA are nothing to worry about. A study published in the journal *Environmental Health Perspectives,* however, suggests that when mice are exposed to low levels of BPA for several days, they develop insulin resistance.[204] What is so alarming about this discovery is that the levels of BPA used in the experiment would be considered safe for humans by the Environmental Protection Agency (EPA). We don't know whether BPA is contributing to the ever-increasing incidence of type 2 diabetes, but we sure wish scientists would find out before it's too late.

Preventing Type 2 Diabetes

No one knows whether reducing high-fructose corn syrup in the diet or limiting BPA exposure will reduce the risk of diabetes. But we do know that there are certain risk factors that make people more susceptible to type 2 diabetes. Changing those conditions may help people avoid this disease.

It is estimated that as many as 40 million Americans might have prediabetes. Their fasting blood sugar is between the cutoff for definite diabetes of 126 milligrams per deciliter (mg/dl) and high normal (110 mg/dl). Some diabetes experts believe that prediabetes should be diagnosed when fasting blood sugar runs at or above 100 mg/dl.[205]

People at risk for diabetes may also be overweight and have high blood pressure, high triglycerides, and low HDL cholesterol. When these conditions occur together, they are labeled *metabolic syndrome.* Anyone who has three of these problems should get motivated to make major changes before full-blown diabetes develops.

METABOLIC SYNDROME[206]

- Waist circumference of more than 40 inches for men and 35 inches for women
- Blood pressure of 130/85 mmHg or higher
- Fasting triglycerides at 150 mg or higher
- Fasting glucose at 110 mg or higher
- HDL cholesterol of less than 40 mg/dl for men and 50 mg/dl for women

---

Almost anyone who has ever tried it knows that losing weight is really hard. Keeping it off for an extended time is even more of a challenge. But when you stop to think that diabetes could cost you your eyesight, your kidney function, your sex life, or your heart, it is worth the effort. A relatively modest weight loss, even just 5 percent of your initial weight, can help lower blood pressure and triglycerides and reduce insulin resistance.[207] This works out to just under 10 pounds for a 195-pound man. Such a loss may even reduce the likelihood that you will need medication. But how can you get the pounds off? Most experts agree that a two-part approach works best: Change the diet, and increase the exercise. See page 403 for strategies for weight loss.

Diet against Diabetes

"Diet" is a dirty word. Basically, it seems to say you can't eat anything you like. What we really mean by "diet," though, is a blueprint for eating. There is some evidence that one very common dietary pattern puts people at higher risk for developing type 2 diabetes. Consuming soft drinks (either sugar-sweetened or diet), refined grains (think bread and pasta), and processed meats increases inflammation in the body and nearly triples women's risk of being diagnosed with type 2 diabetes.[208] In comparison, the diet that does not raise diabetes risk includes plenty of yellow and green vegetables (especially those in the cabbage family, like broccoli and kale) as well as whole grains, coffee, and wine.

In attempting to prevent diabetes, it might make sense to get used to eating as though you already have diabetes. There are a gazillion diets out there, but the one that makes the most sense to us is a low-carbohydrate, high-vegetable diet. This means, of necessity, that it is also relatively high in lean protein, whether from animal or vegetable sources.

Be prepared for some resistance from dietitians. The American Diabetes Association (ADA) has been preaching a low-fat, high-carbohydrate approach for decades. But we have had an opportunity to interview a medical heretic on several occasions, and he has convinced us that his diet plan makes sense.

Richard K. Bernstein, MD, is a medical maverick who has battled the ADA for a long time. He described his low-carb solution in his book *The Diabetes Diet*. Dr. Bernstein himself has diabetes, though not type 2 diabetes. He was diagnosed at age 12 with type 1 diabetes. Back in 1946, there were no tools for measuring blood sugar at home. Even after he finished college, the only home tools were urine tests that detect high blood glucose only when it is so high that it "spills over" into urine.

As an engineer, Dr. Bernstein was fascinated by the first machine that analyzed blood glucose directly. He talked his wife, who is a physician, into prescribing one for him. Then he used it to determine what diet did to his own blood sugar levels. What he found is that carbohydrates raise blood glucose. Despite keeping meticulous records, he could not convince the medical establishment that he knew what he was talking about. He finally went to medical school to help make this information available to other diabetics.

"My fasting blood sugar (glucose) was slightly elevated (top of norm was 99 and mine was 126). My doctor requested I take a repeat test, which consisted of a fasting finger-stick only. This was normal at 99. I told the doctor I would start cutting down on sugar, but he replied, "You really need to watch carbohydrates more than raw sugar." What carbohydrates would you recommend avoiding? I am 76 years old and certainly want to avoid adult-onset diabetes."

Millions of diabetics are confused about what to eat and what to avoid. Dr. Bernstein has developed a list of foods that he believes make the blood sugar level rise. Although we

DR. BERNSTEIN'S NO-NO'S

- Barley
- Beans
- Beets
- Bread and crackers
- Breakfast cereal (including oatmeal)
- Candy (sugar-free also)
- Carrots
- Corn
- Fruits
- Honey
- Juices
- Onions
- Pancakes or waffles
- Pasta
- Potatoes
- Rice
- Rye
- Sweets and sweeteners (except stevia)
- Tomatoes (cooked or in sauce)
- Wheat
- Yogurt (sweetened, low-fat)

cannot promise that eliminating these foods will lower glucose readings, we think this experiment is worth trying.

Dr. Bernstein's main diet plan involves eggs or other protein for breakfast, but no cereal; 2 cups or so of salad and some lean protein such as tuna or salmon for lunch; for dinner, another serving of lean protein such as chicken, a cup of salad, and ⅔ cup of cooked veggies. His list of sanctioned vegetables runs from artichokes to zucchini.

Although Dr. Bernstein is considered to be out of the mainstream of diabetes experts and diabetes educators, his suggestions make sense to us. He urges diabetics to monitor their own blood sugar frequently to determine how their own bodies respond. Initially he recommends 2 weeks of measuring and recording blood sugar first thing in the morning, then right after breakfast, 2 hours after meals and snacks, at bedtime, and before and after exercising.[209] Once you know how you respond to these various conditions, you may not need to measure more than a few times a day.

Share these records of your blood sugar measurements with your doctor so the program can be fine-tuned. When it comes to this disease, one size does not fit all. Each person responds to stress, food, exercise, and medications differently. Finding the most effective strategy for you will require careful record keeping and excellent collaboration with your health-care providers.

People with prediabetes may also find it helpful to limit carbohydrates, especially highly refined foods like bread, pasta, crackers, and cookies. So-called whole wheat bread is no solution, since it too can make blood

SOME BERNSTEIN LOW-CARB FAVES

- Artichokes
- Asparagus
- Beet greens
- Bell peppers
- Bok choy
- Broccoli
- Brussels sprouts
- Cabbage
- Cauliflower
- Celery
- Cheese
- Collard greens
- Eggplant
- Eggs
- Endive
- Escarole
- Fish
- Fowl

- Green beans
- Meat
- Mushrooms
- Nuts
- Okra
- Pumpkin
- Radicchio
- Sauerkraut
- Scallions
- Seafood
- Snow peas
- Soy milk and products
- Spaghetti squash
- Spinach
- Tofu
- Yogurt (full-fat)
- Zucchini

sugar rise. It used to be an old wives' tale that eating sugar would give you diabetes. But as we learn more about diet and metabolism, it becomes clear that rapid spikes in blood sugar and insulin from any source are not good for the body. A breakfast of pancakes, syrup, and orange juice is guaranteed to make blood sugar rise. But so could a "sensible" breakfast of instant oatmeal and skim milk.

Many people find it easier to lose weight on a low-carbohydrate regimen, whether it is the South Beach diet, the Zone, or the Atkins diet. If one of these appeals to you more than the others, it makes sense to follow it.

Those who don't yet have blood sugar in the danger range can probably risk an occasional carrot or serving of fruit that qualifies as a complete no-no on Dr. Bernstein's Diabetes Diet. But there is increasing evidence to support the overall pattern he recommends. A 4-month study of type 2 diabetics put on a low-carbohydrate Atkins-style ketogenic diet showed a significant improvement in blood sugar control, along with weight loss and reduction in the amount of diabetes medications needed.[210] In addition, Swedish researchers report that a low-carbohydrate diet improved blood sugar control and reduced the average insulin requirement in a small group of obese type 2 diabetics.[211] These clinical investigators also had success reversing a 6-year decline in kidney function in one diabetic patient by changing his diet from the usual prudent low-fat, high-carbohydrate diet to a regimen with no potatoes, bread, pasta, rice, or cereal. This 60-year-old man lost weight and stabilized his blood glucose, the progression of his diabetic eye disease was halted, and his kidney function was dramatically improved.[212]

Chocolate and Insulin Resistance

People with insulin resistance may even benefit from eating a bit of dark chocolate once in a while. This certainly won't help anyone lose weight, so caution is advised! Research has shown, however, that cocoa compounds can help improve insulin sensitivity slightly, as well as lower blood pressure.[213] The sugar in chocolate candy might raise blood sugar too much for a frank diabetic, though, so use your good judgment and your blood sugar monitor. Never eat chocolate by itself between meals. It will be better for your health if you have it after a low-carbohydrate meal. And it should go without saying, though many doctors have

> "In summary, a reduced carbohydrate diet is an effective tool in the management of motivated obese patients with type 2 diabetes."[214]
> —J.V. Neilsen and E. Joensson, *Nutrition and Metabolism*, June 2006

said it, that chocolate is no substitute for a careful diet, healthy lifestyle, and medication if it is needed.

Coffee and Diabetes Prevention

Another option for preventing type 2 diabetes may surprise you: Drink coffee. Although diabetics need to be careful about coffee consumption, healthy people who drink a lot of coffee—6 or 7 cups a day—lower their risk of developing type 2 diabetes significantly, by about 35 percent.[215] It's not completely clear why coffee has such an effect, but it doesn't seem to be the caffeine. In fact, caffeine alone reduces insulin sensitivity.[216] Drinking either caffeinated or decaf coffee lowers the likelihood of impaired glucose tolerance in people who don't yet have diabetes. Perhaps it is the chlorogenic acid, a coffee com-

> ★★ **Dark Chocolate**
>
> Dark chocolate, with as little sugar as you can stand, helps to lower cholesterol, triglycerides, blood pressure, and insulin resistance. One brand used in a study was Ritter Sport Dark. A minimum dose was not determined. The study dose was 100 grams.
>
> **Downside:** High in calories and extremely appealing. Too much will derail weight loss.
> **Cost:** Approximately $2 for a "study" dose

ponent that lowers blood sugar and leads to better insulin sensitivity in rats.[217]

Exercise

It may sound boring, but exercise has such an amazing effect on metabolic syndrome and type 2 diabetes that it is surprising that doctors don't prescribe it more often. If the benefits of exercise came in a pill, drug companies would charge thousands of dollars a year for it and doctors would prescribe it like candy. You would see commercials on television for a miracle medicine for fighting diabetes. Exercise truly is the best and least expensive component of effective diabetes care.

In one large, well-designed study, modest weight loss (7 percent of body weight) and 150 minutes per week of exercise were more effective than the prescription drug metformin in warding off metabolic syndrome and type 2 diabetes.[218] Among the group that exercised and lost weight, the incidence of metabolic syndrome dropped by 41 percent, the diagnosis of diabetes was delayed by 11 years on average, and the incidence of diabetes was reduced by 20 per-

cent.[219] Among those who took the medication, in comparison, the incidence of metabolic syndrome dropped by 17 percent,[220] the diagnosis of diabetes was delayed by an average of 3 years, and the incidence of diabetes dropped by 8 percent.[221] Exercise was also a lot more affordable.

If you were to follow this approach, 150 minutes of exercise a week would break down into 30 minutes a day 5 days a week—or, if it fits the schedule better, 50 minutes a day 3 days a week. Vigorous activity is even better than walking at preventing type 2 diabetes, but walking briskly is better than sauntering, and even that is more helpful than no exercise at all.[222]

People who already have diabetes also benefit from regular exercise, because it has a profound impact on a person's ability to control blood sugar. Exercise may even reduce the likelihood of serious complications of diabetes.[222, 223] Physical activity can improve insulin sensitivity and make weight control (at least a little) easier.

People with type 1 diabetes need to monitor their blood sugar closely when they exercise to make sure they don't overshoot and go into the low-blood-sugar condition called *hypoglycemia.* Those with type 2 diabetes have a little more leeway, but still should be monitoring to see how exercise influences their glucose control.[224]

> "Solid evidence exists that vitamin D deficiency is detrimental to beta cell function, leads to glucose intolerance in animal models and humans, and predisposes to type 2 diabetes.... A major practical conclusion that can be drawn from the studies conducted on vitamin D and diabetes to date is that vitamin D deficiency is undesirable, not only for calcium and bone, but also for glucose metabolism."[227]
>
> —C. Mathieu et al., *Diabetologia,* July 2005

Vitamin D

If you can exercise outside and get at least 5 to 10 minutes of sunshine on your face and hands three or four times a week, you will be doing one more valuable thing to prevent diabetes. For those few minutes, don't use sunscreen, because it can block the formation of the "sunshine vitamin," vitamin D. There is growing evidence that lack of this essential nutrient may predispose people to metabolic syndrome and diabetes.[225] Low levels of vitamin D make it harder for the body to make or secrete insulin.

Vitamin D deficiency is far more common than you would imagine. Experts report that the majority of the elderly lack adequate amounts of vitamin D circulating in their bloodstream.[226] That might be understandable. Older people might not drink much vitamin-D-fortified milk because of digestive issues. They probably spend less time outside, especially in the winter, and when they do go out, they bundle up, exposing very little skin to sunlight. They may also be more careful about putting on sunscreen in the summer to prevent skin cancer. This will block 95 to 98 percent of vitamin D formation in the skin.

What is more surprising is that younger people may also be vitamin D deficient. Researchers recruited physicians, medical students, and hospital visitors at Boston University Medical Center and asked them to give blood during a vitamin D awareness program. The investigators discovered that "36 percent of young adults aged 18 to 29 years had vitamin D deficiency at the end of winter."[228] While we cannot prove that a lack of this nutrient is contributing to the diabetes epidemic, we would be surprised if it weren't part of the story.

There is still no proof that getting adequate amounts of vitamin D will prevent diabetes. Nevertheless, we think making sure you get enough of it makes sense for lots of other reasons (osteoporosis, arthritis, and cancer prevention, to name just three). If you cannot go outside three or four times a week for some sun exposure, consider a supplement.

Breastfeeding Protects Mom

Nursing a baby at the breast used to be the normal way of feeding a child until she got big enough to chew and swallow solid food. That changed in the early 20th century, though, as canned milk and infant formula became readily available. Many new mothers were urged to use the "modern" technology of bottle-feeding. Today, breastfeeding is still less common than formula feeding, even though scientists have discovered that it is better for the baby in many subtle ways. But the latest discovery is that it is also better for the mother, especially if she is at risk of developing type 2 diabetes later in her life.

Investigators affiliated with Harvard studied two large groups of nurses (one cohort had more than 83,000 women in it; the other, 73,000) for more than a decade. The longer a woman breastfed her infant, the less likely she

was to be diagnosed with diabetes later. The benefit didn't really kick in, though, until she had nursed her baby for at least 6 months with no formula feedings.[230] Women who breastfed exclusively for at least a year got the most benefit, a 44 percent drop in the risk for type 2 diabetes. Unfortunately, though, lactation did not protect women who had developed gestational diabetes—high blood sugar during pregnancy. These women need to be treated for diabetes during the pregnancy; though their blood sugar may return to normal after delivery, they are at higher risk of developing type 2 diabetes for the rest of their life.

Type 2 Diabetes

If a doctor suspects that a patient has diabetes, she will probably order a blood test. When fasting plasma glucose is 126 mg/dl or higher, the diagnosis is clear. Another approach is to administer a 2-hour glucose tolerance test. In this test, a person's fasting blood sugar is measured and then he or she is given a sugary drink with a standard dose of glucose. Blood sugar is then measured at intervals over the next 2 hours. If it is 200 mg/dl or higher, the doctor will probably diagnose diabetes.

Diabetes treatment is *not* a do-it-yourself project. Because this condition is so serious, it absolutely requires a close working partnership between patient and physician. But it is too important to leave entirely up to the doctor. For the best control, a person with diabetes should be monitoring blood sugar at home and striving to keep it as close to the target range as possible. A daily glucose diary that can be shared with the doctor will help to optimize the treatment program.

Monitoring Blood Sugar

It is sometimes possible to overcome type 2 diabetes with exercise, diet, and weight loss. To follow your progress, it makes sense to get a home blood sugar monitor and learn to use it on a regular basis. Exactly what is regular will vary from one person to another and is something you and your doctor will need to work out. Some people have a lot of difficulty stabilizing their blood sugar and may need to measure it several times a day, both fasting and 1 to 2 hours after meals. Until blood glucose is brought under control, you should plan on measuring it at least twice a day and possibly more often.[231] When blood sugar is consistently at target levels, you might do fine measuring blood glucose just a few times a week.

There are many different blood sugar monitors on the market; you may want to check *Consumer Reports* for a recommendation. Whenever you measure your blood sugar, be sure to record the time of day and the circumstances as well as the value to help your doctor figure out the best treatment plan and evaluate any medications he may have prescribed.

Your physician will also be taking regular blood tests to assess your glycosylated hemoglobin. Having elevated levels of glucose in the blood eventually affects hemoglobin, an oxygen-carrying molecule. The measure is called HbA_{1c}, and it offers a way to assess blood sugar control over several months. This will give you and your doctor a way to tell how well your regimen is working to keep your blood glucose under control. In people without diabetes, HbA_{1c} runs somewhere between 4 and 6 percent and varies slightly from lab to lab. Your doctor will want you to try to keep your HbA_{1c} under 7 percent.[232] Monitoring your blood sugar at home on a regular basis can help you in this endeavor, and might reduce your risk of serious complications like heart attack and stroke.[233]

Diabetes Triggered by Drugs

When you are first diagnosed, you should discuss with your doctor whether your diabetes might have been triggered by a medicine you take. In some cases, your physician may be able to prescribe a different medication and your blood sugar level may drop. In other cases, there is no acceptable substitute for a lifesaving medication. Treating the resultant diabetes could be considered a fair trade for being alive.

It is not always possible to predict whether a medication will cause hyperglycemia (high blood sugar) in a particular patient. People vary enormously in susceptibility to this effect; some people react strongly to a diuretic, for example, while many others are unaffected. Although a very small proportion of women on oral contraceptives may experience this problem, so many women use them that it may add up to quite a few people.

The following list is not complete, but it offers a snapshot of some of the drugs for which this reaction has been reported. If you

DRUGS THAT MAY RAISE BLOOD SUGAR[234,235]

amiloride + hydrochlorothiazide (Moduretic)

amlodipine + atorvastatin (Caduet)

amphotericin B (AmBisome)

amprenavir (Agenerase)

arsenic trioxide (Trisenox)

asparaginase (Elspar)

atovaquone (Mepron)

basiliximab (Simulect)

benzthiazide (Exna)

betamethasone (Celestone)

bicalutamide (Casodex)

budesonide (Entocort)

bumetanide (Bumex)

busulfan (Busulfex IV)

celecoxib (Celebrex)

chlorthalidone (Clopres, Tenoretic, Thalitone)

ciprofloxacin (Cipro IV)

clozapine (Clozaril)

cyclosporine (Neoral)

dexamethasone (Decadron)

diazoxide (Hyperstat IV)

didanosine (Videx)

doxorubicin (Doxil Injection)

emtricitabine + tenofovir (Truvada)

estradiol (Activella, Alora, Cenestin, Climara, Esclim, Estrace, Estraderm, Femhrt, Premarin, Prempro, Vivelle, etc.)

fentanyl (Actiq)

fludarabine (Fludara injection)

furosemide (Lasix)

gatifloxacin

gemtuzumab (Mylotarg injection)

goserelin (Zoladex)

hydrochlorothiazide

hydrochlorothiazide + losartan (Hyzaar)

hydrochlorothiazide + moexipril (Uniretic)

hydrocortisone (Cortef)

indapamide (Lozol)

interferon alpha-2b (Intron A)

leflunomide (Arava)

leuprolide (Lupron Depot)

levalbuterol (Xopenex Inhalation Solution)

lovastatin + nicotinic acid (Advicor)

megestrol (Megace)

metformin + rosiglitazone (Avandamet)

methylprednisolone (Medrol)

mycophenolate (CellCept)

mycophenolic acid (Myfortic)

nicotinic acid (Niaspan)

nilufamide (Nilandron)

octreotide (Sandostatin)

ofloxacin (Floxin)

olanzapine (Zyprexa)

olmesartan (Benicar)

oral contraceptives with 35 micrograms ethinyl estradiol or more (Brevicon, Demulen 1/35, Enpresse, Modicon, Mononessa, Necon 1/35, Norinyl 1+35, Nortrel 1/35, Ortho-Cyclen, Ortho-Novum 1/35, Ortho Tri-Cyclen, Ovcon 35, Sprintec, Tri-Levlen, Tri-Norinyl, Triphasil, Trivora, Zovia 1/35E, etc.)

pegaspargase (Oncaspar)

pentamidine

prednisolone

prednisone

ritodrine (Yutopar)

rituximab (Rituxin)

rosiglitazone (Avandia)

salmeterol (Serevent Diskus)

saquinavir (Invirase)

sargramostim (Leukine)

sirolimus (Rapamune)

sotalol (Coreg)

tacrolimus (Prograf)

tenofovir (Viread)

terbutaline

testosterone (AndroGel)

tiotropium (Spiriva HandiHaler)

torsemide (Demadex)

triamcinalone

triamterene + hydrochlorothiazide (Dyazide, Maxzide)

valganciclovir (Valcyte)

take one of them, *do not stop* the medication on your own. Discuss your concerns with your physician. You may also discover, as some people have reported to us, that medications not on the list, such as the cholesterol-lowering drug Lipitor (atorvastatin) and some other statins, may occasionally raise blood sugar.

Diet Does Count

Your doctor will surely urge you to watch your diet. Here again, we suggest you check out Dr. Richard K. Bernstein's suggestions. In addition to *The Diabetes Diet, Dr. Bernstein's Diabetes Solution* goes beyond diet to total diabetes management, and his suggestions are worth consideration. Our earlier recommendations on diet for preventing diabetes mostly hold for people who already have diabetes as well, with two big exceptions. Once a person has actually developed diabetes, chocolate and coffee may destabilize blood sugar too much in the short term and in many cases should be avoided.

Cinnamon

There are some other unexpected items you might want to include in your diet, though. One is cinnamon. Surprising as it seems, ¼ to ½ teaspoon of cinnamon from the spice rack added to food or a beverage can help lower blood sugar if the rest of the diet is sensible. Cinnamon appears to increase insulin sensitivity.[236] Giving a cinnamon extract to diabetic mice lowered blood sugar, raised HDL cholesterol, and reduced triglycerides.[237]

The benefit appears to be primarily from

★★★★ Cinnamon

Cinnamon can help stabilize blood sugar, and may help control cholesterol and triglycerides. Effects are mild, so cinnamon should not be substituted for medical treatment.

Downside: Heartburn; possible liver damage from coumarin contamination
Cost: $30 to $40 a month for Cinnulin

cassia cinnamon (*Cinnamomum cassia*).[238] Although this is the common cinnamon from the spice rack, some grocery store cinnamon contains a compound called coumarin. With regular use, coumarin could be toxic to the liver. It may also interact with anticoagulants such as warfarin (Coumadin).

People who use cinnamon regularly should be monitored for any potential toxicity. Richard A. Anderson, PhD, one of the scientists doing research on cinnamon, says a water-based extract is effective and safer than plain cinnamon. People can take cinnamon capsules such as Cinnulin PF, or they can put cinnamon in a coffee filter and pour hot water over it to create their own water extract.

The Value of Vinegar

Another dietary addition that is worth consideration is vinegar. This old remedy has been floating around for decades, if not centuries. But if you were to ask most registered dietitians whether vinegar is helpful for diabetics, you would probably get a blank stare. Surprisingly, there is now good science to support the value of vinegar. Researchers in Sweden report that when vinegar is given with white bread, it reduces blood sugar and insulin levels.[239] It also helps people feel fuller up to 2 hours later.

Japanese researchers have found that vinegar can counteract the effect of white rice on blood sugar.[240] And investigators at Arizona State University report that 2 tablespoons of vinegar or a handful of peanuts before a starchy meal can significantly dampen the resulting rise in blood glucose.[241] Pickles may be the most palatable way to consume vinegar; drinking it, even mixed with water, may be difficult for some people.

> **"I suffer with type 2 diabetes. My doctor prescribed Glucotrol for my blood sugar. It helped to a degree, but I have found that by adding apple cider vinegar and cinnamon to a careful diet, I can control my blood sugar even better."**

Oolong Tea

Consider sipping oolong tea with your meal. This type of tea is made from a partially fermented leaf, midway between green tea and black tea. Research from Taiwan indicates that drinking oolong tea (1,500 milliliters per day, or around 6 cups) significantly lowered both blood glucose and fructosamine, a longer-term measure of blood sugar control.[242] (Blood glucose measures sugar in the blood

right now; fructosamine indicates how much sugar has been in the blood over the past 2 or 3 weeks; HbA_{1c} is a signal of blood sugar over the previous 6 weeks or more.) Oolong tea can be an acquired taste, but it's definitely worth a try. It can't hurt, and it might help.

Herbs and Supplements

A huge array of botanical medicines and dietary supplements is offered to diabetics. Although several natural products can help control blood sugar, none is a substitute for a diet designed to keep blood sugar under control. If you decide to try an herb or supplement to help with blood glucose control, be sure to inform your physician and get approval. Monitor your blood sugar carefully and keep good records. That way, you will be able to work with your doctor to adjust the dose of your medicine, if necessary, and you will be able to look back over your notes to evaluate if what you were taking lowered your HbA_{1c}. Because the quality of herbal products and dietary supplements varies widely in this country, keeping close track of how well you do may help you find a more effective or more consistent formulation.

CHINESE HERBAL FORMULAS

There are a number of Chinese herbs that are traditionally prescribed in complex formulas. Several herbs are included to help potentiate and balance the main ingredient or ingredients. An objective analysis of available research evidence by the Cochrane Library found that several of these have been reported to lower blood sugar in controlled trials, but that the quality of the studies is fairly questionable overall.[243] The reviewers suggest that herbal medicines such as holy basil or Bushen Jiang-tang Tang merit further study. We can't dis-agree. Any diabetic who chooses to try traditional Chinese herbs needs two doctors, though: one skilled in traditional Chinese medicine and the other up-to-date on endo-crinology, especially diabetes treatment. It might be challenging to organize their close collaboration, but it is essential.

BITTER MELON

Bitter melon, or *Momordica charantia,* is a plant in the cucumber/squash family that is used as a vegetable as well as a medicine in much of China.[244] It does not increase insulin produc-tion, but it seems to improve sugar uptake by the cells. Bitter melon has been reported to lower fasting blood sugar.[245] It may be helpful not as a substitute for standard diabetes medicines, but in addition to them. Careful blood sugar moni-toring is necessary. Children and pregnant women should not take this herb, because it may be dangerous to them. Some children have died after eating the bright red seed coverings.

> *A family friend told us that bitter melon could help reduce blood sugar. We went to our local health food store and bought a bottle, and it seems to work! My husband takes metformin and glyburide for diabetes. After he added this supplement, his blood sugar level was down considerably.*

CHROMIUM

Chromium is an essential nutrient that is needed in minute quantities. It plays a role in glucose utilization and increases insulin sensi-tivity in tissue culture studies. Chromium pic-olinate, which is often found in supplements, is relatively well absorbed.[246] Questions remain, however, regarding its safety.

Some studies suggest that chromium pico-linate supplements (200 micrograms per day) may improve glucose tolerance in type 2 dia-betics.[247,248] Not all studies have been conclu-sive, however. Like the other supplements, chromium is better as an addition to rather than a substitute for exercise, diet, and medi-cation to control blood sugar. Careful blood sugar monitoring and medical supervision are advised.

FENUGREEK

Fenugreek is a seed used to spice Indian food. It has also been used in traditional medicine to treat symptoms that indicate diabetes. Stud-ies done in humans suggest that it can be used in type 1 as well as type 2 diabetes in addition to prescribed medication. The powdered seed lowered blood sugar and HbA_{1c}.[249]

There are potential side effects, however. Fenugreek can cause diarrhea, flatulence, and allergic reactions. It might, in theory, interact with warfarin (Coumadin) or other anticoagu-lant medicines and probably should be avoided by people who take them. There is always a possibility of hypoglycemia when blood sugar–lowering botanical medicines are added to prescription drugs for blood sugar control, so careful monitoring is essential. The usual dose is around 1 or 2 grams of seeds three times a day, but it may also be taken as a tea.[250]

• • •

Q. *I found a spice in my spice rack that I had never heard of, and I had no instructions on how to use it. I looked up fenugreek as a spice and found that it is a medicinal herb.*

It is used to lower cholesterol and control blood sugar. The only side effect I found is nausea if you take too much. What do you know about this herb?

A. Studies in animals and humans show that fenugreek can lower cholesterol and blood sugar. If diabetics take fenugreek, they should monitor their blood sugar to make sure it doesn't fall too much.

Fenugreek seeds are rich in soluble fiber and can be used to treat constipation. At high doses, this herb can cause digestive distress.

• • •

GYMNEMA SYLVESTRE

This herb comes from India and has been used in traditional Ayurvedic medicine for centuries. Animal studies have demonstrated that it is capable of lowering blood sugar.[251] No serious side effects have been reported, but perhaps the scarcity of well-controlled clinical trials explains that to some extent.

NOPAL *(Opuntia sp.)*

One interesting botanical treatment has only a little bit of research to support it, but it is becoming increasingly popular. We heard several years ago from a physician who said one of his diabetic patients had improved his blood sugar control with prickly pear tea. This cactus, called nopal in Mexico, has been studied primarily in animals. That research indicates that the cactus can help lower blood sugar.[252, 253] Research in humans is preliminary, but it suggests that nopal may also be useful in helping to control blood sugar in type 2 diabetes.[254] Close monitoring and medical supervision are advised.

" *I am a family practitioner and want to share an herbal remedy with you. A 60-year-old male Hispanic diabetic patient has had trouble controlling his blood sugar. Despite intensive diet changes and a prescription for Glucovance, his blood sugar still ran around 160 to 180-plus.*

One day he came in with his diary showing consistent blood sugars of 90 to 100. I asked what he was doing differently and he said in a low voice, "I've got a new girlfriend from Mexico. She makes me tea from nopalito [prickly pear] cactus and has me drink it three times a day. Now my sugars are doing better." "

Finding fresh nopal cactus outside of Mexico or the desert of the southwestern United States could be tricky. When we shared the story about nopalito tea (*nopalito* is a young stem segment from the cactus), we were inundated with questions from readers who wanted to know how they could get some nopal cactus leaves. Short of moving, you might try looking for this natural plant product in your local health-food store (or on the Web). Although it is unlikely you will find fresh leaves, you will be able to locate capsules labeled *prickly pear cactus (*Opuntia*)* or *nopal cactus.*

Careful blood sugar monitoring is essential. One reader who blended cactus with apple juice kept careful track of his cholesterol levels, triglycerides, and glucose. In 6 months, his triglycerides dropped from 191 to 139 and his total cholesterol went from 202 to 169. More interesting, his blood glucose drifted down as well. Here is his account:

" I read your article about nopalito tea, so I started using cactus in April and had good results. My doctor knows about it. I blend one bag of cactus and 3 ½ cups of apple juice into a drinkable liquid. I drink 4 ounces three times a day. Here are my results:

Blood Glucose (average)

Jan	147	no cactus
Feb	143	no cactus
Mar	158	no cactus
Apr	142	with cactus
May	132	with cactus
Jun	126	with cactus
Jul	135	with cactus
Aug	128	with cactus

I write down every food I eat every day and take my test every morning and keep a record of it. I can see which food does what, and I take my medicine as always and my doctor has been kept informed. "

This gentleman is the poster child for responsible blood sugar control. Not only is he tracking his sugar levels carefully, he is also working closely with his physician to make sure what he does is safe and effective.

STEVIA

Stevia (*Stevia rebaudiana*) is a nonsugar sweetener derived from the leaves of a South American shrub. It is not approved as a sugar substitute in the United States but is frequently used in Japan. Some preliminary research suggests that using stevia instead of sugar might have a benefit beyond simply not consuming sugar. A small study in Brazil found that stevia tea could improve glucose tolerance in nondi-

---

★★★ Stevia

Stevia is a natural sugar substitute. In addition to sweetening food and drinks without raising blood sugar, stevia may be capable of improving glucose tolerance. Be sure to monitor your blood sugar when adding this sweetener to a medication regimen.

Downside: In laboratory tests, high doses of stevia interfered with animals' reproduction.
Cost: Approximately 1¢ or 2¢ per serving

abetic individuals.[255] The plant can also lower blood pressure. No significant toxicity has been reported.

Easing Stress

There is a direct connection between your level of stress and your blood sugar. For someone without diabetes, this is probably no big deal, unless you are always under stress. But for a diabetic, anxiety, fear, depression, and emotional pressure will boost blood sugar and make the condition harder to control.[256, 257] Giving a speech, having a fight with your partner, or going in for your annual performance review at work can all affect your stress level and your blood sugar. Doctors often look at diet, exercise, and other physical factors. They are less likely to consider emotions, even though they have such a profound impact on a diabetic's health.

How can a diabetic learn how to manage stress successfully? There is no cookie-cutter answer to this question. Everyone handles stress differently. For some, the only effective strategy might be to quit a highly demanding job and move to a cave. Doing that would stress others out even more. Finding the right approach may take trial and error.

Avoiding people who make your hands cold is a good place to start. Buy a mood ring (a relic of the 1970s). It reacts to skin temperature. Whenever your hands get cold as a response to stress, you should do something different from your current activity to warm them up. Relaxation tapes can be helpful if

you can carve out time to listen. Our favorites are by Emmett Miller, MD. Dr. Miller has been in this business a long time and has a soothing voice. We guarantee that if you listen to his *Letting Go of Stress*, you will be more relaxed afterward.

Some people may benefit from individual psychological counseling or biofeedback training to learn to cope with stress. But others may be able to find a group that is learning stress management techniques.[258] If you need a guide to doing it yourself, we suggest you look for a copy of Richard Surwit's book, *The Mind-Body Diabetes Revolution*. It has some good tips on learning to relax and overcome stress as well as background on the importance of psychological issues in diabetes.

When all else fails, an antianxiety agent can be surprisingly effective at controlling blood sugar in the short term. If, for example, you know that traveling makes you anxious and throws your blood sugar out of kilter, you may want to ask your doctor whether a short course of diazepam (Valium), alprazolam (Xanax), or some similar medicine might help you deal with the hassle of travel.[259] Such drugs can be habit-forming, however, so relying on them for long periods of time is not desirable.

Depression also has a major impact on diabetes and messes up efforts to keep blood sugar where it should be. Everything feels much harder to manage when you're down in the dumps, and your attention to exercise, diet, medication, and self-care may well suffer. Changes in brain biochemistry associated with depression might also contribute directly to a higher risk of diabetes complications.[260] Blood clots leading to heart attacks or strokes are more likely when diabetics are depressed; so are irregular heart rhythms and inflammation. It's just as crucial for a diabetic to be evaluated regularly for depression, and to get treatment when it is needed, as it is for her to get regular eye exams and foot care.

Pills to Lower Blood Sugar

Quite often, diet and exercise alone are not enough to control blood sugar. There is a bewildering array of medicine the doctor may prescribe: metformin, which also is dispensed under the brand name Glucophage; medicine with "glitazone" in the generic name, like pioglitazone (Actos); and old-fashioned blood sugar–lowering drugs similar to chlorpropamide or tolazamide, or their newer cousins glyburide (Micronase), glimepiride (Amaryl), or glipizide (Glucotrol). Newer drugs that stimulate insulin secretion, called nateglinide (Starlix) and repaglinide (Prandin), might be used instead of one of the older blood sugar–lowering drugs. Eventually, if blood sugar and

glycosylated hemoglobin can't be brought down to acceptable levels, even type 2 diabetics may end up using insulin. But it usually makes sense to try oral medicines first.

It is difficult to tell which of these pills would work best for any given patient. As with everything else pertaining to diabetes, people vary in their responses. Some do well on a single drug, while others need a complicated regimen. Only you and your doctor can determine which medication(s) are likely to be safest and most effective for you.

To try to sort out the patterns and give doctors some guidance, scientists at Kaiser Permanente, an enormous HMO in northern California, reviewed the organization's vast database. First they created a registry of the diabetic patients, and then they examined the data to see which drugs were most effective over time. Even though most patients are started on one of the medicines like chlorpropamide or glyburide, this was the least effective treatment for getting HbA_{1c} down to target.[261] The most effective treatment was triple therapy: a "glitazone"-type drug in combination with metformin and a drug like glyburide. Next best after that was metformin together with insulin.

One of the most interesting features of the Kaiser Permanente study was that patient behavior could be used to predict success, aside from the drug used. Patients who monitored their blood sugar frequently and those who kept all or nearly all of their appointments were significantly more likely to get their blood sugar under control and keep it there.[262] Making sure that you are on top of your diabetes treatment, taking your medication, monitoring your blood sugar, keeping track of HbA_{1c}, following a sensible diet and exercise regimen, and controlling your weight as much as possible may be nearly as important as which drugs your doctor prescribes.

Metformin (Glucophage)

A review by the Cochrane Collaboration of most of the world's diabetes literature shows that metformin (Glucophage) alone, if used to keep blood glucose under tight control, is an excellent treatment.[263] Metformin improves blood sugar control by improving the cells' response to insulin and reducing the amount of sugar that the liver makes. Unlike some other oral diabetes drugs, it doesn't lead to weight gain and may even help people get their weight under control.

It can be dangerous, however, for people with kidney disease. They should not take the drug, and everyone on metformin should have their kidney function monitored regularly (at least once a year). People with congestive heart failure should not take metformin, either.

Metformin has two nasty side effects that patients must know about. One, lactic acidosis, is rare, but it is a medical emergency if it occurs. Lactic acidosis can be lethal. People with kidney disease or congestive heart failure are more susceptible to this problem, which is why they must not take metformin. Otherwise healthy diabetics might also develop lactic acidosis

---

> ## SYMPTOMS OF LACTIC ACIDOSIS
>
> - Muscle aches or weakness
> - Shortness of breath
> - Stomachache, nausea, or vomiting
> - Lethargy or drowsiness
> - Irregular heartbeat
> - Feeling generally awful

---

on metformin, especially if they drink alcohol.

What makes metformin so tricky is that patients frequently experience digestive tract distress when they first start taking this medicine. Side effects can include diarrhea, nausea, vomiting, indigestion, and stomachache. After several weeks, however, these side effects should fade away. If digestive symptoms recur, they must be brought to the doctor's attention immediately since they might be symptoms of lactic acidosis.

The other side effect is depletion of vitamin B_{12}. Because this vitamin is stored in the body, the depletion is gradual and the symptoms either may not be noticed or may be attributed to some other cause. The physician should test for methylmalonic acid (MMA) as well as for vitamin B_{12} levels. Fortunately, it is easy to treat vitamin B_{12} deficiency with supplements. The vitamin does not need to be injected in such cases; oral supplements of around 1 milligram daily (a large dose of vitamin B_{12}) will work. Do check with your doctor to find out if this is appropriate for you.

> *I am a retired physician with type 2 diabetes. Metformin has kept my blood sugar in the normal range for 10 years. Despite good control of my blood glucose and glycosylated hemoglobin, my foot numbness was getting worse. I was also a little unsteady on my feet, though it was very subtle.*
>
> *I reviewed the medical literature and discovered that metformin interferes with vitamin B_{12} absorption. I suspected I might be deficient in this vitamin, and I started taking oral vitamin B_{12}.*
>
> *Within a week, I noticed that my mental capacity was sharper. I had not realized before this that I was having any cognitive problems. I stopped having any trouble walking, and my foot numbness has decreased.*
>
> *Many older diabetics take metformin. If they developed subtle neurological and mental deficits as a result of lack of vitamin B_{12}, these problems could be treated but may well be overlooked.*

Pioglitazone (Actos)

Pioglitazone (Actos) is a newer diabetes medicine that increases insulin sensitivity and decreases insulin resistance. These actions reduce the amount of insulin in the bloodstream and should lower HbA_{1c}. Not only can this medication bring fasting blood sugar down, it can also help control blood sugar levels after meals.[264] In the Kaiser Permanente study mentioned above, drugs in this class were the medications most likely to get HbA_{1c} down to normal range by themselves.

Actos has received a lot of attention from doctors who specialize in treating diabetes because it has a favorable impact on some blood lipids. It doesn't seem to do much for bad LDL cholesterol, but it raises good HDL cholesterol (no mean feat) and lowers triglycerides.[265]

No one knows if these improvements in blood fats will result in a lower risk of heart attack or other cardiovascular complications in the long run. That, after all, is the really important issue, since diabetics are at such high risk of cardiovascular catastrophes. But Actos is fairly effective in preventing the closing up of a cardiac stent after it is put into a coronary artery.[266] And a head-to-head study of Actos and Avandia (a similar medication)

★★★ Metformin (Glucophage)

Metformin improves insulin sensitivity. It may control blood sugar alone or be combined with other diabetes drugs to improve blood sugar control. Common side effects include diarrhea, nausea and vomiting, flatulence, fatigue, indigestion, and headache.

Avoid guar gum in low-fat foods (salad dressing, frozen desserts, etc.), because it reduces metformin's absorption and effectiveness.

Downside: Lactic acidosis, a rare reaction, requires emergency medical attention and can be fatal.

Cost: Approximately $90 to $120 per month; generic $65 to $100

---

showed that Actos has a better effect on several measures of cholesterol and blood lipids.[267] If this translates down the road into reducing the likelihood of a heart attack or stroke, it would certainly be worthwhile.

Pioglitazone can cause fluid retention and as a result is not appropriate for use by patients with congestive heart failure. Side effects include a greater susceptibility to sore throats, colds, bronchitis, and the like; headaches; toothaches; sinusitis; and muscle pain. A competing drug, rosiglitazone (Avandia, Avandamet), has also been linked to fluid retention. More worrisome, though, is the possibility that this drug may contribute to fluid accumulation in the back of the eye. This macular edema could lead to blurred vision and eye damage.

Repaglinide (Prandin)

The goal of treating diabetes is to keep blood sugar within the normal range, because that reduces the likelihood of serious complications. If you can't achieve this with metformin or one of the "glitazones," the doctor may add

---

★★★★ Pioglitazone (Actos)

Pioglitazone improves insulin sensitivity and decreases insulin resistance. It lowers triglycerides and raises HDL, which might result in a lower risk of cardiovascular problems. It is taken once a day.

Downside: May interact with oral contraceptives to make them less effective

Cost: Approximately $100 to $115 per month

---

a medicine to stimulate the secretion of insulin. Two drugs, nateglinide (Starlix) and repaglinide (Prandin), make beta cells in the pancreas pump out more insulin at mealtime.[268] This helps keep blood glucose levels from going too high after eating.

Some studies have compared these two medicines alone or in various combinations. The results aren't definitive, but comparing nateglinide alone to repaglinide alone suggests that there is an advantage to repaglinide.[269] Prandin lowered HbA_{1c} significantly more than Starlix did; it brought down fasting blood sugar better; and more than half (54 percent) of the patients on Prandin were able to get their HbA_{1c} below 7 percent, whereas fewer than half (42 percent) of those on Starlix managed that. Of course, there's a price. Patients on Prandin were more likely to suffer from hypoglycemia (low blood sugar). They also gained more weight (almost 4 pounds in 4 months), a discouraging side effect.

These drugs are more effective in combination with metformin than they are on their own.[270, 271, 272] Side effects of repaglinide include headache, joint or back pain, and upper respiratory infection. Drugs such as ketoconazole (Nizoral) and clarithromycin (Biaxin) boost blood levels of repaglinide, and that could increase the likelihood of unpleasant reactions. Grapefruit affects the same enzyme (CYP3A4) and might have a similar effect.

Exenatide (Byetta)

Exenatide (Byetta) is another treatment option for type 2 diabetics. It has an interesting his-

Repaglinide lowers blood sugar by stimulating insulin release and is especially effective for reducing blood sugar following a meal. Repaglinide is taken before meals, usually within 15 minutes before beginning to eat.

Downside: Blood sugar may fall too much (hypoglycemia). Repaglinide may contribute to weight gain.

Cost: Approximately $130 to $140 per month

tory, because it got started with research into the saliva of a poisonous Southwestern lizard called a Gila monster. Byetta is injected and is used in combination with metformin or a blood sugar–lowering drug like glyburide. Byetta reduces the bump in blood sugar after meals and can help diabetics lose weight.

The most common side effect is nausea, but the most serious is hypoglycemia. Adding Byetta to a medicine like glyburide increases the risk of a dangerous drop in blood glucose level. Patients using Byetta must learn what to do if blood sugar drops too low. Other side effects include vomiting, diarrhea, dizziness, jitters, headache, and indigestion. Byetta should not be given to people with kidney problems or serious digestive disease.[273]

Conclusions

By now, we hope you appreciate the importance of controlling blood sugar. Diabetes is common (some diabetologists believe it will soon affect nearly half the population), and its complications are devastating. We have tried to give you a variety of strategies to prevent or control this disease. Remember, though, that whatever tactics you adopt, you must work in close collaboration with your health-care providers.

Below you will find an overview of our recommendations in this chapter.

• Preventing diabetes is possible. Keep your weight under control, emphasize nonstarchy vegetables over pasta or bread, and avoid soft drinks, fruit juice, and processed meats.

• Get plenty of exercise, preferably including some time outdoors so you have 10 to 15 minutes of sunshine on your face and hands several days a week. If you don't get outside, take 800 to 1,200 IU of vitamin D_3 daily.

• If you are diagnosed with diabetes, learn to monitor your blood sugar. Keep track of how exercise and food affect it. Consider cinnamon or vinegar to help smooth out blood sugar in reaction to a carbohydrate meal.

• If you're considering using herbs or dietary supplements such as chromium, bitter melon, fenugreek, *Gymnema sylvestre*, or nopal, check with your health-care providers before taking them. Monitor your blood sugar carefully.

• If medication becomes necessary, make sure that you and your physician find the safest and most effective option for you. You shouldn't have to suffer with dreadful side effects to keep your blood sugar under control.

ECZEMA

• Apply moisturizer immediately after washing skin.	★★★
• Take probiotic supplements such as viable *Lactobacillus GG*	★★★
• Try hemp seed oil capsules	★★
• Season your food with salsa	★★
• Sip oolong tea	★★★
• Take vitamin E capsules daily	★★★
• Smear Noxzema (original) on itchy skin	★★★★
• Try nonprescription hydrocortisone cream	★★★
• Apply CamoCare Soothing Cream to itchy areas	★★★
• Follow doctor's instructions for using prescription steroid creams	★★★★
• Consider prescription Atopiclair	★★★
• Ask the doctor about Protopic or Elidel as a second-line prescription treatment	★★

Eczema is one of those old-fashioned words, like *apoplexy*, that sounds as though it should have become obsolete. Unfortunately, the condition it describes is still very much in evidence, now perhaps more than ever. Dermatologists estimate that the red itchy rash of chronic eczema may affect as much as 20 percent of the population in Scandinavia, Australia, and England.[274] The United States has similar figures, compared to only about 2 percent of the population in places like Iran and China.

Scientists don't know why the rate of eczema varies so widely from one place to another. A lot of other things are still pretty mysterious about eczema, too. The researchers who study it have not come up with a single unified measure of eczema severity, so it is sometimes difficult to compare studies. In fact, when dermatologists discuss eczema, they frequently use the term *atopic dermatitis* instead. It means

the same thing: a nasty, itchy rash, especially in places where the skin creases (like inside the elbows and on the backs of the knees). It may be associated with dry skin, redness, and irritation on the cheeks or forehead, as well as asthma or hay fever.

Very young kids with eczema may have family members with asthma or hay fever. Atopic dermatitis is pretty common in children and may start early, at as young as 2 or 3 months of age.[275] If it is severe, the itching can drive the sufferer crazy and even keep him or her awake at night. It is no wonder patients and their parents are anxious to get relief.

Skin Care Basics

There is a huge overlap between eczema and dry skin, so it makes sense that the very first things to try for eczema are recognized as elementary care for dry skin.

Especially in adults, eczema frequently affects the hands. Avoid soaking your hands in water. If they are dirty, by all means wash them. But if you need to do the dishes or wipe off the counters, wear waterproof gloves. Likewise, if you are working out in the yard, wear garden gloves. Apply a moisturizer you like as soon as you finish washing your hands. (We're fond of Udder Cream.) You might even consider applying a heavy-duty ointment-type moisturizer at night and wearing cotton gloves to bed, so the sheets are protected and the ointment really gets a chance to sink in.

What about rashes that affect other parts of the body? Basically, follow the same principles. Bathing or showering are okay, but shouldn't be prolonged. Don't use soap or detergent, if you can avoid it; instead, use a gentle, nonsoap cleanser such as CeraVe or Cetaphil. Gently pat your skin dry and apply moisturizer as soon as you step out of the tub or shower stall.[277]

Moisturizers don't actually make eczema better by themselves.[278] What they do is improve the symptoms of dry skin, so the skin looks better and itches less. In addition, a topical medication may work better on skin that is properly moisturized. So, there are reasons to start with a moisturizer, although it's unlikely to be enough of a treatment on its own.

Dietary Approaches

The connection between eczema and other allergies has inspired people to search for the source of the allergies and try to avoid them. Avoiding one of the most common allergens, dust mites, is very difficult. Dust mites live in bedding, furniture, carpets, and even stuffed animals. As it happens, though, even extreme measures such as encasing the mattress in plastic don't reduce eczema in adults.[279] We don't have good research on whether this would help in babies or young children.

Dietary recommendations are aimed at reducing a child's exposure to foods that could be triggering eczema. One trap that parents sometimes fall into is restricting the diet too much, so that the child isn't getting enough nutrients. Scientists say that most of the time, dietary restriction isn't very helpful for improving eczema. If a child reacts to eggs, though, avoiding them is likely to help clear up the

★★★ CeraVe Cleanser and Moisturizer

These skin products contain no fragrances, soap, or detergent. The cleanser is an emulsified formulation that contains cetearyl alcohol, one of the primary ingredients in Cetaphil cleanser. But both the moisturizer and the cleanser also contain ceramides. (So does Dove Facial Lotion.) Skin with eczema is depleted of ceramides,[276] and the CeraVe products are supposed to restore these natural skin fats and keep skin from drying out.

Downside: No real downside, but other products may be less expensive.

Cost: A 12-ounce bottle runs about $12 and should last several months.

skin.[280] Switching a baby from cows'-milk formula to soy-based formula is often advised and occasionally helpful.

Luckily, kids often "outgrow" their food allergies as they get older. The big exception is peanuts. Children who are allergic to peanuts need to avoid them scrupulously, and will probably need to do so indefinitely.

> **"** *I've had eczema since childhood, and it had been getting worse, despite applying steroids three times daily. I had read advice about cutting back on trans fats and adding omega-3 fats but I had no success until I tried completely eliminating trans fats. Since getting hydrogenated oils out of my diet, my eczema has nearly disappeared and I have discontinued the steroids for the first time in 3 years. The trans fats that apparently caused this problem were coming from one or two servings of packaged cookies per day.* **"**

Probiotics

Most Americans are familiar with the idea of using antibiotics to kill germs when there is an infection. But probiotics are not nearly as popular in the United States as they are elsewhere in the world, especially in Europe. Probiotics are beneficial bacteria that are used in an attempt to colonize the gut with "good guys" and crowd out dangerous bacteria.

There is evidence that babies with eczema may benefit from treatment with probiotics, particularly if they have evidence of allergic-type immune-system activation. Doctors determine this by measuring the amount of an immune globulin, IgE, in the blood. It is usually elevated in people who are experiencing an allergic reaction. Adding probiotics such as *Lactobacillus fermentum* or *Lactobacillus GG* to formula helped ease the condition in very young children with severe eczema.[281,282,283]

We don't know why probiotics can make eczema better, but some researchers speculate that they may cause a low level of inflammation that stimulates the immune system in a different direction from allergy.[284] More research is needed before that hypothesis can be confirmed—or tossed out. For adults, many probiotics are considered relatively safe,[285] although there are some theoretical risks whenever living microbes are introduced into the body.[286] For very young children, it would be sensible to follow the pediatrician's recommendation.

★★★ Probiotics

Beneficial bacteria such as *Lactobacillus GG*, *Lactobacillus reuteri*, or *Lactobacillus fermentum* seem to reduce the severity and extent of eczema in young children. This approach is reasonably safe[287] and might be worth a try.

Downside: Probiotic products are sold as dietary supplements, so the quality is not regulated. Check www.consumerlab.com for quality evaluation and price information. It is important that the supplement contain viable organisms.[288]

Cost: Approximately $10 to $30 per month

Oil Supplements

We already mentioned that the connection between eczema and diet has led to research investigating various dietary restrictions. For the most part, a really restricted diet just makes life more difficult without any payoff for the skin. (One big exception is in the case of celiac disease. This intolerance of gluten can cause a distinctive skin reaction—herpetiform dermatitis—along with a wide range of other symptoms. For a person with celiac disease, avoiding gluten completely not only clears up the skin, but also has many additional health benefits.)

We have heard from many eczema sufferers who have found that various supplements have helped to clear up their rash, at least for a while. Borage oil and black currant seed oil are among the most popular supplements. They supply fatty acids, especially gamma-linolenic acid, that may be underrepresented in the typical American diet.

I have been plagued with persistent eczema. The skin on my hands was always red, itchy, cracked, and often bleeding. My hands were always covered with bandages.

Dermatologists prescribed cortisone creams of increasing strength, but none was helpful over the long-term. An allergist I saw for an unrelated problem was concerned that the open wounds on my hands put me at risk of infection. He suggested borage oil.

I tried it (one capsule after breakfast and one before bed), and within a few months the eczema on my hands disappeared completely. While I still have some outbreaks behind my ears, the condition is now only a minor annoyance. What a difference!

Although some individuals have found gamma-linolenic sources such as borage oil, evening primrose oil, and black currant seed oil helpful, scientifically controlled studies of these supplements are disappointing.[289] They do seem to be safe, but overall they don't reduce the rash or itching any more than placebo capsules do.[290]

One possible exception is hemp seed oil. It contains omega-3 as well as omega-6 fatty acids, including gamma-linolenic acid. One placebo-controlled study found that hemp seed oil capsules reduced itchiness and dryness in skin. (The placebo capsules contained olive oil.) Patients on the active supplement used less topical medicine for their dermatitis during the 5 months the trial lasted.[291] We

---

★★ Hemp Seed Oil

Hemp seed offers a balance of omega-6 and omega-3 fatty acids. One study demonstrated that it reduces eczema symptoms significantly more than olive oil does.

Downside: A single study is not enough for a full evaluation of the supplement's benefit. Another, larger study might not show a significant effect.

Cost: Approximately $5 to $15 per month

---

hope other dermatologists will continue to study this treatment to see if it stands up to further investigation.

Low-Carb Diet

One of the most unusual testimonials we have received about controlling eczema with diet was from a woman who adopted a low-glycemic-index diet for other reasons. She found that it helped clear up her itchy rash. Cutting sugar, white bread, and pasta out of the diet may well have other health benefits. Most dietary experts agree that these foods are not very nutrient-dense. Your body won't miss them, even if your taste buds do.

● ● ●

Q. *I used to get urinary tract infections or yeast infections every other month. Then I changed my diet and cut out sugar, white flour, and starches like potatoes or rice. Since then I have had only one urinary tract infection.*

I've lost 20 pounds and my eczema is 99 percent better. I have a flare-up only when I eat cake or milk chocolate.

I was surprised that diet could have such an effect on my system. Other people with eczema or seborrheic dermatitis might benefit the way I did.

A. There is next to no research linking a high-carbohydrate diet to urinary tract infections or eczema. On the other hand, reducing the amount of sugar, starch, and refined carbohydrates seems like a simple enough experiment. If it works for some people with such hard-to-treat conditions, it might be worth the trouble. Thanks for sharing your interesting story.

● ● ●

This approach has not been well studied, to say the least. German researchers have investigated a sugar-free diet in 29 patients.[292] After 1 week of a strict sugar-free diet, they were given a food that contained either sugar or an artificial sweetener. There was no discernable difference between the reaction to sugar and the reaction to an artificial sweetener.

You may feel that this study was small and perhaps didn't give the diet enough of a chance. If so, go ahead and conduct your own personal study. It won't have scientific significance for anyone else, but if it helps your skin, that's all you really need to know.

Hot Salsa

Believe it or not, some people have done their own experiments on one dietary staple. After one person reported that his increased consumption of salsa had been correlated with a decrease in the severity of his lifelong psoriasis, other people decided to try salsa or hot chili peppers for eczema. At least a few of them have found capsaicin consumption helpful. (Capsaicin is the compound in chili peppers that makes them hot. We have no idea if eating it has any role in making eczema better.)

> *I read your column about eating salsa for a skin condition. I tried it and it worked for me. For over a year I've been free of the eczema I had for 8 years before that. I ate salsa daily for about a month.*

Capsaicin is an ingredient in some topical liniments or rubs designed to alleviate arthritis pain. Usually, there is a warning for such products not to apply them to broken skin. For one thing, capsaicin on a cut or sore would hurt horribly. There is also no evidence that capsaicin cream would be effective for eczema. A review of the evidence in veterinary medicine concluded that more studies are needed to see if topical capsaicin works for dogs with itchy spots.[293] If more data are needed for dogs, you can well imagine how much more evidence is needed for humans!

★★ Salsa

The People's Pharmacy has received a number of testimonials claiming that eating salsa eased eczema. No clinical trials have been conducted as far as we know.

Side effect: Sore mouth
Downside: Not everyone likes salsa.
Cost: $6 to $10 a month

Oolong Tea

If you think that salsa is on the strange side, you might be nonplussed by oolong tea. It has one major advantage over salsa, though: A study of people with atopic dermatitis showed that it helped to reduce their symptoms.[294] People with severe eczema that had not responded well to standard treatments were given tea bags and told to make and drink a liter (about a quart) of oolong tea daily. Their symptoms were recorded. Although there wasn't any placebo tea, researchers and almost two-thirds of the patients noticed an improvement within a couple of weeks. The improvement, which lasted for the entire 6 months of the study, might have been due to the anti-allergy activity of the polyphenol compounds in oolong tea.

• • •

Q. *Thank you for your advice to try oolong tea for eczema. It's been like a miracle.*

I've had eczema on my scalp for most of my life. I would have terrible itching and scaling on my scalp that would usually bleed and scab over. It's worse around the hairline and is embarrassing as well as painful.

I had tried everything my doctor prescribed: Nizoral, Elidel, topical steroids in oils and shampoos, and even an injection. Nothing worked until the tea. I've been drinking it for about 2 weeks now and I'd say there's been at least an 85 percent improvement.

A. You aren't the only reader to find oolong tea helpful. One person with hard-to-treat eczema reported: "The last time I had an outbreak, I tried oolong tea and the results were amazing. Within 24 hours, the itching and inflammation were gone. It took a couple of days, but the lesions disappeared and didn't leave scars."

• • •

Oolong tea is available in many grocery stores, although black tea and green tea are better known in the United States. All three teas are made from the same plant, but the leaves are processed differently. Green tea leaves are processed very little; black tea

★★★ Oolong Tea

Oolong tea is a popular beverage in China and Japan. More than half of the patients in the only study that has been done had good improvement that lasted 6 months.

Side effect: Oolong tea, like other tea, contains some caffeine and could be stimulating.

Downside: American taste buds need to get used to the flavor.

Cost: $3 to $5 a month

leaves are "fermented" and oxidized; and oolong tea leaves are partially oxidized. It's an acquired taste, but it could be a taste worth acquiring.

Over-the-Counter Remedies
Vitamin E

Vitamin E, once considered a potential super-nutrient, has fallen out of favor as a preventive for heart disease or cancer. But back when it still looked ever so promising, a group of Italian dermatologists conducted a study to see if vitamin E could improve symptoms of eczema.[295] It was single-blind; that is, the patients did not know who was getting the active treatment, but the doctors did. The patients ranged in age from 10 to 60 years old, and all had itching that had not been well controlled by their previous therapies.

The study lasted 8 months, and over the course of that time, the skin of fewer than 10 percent of the people taking vitamin E (400 IU daily) got worse. The skin of more than three-fourths of those on placebo had worsened. Conversely, almost half of the patients on vitamin E had excellent improvement, compared to only 1 (of 46) of those on placebo. The investigators noted that the patients who had good results clinically also had marked reduction in the IgE levels that indicate allergic arousal of the immune system. They concluded that vitamin E might prove to be an excellent therapy for atopic dermatitis. Unfortunately, there are no other studies to confirm or refute these findings.

★★★ Vitamin E

This fat-soluble vitamin has been disappointing in studies of cancer or heart disease prevention. The natural form of vitamin E used in this study (alpha-tocopherol at 400 IU daily) was surprisingly effective in reducing the lesions and itching of eczema.

Side effects: Minor digestive upset is possible, but unlikely.

Downside: There has been only one study of this therapy for eczema. Although vitamin E is inexpensive and relatively nontoxic, more studies to substantiate the benefit would be desirable.

Cost: Approximately $3 to $8 a month

Topical Creams

Over the years, we have learned of a number of surprising remedies for itchy eczema. One is the old-fashioned moisturizing cleanser Noxzema. Many people have written to say they had success easing the itching and even clearing up the rash after applying Noxzema to their eczema. Of course, nothing works for eczema all the time. But Noxzema is relatively low risk. We suspect the herbal oils it contains may contribute to its effect. According to the manufacturer, camphor, menthol, and eucalyptus have given Noxzema "its redolent signature since 1914."

• • •

Q. *I just had to let you know the success I've had with your suggestion to use Noxzema for eczema. My 3-year-old son has suffered with this skin condition on his legs and feet for 2 years.*

We treated it successfully with the prescription drug Elidel, but after learning of safety concerns, we checked with his doctor and stopped using it.

I tried many moisturizing creams to soothe his skin, but he cried and said they hurt. I started using Noxzema the day I read your article, and there were no tears.

His skin responded quickly and after 3 weeks almost all traces of eczema are gone. This advice has changed my young son's life.

★★★★ Noxzema

The brand now includes a number of different cleansers, but the one you want is the original, in the blue jar. Apply it to the affected areas like you would a moisturizing cream. The herbal ingredients, camphor, menthol, and eucalyptus, may be helpful against itch, and the base cream is a good moisturizer.

Side effects: Uncommon. Discontinue use if it irritates the skin.

Downside: There's no scientific proof that this product will help eczema.

Cost: Approximately $4 to $6 for 14 ounces

A. We are certainly pleased to learn of your success. Lore has it that the name *Noxzema* was given after the product helped an early customer "knock" her eczema.

● ● ●

The mainstay of eczema treatment is a topical corticosteroid. In most cases, the doctor will prescribe a mild cream for use on the face and a more potent one for use elsewhere on the body. Hydrocortisone 1 percent is available without a prescription and can be used for eczema. We don't suggest long-term use without checking in with the doctor, though. Even though the nonprescription cream is not very strong, it could still cause some thinning of the skin if it were used for many months.

Those who would prefer to avoid hydrocortisone cream may want to check out a product called CamoCare Soothing Cream. It contains extract of chamomile flowers in an emollient base and has been helpful against eczema in one study.[296] Apparently, it has an effect comparable to low-dose hydrocortisone cream (0.25 to 0.5 percent), although it does not contain any steroid.

Another nonprescription ointment that has been put through a clinical trial is a homemade mixture of honey, beeswax, and olive oil.[297] This study was not as rigorous as we would like—not by a long shot. And honey, beeswax, and olive oil might just be too messy to be practical. But the Dubai dermatologist who ran the trial found that it had benefit for about 80 percent of the patients with eczema. That is almost the same as the percentage who respond well to topical steroid creams. So if you are in the mood for an experiment, get

---

★★★ Topical Hydrocortisone 1 Percent

Topical corticosteroid lotions, creams, and ointments are the mainstay of eczema treatment. This is the one that is available without a prescription, because it is less potent than prescription products. It probably will help mild eczema. It may not be strong enough for moderate or severe conditions.

The best way to use this lotion or cream is to apply it conscientiously for 3 to 7 days at a time. Then take a break for several days.

Side effects: Uncommon, but burning, itching, irritation, or dryness could occur where the product is applied.

Downside: Long-term use could lead to thinning of the skin. This is a small risk with the over-the-counter creams, but it should be kept in mind.

Cost: Approximately $3 to $8 for a 1-ounce tube

★★★ CamoCare Soothing Cream

This cream apparently was developed in Germany and is better known in Europe than in the United States. German chamomile (*Matricaria chamomilla*) contains an oil called *bisabolol* that has been shown to have powerful anti-inflammatory action, comparable to that of the drug indomethacin. That might explain its improvement of skin irritation.

Side effects: Some people are allergic to chamomile. Since individuals with atopic dermatitis may be especially susceptible to developing allergies, discontinue use immediately if the rash gets worse.

Downside: We know of only one study of CamoCare for eczema. In addition, it is relatively expensive.

Cost: Approximately $10 to $14 for a 1-ounce tube

out the blender and mix together equal amounts of honey, beeswax, and olive oil. Then see what it does for you. It should have no side effects, other than being sticky. And it should not be overly expensive.

Prescription Options

Doctors are most likely to prescribe some form of corticosteroid (cortisone-like) cream or ointment for eczema. That's because around 80 percent of patients with atopic dermatitis seem to respond well to these prescription creams. Fewer than 40 percent of those patients improve on a placebo cream or oint-

ment.[298] That's why topical corticosteroids are so widely used.

If your doctor has given you a prescription for a corticosteroid, be sure to get the details on how to use it. Using too strong a preparation on the face can have negative consequences. The skin may become thin and tear or bruise easily, and blood vessels may become prominent. In fact, some people with eczema

★★★★ Topical Steroids

One or more topical steroid preparations—a cream or an ointment—will probably be the dermatologist's first choice to control eczema. It helps significantly in most cases.

Follow the directions carefully. The cream may need to be applied two or three times daily. Do not put a strong steroid on the face, or any steroid cream near the eyes. Ask your doctor about "pulsing" the use of cream—applying it for 3 to 7 consecutive days and then stopping for several days. Adults may be able to use such products for just a few days a week.

Side effects: Stinging, burning, irritation, itching, peeling

Downside: Long-term use or application over a large part of the body, especially under a close covering, could thin the skin, lead to marks on the skin, or (most serious) result in side effects similar to those from oral prednisone.

Cost: Depends upon the specific steroid the doctor selects. These drugs can be expensive. Inquire about a generic version, which may cost much less.

need two different formulations—a fairly strong one for hard-to-treat areas like the hands and a relatively mild one for eczema on the face. Keep in mind, too, that overuse of topical corticosteroids can thin the skin.

People sometimes worry about steroid side effects from such creams. It's not impossible that side effects typically associated with steroid use might occur, but it is very unlikely unless the area treated is large and has been covered with some kind of bandage or "occlusive dressing." Be very careful in applying this kind of treatment. It may indeed help the skin, but it must not be overdone.

Atopiclair

In 2005, the FDA approved a nonsteroidal cream for eczema. Atopiclair is a prescription product that contains a number of botanical extracts in an emollient base. Like CamoCare, it contains bisabolol, but Atopiclair also contains a vitamin E–like compound, a licorice

> ### ★ ★ ★ Atopiclair
>
> This nonsteroidal cream is significantly better than a simple moisturizer at alleviating itch and reducing rash. It should be applied two or three times a day.
>
> **Side effects:** Local irritation
> **Downside:** People allergic to any of the ingredients, including nuts, should avoid Atopiclair.
> **Cost:** Approximately $85 to $95 for 100-gram tube

root derivative, and an extract of grapeseed, along with shea nut butter. A gel containing licorice extract had earlier shown promise for treating atopic dermatitis.[299]

Elidel and Protopic

The frustration of trying to control eczema, a condition that may not respond to the usual anti-inflammatory treatments, has led doctors to explore other treatment options. The development of immune-modulating treatments to prevent the rejection of transplants led some dermatologists to think about modulating the immune reaction at the level of the skin. After all, eczema does seem to be linked to an immune reaction gone a bit haywire, comparable to hay fever. It turns out that there are two compounds that can be applied topically to dampen the immune response. They are Elidel (pimecrolimus) and Protopic (tacrolimus).

Parents of children with eczema were very pleased to have these effective treatments made available so they would not have to rely so heavily on potent corticosteroid creams to keep their youngsters comfortable. They were alarmed, however, when the FDA issued a warning that these immune-suppressing drugs might increase the risk of children developing cancer, especially lymphoma. Such cancers are rare in kids, so it will probably be years before it is possible to assess how serious this potential risk really is. But weighing red, itchy skin against a potentially lethal disease suggests that these drugs should be used only when

★★ Protopic (tacrolimus)

This immune-suppressing cream is significantly better than a simple moisturizer. It is approved for use in adults and in children older than age 2.

Side effects: Local irritation, burning, stinging, itching, infections, seizures
Downside: Long-term use is discouraged because there is a possibility that it increases the risk of cancer. When application of the cream is discontinued, however, a high proportion of patients regress to pretreatment condition.
Cost: Approximately $65 to $80 for a 30-gram tube of 0.03 percent ointment, the only strength approved for use in children

other treatments have not worked.

Another topical cream for treating eczema is called MimyX cream. It is available by prescription, but does not contain a steroid. Clinical trials showed that it can reduce the size of areas affected by eczema and extend the period between flare-ups. Side effects appear to be local, such as irritation or itching. The manufacturer, Stiefel Laboratories, suggests that MimyX could be used on a regular basis without danger. Because it was approved relatively recently, however, there are no good long-term safety data.

Other Approaches

A number of other possible treatments may have some benefit for people suffering from atopic dermatitis. Some of them are pretty straightforward and well accepted, whereas others are on the wacky side. Here's a brief summary:

1. **Heliotherapy.** This means: Get some sunshine on your skin. Sunburn is bad, of course, but a couple of weeks of moderate sun exposure seems to make eczema better.[300] This almost sounds like a prescription for a tropical vacation! Be forewarned, though, that some of the medicines used to treat eczema could make skin more sensitive to sunburn. This is a worry particularly with Elidel and Protopic.

2. **Ultraviolet light therapy.** This probably explains why sunshine is beneficial. Exposure to ultraviolet A in the dermatologist's office can help alleviate eczema symptoms. Stubborn cases may improve with the addition of a psoralen gel or bath before the light exposure. This is similar to a standard treatment for psoriasis. The dermatologist will probably recommend it if she thinks it will be helpful. Although it is usually administered in the office or hospital, a portable unit used at home can be equally effective.[301]

3. **Balneotherapy.** Immersion in salts derived from the Dead Sea, followed by

exposure to ultraviolet B, can be helpful, especially if eczema is chronic and widespread. This effect was first observed in people actually bathing in the Dead Sea, but it is no longer necessary to go there. Some dermatologists offer this type of therapy in their treatment suites. One big drawback is that it takes a lot of time.[302,303]

4. **Hypnotherapy.** Both hypnosis and self-hypnosis can help people cope with eczema, especially with its terrible itch.[304]

5. **Music.** Listening to Mozart—but, oddly enough, not to Beethoven—reduced the size of a wheal that rose on the skin in response to a specific allergen challenge in people with eczema and latex allergy.[305] This is probably the most peculiar of the therapies we have come across, but the study used quite objective measures (IgE production, size of wheal) that presumably are not easily manipulated.

Conclusions

Eczema, or more precisely atopic dermatitis, is an itchy skin condition that is often chronic. Besides the itch, skin affected by eczema may develop a rash with liquid-filled bumps. Skinfold areas, such as the back of the knees, seem to be especially susceptible to the rash. Eczema is often accompanied by generalized dry skin, and the patient may also have asthma or hay fever.

There's no cure for eczema, although sometimes it does go away for a period of time. No treatment works all the time or for everyone, so people are understandably on the lookout for something that might work better than what they have already tried. Eczema is quite common in young children, and parents need to be especially vigilant in weighing the benefits against the risks of various therapies they might use for their kids.

- Avoid prolonged exposure to water or any irritating chemicals, including soap or detergent. After washing hands or bathing, apply a moisturizer within 3 minutes of patting the skin dry.
- A person with a documented food allergy that makes eczema worse should avoid that food. Eggs may be a culprit for young children.
- Probiotics can help in some instances. Look for a high-quality supplement with viable organisms. *Lactobacillus GG* and *L. fermentum* have done well in studies.
- Fatty acid supplements providing gamma-linolenic acid (such as evening primrose oil, borage oil, or black currant seed oil) help some individuals, but have not performed well in clinical trials. One exception is hemp seed oil, although the data on it are limited to one study. It might be worth a try.
- Cut table sugar and simple starches out of your diet. A low-glycemic-index approach might be worth trying, though there is no scientific evidence that it will control eczema.

- According to anecdotal reports, eating salsa may ease eczema symptoms. If you like spicy foods, go for it.
- Drinking 4 cups of oolong tea daily was shown in one study to help eczema that wasn't responding to other treatments. It is easy and nontoxic, so it would be worth a try.
- Vitamin E capsules did very well in one study of people with atopic dermatitis. Check with your doctor first if you are a smoker or at high risk of heart disease; some large studies suggest vitamin E might increase your risk of serious complications. For others, there is very little risk in a short-term personal trial to see if it helps your skin.
- Apply Noxzema—the original formula in the blue jar—to the affected areas. The herbal ingredients, camphor, menthol, and eucalyptol, may soothe itching. Be alert for increased irritation, though.
- Over-the-counter hydrocortisone cream (0.5 or 1 percent) may help if the eczema is mild.
- CamoCare Soothing Cream is available without a prescription and may ease itching, redness, and inflammation.
- Blend up a batch of honey, beeswax, and olive oil for a homemade salve that may help. It sounds sticky, though.
- Use prescription steroid creams according to the physician's instructions. Don't use a potent steroid on the face, or for too long a time. "Pulsing" the dose—applying the cream for 3 to 7 days straight, then not using it for a time—may help. Ask your doctor.
- Drugs such as Protopic (tacrolimus) or Elidel (pimecrolimus) may be helpful as back-up treatment if the steroid creams stop working or don't work well enough. Don't overuse these creams in young children (and don't use them at all in kids under 2) because the immune suppression they induce may increase the risk of infection and even cancer.
- Experiment with other approaches such as light therapy or hypnosis. Work with your physician to coordinate a safe and effective regimen.

FOOT ODOR

• Soak feet in a solution of Epsom salts	★★★
• Brew strong black tea for a foot bath	★★★
• Ask about a prescription for Drysol	
• Sprinkle socks and shoes with alum, baking soda, or Zeasorb	★★★

Some people really suffer with smelly feet. Any time they take their shoes off, family and friends complain. Sometimes, they complain a lot. This makes the tiresome routine of removing one's shoes to go through an airport security check even worse for these folks—and everyone else around them.

We don't know why some people have little or no problem with foot odor their entire lives while others are constantly fighting against it. Foot odor is probably linked to another problem, sweaty feet. Most likely the folks who are suffering with stinky toes are playing unwilling host to bacteria and possibly some fungi that feast on sweat and dead skin cells, producing a horrific aroma.

● ● ●

Q. My 12-year-old daughter is a ballet dancer and has started pointe. Her feet smell so bad that we gag if she takes her shoes off. Do you have any remedies for foot odor?

A. Foot odor seems to be a common problem among young ballerinas. The mother of a 20-year-old dancer offered this advice:

"First, get some 'shoe dogs.' These are cedar-filled bags that absorb the moisture in the shoe and help with the odor.

"Second, ballet students also wear classic soft ballet slippers. Canvas slip-

pers are better than leather, since the canvas kind can be washed every other week if need be. With daily classes, shoes don't dry out, so purchasing a few pairs will help. They should be stored in mesh bags, not plastic, and outside the dance bag, not in it.

"Third, try a dry rub-on antiperspirant on the feet once a day. This also helped my son with his sweaty, smelly soccer feet."

● ● ●

Scientists estimate that an average foot produces a quarter cup of sweat each day. When the weather is warm or the person is active—dancing, jumping rope, playing soccer or basketball—the amount of sweat produced increases significantly, to as much as a cup. A person with excessive sweat gland activity in the feet could produce even more.

All this sweat, combined with the protein from dead skin cells on the surface of the feet, can feed six trillion bacteria. If some of the bacteria produce isovaleric acid, which has an odor like ripe Limburger cheese, you have a real smelly foot problem! The solution is to either control the sweat or kill the bacteria.

For some reason, scientists have not devoted a lot of attention to stinky feet. Double-blind, placebo-controlled trials are few. After all, this isn't a life-threatening condition. However, it can be embarrassing and unpleasant.

Selecting Shoes

One factor that contributes to smelly feet is shoes that trap moisture. Going barefoot whenever it is practical can help prevent odor. In addition, dermatologists often recommend shoes that "breathe." In the summertime, sandals work well, as long as they are not made of plastic, like "jellies." At other times of the year, look for shoes with leather uppers, or canvas shoes that can be thrown into the washing machine.

Shoe manufacturers, especially those that specialize in sports shoes, are aware of this issue. They are looking to high-tech materials that will wick moisture away from the foot. The maker of Merrell shoes and hiking boots (a division of Wolverine Worldwide) is using Polartek fleece to line boots. Nike is investigating Gore-Tex for some of its sneakers.

Whatever shoes you choose, you need more than one pair. The shoes should dry out for at least a day, and preferably 2 or more days, between wearings. Several readers have suggested spraying them with rubbing alcohol or soaking a paper towel with rubbing alcohol and stuffing it into the shoe overnight to try to "disinfect" it a bit. If the shoes are washable, they ought to be washed every so often as well, to get rid of the bacteria causing the problem.

• • •

Q. *My 10-year-old daughter has terribly smelly feet. When she takes her sneaks off, the odor is overwhelming. Her brother teases her mercilessly, and she is becoming self-conscious. Is there anything that will help cut down on the smell?*

A. It's time to drop the sneakers in the wash or the garbage. Feet smell because of a buildup of moisture and bacteria in shoes. Sweat is a wonderful medium for these bugs to flourish in.

Your daughter needs a couple of pairs of shoes that can breathe. Have her switch off between them and wear sandals when she can. Make sure her socks are made of cotton, and have her change them daily.

• • •

Technology has produced improvements on the all-cotton sock, which tends to soak up sweat and stay soggy. Investing in some moisture-wicking socks made of Coolmax or a similar material would be a smart idea for anyone who suffers with foot odor.

Home Remedies

Since science hasn't offered much help, people have taken matters into their own hands. We have heard about quite a few different soaking solutions that seem to help reduce foot odor considerably. One is the familiar Epsom salt soak that is a popular remedy for sore muscles and infected cuts and hangnails.

> *When I read about the lady whose daughter had smelly feet, I thought you should know about the best remedy. Soak the feet several nights in a row in very hot (but not burning) water containing a generous handful of Epsom salts. The feet will be dry and without odor for a long time.*

Another popular soaking solution is baking soda or plain table salt dissolved in warm water. The baking soda formula is 2 tablespoons of baking soda in 2 quarts of water. The instructions are to soak the feet for 30 minutes each night for a month. This simple kitchen supply (sodium bicarbonate) may have an effect similar to that of the magnesium sulfate in Epsom salts.

> *When I was a kid my feet sweated and smelled something awful. My barber gave me the solution. I'd love to pass it on, as this is one of the worst odors I have ever smelled.*

★★★ Epsom Salts

Add a handful of Epsom salts (magnesium sulfate) to a pan of very warm water and soak your feet for 20 to 30 minutes for several evenings in a row.

Side effects: Irritation is theoretically possible but unlikely.
Downside: No scientific studies support this use.
Cost: Approximately $3 for 64 ounces

★★★ Tea Soak

Steep 5 tea bags in a quart of hot water for 10 to 15 minutes. Allow the brew to cool, then soak the feet for 30 minutes. This may be repeated daily or every other day.

Downside: The feet may be stained brown.
Cost: Approximately $5 for 100 bags (of Lipton tea), or about 25 cents per treatment.

> *Take a pan big enough for your feet and fill it with water as hot as you can stand. Put 2 tablespoons of plain old baking soda in the water and soak the feet for 30 minutes for 30 nights.*
>
> *Throw away synthetic sneakers. They hold in the moisture. Leather or canvas shoes with a clean pair of socks each day will breathe better. I'm 72 and my feet don't sweat. I feel at ease if I have to take my shoes off for any reason.*

Don't forget that reducing sweat is an important part of treating smelly feet. (You'll find more about that on pages 307–314.) Soaking them in a strong tea solution will often help with that and ease the odor as well. The tannic acid in tea is astringent, which helps close down those sweat ducts. This soak is readily available, simple to prepare, and inexpensive.

Nonprescription Treatments

If soaking the feet in baking soda, Epsom salts, or strong tea doesn't eliminate the odor, it's time to investigate more powerful antiperspirants. Nonprescription Certain Dri, with 12 percent aluminum chloride, is an effective treatment to reduce excessive sweating. It should be applied to clean, dry feet in the evening. It's best to put it on every night for about 2 weeks to see if it will work. If the foot dampness and odor continue after that treatment, it may be time to talk with a doctor about something similar but stronger. (Prescription Drysol is 20 percent aluminum chloride hexahydrate. Xerac AC, also available by prescription, contains 6.25 percent aluminum chloride hexahydrate. You can find out more about all of these treatments on page 311.)

• • •

Q. *I have a fabulous home remedy for sweaty feet and bug bites all rolled up into one. Antiperspirants (any brand with aluminum) will keep feet from sweating. If you put it on right away it will also take the sting out of insect bites.*

A. Aluminum is the mainstay ingredient in most antiperspirants. We have heard from other readers that it can also help sweaty feet, but the bug bite application is new to us.

People who have a serious sweating problem (underarms or feet) may wish to try an aluminum chloride solution. It is one of the most powerful antiperspirants available.

• • •

Foot powder can be helpful against foot odor. So can powdered alum shaken into the shoes or socks, according to a number of readers. You'll find alum on the spice shelf at your supermarket. (You also might try adding it to warm water to make a footbath.)

One reader urges others to sprinkle baking soda in their shoes as soon as they are removed. She has found that this controls the odor in her kids' shoes. Keeping the feet clean is essential, and she has them use baking soda as a dusting powder on their feet before they put on their clean socks.

Zeasorb powder can help absorb sweat and prevent smell from developing. As an alternative, you can ask your pharmacist to mix up a concoction of equal parts fluffy tannic acid, talc, and bentonite. Put it in a shaker can and sprinkle it on dry feet before donning socks and shoes, or put it directly in your shoes.

One other remedy that may be helpful for smelly feet is available for free anywhere you go.

★★★ Zeasorb

The powder contains cellulose, talc, and other absorbent ingredients. One version, Zeasorb-AF, also contains an antifungal drug called miconazole. It is sold for athlete's foot, but it works well to sop up sweat and minimize odor. If you can find plain Zeasorb without the miconazole, it should work too.

Downside: Easy to get powder all over
Cost: $12 to $15 for 11 ounces

Perhaps that is why it seems to be popular with the Armed Forces. Fighting men and women must keep their feet in boots for long marches, and they may not have ready access to laundry facilities for clean socks. We first heard about the benefits of applying urine to bare feet from an elderly woman several years ago. We have since heard it from soldiers and ex-soldiers of varying ages and military experiences.

• • •

Q. *For years I have sympathized with your readers who complained about smelly feet. I wondered if I had the nerve to write to you and if you would have the nerve to publish the surefire remedy for their complaint.*

I have known about this cure for over 50 years and have passed it on to people I knew who had this problem. During World War II, the men in the military complained of smelly feet, and an older man told these fellows to urinate on their feet in the shower. They said it worked, and so has everyone else who has tried it. This is no hoax. I'm a great-grand-mother and I wouldn't pull your leg.

A. This is definitely the most unorthodox home remedy for foot odor that we have come across. We expect readers will let us know whether it is effective for them.

• • •

66 *A few years back my teenage son suffered terri-ble foot odor. My husband and I would not let him bring his sneakers into the house, nor would we let him put his dirty socks in the hamper! His worst experience was a high school trip to Europe when he shared a room with two other boys. They made my son keep his sneakers in the closet.*

I then read in your column a solution to elim-inate foot odor: Urinate on your feet in the shower! I mentioned the column to my son and then kept quiet. Within a day, the odor was elim-inated. I thought that during the next few years you would mention this remedy again but I haven't seen it. I think there are many, many high school and college students who might benefit from the suggestion of urinating on your feet in the shower. 99

Dietary Supplements

As far as we know, there is no medicine you can take by mouth that will magically elimi-nate foot odor. That doesn't mean, though, that people haven't tried dietary supplements of various sorts. Some of them might work, although none has been extensively studied.

One of the most popular is green: A num-ber of readers are enthusiastic about the power of chlorophyll. The deodorant activity of chlo-rophyll was a popular idea in medicine around the middle of the 20th century, but no recent research supports it.

66 *I could sympathize with the lady who wrote to you about her daughter's smelly feet. I too suf-*

fered but found that when I cut down on sweets and take two chlorophyll tablets daily I no longer have any trouble."

One way people may get chlorophyll is in parsley. Many people are convinced that eating parsley will counteract bad breath from onions or garlic. Some are also quite sure that parsley can alleviate the stink of smelly feet. Here again, there is no scientific evidence to support the claim, but it is relatively inexpensive. People who are allergic to parsley obviously should avoid it; so should those with allergies to fennel, celery, or carrots, because they can cause cross-reactions. Besides that, we can't think of any serious downside to this remedy.

● ● ●

Q. *I felt so sorry for the person who wrote to you about smelly feet. When I married my husband 50 years ago, he had very smelly feet. He suffered and so did I. But we found the solution: It's parsley.*

He takes parsley pills every day. Within a few months, a miracle happened. Not only did his feet stop smelling bad, but his prematurely gray hair grew back in its natural color.

A. We have collected all sorts of home remedies for sweaty and smelly feet, but this is the first time we ever heard of parsley. We could find no scientific evidence that parsley pills would be effective for smelly feet, much less turn gray hair back to a natural color. On the other hand, parsley appears to be safe, though pregnant women and those allergic to fennel, celery, or carrots should avoid this herb. Parsley pills can be found in many health-food stores.

● ● ●

Some families are quite enthusiastic about zinc tablets as a way to control foot odor. We could find no investigations of this particular property of zinc, but there is enough other research to suggest a hypothesis that should be tested. Norwegian scientists interested in bad breath[306] have established that zinc compounds can bind to sulfur and prevent the formation of stinky "volatile sulfur compounds" that are the main culprits in bad breath. If you need a reminder of what those volatile sulfur compounds smell like, just conjure up the aroma of a rotten egg: hydrogen sulfide.

● ● ●

Q. *You offered a desperate parent advice regarding a daughter who came home from college complaining of foot odor. I read years ago that this problem can be caused by insufficient zinc in the* *system, and that zinc supplements have cured foot odor problems for many. It is probably worth a try.*

A. You are not alone in suggesting this remedy for smelly feet. We heard from another reader: "Several members of my family had the same problem until they discovered that zinc will alleviate the odor. Whenever we hear of someone with this problem, we suggest to the offending party, 'Don't stink—take zinc!' Usually 50 to 100 milligrams per day will solve the problem in less than 30 days."

We caution readers not to exceed the high dose of 100 milligrams daily or the treatment period of 30 days. Otherwise, zinc could reach toxic levels.

• • •

It's a long way, you may be thinking, from the mouth to the toes, and of course you are right. We've no idea whether zinc tablets release enough of the right kind of zinc compounds to the skin to keep any volatile sulfur compounds that might be contributing to foot odor out of harm's way. But another group of scientists tackling the difficult problem of dog flatulence also found that zinc had some benefit.[307] Our conclusion: We don't know if zinc will work, but it's worth a try. Don't take high doses of zinc for an extended period of time, though, as it could cause copper deficiency and blood disorders, especially in children.[308]

Conclusions

Most foot odor is probably due to bacteria producing stinky stuff like isovaleric acid and volatile sulfur compounds as they digest sweat and proteins from dead skin cells. To control the smell, reduce the sweat or kill off the bacteria.

• Go barefoot, or choose shoes that breathe and let them air out for at least a day between wearings. Treating them with rubbing alcohol may be helpful. Wear socks designed to wick moisture away from the feet.
• Soak feet in a solution of Epsom salts, baking soda, alum, or regular table salt. The soaks may need to be repeated until the feet stop sweating and smelling bad.
• Brew a strong tea solution to use as a footbath, or treat feet with a tannic acid gel.
• Control sweating with an aluminum chloride antiperspirant such as Certain Dri, Xerac AC, or Drysol. Apply to dry skin at bedtime.
• Sprinkle powdered alum, baking soda, or Zeasorb powder in socks and shoes to absorb sweat and minimize smell.
• Urinate on feet in the shower to control odor.
• Take a zinc supplement for a few weeks or a month to see if it helps.

GAS (FLATULENCE)

• Try Beano with beans and vegetables	★★★★
• Wear carbonized undergarments to trap odors	★★★★
• Take Pepto-Bismol for smelly gas	★★★★
• Experiment with probiotics to supply good germs	
• Sip fennel seed tea three times a day	★★★
• Try Angostura bitters in club soda	

We're not supposed to utter the *F* word in polite company. Physicians gussy it up by calling it flatus. Grandmothers use the euphemism "breaking wind." But adolescent boys love the word *fart*. And why not? It is what comes to mind when you pass gas. Almost 30 years ago we stumbled across a letter to the editor of the *New England Journal of Medicine* titled "Speaking the Unspeakable." W.C. Watson, MD, voiced his strong support for wider use of the F word.

So, dear reader, we shall take Dr. Watson's advice and refer to flatulence as farting. Regardless of what you call it, passing gas is not a particularly pleasant pastime. We actually think intestinal *GAS* stands for *Gross And Smelly*. But

seriously, is there anything more embarrassing than riding to work in a car pool and letting out a noisy, malodorous fart? There's no place to hide, and you can't blame it on the other guy.

SPEAKING THE UNSPEAKABLE

"This letter is to make it official. The word fart was used factually, without embarrassment at 1310 hours on Wednesday, May 17, in Lecture Room B, University Hospital, during a lecture to the second year medical class on "Gaseousness." I was encouraged to use the term by recent correspondence on the matter in the *Journal*.

I am essentially a God-fearing man, an avoider of obscenities, and a lover of the English language. On due reflection I was persuaded of the intrinsic value of this word and of its non-offensiveness. The students have been encouraged to use it freely where clinically appropriate. Not unnaturally, there were a few titters; indeed it would be true to say there were even a few guffaws at first. But once the word had been used a few times, it came to sound natural and as unremarkable as any other suitable clinical term.
I hope that all other clinicians, men of honor and upright standing, will follow this lead. A spark has been struck, a torch has been lit. Let it shine forth and illuminate the dark recesses of what has hitherto been that unspeakable thing. I am acknowledging the encouragement of the *Journal* with fart healt thanks.[309]

W. C. Watson, MD
Victoria Hospital
London, Ontario, Canada

• • •

Q. *I feel sorry for my sister's husband. When they are together in a moving car, he can't jump out to escape her horrible gas odor. It sounds funny, but being trapped in a closed space with her is no joke. Everyone in the family has been a victim at one time or another, so we all try to keep her away from the foods that make it worse. Do you have other suggestions?*

A. Your sister might want to try a Flat-D seat pad. This activated charcoal cloth pad traps 60 percent of unpleasant odors. Then she would not need to worry so much about offending family members. Order information is available from Flat-D Innovations on the Web at www.flat-d.com or by phone at 866-354-0056.

• • •

Some people are better able to control their sphincter than others. They can pass gas semi-surreptitiously (unless it is smelly). Holding gas in, however, is not necessarily a good thing. Self-restraint leads to gas retention.[310] That can cause symptoms such as pressure, bloating, cramping, or colic. Some people are so embarrassed about passing gas that they become hermits. Women may be especially vulnerable because they believe it is not lady-like to fart. Well, we would like to clear the air. It is time to stop suffering in smelly silence and let them out. Let the fight for the fart begin!

" *Flatulence is very stressful and embarrassing for me. I worry that I may not be able to control myself when I am out in public. I watch what I eat and even skip meals because I worry about this so much. I have tried lots of over-the-counter medications, like Mylanta, Gas-X, Tums, and others. No matter what I do I still pass stinky gas. It's gotten so that I don't want to go out anymore. I am desperate for help.* "

Physician Phlatulence

Flatulence has not received the respect it deserves from the medical establishment. Dr. E. M. M. Quigley of Cork University Hospital in Cork, Ireland, chastised his colleagues thus: "Long the sole preserve of the music hall and the stand up comedian, the application of serious science to the area of intestinal gas has been long overdue. It is also regrettable that these symptoms have tended to be trivialized and dismissed as imaginary by the medical practitioner."[311]

Most doctors would never cop to causing flatulence. And yet many of the medications they recommend can actually contribute to gassiness. When was the last time a doctor warned you that the drug he just prescribed might make you fart? We suspect that a lot of folks have been blaming their gas problems on dietary indiscretion while ignoring the pills they pop every day. Some medications contain lactose (milk sugar) as a filler. People who are lactose intolerant could experience gas and other digestive symptoms from even a small amount of lactose.

• • •

Q. I'm becoming a social recluse because of embarrassing digestive problems. Over the last 6 months I have become constipated and produce a great deal of gas.

These problems first cropped up after I started some new prescriptions, Actonel for osteoporosis and Paxil for anxiety. Could they be responsible? My doctor says the medicines wouldn't cause gas and told me to keep track of foods that cause trouble.

Controlling the gas has become so difficult that I don't want to go out with friends, attend church, or even visit relatives.

A. It's always a good idea to keep a record of foods and of "flatus events" so you can figure out which foods to avoid. But medications can be an overlooked source of both flatulence and constipation. Both Actonel and Paxil have been linked to these side effects. Perhaps your doctor could consider alternate drugs. Constipation itself can contribute to flatulence, so solving that

problem (see page 102) might ease the discomfort.

• • •

Hundreds of drugs can cause flatulence, directly or indirectly. We were surprised to learn that the Climara (estradiol) skin patch prescribed for menopausal symptoms might contribute to gas problems. So can hormone replacement drugs like the conjugated estrogens Premarin and Prempro and osteoporosis medications such as Actonel (risedronate) and Fosamax (alendronate). Other potential offenders include the antidepressants Paxil (paroxetine), Prozac (fluoxetine), and Zoloft (sertraline) and the cholesterol-lowering medicines Mevacor (lovastatin), Lipitor (atorvastatin), Crestor (rosuvastatin), and Zocor (simvastatin).

We can provide you with only a partial list of suspected fart producers. If you are watching what you eat, taking other precautions, and still suffering, you may want to discuss this issue with your physician. He might be surprised to learn that he is turning you into a gasbag.

Over the years physicians have tried to solve flatulence complaints with several silly strategies. For example, the farty fellow who passed a prodigious quantity of gas was told that his problem was attributable to swallowing air. He was counseled to eat more slowly with his mouth closed and to reduce the pace of his life. He was also given a variety of medications. This advice was worthless.

FARTY DRUGS*

GENERIC	BRAND
Alendronate	Fosamax
Anagrelide	Agrylin
Bevacizumab	Avastin
Colesevelam	WelChol
Conjugated estrogens	Premarin
Fenofibrate	Tricor
Imatinib	Gleevec
Lovastatin	Mevacor
Naproxen	Aleve, Anaprox, Naprosyn
Orlistat	Xenical
Oxybutynin	Ditropan
Pantoprazole	Protonix
Paroxetine	Paxil
Reloxifene	Evista
Risedronate	Actonel
Sertraline	Zoloft
Thalodomide	Thalomid
Venlafaxine	Effexor

*This is a partial list. Hundreds of drugs can cause flatulence.

> *I used to have a problem with terrible smelly gas that affected my life in every aspect. I couldn't exercise near others. Work was stressful because I never knew when I'd 'erupt.' Sex also had embarrassing surprises.*
>
> *"Last year I went on a low-carbohydrate diet, cutting out wheat and pasta, potatoes and starches. Within a week my horrendous flatulence was gone. I changed jobs and now work closely with others. I also go out dancing, dating, and exercising and feel like I have a new life."*

Although it is true that swallowed air may contribute some gas to the overall system, it is usually trapped in the stomach. Farts, especially the smelly kind, generally originate in the large intestine. Experts estimate "that almost three-quarters of the flatulence is made of bacterial gases."[312] It is these germs feasting on leftover carbohydrates and sugars that really contribute to gas production. There is a growing recognition that we each have our own unique population of colonic bacteria.[313] That may be why some folks are more vulnerable to certain foods than others are.

The Fart Chart

Everyone makes gas. Most folks average about 14 farts a day.[314] Michael Levitt, MD, one of the world's foremost flatologists, has declared that anything less than 22 flatus passages per day is "normal" and requires no "therapeutic manipulation."[315] Just let 'em rip.

Some people are regular fart factories, though, producing over 100 "events" daily. Dr. Levitt shared the story of one poor fellow who recorded "70 passages in one four-hour period."[316] That means he was farting on average every 3.4 minutes for four hours. Which brings us to the importance of a "fart chart." Doctors used to call it a "flatographic" record or a "flatulogram." By creating a fart chart, this gentleman was ultimately able to link milk to his flatulence. When he eliminated dairy products from his diet he was able to reduce, though not eliminate, his fartiness. He was also susceptible to foods like brussels sprouts, beans, bacon, raisins, celery, and onions. We highly recommend keeping a food diary and a fart chart so you can attempt to identify the particular foods that give you trouble.

> *People who have problems with gas may benefit from my experience. I read that 'Bananas are notorious gas producers.' Though I was incredulous, I cut them out of my diet. That was the end of the problem!*

The Celiac Culprit

A surprising source of gas trouble is nearly ubiquitous: the grains wheat, rye, and barley. It turns out that celiac disease is one of those mysterious conditions that affects many more people than previously recognized. Medical students once were taught that only 1 out of 5,000 people was afflicted. Now we suspect it is more like one in 100 or so, and in susceptible families it may be one in 22. That means millions of people are affected and don't even know it. Celiac expert Peter Green, MD, believes 97 percent of patients go undiagnosed.

In celiac disease, the gluten in the aforementioned grains leads to an immune reaction that destroys cells in the small intestine. This can cause all kinds of mischief (stomachache, gas, diarrhea, itchy rash, nerve pain, and anemia) and make it hard to absorb calcium,

---

SIGNS AND SYMPTOMS OF CELIAC DISEASE

- Abdominal pain and stomach cramping
- Anemia (iron deficiency)
- Bloating
- Bruising
- Dementia
- Diarrhea or runny stools
- Fatigue
- Gas and flatulence
- Headaches or migraines (frequent)
- Heartburn
- Itchy skin rash
- Numbness or tingling (hands and feet)
- Osteopenia
- Osteoporosis
- Peripheral neuropathy
- Reflux

---

magnesium, iron, and other essential nutrients from food.[317]

> *I had a terrible time with gas until I discovered that I was unable to eat foods that contained gluten. Once I eliminated everything with wheat, barley, and rye, my flatulence went away.*

Many physicians practicing medicine today never learned about the range of problems celiac disease can cause, including frequent migraines, peripheral neuropathy, fatigue, and dementia. Peripheral neuropathy is a condition in which nerves that detect pain may go haywire, resulting in tingling, burning, or numbness in the hands or feet and legs. With evidence mounting that celiac disease is common, patients deserve to be tested. If you have several of the symptoms listed, ask your doctor for EMA (endomysial antibody) and tTG (tissue transglutaminase) blood tests. Anyone with celiac must avoid all foods containing gluten (such as wheat pizza, bread, bagels, pretzels, pasta, and beer). A strict gluten-free diet can prevent most complications of celiac disease, including excessive gas.

We cannot possibly tell you which foods are likely to cause you gas grief. Some people are susceptible to bagels, bran, or broccoli. Others react to apples, cabbage, cauliflower, pretzels, or prunes. Fructose, a sweetener used in soft drinks, fruit juices, yogurt, and many other foods, can be a hidden culprit for many. Milk or other dairy products can be deleterious for folks with lactose intolerance. And almost everyone will react to beans.

Giving up beans, lentils, and other legumes would be a terrible tragedy. These are high-quality foods. Ditto for vegetables like broccoli, kale, and cauliflower. We have been told by just about every nutrition expert on the planet that we need to eat many more servings of fruits and vegetables each day to prevent a variety of chronic conditions. So how do we eat heart-healthy foods without being consumed by flatulence?

Beano

Despite all the products on the market that claim to provide relief from gas, there is

---

★★★★ Beano

The enzyme in Beano (alpha-galactosidase) breaks down the sugars in beans, vegetables, and grains that contribute to flatulence. Some people swear by Beano and wouldn't eat gassy foods without it. Others find it is only marginally effective. Take Beano with farty food and don't skimp on the dose. The usual amount is about 3 to 4 Beano pills or 15 drops of liquid with a meal.

Downside: Does not work for everyone. Anyone with galactosemia (a metabolic disorder) should check with a physician before using Beano. Allergic reactions (rash and itching) are rare.

Cost: Approximately $12 to $15 for 100 pills, enough for about 2 to 4 weeks, depending upon diet and dose

---

remarkably little research to support the ads. One that does have some scientific support is Beano. This product was developed by Alan Kligerman, an entrepreneurial genius. He grew up in New Jersey, delivering milk for the family dairy. One of his first big breakthroughs was Lactaid. It contains the enzyme lactase, which breaks down milk sugar. For people who are lactose intolerant, exposure to dairy products can cause bloating, abdominal discomfort, gas, and diarrhea. Lactaid makes milk digestible for millions of people.

Kligerman's next big project was Beano. It contains the enzyme alpha-galactosidase, which helps break down complex sugars found in beans and many vegetables such as cabbage and cauliflower. One small double-blind, placebo-controlled trial reported some success with Beano. Another study confirmed that Beano counteracted the gas-producing effects of a diabetes drug called acarbose (Precose).[320]

We cannot guarantee that Beano will work for everyone. Some people report that it really helps control flatulence. Others tell us it doesn't do much, if anything. You will have to be your own judge. Make sure you use an adequate dose before giving up on Beano.

Simethicone or Charcoal?

Simethicone has been one of the most widely advertised ingredients in anti-gas products. A defoaming agent, it works by reducing the surface tension of bubbles. Theoretically, this would turn lots of little gas bubbles into "larger gas collections." According to flatologist-in-chief Dr. Levitt, "Why this should be beneficial is not obvious; however one could speculate that the large gas collection might be more effectively propelled through the gut and expelled per rectum. Such an effect has not been demonstrated, and to the contrary, there are claims that simethicone ingestion actually decreases the amount of gas passed per rectum."

There is another over-the-counter remedy that is supposed to reduce the amount of gas that is passed. When you hear *charcoal*, you think barbecue, right? But activated charcoal is used in water filters, gas masks, and air filters to suck up noxious chemicals. Charcoal capsules have been sold for years to relieve intestinal gas. Their effectiveness, however, remains controversial. One older study suggested that oral charcoal might reduce "flatus events," whereas newer research concluded that "commonly employed doses of activated charcoal do not appreciably influence the liberation of fecal gases."[322,323] Charcoal can interact with quite a few medications, so it should never be taken within several hours of aspirin or many pre-scription medicines. Since they are questionable at best, we would probably skip the charcoal pills.

What about charcoal-containing pads or cushions? Did you know that there are several products on the market that purportedly trap gaseous odors before they can escape your personal space? Dr. Levitt and his colleagues have tested seven such products and found a couple that performed surprisingly well.

These experiments were somewhat diabolical and we won't go into great detail. Suffice it to say, they simulated the natural situation by getting volunteers to allow the scientists to infuse "two malodorous intestinal gasses, hydrogen sulfide and methylmercaptan . . . at the anus over a 2-second period." They then measured how successful the various pads, underwear, and cushions (GasBGon, Flat-D, and Flatulence Filter) were at trapping odors.

Pepto-Bismol

Another solution for obnoxious odors is that old-fashioned pink medicine, Pepto-Bismol. Dr. Levitt and his colleagues at the Minneapolis Veterans Affairs Medical Center discovered that bismuth subsalicylate (the active ingredient in P-B) provided "effective therapy for flatus odor."[324] They discovered that Pepto reduced colonic hydrogen sulfide by more than 95 percent.[325] We would not take Pepto-Bismol on a regular basis, however. Too much absorption of the mineral bismuth can lead to bismuthism, which is not a good thing.

★★★★ Pepto-Bismol (bismuth subsalicylate)

For occasional use, say, after a meal of baked beans, Pepto-Bismol could rescue you from embarrassing odors. The dose that was tested and shown to be 95 percent effective was two 260-milligram tablets four times daily. A lower dose might also work for you.

Downside: Only for occasional use. Too much bismuth subsalicylate can be toxic. Pepto-Bismol will turn your stools black, but this is not a cause for concern. Do not combine with blood thinners like warfarin (Coumadin), aspirin, or certain antibiotics. Be alert for ringing in the ears or loss of hearing.
Cost: Approximately $6 to $8 for 48 tablets, about a week's worth

---

Symptoms of bismuth poisoning include nausea, vomiting, stomach pain, diarrhea, mouth ulcers, skin rash, and kidney damage. So, please be moderate in your use of it and follow the instructions on the label.

Probiotics

If gazillions of bacteria in the lower intestine are largely responsible for the production of the gas, then it only stands to reason that if we could modify the population of our colon buddies, we might be able to affect their output. This may be far easier in theory than in practice. Nevertheless, a few small studies have reported that probiotics (good bacteria) can reduce pain, bloating, and flatulence for some patients. One study was a double-blind, placebo-controlled trial involving *Lactobacillus rhamnosus* of the GG strain (LGG).[326] Another involved *Lactobacillus plantarum*.[327]

> *Ever since childhood, I've been a bloated and gassy person, which caused me much discomfort and embarrassment. I couldn't pinpoint one type of food because almost anything would make me gassy.*
>
> *Finally, a couple of years ago, I discovered something which has set me free:* Lactobacillus GG *in capsule form. Culturelle is the brand name.*
>
> *My naturopath prescribed it for me when I had an intestinal infection to help recolonize my digestive system. After a couple of weeks I noticed the bloating and constant gassiness were gone! I was so happy that I have taken it as a daily supplement ever since.*

Fennel

One common herb that has traditionally been used to treat gas is fennel seed. It has a pleasant licorice-like aroma, although it is not licorice and does not have the same medicinal action as licorice. Many Americans are not familiar with fennel seed as a seasoning, but you can find it on the spice shelf of most supermarkets. You may taste it in Italian sausages. No, we're not suggesting you eat sausage to tame your farts. Both fennel seed tea and fennel seed capsules (try the health-food store) are easy ways to get this antifart herb.

To make fennel seed tea, take 1 teaspoon of fennel seeds. Smash them with the back of a spoon to crush them slightly. A mortar and pestle certainly works but is not necessary.

★★★ Fennel Seed (*Foeniculum officinale*)

Fennel is a member of the celery family, which also includes other culinary herbs like anise, caraway, and dill. It was traditionally used for indigestion and flatulence. A laboratory study suggested that it may counteract spasms of smooth muscle in the intestines.

Fennel seed capsules and fennel seed tea should ease gas.

Downside: There is little if any scientific evidence to support this claim.
Cost: Approximately $3 to $5 for 4 ounces, enough to make many cups of tea

Cover the "bruised" seeds with 8 to 10 ounces of boiling water and allow the brew to steep for about 5 minutes. Discard the seeds, sweeten the beverage if you wish, and drink it. You can have up to 3 cups a day.

• • •

Q. *Some time ago you offered a solution to a long-standing problem I've had. I've had explosive flatulence during my workday.*

I tried the crushed fennel seed tea three times a day for the past week. It's proven an almost instant cure. Thanks so much for sharing the tip. Now that I know it works, I wonder if you have any idea how.

A. Fennel originated in southern Europe and western Asia, but it was widely known in the ancient world, from China to Greece. For centuries it has been used to treat indigestion and flatulence. How it relieves gas, however, remains mysterious. We're glad you got such great results.

• • •

Other herbs in the same family as fennel may also be helpful. These include anise (which has an even more pronounced licorice-like aroma and flavor), caraway, dill, and parsley. Caraway may be most commonly used for this purpose.

• • •

Q. *My mother's remedy for gas cramps was caraway tea. Just steep some caraway seeds in hot water. Caraway always helps with gas build-up, which is why we Germans add it to sauerkraut.*

A. We've heard fennel tea is good for gas. Since caraway is related, we are not surprised that it might help.

• • •

Other Herbs and Spices

Many other botanicals that are usually considered spices for food have also been used to combat gas. In fact, there are some herbal mixtures called "bitters" that are designed specifically to ease various digestive complaints. A number of people have found that Angostura or Swedish bitters can be quite helpful against gas as well as indigestion.

• • •

Q. *Do you have a suggestion for someone with frequent, odorous flatus? One of my sons has this problem and besides causing lots of laughs, it also causes the rest of us to groan.*

A. We recently received a suggestion from a reader on this very topic: "Has anyone suggested Angostura bitters for gas? When I was a waitress and had that problem, someone suggested a teaspoon in a glass of 7-Up or just club soda. It worked immediately."

Angostura bitters have been sold for more than a century as a digestive aid. The label suggests taking 1 to 4 teaspoonfuls after meals to combat flatulence. Bartenders use this herbal flavoring in mixed drinks, and cooks use it in sauces. It can be purchased in grocery stores.

• • •

Other spices that have been used with success include ginger and turmeric, the rhizomes so popular in Indian cooking. Ginger in particular has had a reputation for hundreds if not thousands of years as being beneficial for digestive problems of all sorts. It may be most noted and best studied for preventing nausea due to motion sickness, but it is also a traditional remedy for gas.

• • •

Q. *Whenever we cook beans we include a small piece of fresh ginger root. It adds flavor and avoids the problem with gas. Maybe it will help someone else.*

A. Ginger has a long tradition as a digestive aid and antiflatulent. Thanks for sharing your home remedy.

• • •

Besides being a staple of South Asian cooking, turmeric (*Curcuma longa*) has been used in the traditional Ayurvedic medicine of India for thousands of years. It also is an ingredient in yellow mustard. It has recently gotten a lot of scientific attention for its anti-inflammatory properties. Some of our readers report that it is also helpful against gas.

• • •

Q. *I have found that eating more than one hard-boiled egg produces bloating and gas with an unpleasant sulphurous odor. Adding mustard to the eggs before consuming them seems to eliminate this problem. I can eat a dozen deviled eggs without trouble. Is the turmeric in yellow mustard the key ingredient?*

A. A dozen deviled eggs is a lot of eggs! Turmeric, a yellow root in the ginger family, has been used historically in Chinese medicine to treat flatulence and other digestive upset.

• • •

A number of other herbs also have a reputation for fighting off farts. They may be too numerous to name, but we'll mention two of the best known. Peppermint (*Mentha piperita*) is said to be quite helpful. A cup or 2 of peppermint tea is said to settle the stomach and also help relieve smelly gas. Another that is well known in Mexico and the Mexican-American community is epazote (*Chenopodium ambrosioides*). The leaves of this herb are added to black beans while they are cooking to make them more digestible and less flatulogenic. They also give black beans a special flavor.

• • •

Q. *Many years ago I started using a rather unusual method for degassing beans. When it is time to soak the beans overnight I use Sprite or its generic equivalent instead of water. I then rinse the beans with water prior to cooking.*

This method virtually eliminates the gas problem and there is no difference in the taste. This is one way to enjoy a good bean soup and not have to worry about the after-effects.

A. You offer an interesting twist on a familiar practice. Indigestible sugars in the coating of the beans are responsible for most bean-related flatulence. To minimize these compounds, soak beans in water that has been brought just to the boil, then discard the soaking water. Your technique is a variation.

Another reader suggested a different approach: "Add a potato while cooking dried beans. This works for me every time."

Several culinary traditions also have hints that may help. Mexican cooks add the herb epazote to black beans, both for the taste and the anti-gas effect. The spices hing (asafoetida) and ginger are used in India.

• • •

Conclusions

We all fart, some more than others. If you average less than 22 events a day, the experts tell us that there is nothing to worry about. Trying to reduce that number is a losing battle. If, on the other hand, your flatulence is affecting the quality of your life or restricting your social activities, there are some things you can try.

• Keep a fart chart. This is a diary of the foods you eat and the gas you pass. Track trends to see whether there are special foods that foment flatulence. Consider wheat, rye, and barley as possible culprits (in which case you might have undiagnosed celiac disease). Don't forget dairy. Lactose intolerance is a common cause of gas.

• Consider your medications as possible contributors to a gas problem. A surprising number of drugs can cause flatulence.

• Try Beano (or Lactaid if you are lactose intolerant). These digestive enzymes can minimize the sugars that bacteria use to produce gas.

• To diminish offensive odors, invest in a pair of carbonized undies. They can trap unpleasant smells.

• Pepto-Bismol is a proven antidote to malodorous flatulence. Don't overdose, though, as it can become toxic.

• Probiotics may reestablish a healthier bacterial environment in your lower digestive tract. This may reduce the amount of gas that is produced.

• Consider fennel seed tea or capsules. This herbal remedy has been used to treat digestive woes, including gas, for centuries.

• Other herbal approaches may include ginger, turmeric, peppermint, caraway, or a combination like Angostura bitters.

HEADACHES AND MIGRAINES

• Take aspirin or acetaminophen for an occasional tension headache	★★★★★
• Don't overuse headache medication	
• Consult a doctor if headaches are frequent or severe	
• Experiment with riboflavin or feverfew for natural migraine prevention	★★
• Try acupuncture treatments to reduce migraine frequency	★★★
• Treat a migraine as early as possible	
• Use Excedrin Migraine for mild migraines	★★★★
• Ask your doctor about a triptan for more severe migraines	★★★
• Discuss topiramate (Topamax) with your MD if you suffer frequent migraines	★★
• Prevent menstrual migraines with NSAIDs	
• Prevent sex headaches with NSAIDs	

Headaches are extraordinarily common, number seven on the list of reasons why people see their doctor. It is estimated that 45 million people suffer from chronic head pain. That doesn't begin to include those who have occasional headaches. Yet for all that, the exact causes of head pain are not all that clear.

According to Joel Saper, MD, director of the Michigan Head Pain and Neurological Institute, the brain itself doesn't feel pain. That's why neurosurgeons can operate on the brain tissue while a patient is wide awake. So, a headache isn't exactly the result of pain in the brain. We perceive head pain that may originate from the scalp, the skull, or the coverings of the brain. Muscles and nerves in the neck can also create discomfort that is perceived as a headache.

An occasional mild headache does not usually pose a serious problem. But a more severe headache, even if it occurs only once in a while, or a chronic headache, even if it is not extremely painful, deserves medical evaluation. Popping a couple of aspirin or acetaminophen pills just isn't a good idea when the headache occurs several times a week. In fact, Dr. Saper says that using such over-the-counter (OTC) analgesics too frequently can actually cause the headaches you're trying to treat. It takes an experienced headache doctor to help someone out of such a vicious cycle.

" I have suffered from headaches all my life. For the past 30 years, I've taken from 25 to 35 aspirins daily, in addition to sinus medication. My doctor doesn't know about these large doses, but regular checkups reveal no damage to my liver or kidneys. "

The trouble is that many physicians are not aware of how serious this problem can be. John Edmeads, MD, editorializing in the journal *Headache*, noted that "the daily use (or, more accurately, abuse) of analgesics actually worsened and perpetuated headaches." He bemoaned the fact that so few physicians "know that chronic analgesic abuse causes chronic headaches."[328]

The diagnostic dilemma for doctors is that they must distinguish between headaches brought on by overuse of pain relievers, headaches caused by some other medical condition, and headaches caused by a change in brain chemistry. If the headache is a consequence of an underlying condition like the flu, it will go away when the infection runs it course. Celiac disease is one condition that can cause recurrent headaches, among many other symptoms, although the underlying issue is actually a reaction to gluten in the small intestine. The treatment is to avoid any foods that contain gluten (wheat, barley, and rye).

" I suffered from migraine headaches for more than 10 years. I saw several neurologists, but my intense headaches forced me to take early retirement.

In the fall of 2002, I went from three headaches a week to almost nonstop. That November, I had only 3 days without headaches. I took migraine meds like Frova, Maxalt, and Imitrex, but I mostly lay in bed in a dark room.

I was at my wit's end. Then my family doctor suggested a gluten-free diet. Gradually my headaches became less frequent, and after several months I was 98 percent headache-free. I feel I have been given a new life! ''

Caffeine Withdrawal Headache

By now, many people recognize that daily use of caffeine can lead to a dependence on it. Stopping the caffeine—for example, by not drinking coffee on the weekends—can lead to a caffeine withdrawal headache, accompanied by irritability and fatigue. Probably the best way to deal with this type of headache in the short term is to get a little caffeine. In the longer term, though, a more gradual withdrawal from coffee, soda, or caffeine-containing medications will allow a person to drop the use of the drug without the wicked headache.

• • •

Q. *I am a healthy person and rarely take any medicine. I quit smoking 14 months ago and am trying to stop drinking coffee. Lately I've had trouble with fatigue and tension headaches in the afternoon. If I take Extra Strength Excedrin with a Coke on my break, the headache goes away like magic. Regular aspirin doesn't work as well. Why is Excedrin more effective?*

A. Each Extra Strength Excedrin contains aspirin (250 mg), acetaminophen (250 mg), and 65 mg of caffeine. That means that a standard two-caplet dose will provide you with 130 mg of caffeine. Together with your cola, this probably provides as much caffeine as two mugs of coffee.

It is conceivable that your afternoon slump and headaches are due to caffeine withdrawal. People who customarily drink as little as 2½ cups of coffee can experience symptoms such as lethargy, headache, and anxiety when they stop.

By taking a pain reliever that contains caffeine, you could be easing your withdrawal. An alternate solution is to try to reduce your caffeine intake gradually until you are completely weaned.

• • •

Tension Headache

Experts used to pigeonhole headaches into separate categories: tension headache, sinus headache, migraine, and so forth. While some categories may be useful, the separations between them have blurred. Trying to tell a tension headache from a migraine is not for amateurs.

Although tension headaches are said to be far more common than migraines, much of the research lately has focused on migraine prevention and treatment. How should you handle recurrent tension headaches, then?

As long as the headache does not occur more often than once a week, there is no problem with using the regular OTC headache pills or powders. These may contain aspirin, acetaminophen, or a nonsteroidal anti-inflammatory drug (NSAID), usually ibuprofen. All of these have been shown to ease headache pain. For this type of occasional use, the only reason to prefer one instead of another is based on your own experience of pain relief. If aspirin doesn't seem to help but Tylenol does, go with the acetaminophen—and vice versa.

Adding caffeine to the analgesic may help it work better. You can buy a pill that already contains caffeine, or you could take your aspirin, acetaminophen, or ibuprofen with iced tea or a cup of coffee.

Readers have suggested a few unique approaches that might be worth consideration, though we don't have any good evidence that they work. They are, at least, inexpensive and low risk and will not perpetuate headache even if someone gets carried away and uses them too often.

People have tried applying a dab of peppermint oil to the forehead. Others have put Vicks VapoRub on their temples. Using Vicks for a headache is strictly an "off label" use, just like so many of the other creative uses people have invented for VapoRub. It contains menthol as one of its ingredients; peppermint oil also contains menthol. We're not aware that menthol has special properties to help ease headaches, but it has been shown to alleviate the pain of sore muscles. Perhaps it is doing something similar for a tension headache.

> ❝ *I have enjoyed your columns about Vicks Vapo-Rub for a variety of uses. Here's one you may not have heard before. A friend had a headache that would not go away. I told her to rub a dab of Vicks on her forehead. She thought I was nuts, but it worked. She has been using it ever since.* ❞

★★★★★ Aspirin

Plain old generic aspirin, 650 milligrams (two tablets), will ease the pain of an occasional tension headache in most cases. The danger is if the headache becomes more frequent. Aspirin overuse increases the possibility of stomach irritation or ulcers and can also be associated with "rebound headache." Regularly using aspirin (or acetaminophen) at least 2 days a week may increase the risk that the headache will become chronic because of the medication.

Side effects: Digestive tract upset, including ulcers
Downside: People who are allergic to aspirin must avoid it completely.
Cost: Inexpensive, about 5 cents a dose. More if you buy a brand name.

Some headache specialists have used relaxation training for people who suffer from chronic or recurrent headaches. This can help individuals who are willing to practice the technique, including teenagers who have frequent headaches at school.[329]

One very important point for people who suffer frequent headaches of any sort: Overusing pain relievers can actually cause chronic headache. This is a very difficult problem to handle alone, so a person who is using painkillers for a headache more than 2 days a week on a regular basis should get help from a headache specialist.

Migraine Headache

Experts estimate that 28 million to 30 million Americans suffer from migraines.[330] Many more migraine sufferers are women than men. As we have pointed out, trying to distinguish between a migraine headache and some other cause of head pain is generally a job for an expert. Usually, though, if the headache is accompanied by exceptional sensitivity to light or noise or by nausea, or if it is preceded by an aura of flashing lights or blind spots, a person should be evaluated for migraine. Other tip-offs might be pain on just one side of the head or pain that throbs, especially when you move.

We tend to think of migraines as crushingly painful. That's not always the case. But if it is a migraine, there are ways to treat it that should help get the pain under control, whether it is simply annoying or completely incapacitating.

• • •

Q. *I am 20 years old and have suffered with severe headaches for as long as I can remember. Recently I asked my doctor about them, and he told me as long as I could stop them with an OTC pain medicine I shouldn't worry about them.*

I am concerned about the frequency of the headaches and the fact that the pain is always on the left side of my head. I suffer from at least one a week, usually more. Which pain reliever is best?

A. Please check in with a headache center. A one-sided headache could be a symptom of migraine. If that is your problem, a prescription migraine medication might be helpful.

According to Joel Saper, MD, one of the country's leading experts on headache, using any OTC pain reliever more than 2 days a week might aggravate the problem by causing rebound headaches.

• • •

If you are diagnosed with migraines, you will want to know what stimuli jump-start them so you can avoid them to the extent possible. The migraine-prone brain likes to have a certain amount of routine. Disrupted sleep, dehydration, missed meals, secondhand smoke,

MIGRAINE TRIGGERS

Alcohol (including but not limited to red wine)

Aspartame (found in many "light" sugar-free foods)

Caffeine withdrawal

Chocolate

MSG (monosodium glutamate, found in many processed foods, including peanuts)

Nitrates (found in processed meats like hot dogs and salami)

Tyramine (found in aged cheese, chocolate, nuts, sour cream, and yogurt)

perfume, and a number of different foods or ingredients are common triggers.[331] Keeping a headache diary is a good way to figure out what things get your migraine going. In it, you record details like meals, exercise, sleep schedule, and so forth, as well as your migraines, so you can track back for any patterns.

The validity of some of these suspected triggers has been questioned. The manufacturer of aspartame has produced data demonstrating that aspartame does not cause headaches. One double-blind study using carob candy as a placebo for chocolate found that women with recurrent migraines were no more likely to develop headaches when given chocolate than when given placebo.[332] This news was greeted with relief bordering on glee in some circles.

• • •

Q. *My wife loves chocolate, but she read that it can trigger headaches. Now* she won't eat it, even on special occasions. I used to buy her great chocolate for Valentine's Day and her birthday and she really enjoyed it.

I never remember her getting a headache right after eating chocolate, but she does occasionally suffer from migraines. Can you tell me why chocolate is a problem?

A. Chocolate has long been blamed for triggering headaches because it is high in tyramine. This substance is thought to release serotonin and make blood vessels contract and expand. But research shows that most headache sufferers may not be susceptible to chocolate.

In a carefully designed study, 63 female headache sufferers were given either carob or chocolate bars (both mint flavored to disguise the obvious difference). There was no significant association of headaches with chocolate bar consumption.

Your wife might perform her own experiment to see if she really is sensitive to chocolate. She may be depriving herself needlessly.

• • •

Some scientists doubt that cheese, chocolate, and nuts are actually migraine triggers. Even if they are not migraine triggers for most people, some individuals may react to aspartame, chocolate, cheese, or any of a number of other foods.

> *Have you ever heard of sipping beer to stop a migraine? I went to a doctor in a little town in Louisiana, and he asked if I get an aura. Before my head starts to hurt, my vision changes and I see little blinky lights.*
>
> *The doctor said I should drink a can of beer (not wine or liquor) as soon as I start to see the lights. Over the last 20 years, this remedy has worked almost every time. I thought some other migraine sufferers would like to know.*

There is no way to predict what foods will trigger a migraine for one person or be helpful for another. Beer is thought to cause headaches for some people. But we heard from one woman that if she drank a beer at the very first sign of trouble, the headache never materialized. She even traveled with an emergency can for medicinal purposes. The headache diary we mentioned will help you sort out what foods create problems for you.

> *I have suffered with migraines all my life, but in the last few years they got worse. My medicine stopped working and I had headaches every day.*
>
> *I was desperate, so when someone suggested I see an allergist I did. I discovered I am allergic to a lot of foods I ate every day, including coffee, wheat, rice, oats, eggs, and tomatoes.*
>
> *Now that I have changed my diet, my head is much better. Some recurrent migraines warrant seeing an allergist.*

Natural Remedies

The real action in migraine treatment is with the "triptan" prescription drugs that have been developed over the past decade. There is also an interesting advance in a prescription drug to be taken preventatively by those who suffer chronic migraines. But some herbal remedies and dietary supplements have shown promise in preventing migraines, too.

RIBOFLAVIN

> *I've had migraines for many years. I think I've taken every migraine drug on the market and even ended up in the emergency room a few times.*
>
> *I was finally sent to a neurologist who told me to take vitamin B complex (B-100). I can honestly say I have not had a migraine headache in 2 years. I couldn't believe after so much time taking drugs that all I needed to do was take a vitamin.*

Riboflavin, a B vitamin (B_2), has been reported to help prevent migraine recurrences. One study found that 400 milligrams of riboflavin per day was able to reduce headache frequency markedly, from 4 days a month to 2 days a month.[333] This is a very high dose, however. Another study compared a product that combined 400 milligrams of riboflavin with 300 milligrams of magnesium and 100 milligrams of feverfew extract to a "placebo" of 25 milligrams of riboflavin.[334] The researchers found no difference between the placebo and the combination product. Nevertheless, the scientists weren't disappointed because both groups had fewer migraines and less overall discomfort than they had had before starting the study. The investigators hypothesized that 25 milligrams of riboflavin might have been enough to help reduce migraines, which would have explained the lack of difference between the placebo and the tested preparation.

• • •

Q. *I've read that riboflavin, feverfew, and magnesium can help prevent migraines. But finding all these things and taking multiple products can be difficult. All three are contained in an OTC product called MigreLief.*

I am a 31-year-old female who has suffered from migraines for many years. Two or three migraines a week really interfered with my life. I would make plans and then at the last minute I would have to cancel due to another migraine.

This was an ongoing problem. Even after numerous doctor visits and many prescription medicines, I never got relief.

When I decided to try MigreLief as a more natural approach, I had fewer headaches within a month. In a couple of months my migraines disappeared almost completely.

A. Thank you for bringing this product to our attention. The manufacturer, Quantum, points out that MigreLief is intended only for headache prevention and not for immediate pain relief. We have not seen a placebo-controlled trial of this combination product, although there is some research to support the use of each of the ingredients for migraine prevention.

• • •

FEVERFEW

Feverfew (*Tanacetum parthenium*) has a history of use by healers that goes back to the ancient Greeks. Seventeenth-century English settlers brought it with them to the colonies and used it to treat fever, vertigo, depression, and headaches. Although it fell out of favor by the 19th century, it has experienced a revival in the last decade or so. Studies have shown that it can indeed help headaches, but it is used primarily for migraine prevention rather than for treatment.

Feverfew is used more often in Europe and Canada than in the United States, perhaps because their regulatory bodies have authority over herbal products. In Canada, feverfew products must by law contain a minimum of 0.2 percent parthenolide. In France, the minimum is 0.1 percent. Animal studies have confirmed that parthenolide is the active ingredient.[335] For migraine prevention, the herb is taken daily for at least 2 months.

A rigorous review of double-blind, placebo-controlled trials involving feverfew found that the results were mixed. Not all the studies supported the efficacy of the herb as a migraine preventive.[336] The reviewers did conclude, however, that feverfew appears to be safe. A more recent German study demonstrated that a supercritical carbon dioxide extract of feverfew was more effective than placebo in reducing the frequency of migraine headaches.[337] In this study, side effects were equally uncommon with the feverfew extract and the placebo.

Feverfew is generally thought not to be effective for treatment once a migraine headache has begun, but a small preliminary study had patients take a product called GelStat Migraine under their tongues as soon as they had an inkling that a migraine was about to occur.[338] This nonprescription product contains both feverfew and ginger. A majority of patients who used it got relief, but the study was not placebo-controlled, and further research is needed to confirm these results.

BUTTERBUR

Butterbur (*Petasites hybridus*) is another old-fashioned herb that has just resurfaced. In Europe, it is sometimes referred to as "plague plant," despite a lack of any evidence that it was effective against the plague. There is evidence that butterbur can be useful in preventing migraine headaches, but only a few randomized, double-blind studies have been reported.[339, 340] One study without placebo control found that butterbur root extract can reduce migraine frequency in children and adolescents.[341]

Questions have been raised about the long-term safety of some butterbur products because the plant contains pyrrolizidine alkaloids, which are toxic to the liver. The manufacturer of the patented butterbur root extract used in one of the trials, Petadolex, has reported that the studies conducted on this product confirm its safety for humans.[342] The supercritical carbon dioxide extraction process leaves behind the dangerous pyrrolizidine alkaloids.[343]

A product intended for prevention is taken on a daily basis for a long time. If you decide

---

★★ Feverfew

A feverfew extract with at least 0.1 percent parthenolide might be helpful in preventing migraines. It is taken daily. Look for a standardized product such as the Canadian non-prescription medicine Tanacet.

Side effects: Canker sores, mild indigestion, and flatulence

Downside: May interact with anticoagulant medicines. Pregnant women should avoid this herb. Discontinuation should be done gradually; stopping abruptly has been associated with a "rebound effect" of severe migraines and sleep disturbance.

Cost: Approximately $3 to $4 for a month's supply

---

to try butterbur, we suggest you stick with one that is extracted with supercritical carbon dioxide and check in with your doctor.

Acupuncture

Quite a few studies have evaluated acupuncture for treating migraine headaches. The majority of them demonstrate that acupuncture is helpful in alleviating the pain, whether it is used as a preventive measure or in treating an acute headache.[344] In one large British study, patients undergoing acupuncture took fewer sick days and used less pain medication than they had before treatment.[345]

Oddly enough, acupuncture seems to achieve these goals even though a properly randomized trial, with sham acupuncture serving as the placebo treatment, couldn't distinguish between the benefits of real Chinese acupuncture and those of fake acupuncture.[348] Both "acupuncture" treatments were clearly superior to doing nothing, as shown by the results from patients in a second control group, who received no treatment during the study. Both were also equal to standard preventive drug treatment in another well-designed study.[349]

Not everyone responds to acupuncture, but for those who do, it appears to be a reasonable way to cope with migraine headaches, with a minimal risk of side effects. For treating an acute headache, acupuncture is better than placebo, but not quite as good as sumatriptan (Imitrex).[350]

★ ★ ★ Acupuncture

In general, acupuncture seems to be a safe way to reduce the frequency of migraines and help sufferers cope with them better. Despite research showing that sham acupuncture works just as well, we suggest that you consult a doctor who has been formally trained in acupuncture technique and is experienced in its use for migraine.

Side effects: Serious side effects are rare.[346] Minor pain or bruising at the needle site is fairly common.[347]

Downside: Not everyone responds to acupuncture. Some studies suggest the effect is essentially a strong placebo reaction.

Cost: Approximately $60 to $120 per session. May be covered by insurance.

Other Nondrug Approaches

As limited as it is, the research literature on herbal products like butterbur and feverfew is almost extensive in comparison to a few other approaches that pop up in medical journals here and there. A Brazilian study suggests that melatonin (3 milligrams daily) is effective in preventing migraines.[351] Another study, this one carried out in Switzerland, found that coenzyme Q_{10}, given at a dose of 100 milligrams three times a day, was superior to placebo.[352] Both of these treatments are readily available without a prescription and reasonably safe. Coenzyme Q_{10} probably should be avoided by people taking the anticoagulant Coumadin (warfarin), however, because of the potential for interaction between the two.

Since the age of 23 I have had frequent migraine headaches. Over the years, many doctors have prescribed medicines to prevent them, but none has worked. Drugs can stop the migraine if I take them early enough, but they shouldn't be taken too often.

I was told the headaches would disappear at menopause, but instead they got worse. For the past 10 years I have awakened three or four times a week between 2 and 4 a.m. with a migraine. I look at my bedside clock when the headache wakes me.

I read an article about people taking melatonin for jet lag and wondered if my headaches were due to a body clock problem. The article didn't say anything about migraines, but I tried an experiment. I started taking one 3-milligram melatonin tablet each evening, and I stopped waking up with a headache in the wee hours.

For years I have been avoiding all sorts of foods that might be migraine triggers. The success with melatonin made me brave and I ate some of them. No headache, as long as I take the melatonin. I consider myself lucky and want to share my discovery.

Another treatment that seems to be both safe and fairly effective is biofeedback to help people learn to warm their fingers. Presumably this activity also affects the blood vessels in the head that are believed to be involved in migraine. This type of biofeedback has been studied and found helpful in children and adolescents.[353] Finding a professional to supervise biofeedback training and maintaining practice in the biofeedback technique might be a challenge for families.

We have heard from a number of people who have used hot, spicy soup to stop a migraine quickly when they feel one coming on. There's not much research on this approach but no harm in trying it, either.

• • •

Q. *I have enjoyed reading about spicy gumbo and hot and sour soup for migraine and cluster headaches. No one can imagine how terrible cluster headaches can be. Anything that could help stop the cycle of pain would be a blessing.*

A. People have described cluster headaches as feeling like a blowtorch applied to the eye or a red-hot poker being thrust into the skull. To make the agony worse, cluster headaches may recur a few times a week or even several times in a day.

People tell us that hot peppers in a variety of forms can be helpful in cutting the cycle short. One fellow prefers a spicy Chinese tofu dish called *mapo dofu*, but he says anything with enough hot sauce works for him.

Another man relies on Tabasco sauce under his tongue. He chases this "strong medicine" with a glass of ice water and reports relief "in 5 minutes max."

The active ingredient in hot pepper is capsaicin. Though it may not work for everyone, sipping spicy soup seems worth a try.

● ● ●

None of these approaches is a substitute for regular medical care. A person with migraines should be under the care of a health-care provider, usually a physician, who can diagnose the problem and supervise the treatment. That is doubly true for anyone whose headaches are so frequent that prevention is an appropriate strategy. If you are interested in nondrug approaches to headache prevention, find a doctor or nurse practitioner who is comfortable discussing them with you and keep that person informed of what treatment you are using and how well it is working.[354] There are a number of drugs that can be effective both for preventing and treating migraine headaches.

Migraine Medications

There are no advantages to having migraine headaches. By all accounts, it is a miserable experience. But a person who is tuned in to her body may have an advantage in outflanking the migraine: Sometimes there are early warning signs—the so-called aura—that tip a person off that a migraine is on its way. These sensations can range from "little blinky lights" (as one caller described them on our radio show), to tingling in the fingers, to a hint of nausea. (Full-blown nausea and even vomiting are frequent components of a migraine.)

If you are a migraine sufferer, get to know your own warning signals of an oncoming headache and act immediately. Any kind of medicine used to treat a migraine works best if it is taken at the earliest possible stage,

★★★★ Excedrin Migraine

This widely available nonprescription medicine contains acetaminophen, aspirin, and caffeine. The caffeine may help it take effect quickly. It works better than placebo and also better than nonprescription ibuprofen and prescription sumatriptan pills.

This medicine is not intended for the most severe migraines. The dose of two tablets should be taken as soon as a migraine sufferer suspects a headache is on its way.

Side effects: Uncommon, but nervousness and nausea have been reported.
Downside: If this medication is overused, an occasional migraine could become chronic. At that point, the potential side effects of liver and kidney problems would be worrisome. If you find you are using this medicine more than twice a week, seek professional help for your headaches.
Cost: Approximately 10 to 15 cents per dose

before the headache has really taken hold. Don't wait to see if your early warning was accurate; assume it was and take action.

Over-the-Counter Painkillers

Because migraines are heavy-duty headaches, we tend to think of treating them with prescription medicines. That may be completely appropriate for people whose headaches often include nausea or frequently drive them to take to their beds. But for less incapacitating headaches, an OTC combination drug containing acetaminophen, aspirin, and caffeine (Excedrin Migraine) is surprisingly effective.

OTC ibuprofen has also been tested for the treatment of migraines. Randomized, double-blind studies have shown that both Advil Migraine liquigels and Motrin Migraine Pain tablets are better than placebo.[355,356] But Excedrin Migraine outperformed ibuprofen in a head-to-head trial.[357] What's more, the acetaminophen-aspirin-caffeine combination also beat out the prescription drug sumatriptan (Imitrex) in reducing pain and associated symptoms and reducing the amount of additional pain medication that study subjects needed.[358]

Prescription Migraine Medicines

TRIPTANS

The biggest advance in the treatment of migraines has been the development in the last decade and a half of medicines called "triptans." These selective serotonin receptor agonists are now the mainstay treatment for

---

TRIPTANS

- Almotriptan (Axert)
- Eletriptan (Relpax)
- Frovatriptan (Frova)
- Naratriptan (Amerge, Naramig)
- Rizatriptan (Maxalt)
- Sumatriptan (Imitrex, Imigran)
- Zolmitriptan (Zomig)

---

severe migraine headaches. Taken early in an attack, they reverse the chemical changes that lead to migraines and actually stop the headache pain in many cases.

The first triptan to be developed was a self-administered injection of sumatriptan (Imitrex), but before long both Imitrex and other triptan compounds became available as oral medicines. The injection may still be very helpful for some individuals who become so nauseated at the onset of a migraine that pills won't stay down.

The triptans are available only by prescription. In studies that have compared them to the older migraine medicine, ergotamine and caffeine (Cafergot), the triptans have done well, relieving the headache pain more quickly and effectively without significant side effects.[359,360]

The doctor will need to know about certain aspects of your health and medical history that might make one of these medications too dangerous. For example, there have been some

WHAT THE FDA KNEW

After a woman in Kansas City died following an injection of Imitrex, we followed up on a lead from reporter Kelly Garbus in the *Kansas City Star*. Through a Freedom of Information Act request (Number F95-00866), we discovered that the FDA was aware of this risk even before the drug was approved. These lines were included in a memo from Paul Leber, MD, who headed the section that reviewed the drug, to Robert Temple, MD, director of the FDA's Office of Drug Evaluation I:

"Used appropriately, Imitrex is reasonably safe; used in the patient with pre-existing cardiovascular disease, however, it may be dangerous, even deadly. . . .

"The division's recommendation to approve the Imitrex NDA [New Drug Application] reflects a risk benefit assessment which, in common with all such determinations, turns as much on personal values and implicitly held private assumptions as it does on evidence and reason . . . .

"In sum, a case can be made that, from the viewpoint of the public health, the benefit accruing to the population of migraineurs is outweighed by the injury and fatalities that Imitrex's marketing seems certain to cause."[361]

Dr. Leber had advanced this argument just for the sake of thorough consideration of every angle and titled it "Alternative Perceptions of Imitrex's Risks and Benefits." This memorandum makes clear, however, that the FDA knew before approval that the drug was likely to kill some patients.

unanticipated heart attacks among people taking one of these drugs during a migraine, so the prescriber will want to know about your risk of heart attack. Do you have high blood pressure, diabetes, or high cholesterol? Is there a family history of heart attack or stroke? Such serious reactions, fortunately, are rare, but make sure your physician gets all the relevant details. It's your life at stake.

One possible benefit of the extremely high price tags on most of the triptans is that it would discourage anyone from overusing these medications. Of course, without insurance that covers prescription drugs, a migraine sufferer might find it difficult to afford them at all. If cost is an issue, ask your doctor whether an older, less expensive drug such as ergotamine and caffeine (Cafergot) might work for you. Ergotamine is not appropriate for people with a history of heart disease and should not be taken by pregnant women because of a risk of birth defects.

TOPAMAX

A migraine sufferer who discovers that she needs to use her migraine medicine to stop a headache more than 2 days a week on a regular basis should definitely schedule an appointment with the doctor.[362] Frequent use of any migraine medicine has risks, not the least of which is a "rebound" that makes headaches more frequent. If headaches are coming that fast and furious, a preventative medicine could make more sense.

The most recent drug to be approved for migraine prevention is topiramate (Topamax). It was originally developed as an anticonvulsant, but the FDA has approved it for preventing migraine headaches as well. It works better than placebo to ward off migraines in children and teenagers.[363] Adults who take 100 milligrams of Topamax daily have roughly two fewer migraines per month.[364] This is similar to the results achieved with other preventive medicines and significantly better than placebo.[365] Side effects with Topamax include tingling and numbness (paresthesia), confusion or mental fuzziness, and weight loss.[366]

There are other, older medications that the doctor may prescribe for migraine prevention if topiramate is not appropriate. A different anticonvulsant, divalproex, is prescribed for this purpose. Even before doctors started using anticonvulsants to prevent migraines, though, they had found that beta-blockers could be helpful. Propranolol and atenolol are the two that are most often used, and because they are available in generic form, they are

★★ Topiramate (Topamax)

Topamax is taken on a daily basis to prevent migraines. In clinical trials, nearly half of the patients taking Topamax were able to cut their migraine frequency in half. This averages out to reducing migraines by two per month.

Side effects: Numbness (paresthesia), cognitive dysfunction, weight loss, tiredness
Downside: In rare cases, topiramate can cause a serious metabolic problem, with a buildup of ammonia in the body. It may also cause visual problems and glaucoma.
Cost: Approximately $150 to $175 per month

quite affordable. This use is distinct from their use for heart problems or high blood pressure.

In addition, a small study found that people who have both frequent migraine headaches and elevated blood pressure can benefit from the blood pressure medicine olmesartan (Benicar).[367] A few patients felt dizzy, but the drug was well tolerated otherwise.

Headache specialists are experimenting with Botox injections for migraine prevention. Double-blind studies have been somewhat promising.[368, 369, 370] Although the experts have still not figured out exactly who is the best candidate for this type of preventive treatment, it is generally well tolerated and far less invasive than a type of heart surgery that is also now being studied as a way of preventing persistent, recurrent migraines.

For Women Only: Menstrual Migraines

Women far outnumber men as migraine sufferers, and menstrual migraines might be part of the reason. Within the past few decades, clinicians have recognized that many women's periodic migraines are tied to their menstrual cycles and are presumably triggered by regular hormonal fluctuations. Estrogen and progesterone both affect the brain chemicals that are believed to be important in the development of migraine headaches.[371] Migraine attacks, especially migraines without aura, are about twice as common during the first few days of menstruation as at other times of the cycle.[372]

Knowing when the migraine is likely to strike can allow for a preventive strategy. Women susceptible to menstrual migraines are often advised to take a nonsteroidal anti-inflammatory drug (NSAID) such as mefenamic acid (Ponstel) for several days prior to the expected start of menses and continuing for a few days.[373] An OTC NSAID such as naproxen (Aleve) or ibuprofen (Advil, Motrin) might also work. The most common side effect of such pain relievers is digestive upset.

Another treatment that may be useful in preventing menstrual migraine is the mineral magnesium. A placebo-controlled study found that taking 360 milligrams of magnesium daily starting on day 15 of the cycle through the start of menstruation reduced the number of headache days and the severity of pain.[374] There are also a few small studies showing that soy isoflavones taken daily can help prevent menstrual migraines.[375, 376]

> *For the last few years I have been plagued with migraine headaches during the last week of my cycle, when my birth control pills contain no hormones.*
>
> *I discussed this problem with my doctor, and she prescribed Mircette. This brand of birth control pill is supposed to have hormones during the last week. Unfortunately, I still suffered terrible headaches during that week. I was at my wits' end because I could hardly function.*
>
> *I bought soy isoflavones containing "natural hormones." I began taking these capsules three times a day during the last week of my next packet*

of pills. For the first time in many years, I had no headache! I dreaded the next month, fearing the success of the soy isoflavones had been a fluke, but it has worked for 3 months in a row. "

Doctors have also experimented with longer-acting triptans, particularly Amerge, Frova, and Naramig. These drugs are frequently used to stop a headache once it has begun, but they also can be used when a headache is anticipated to prevent the menstrual migraine.[377] In some women, oral contraceptives will help prevent menstrual migraines, especially those that limit the number of menstrual periods to just a few each year.[378]

Not Tonight, Dear: Sex Headaches

The term *sex headache* sounds like an elaborate excuse or maybe a setup for a stand-up comic, but they are no laughing matter. These are headaches, often severe, that occur at or just before orgasm.

• • •

Q. *I have a problem my doctor and neurologist can't help. I am hoping you can give me a hint as to what to do.*

Whenever I strain in heavy lifting or in hanky-panky (don't laugh), I get severe pounding headaches lasting 5 to 15 minutes. They are incapacitating. My neurologist says they are "benign sex headaches" caused by my blood pres-sure going high, but I'm on Accupril for hypertension. Do you have any ideas?

A. Two kinds of headache are associated with sexual activity and exertion. One develops gradually with a dull, throbbing ache at the back of the head. The other type is explosive and excruciating, starting just before or during orgasm and lasting 5 to 15 minutes.

Neurologists often prescribe NSAIDs (nonsteroidal anti-inflammatory drugs) such as ibuprofen (Advil, Motrin IB), naproxen (Aleve), or indomethacin (Indocin) to be taken prior to lovemaking. An alternate approach is the blood pressure pill propranolol (Inderal) as a preventive measure. Consult a headache specialist to find out if such treatment would be appropriate in your case.

• • •

The first important step to take if such a headache strikes is to schedule an appointment with the doctor without delay. There are several potential causes of sex headache, and some of them require treatment to prevent great harm. If a workup eliminates the possibility of a serious underlying problem, a nonsteroidal anti-inflammatory drug such as ibuprofen, naproxen, or the prescription drug indomethacin usually works well for preventing or relieving the pain of a sex headache.

• • •

Q. *My doctor thought I was nuts when I complained of a sex headache. It happens only when I'm on top. This position gives me the most pleasure, but I have been avoiding it for fear of a stroke. The only other time I had such a headache was after going down a steep water slide. My kids and husband were terrified I was dying.*

I have high-normal (130/80) blood pressure. I take naproxen for arthritis and Zyrtec for allergies. The headache is explosive and excruciating. Your article on sex headaches vindicates me and assures me I am not alone!

A. Have a specialist evaluate your headaches. If they are "benign sex headaches," there are a number of treatments. For example, the naproxen you use for arthritis may prevent such headaches if taken before lovemaking.

It is extremely important to rule out other potential causes of severe headaches. One woman responded to the same article:

"I read with great concern your column about the man who asked for help with headaches that occurred with exertion or sexual activity.

"When my husband was 25, he had a very similar headache while having sex. The doctors told him it was viral. After a week of bed rest and Tylenol he felt better and went back to work. The next week while having a bowel movement it recurred, but this time the headache was fatal. He had a ruptured aneurysm in his brain. Please tell your readers to rule out all possibilities of problems with blood vessels."

• • •

Sex headaches appear to be similar to headaches caused by exertion or even cough.[379] Although such headaches may be very intense, they don't last very long. Anyone suffering a headache of this sort should have a thorough workup to rule out an aneurysm or another serious problem. In fact, any sudden, severe headache deserves medical attention. A headache that begins with a feeling as though someone has kicked you in the back of the head could herald a medical emergency and should be treated as one.

Conclusions

Headaches are extremely common. Occasional uncomplicated ("garden-variety") headaches respond well to self-treatment with OTC analgesics. Severe or recurrent headaches deserve medical attention. A number of approaches have been developed to treat migraines, so it should be possible for most sufferers to get relief.

Anyone who is using a headache medicine of any type more than 2 days a week on a regular basis is flirting with the danger of converting a frequent headache into a chronic headache. This holds true whether the drug is an OTC pain reliever or a prescription migraine medication. In such a situation, the help of a headache specialist may be needed to break the vicious cycle and help find a headache management plan that works.

- Consider phasing off caffeine intake gradually to avoid caffeine withdrawal headaches.
- Try relaxation techniques for a tension headache.
- If you regularly take headache medicine more than 2 days a week, see a headache specialist for help. Such frequent use of medication can cause rebound headaches that become chronic.
- Keep a headache diary to discover your migraine triggers. Include details on exercise, sleep, diet, and weather.
- Experiment with riboflavin, magnesium, feverfew, or butterbur for natural ways to prevent migraine.

- Acupuncture may help reduce the frequency of migraines.
- Sip hot, spicy soup to stop a migraine that has just begun.
- For best results, treat a migraine as early as possible. Don't wait to see if it will really turn into a headache.
- For mild to moderate migraines, try OTC treatment.
- Try a prescription triptan drug for moderate to severe migraines.
- Use prescription Topamax to prevent frequent migraines.
- Prevent menstrual migraines by taking NSAIDs for several days before the expected onset of menses.
- See a doctor if you experience a headache during sex or upon exertion. Serious problems need to be ruled out.
- Take an NSAID before making love to prevent benign sex headache.

HEARTBURN

• Try limiting high-carb foods	
• Stimulate saliva with gum	★★★★
• Sip chamomile or ginger tea	★★★★
• Swallow a little mustard or vinegar	
• Drink baking soda dissolved in water	★★★★
• Chew calcium carbonate antacid	★★★★
• Control acid with Pepcid Complete	★★★
• Suppress acid with Prilosec OTC	★★★

Humans have suffered from heartburn for all of history. Hippocrates warned in 400 BC that eating cheese after a full meal could cause indigestion, especially if accompanied by wine.[380] Centuries ago, doctors called it *dyspepsia*, from Greek words meaning *difficult to digest*. These days, drug companies stress an even scarier name: gastroesophageal reflux disease (GERD).

Whatever you call it, heartburn is unpleasant. It can ruin the memory of a great dining experience. And trying to sleep with a burning sensation in the middle of your chest can be difficult at best and impossible at worst. Reflux can also lead to more serious conditions. The longer irritating stomach contents stay in contact with the delicate tissue of the esophagus, the more damage they do. Repeated exposure to this noxious nastiness can cause scarring, stricture, and abnormal cell growth. Most worrisome of all is the risk of esophageal cancer.

Let's be perfectly clear. Anyone who experiences prolonged bouts of heartburn must be

COMPLICATIONS OF GERD

- Esophageal narrowing (stricture)
- Chronic cough
- Laryngitis
- Asthma
- Pneumonia
- Barrett's esophagus (scarring)
- Esophageal cancer

HEARTBURN OR HEART ATTACK?

Although heartburn is rarely considered a life-threatening condition, there are times when vague upper gastrointestinal tract symptoms indicate a heart attack in progress. This may be especially true for women, who do not always experience "classic" heart attack discomfort. If you have any reason to suspect you're having a heart attack, call 911 and hightail it to the hospital.

seen by a competent gastroenterologist for a thorough workup. This is not a do-it-yourself project!

The underlying cause of GERD is more mysterious than you would think. Commercials for antacids or powerful prescription reflux drugs often blame heartburn on excess stomach acid, as if Mother Nature made a giant mistake. But we're supposed to have acid in our stomachs. Starting some 350 million years ago, virtually all animal species evolved sophisticated systems for creating strong stomach acid.[381] Halibut make hydrochloric acid in their stomachs. So do dogs, cats, cows, birds, frogs, snakes, and salamanders. Just because drug companies have figured out ways to shut down acid production with medications such as omeprazole (Prilosec), lansoprazole (Prevacid), and esomeprazole (Nexium) does not mean this is the only way to combat heartburn.

Stomach acid is essential for digesting food

and facilitating the absorption of certain nutrients. The acid environment in the stomach also creates a barrier against infection. We swallow germs every day from our food and other sources. But it is hard for bacteria to survive in the stomach if there is a hostile acidic environment. Trying to prevent the creation of stomach acid is like fighting back the tide. We're not at all certain that long-term acid suppression is always such a good idea.

Lazy LES

The real cause of heartburn is a lazy muscle at the end of the esophagus (food tube), just above the stomach. Normally, food is chewed, swallowed, and pushed into the stomach past a one-way valve called the lower esophageal sphincter (LES). This muscular sphincter is not supposed to let food or gastric juice (which contains hydrochloric acid and digestive enzymes) back up into the esophagus, where it does not belong.

Imagine that you are holding a balloon filled with air. Just like your stomach, there is more pressure inside the balloon than outside. As long as your fingers tightly pinch the little neck end of the balloon, no air can escape. But if you loosen your grip, air begins to seep out. In the same way, if the LES relaxes, stomach contents can escape into the esophagus. For reasons that are not completely understood, this muscle can lose its contractility and allow reflux to occur. Many medications, including diazepam (Valium), nitroglycerin, and progesterone, may contribute to LES laziness.

Food Fight

People are frequently given lots of advice about what *not* to eat to avoid heartburn. Dietary dogma has it that fatty food is bad news. Cheese, for example, is considered a major problem, just as Hippocrates suggested back around 400 BC. The trouble is, there just haven't been any good studies to prove that fatty foods should be forbidden. Investigators who actually performed a study to determine if a high-fat meal was a culprit came up empty:[382]

> *In summary, our study did not provide evidence for an increase in gastro-oesophageal reflux after fatty foods, at least for the first 3 postprandial [after eating] hours, suggesting that the relationship between fat and induction of heartburn in reflux disease is more complex than commonly thought.*[383]
> —R. Penagini

So fatty foods may not really be as bad as everyone thought, at least in terms of heartburn. Doctors have long believed that many other foods can also make the LES relax and contribute to GERD. But a thoughtful review of the medical literature now calls this belief into question. People suffering from heartburn have been warned to avoid spicy foods, citrus fruits, chocolate, mint, coffee, tea, and alcohol. There is, however, little scientific evidence that avoiding these foods and beverages reduces reflux.[384] If you find that mint or coffee causes you distress, by all means avoid it. If it doesn't bother you, relax and enjoy it. Each person is different, so you may have to keep a food diary and a record of your symptoms to identify your particular nemesis.

Despite the lack of solid scientific evidence, many people maintain that highly acidic foods make them uncomfortable. Things like coffee, tomatoes, citrus juices, colas, sauerkraut, and wine may produce irritation of the stomach and esophagus as well as urinary tract discomfort. Not surprisingly, many folks give up some of their favorite foods because of the unpleasant consequences. Prelief (calcium glycerophosphate) reduces the acid content of such foods and provides elemental calcium. In addition, it may help relieve bladder symptoms associated with acidic foods. Losing weight may also be important in preventing reflux.

Although most physicians warn against fatty foods, they rarely mention carbohydrates. But we have heard from many readers that a typical American high-carb diet can also cause gastric grief.

“Years ago, I was overweight and had high blood pressure. So my doctor put me on a diet. When I reached a plateau, the doctor told me to cut out bread. It worked. I lost the desired amount and my blood pressure normalized.

During this diet, I found that I could eat corn or wheat chips in place of bread and continue to lose weight. I love them, so I ate lots.

Looking back, I began having indigestion about the same time, though I didn't make the connection. This indigestion occurred nearly every evening for several years.

Recently I developed borderline high blood sugar, and my doctor recommended that I cut down on carbohydrates. I cut out the chips completely, and my indigestion disappeared. I don't mean it diminished, I mean it totally stopped. I have not had indigestion since.”

We do not think this reader was imagining things. Many people have told us that when they go on an Atkins- or South Beach-type diet their heartburn disappears. If you search the medical literature, you will discover that as far back as 1972 researchers reported that a low-carb diet was far superior to a “gastric” diet for heartburn relief.[385] In those days a gastric diet was likely bland: low in fat, low in acid, and restricted in coffee and alcohol.

Another small study (2001) confirms these observations. Duke University physicians carefully observed several patients on a low-carbohydrate diet. They reported that “carbohydrates may be a precipitating factor for GERD symptoms and that other classic exacerbating foods such as coffee and fat may be less pertinent when a low-carbohydrate diet is followed.”[386] Follow-up research has produced more provocative data suggesting that a low-carb approach reduces acid splash-back into the esophagus and eases GERD symptoms for overweight patients.[387]

Treating Heartburn

The saying goes that when all you have is a hammer, everything looks like a nail. Drug companies have been very good at developing acid-suppressing drugs, so they have decided that heartburn is a disease of excess acid. Never mind that stomach acid is important in digesting food and serving as a barrier against bacterial infection.

There's another thing drug companies don't mention. Acid is not the only irritating chemical in your stomach. Gastric juice contains a witches' brew of compounds. A digestive enzyme called *pepsin* can be irritating to delicate tissue in the esophagus. Bile acids that aid in digestion get into the esophagus during reflux and can also be quite irritating.[388] And bacteria that flourish in the stomach during acid suppression may create carcinogenic chemicals such as nitrosamines and acetaldehyde.[389]

Since we don't have drugs to neutralize these chemicals, they continue to affect the esophagus during reflux. Because you may not "feel" these nasties the way you feel acid, they are left to silently do damage during usual drug treatment. If the real goal, however, is to keep all these irritating contents of the stomach out of the esophagus, perhaps there are some other tricks to try.

There used to be an interesting drug called cisapride (Propulsid). It worked reasonably well to increase the strength of the lower esophageal sphincter. In addition, the drug helped the stomach empty. These two actions made cisapride a logical choice to fight reflux by keeping stomach contents out of the esophagus. Unfortunately, this medicine had a fatal flaw. It could occasionally cause life-threaten-ing heart rhythms (torsades de pointes), especially when taken with certain other medications. Because the FDA was unsuccessful at keeping physicians and pharmacists from prescribing and dispensing incompatible drugs with cisapride, the feds decided that this heartburn drug needed to be removed from the market.

Another medicine with a somewhat similar effect that has been prescribed for reflux is metoclopramide (Reglan). Unfortunately, it also has some nasty side effects, including drowsiness, dizziness, mental depression, suicidal thoughts, confusion, fatigue, insomnia, headache, hallucinations, and involuntary muscle movements that may sometimes be irreversible. Not surprisingly, Reglan is not one of our favorite drugs.

There is a new prescription heartburn medication that we are quite excited about, though. At the time of this writing it has not been approved for sale in the United States, but it is very popular in Japan and India. Itopride (sold in India as Itoz) appears to be quite effective against symptoms of indigestion (bloating, nausea, fullness, and pain) as well as heartburn.[390, 391]

We are intrigued by this drug because it is a "prokinetic" agent. That means it speeds emptying of food from the stomach and may also enhance muscle tone in the esophagus, helping clear out acid and preventing it from splashing back. It may turn out to be especially beneficial for diabetics, who often have difficulty with "gastric emptying." Unlike cisapride, itopride does not appear to cause irregular heart rhythms. Other side effects are relatively rare, and the drug appears to be well tolerated.

Soothing Heartburn with Saliva

One of the cheapest and most effective remedies for heartburn is produced by our own bodies. It is as simple as spit. We stumbled across this approach in 1984, when researchers reported in the *New England Journal of Medicine* that "residual acid [in the esophagus] is neutralized by swallowed saliva."[392] Not only does saliva buffer acid, swallowing also increased the muscular contractions of the esophagus, moving acid (and other unpleasantness) back into the stomach where it belongs.

Scientists have looked for easy ways to increase saliva production. What they came up with is as simple as chewing sugarless gum.[393,394] More important, however, is whether chewing gum can relieve heartburn. British researchers discovered that chewing

---

★★★★ Saliva

Saliva is free, helps neutralize acid, and washes irritating stomach contents out of the esophagus and back where they belong. There are no side effects or downsides.

Ways to stimulate saliva production: chew sugarless gum or suck on lozenges or something sour.

---

gum could double the flow of saliva and shorten the amount of time the lower esophagus is bathed in acid. They concluded that "chewing gum might be a non-pharmacological treatment option for some patients with symptomatic gastro-oesophageal reflux."[395]

> **Yeah! I finally found out why my "home remedy" works.**
>
> **I'm a nurse and have often given chewing gum to a patient who complains of indigestion. I'd tell them this helps me. It often seemed to help them. Now you've told me what's behind it—thanks!**

Another group of researchers asked patients who suffered from symptoms of heartburn to chew sugarless gum (Orbit) for 30 minutes after eating a high-fat meal. They found that acid was washed out of the lower esophagus much more quickly when people chewed gum. Two-thirds of these patients had significant improvement in their heartburn symptoms. The researchers concluded that "the use of chewing gum with other conservative measures could provide a comparatively safe and effective method of controlling acid reflux and symptoms."[396]

Most people do not know about this incredibly easy and inexpensive remedy because there are no TV commercials promoting the benefits of a pack of gum against heartburn. Chewing gum makers cannot advertise this benefit because they would run afoul of the FDA. And drug companies certainly have nothing to gain if people use chewing gum instead of high-priced acid suppressors. Doctors may not know about the substantial research supporting this home remedy. It may seem wimpy compared to prescribing potent and pricey drugs.

If you walk and chew gum at the same time, you may get a little added benefit. Investigators found that walking after a study breakfast of bacon, eggs, toast, and coffee helped reduce heartburn symptoms among those with reflux.[397] Chewing gum for 1 hour, however, worked even better and the effect lasted longer—3 hours compared to 1 hour for walking. Although the researchers did not combine the two, we think it might be a very sensible approach to take a walk after eating and chew gum at the same time.

Sucking on hard candy also stimulates saliva production. If you really want to liven up your taste buds and create astonishing amounts of saliva, search out the cough lozenges called Fisherman's Friend. These lozenges have been made by Lofthouse of Fleetwood in Lancashire, England, since 1865 (www.fishermansfriend.com). They are all natural and contain menthol, capsicum (essence of hot peppers), eucalyptus oil, and natural licorice. This is an acquired taste, however, and will not be to everyone's liking. Too much licorice for a long time could have negative health consequences. We don't know how much licorice is in Fisherman's Friend. The company also makes a menthol eucalyptus sugar-free chewing gum that might be worth a try.

Tea for Tummy Trouble

Anything that washes stomach acid and other digestive juices out of the esophagus is beneficial. Sipping tea slowly might be just the ticket, especially if the tea is herbal and has calming properties. People have used all sorts of preparations to soothe an upset stomach, including anise seeds, caraway seeds, catnip, lemon balm, licorice, and sage. But our two favorite herbs are chamomile and ginger. They have been used for centuries all around the world to relieve indigestion.

Ginger for the GI Tract

Ginger tea is another excellent option for heartburn. Like chamomile, ginger has a long history of easing nausea and upset stomach. You can make your own pungent brew by getting fresh ginger root and shaving off approximately 1 inch of the "skin." Then grate the

---

★★★★ Chamomile Tea

Renowned for relieving digestive distress, chamomile tea, when sipped slowly, should help rinse away stomach acid and relieve heartburn.

Side effects: Uncommon, but an allergic reaction could lead to rash, stomach cramps, or difficulty breathing
Downside: Allergy to ragweed or chrysanthemums precludes use of chamomile, since it is in the same family.
Cost: Approximately $5 for a month's supply

---

shaved ginger into a mug. Pour boiling water over it and let steep for a few minutes. Strain the liquid through a sieve to remove the grated ginger. Add sweetener and lemon to taste to the tea. If you sip it slowly, this ginger tea will definitely stimulate saliva production and also help wash down any residual acid in the esophagus.

If making your own ginger tea from fresh ginger root sounds like too much work, you might want to try what this reader used:

> *I started having acid reflux in my late fifties. (I am now 64.) For a while, I took over-the-counter acid-controlling drugs with moderate success. After reading in your column about the benefits of ginger tea, I tried a tea I found in the health-food store. Tazo Chai organic spiced black tea contains ginger root, cinnamon bark, black pepper, cardamom seed, cloves, and star anise seed.*
>
> *I drink 1 or 2 cups a day, and the results are phenomenal. I have not had an episode of gastritis or acid reflux in 2 months. In addition, I eliminated alcohol from my diet except for an occasional beer. I also watch what I eat. Your column set the wheels in motion for me.*

Another reader wrote this:

> *My reflux became really bad when I stopped hormone replacement therapy. Acid-suppressing drugs worked great, but after 2 months I couldn't stop them without the heartburn recurring.*
>
> *One night, I took colleagues to dinner at a Korean restaurant. Someone ordered Persimmon Punch, a concentrated cinnamon-ginger drink, for dessert. A few sips later, I felt fantastic.*
>
> *After 1 month of adding about 3 tablespoons of the cinnamon-ginger drink to my tea in the morning and at night, my low-density lipoprotein cholesterol levels had dropped 30 points, blood sugar dropped 10 points, and the heartburn was in control.*
>
> *This cinnamon-ginger tea has sugar, unfortunately. A simpler alternative is to add a piece of candied ginger to tea.*
>
> *The ginger is amazing for heartburn and the Chinese have used it for centuries for motion sickness.*

If tea is not your thing, you may want to opt for other forms of ginger. Readers have shared

★★★★ Ginger

Chinese healers have used ginger for thousands of years. Studies show that it can relieve symptoms of nausea and vomiting associated with motion sickness. It works best if you sip it slowly as a tea or in real ginger ale (Carver's Original or Blenheim). Ginger cookies and candied ginger may also do the job.

Side effects: Allergy is uncommon.
Downside: Those taking blood thinners like warfarin (Coumadin), Plavix, or even aspirin may be more vulnerable to bleeding.
Cost: Approximately $5 to $8 for a month's supply of ginger tea

that candied ginger relieved reflux and "stomach burn" just as well as acid-suppressing drugs. And while we cannot endorse eating the carbs found in cookies, we found this report intriguing: "Since I have had a problem with Prevacid, I tried ginger, both in ginger snaps and as crystallized ginger. It's been working like a charm."

Mustard for Heartburn?

Just about the last thing we would ever consider for heartburn is mustard. It seems like a spicy food would only make matters worse. And yet enough people have shared their enthusiasm for mustard that we cannot ignore this odd remedy.

> *My husband and I use a teaspoon of yellow mustard to relieve heartburn. I was in a chat room a while ago when one of the chatters complained about her heartburn. Another said, "Try mustard." We all thought this was ludicrous, but she did try it and it helped.*
>
> *The next time my husband had one of his terrible roll-on-the-floor-in-agony bouts of heartburn, I suggested mustard. I figured it couldn't hurt any more than what he already had. Amazingly, it worked, faster than Tums or DiGel. Our friends have had good results also.*

Some folks are not going to be able to stomach mustard. The spiciness is just too much for them. But mustard may stimulate saliva and work in a similar manner as chewing gum. When we checked with one of the world's leading experts on herbs, James Duke, PhD, he suggested that turmeric, the spice that makes mustard yellow, has ingredients that are beneficial for the digestive tract.

• • •

Q. *I was interested in your column about the person who used yellow mustard for indigestion. I want to provide some positive feedback: I tried the mustard remedy for indigestion over the last couple of days and am amazed and delighted that it works!*

A. You are not the only one who has remarked on this home remedy:

"I was fascinated to read that someone else takes yellow mustard for heartburn. I stumbled onto this remedy myself years ago: I noticed several things that often caused me heartburn. But when I put mustard on them, I was fine. Now when I experience heartburn, I put some yellow mustard on Saltines and get relief."

• • •

Vinegar

If you think mustard makes no sense for heartburn, then you will think we are totally crazy to mention vinegar. After all, drug companies have been promoting antacids and acid-suppressing drugs for decades. Consuming acid (vinegar is acetic acid) would seem like the last thing one would want to do when dealing with heartburn. Of course, that assumes that acid somehow contributes to reflux. But if the theory is wrong, then perhaps this remedy might have some merit.

> *A doctor advised a family friend to take a tablespoon of vinegar for heartburn relief. I tried 2 teaspoons of apple cider vinegar and it worked. It tastes strong for a few minutes and I thought the heartburn was worse. Then the pain went away for good.*

We admit that it sounds strange, but others have shared similar success. We would discourage anyone from sipping pure apple cider vinegar however. It's just way too strong. Perhaps diluting it in water would make it easier to swallow. One reader offered something even more bizarre than dilute vinegar. She combined vinegar and baking soda, which seems counterintuitive. But who knows, it might help someone.

• • •

> **Q.** *I used to have real bad heartburn until I remembered a home remedy my mother used to make. I mix a couple ounces of water, an ounce of apple cider vinegar, and a teaspoon of sugar until the sugar dissolves. Then I add half a teaspoon of baking soda, stir it briefly and drink immediately. This offers fast relief.*

A. Thanks for an inexpensive remedy for heartburn. Baking soda is a time-honored approach to neutralizing stomach acid that has splashed into the esophagus and is causing heartburn.

• • •

If apple cider vinegar seems just too strange for you, maybe an apple a day could keep reflux at bay. At least that's what we have heard.

> *Recently I have had terrible episodes of acid reflux. I have tried raising the top of our bed, not eating 3 hours before going to sleep, and cutting out citrus, tomato products, caffeine, and alcohol. But nothing worked.*
>
> *My doctor gave me a prescription for Nexium, but before I tried it, someone told me that an apple helps acid reflux. I had a bag of apples in my refrigerator, so I decided to try this approach. I ate the apple with the peel right after dinner and to my amazement I did not have any heartburn that night. I have been eating an apple every night for the past 10 nights and have not had one episode of heartburn.*

We have no scientific explanation for why apples, apple cider vinegar, or even lemon juice in water might be helpful against heartburn. They probably won't work for everyone, but some people report benefit. They are inexpensive and worth a try just on the off chance that they might do the trick.

Hot Peppers for Indigestion?

If mustard and vinegar seem too scary for you, please skip this section. Although people who frequently suffer from indigestion are usually advised to avoid spicy food, some pepperheads maintain that hot peppers don't trigger stomach upset. They insist that the "burn" may actually be beneficial. And they may be right. There is some research suggesting that capsaicin (the hot stuff in hot chile peppers) can protect the stomach lining.[398]

• • •

Q. *My brother-in-law is addicted to hot peppers. He puts Tabasco on everything, and I can't figure out how he avoids heartburn. Spicy foods give me indigestion, but he claims hot peppers are good for the stomach. Is he nuts?*

A. Your brother-in-law actually has some science on his side. Italian researchers wrote a letter to the *New England Journal of Medicine*[399] reporting that red pepper powder in capsules reduced indigestion symptoms (stomachache, fullness, and nausea) by 60 percent. In this small, double-blind, placebo-controlled study, a look-alike placebo reduced these symptoms by only half as much. The researchers concluded that "although larger trials with standardized materials are needed, capsaicin could represent a potential

therapy for functional dyspepsia."[400]

Capsaicin is the ingredient in hot peppers that is believed to be responsible for this effect. It is used in topical creams to relieve pain. A study in rats demonstrated that capsaicin can reduce damage to the stomach lining that aspirin or alcohol causes.[401]

• • •

Baking Soda

One of the oldest, cheapest, fastest, and most effective treatments for heartburn is plain old baking soda. The chemical name is *bicarbonate of soda*, and it has been used for thousands of years as a leavening agent to make bread rise.

★★★★ Baking Soda

The label on the familiar Arm & Hammer Baking Soda box recommends that you dissolve ½ teaspoon of powder in ½ glass (4 ounces) of water and take every 2 hours, or as directed by a physician. Do not take more than 7½ teaspoons in 24 hours. If you are over 60 years of age, do not take more than 3½ teaspoons in 24 hours. Do not use the maximum dosage for more than 2 weeks.

Downside: High in sodium (616 milligrams in ½ teaspoon). Not safe for those with high blood pressure or congestive heart failure or for anyone on a sodium-restricted diet.
Cost: Approximately 1 cent per dose. A 2-pound box contains roughly 373 doses.

That's because it is alkaline and reacts with acid to produce carbon dioxide. The antiacid action is why "bicarb" also helps ease symptoms of "sour stomach" or indigestion.

As long as you are not on a low-sodium diet, it is hard to beat baking soda for treating occasional indigestion or heartburn. One big warning, though. *Do not use* baking soda if you have really stuffed yourself. There are several reports in the medical literature of "spontaneous rupture of the normal stomach after sodium bicarbonate ingestion."[402]

We will never forget the story of the man who blew a hole in his stomach after swallowing baking soda. He had eaten a large Mexican meal and followed it with bicarb. The resulting buildup of carbon dioxide gas had no place to go because his stomach was too full. He survived after emergency surgery, but we do not want anyone else to repeat his experience.

• • •

Q. I have tried almost every nonprescription product for occasional acid reflux, and have also taken Prilosec. Nothing works as quickly and dependably as plain baking soda in water.

I've been told that regular use of this remedy can be harmful, but a medical newsletter I read recommends it. If it is not good to use regularly, can you use it occasionally?

A. Baking soda (sodium bicarbonate) is one of the cheapest, fastest, and most effective antacids available. It has been used to relieve heartburn for more than 100 years.

Its one drawback is its high sodium content. For salt-sensitive individuals, this can raise blood pressure. That's why baking soda should be reserved for occasional use.

• • •

Alka-Seltzer

We used to think that Alka-Seltzer was one of the more irrational remedies in the drugstore. That is because it contains both aspirin and bicarbonate of soda. In the original edition of *The People's Pharmacy*, published more than 30 yeas ago, we said, "If you have indigestion or upset stomach, the last thing you want is aspirin included in the tablet. That is like trying to put out a fire with gasoline."

We may have been wrong. It's not just that millions of people have used this product successfully for decades. This tablet of aspirin (325 milligrams), bicarbonate of soda (1,916 milligrams), and citric acid (1,000 milligrams) is converted into sodium citrate when it fizzes in a glass of water. This antacid seems to provide fast and effective relief of "acid indigestion, upset stomach, and heartburn." What we don't know is whether Alka-Seltzer is any more effective than a half-teaspoon of baking soda in 4 ounces of water when it comes to heartburn symptoms.

Q. *Allow me to tell you about my experience with heartburn, which I have had for a very long time. Last year I started using a toothpaste which contains baking soda. Since then my heartburn is gone. If I change toothpaste the heartburn comes back, so it's not a coincidence.*

I brush my teeth three times a day. Even though I don't swallow the toothpaste I think a little of it gets into my stomach and the baking soda neutralizes the stomach acid. Could that be true?

A. Baking soda (half a teaspoon in 4 ounces of water) is a tried and true remedy for heartburn. Alka-Seltzer, long used for stomach upset, contains sodium bicarbonate, the compound in baking soda. Whether you'd get enough baking soda from your toothpaste to actually neutralize stomach acid is hard to tell, but thanks for sharing your success.

• • •

Antacids

For the occasional bout of heartburn, antacids work surprisingly well. In fact, they may be better than pricey acid suppressors. That's because it takes hours to shut down acid production. If you go to the ballpark and gobble down two chili dogs, chase them with beer,

★★★★ **Calcium Carbonate**

Calcium carbonate is inexpensive, fast-acting, and effective. In addition, you get extra calcium.

Downside: Constipation is fairly common if used regularly.

Cost: A bottle containing 160 tablets of Tums Ultra (1,000 mg calcium carbonate per pill) costs $8 to $10. That should be enough to last 2 to 3 months or much longer if used occasionally.

and have Cracker Jack for dessert, you don't want to wait hours for your acid suppressor to go to work. Popping a Tums E-X, Maalox Quick Dissolve, or Rolaids Extra Strength can be safe and effective. That's because they all contain calcium carbonate, which neutralizes stomach acid. There are lots of such products to choose from, so pick something that tastes tolerable and isn't too pricey.

• • •

Q. *I have never seen you recommend calcium carbonate for heartburn. Why? You keep suggesting sodium bicarbonate, even though it introduces too much sodium into the body. Calcium carbonate, on the other hand, provides much-needed calcium. What is your problem?*

A. We agree that calcium carbonate (Caltrate, Titralac, Tums, etc.) is an

excellent, inexpensive antacid that can quickly ease heartburn and supply extra calcium. We've recommended it for decades.

• • •

Don't forget Pepto-Bismol. We think the familiar pink liquid also has some benefit. The active ingredient, bismuth subsalicylate, can be found generically in store brands and in Maalox Total Stomach Relief Liquid. While not a very powerful antacid, Pepto does seem to calm the fire of heartburn through mechanisms we may not understand very well. Perhaps it coats the esophagus and helps reduce the irritating effects of acid reflux. There are even decent data to suggest that bismuth subsalicylate can help against traveler's diarrhea. When it is combined with antibiotics, Pepto-Bismol can help fight infection by the bacterium *Helicobacter pylori*, which leads to gastritis and stomach ulcers.

Acid Suppressors

The mainstays for treating indigestion or heartburn are acid suppressors. That's because pharmaceutical companies have become extremely adept at creating such drugs. In the 1960s a team of scientists led by an extraordinary researcher (Sir James Black) hypothesized that if they could block specialized histamine receptors (H_2 receptors) in the stomach, they could reduce acid production.

Histamine$_2$ Antagonists

When drug companies thought about antihistamines, they focused on relieving allergy symptoms in the nose. But Sir James thought he could come up with a new kind of antihistamine that would work primarily in the stomach. In 1972 the breakthrough was announced, and in 1977 cimetidine (Tagamet) became the first H_2 antagonist launched in the United States. It went on to become one of the most successful drugs in history. Like its successor ranitidine (Zantac), Tagamet was one of the first billion-dollar babies (with annual sales of greater than $1 billion).

Although these acid suppressors were initially prescribed to help heal stomach ulcers, they rapidly became popular as super antacids. Any amorphous abdominal pain was treated with an H_2 antagonist. Their success was noted by other drug companies, and "me-too" drugs like famotidine (Pepcid) and nizatidine (Axid) soon appeared. Such drugs were perceived as so safe that once they lost their patent protection, the FDA approved them for over-the-counter sale. Although these drugs can relieve heartburn by making stomach contents less acidic, they are not as fast-acting as antacids.

• • •

Q. *I had two hip replacement surgeries in my mid-forties. I was given cimetidine (Tagamet) to prevent stress ulcers post-op for the first one and it gave me* *very nasty hallucinations. I had already withdrawn myself from the pain medications, and the staff assured me nothing I was taking could induce these things. When the surgeon stopped the Tagamet, the nasties went away.*

For the second operation, I listed cimetidine as a drug problem, but they gave it to me anyway. I knew within an hour something was seriously wrong and fortunately didn't have to take any more.

I was assured that the incidence of problems is low, but I'd hate for others to go through what I experienced.

A. Cimetidine (Tagamet) has been linked to hallucinations, depression, confusion, and disorientation. Such psychological side effects are relatively rare, but people need to know that they can occur.

● ● ●

There are not enough data to recommend one H_2 antagonist over another. They are all roughly comparable in effectiveness. Side effects are generally uncommon. Cimetidine may cause a slightly higher incidence of headache, sexual difficulties, and mental confusion or disorientation than some of the other drugs in this class. This usually only happens at high doses or in older or sicker patients. Other possible side effects associated with H_2 antagonists

may include dizziness, fatigue, diarrhea, and constipation.

Interactions are a bigger issue with medications like cimetidine. This acid suppressor can cause mischief when combined with many other drugs, including alcohol. It is crucial that anyone using such acid suppressors check with both a physician and a pharmacist for any incompatibilities.

● ● ●

Q. *I have been on either Tagamet or Zantac for years. I have a hiatal hernia that causes severe heartburn.*

Over the last 2 years I find that I start to feel "tight" after a single beer. I used to drink two or even three beers on a hot day after 18 holes of golf with no problem. Now with just one beer I feel too impaired to drive.

Could these heartburn medicines have that effect? I used to be able to hold my booze with the best of them. Because of this I am loath to even take a drink at a party.

A. You have raised a fascinating issue. More than a decade ago, alcohol expert Charles Lieber, MD, reported that cimetidine (Tagamet) and ranitidine (Zantac) could increase blood alcohol concentrations in susceptible people. He told his colleagues that such interactions "may result in unexpected impairment to perform complex tasks, such as driving. Thus, patients treated with these drugs should be warned of this possible side effect."[403]

More recently Dr. Lieber warned, "Under conditions mimicking social drinking, ranitidine increases blood alcohol to levels known to impair psychomotor skills needed for driving."[404]

• • •

If we had to pick one over-the-counter (OTC) acid suppressor to relieve heartburn, we would probably opt for Pepcid Complete. The reason is that this medication combines the H_2 antagonist famotidine (10 milligrams) with calcium carbonate (800 milligrams) and magnesium hydroxide (165 milligrams). Putting these three ingredients together means that you get the immediate benefit of fast-acting antacids (calcium carbonate and mag-

nesium hydroxide) plus longer-acting acid suppression with famotidine.

Proton Pump Inhibitors (PPIs)

The most powerful acid suppressors available are called proton pump inhibitors (PPIs). This class of medications has been incredibly successful for the pharmaceutical industry, which has done well with graphic commercials featuring a cartoon stomach or "The Purple Pill." Over 70 million prescriptions are written annually for these drugs at a cost of almost $10 billion.[405]

Starting with omeprazole (Prilosec), drug companies have created a series of compounds that are capable of dramatically changing the acid environment of the stomach. Such action is extremely helpful for curing ulcers. It can also help relieve reflux. But there is growing concern that long-term acid suppression may have some unexpected and potentially unpleasant consequences.

Acid is important in the stomach. For one thing, it creates an inhospitable environment. Germs have a hard time surviving in acid.

★★★ Pepcid Complete

Pepcid Complete combines immediate action with longer-lasting acid control.

Downside: Side effects are uncommon but nevertheless, be vigilant for allergy, jaundice, headache, constipation, dizziness, or diarrhea. **Cost:** $17 to $20 for 50 pills. Should last several months. Short-term use should be safe. Long-term use should be approved and monitored by a physician.

PROTON PUMP INHIBITORS

- Esomeprazole (Nexium)
- Lansoprazole (Prevacid)
- Omeprazole (Prilosec)
- Pantoprazole (Protonix)
- Rabeprazole (Aciphex)

★★★ Prilosec OTC (omeprazole)

For years Prilosec was the most prescribed drug in the country. The active ingredient, omeprazole, did not lose its effectiveness when it went over the counter.

Downside: Side effects are uncommon, but headache, diarrhea, rash, cough, and upper respiratory tract infections have been noted. Rare but very serious side effects may include blood disorders, inflammation of the pancreas, liver problems, and severe skin reactions.

Special Cautions: Use Prilosec OTC for only 2 weeks at a time. According to the information on the label, you can repeat another 14-day course after 4 months have elapsed. Prolonged use of prescription proton pump inhibitors may require vitamin B_{12} supplementation (up to 1 milligram daily). Extra vitamin C (500 milligrams) and vitamin E (200 IU) may reduce the possible formation of carcinogens (nitrosamines).

Cost: $30 to $40 for 42 pills (1 year's supply)

Studies published in the *Journal of the American Medical Association* have suggested that constantly suppressing stomach acid may increase the risk of pneumonia and severe infectious diarrhea.[406,407] Presumably, this is because bacteria not killed by stomach acid can work their way up through the esophagus and get into the lungs or work their way down and infect the lower digestive tract. Such serious infections can be life threatening.

PPIS AND CANCER

The really big elephant in the room with the PPIs is a fear of cancer. For years there has been a quiet controversy brewing regarding a possible relationship between acid suppression and the risk of cancer. In 1985 we wrote: "Scientists fear that if bacteria set up housekeeping in your stomach, they can go to work converting nitrate to nitrite. . . . Nitrate is a chemical which can come from food, water, or even saliva; by itself it probably does little harm. But if nitrate is turned into nitrite by bacteria, all hell can break loose, because the end product can be something very bad indeed—nitrosamines. Nitrosamines are among the most potent cancer-causing chemicals known."[408]

Over the last several decades there has been an alarming increase in what was once a rare kind of esophageal cancer. Adenocarcinoma of the esophagus has turned into an epidemic.[409] Gastroenterologists are mystified about the causes of this deadly condition. Some have told us that it's brought on by the American diet. Others blame it on reflux and insist that PPIs can solve the problem by reducing acid exposure to delicate tissues. Has reflux really increased that much in the last couple of decades, and if so, why?

A provocative editorial that appeared in the *American Journal of Gastroenterology* entitled

"Acid Suppression and Adenocarcinoma of the Esophagus: Cause or Cure?" lays out the confusion and the contradictions.[410] Thomas Schell, MD, points out that "decreasing acid reflux by the use of PPIs might help to slow or halt this deadly progression." But he also reminds his colleagues that lack of acid in the stomach (*achlorhydria*) "is a known risk factor for adenocarcinoma of the stomach." Dr. Schell notes that nitrosamines formed by bacteria in the stomach "would also expose the esophagus to these carcinogens."

There are three other disconcerting problems linked to long-term use of PPIs. When the stomach ceases to produce acid, it senses that something has gone terribly awry and it tries desperately to get acid-producing cells working again. It does so by making a compound called gastrin, which aids in digestion and also triggers the production of stomach acid. When acid levels do not rise, gastrin production continues indefinitely, often at very high levels.

Imagine that the float device in your toilet was stuck in the "on" position. The water would keep running forever, which is what happens with gastrin in your stomach. There is no acid "float" to turn off the gastrin supply.

Too much gastrin is not a good thing. In fact, there is increasing concern that gastrin may stimulate abnormal cell growth throughout the digestive tract, increasing the risk of cancers of the stomach, pancreas, and colon, as well as the esophagus.[411,412]

Another concern about long-term treatment with PPIs has to do with nutrient absorption. It is harder to absorb vitamin B_{12}, iron, and calcium when there is not enough acid in the stomach. Older people may have some trouble getting enough vitamin B_{12} or iron under normal conditions. With a PPI on board, this may be an even greater challenge.[413] A vitamin B_{12} deficiency can lead to some very serious consequences. Symptoms may include anemia, fatigue, nerve damage (burning, tingling, weakness, or numbness in the hands and feet), difficulty in sensing vibration, unsteadiness, shortness of breath, and psychological side effects. Depression, confusion, and poor memory may be mistaken for early-onset Alzheimer's disease.

●●●

Q. *I have taken Prilosec and then Prevacid for years to treat severe heartburn. When I began to suffer weakness and confusion, I started taking 1,000 micrograms of vitamin B_{12} daily. Within a relatively short time, the horrible symptoms began to subside.*

My doctor does not really see the relationship, but I sure do! What can you tell me about this side effect?

A. Long-term suppression of stomach acid can sometimes interfere with efficient absorption of vitamin B_{12}. This nutritional deficiency can cause ner-

vous system problems, which may show up as insomnia, memory problems, depression, burning tongue, sore mouth, difficulty walking, and tingling or numbness in feet or fingers.

One reader reported a conversation with a nurse who noticed an amazing improvement in a woman with dementia after a vitamin B_{12} deficiency was discovered and treated.

• • •

This vitamin deficiency often appears very gradually. Patients may describe complaints such as mental fuzziness, a sensation of burning on the tongue, or poor coordination for months or even years before a proper diagnosis is made. Anyone who has been on PPIs for many months (or years) should request a blood test for iron and vitamin B_{12}. It's not enough to just look for vitamin B_{12}, though. Be sure to be tested for serum cobalamin (that is vitamin B_{12}) and methylmalonic acid (MMA). When MMA is elevated and cobalamin is low, that is an indication of a probable vitamin B_{12} deficiency.

PPI ADDICTION?

Another unspoken concern among some gastroenterologists is PPI-induced "physical dependence."[414] That's a nice way of saying addiction. Now, no one is getting high on PPIs. But some people may find it difficult to quit taking such medications once they start down the long and winding road of acid suppression.

Here's the sad story. Proton pump inhibitors like omeprazole (Prilosec), esomeprazole (Nexium), and lansoprazole (Prevacid) are so effective at shutting down acid production that the body seems to rebel. As previously noted, gastrin is produced in large quantities, and it stimulates cell growth. These are cells that want to make acid, but PPIs prevent them from doing their job. They proliferate, though, and if the PPI is stopped, they start churning out acid to make up for lost time. The consequence is something called "rebound acid hypersecretion." This means the body really starts generating excess acid when these drugs are discontinued.

What's so insidious is that it takes several days for the effect to show up. So someone might be fine for a while, but within 2 weeks of stopping a PPI there is maximal acid production from stomach cells.[415] And here's the kicker. This rebound hyperacidity effect lasts for more than 2 months.[416]

Dear reader, this is nothing short of astonishing. Think about it for just a moment. Tens of millions of people have spent billions of dollars on acid-suppressing medications for years and years to soothe the fires in their upper gastrointestinal tract. But Mother Nature does not forgive or forget. No sooner are the drugs discontinued than she turns on the acid-making machinery and puts the pedal to the metal for months.

Within a few days of stopping the medicine, someone with indigestion or heartburn is likely to feel the effect. Not surprisingly, the first thing people experiencing rebound hyperacidity are likely to do is reach for their PPI. According to Norwegian researchers, "Discontinuing treatment may prove difficult in some patients even if the dose of proton pump inhibitor is slowly tapered. . . . In these cases the use of high doses of H$_2$-receptor antagonists or antacids should be considered."[417] From a drug company's perspective, PPIs could be the perfect pills. As long as people take them, they feel pretty good. But if they stop, they could be punished for a very long time. That's strong motivation to beg the doctor for more medicine—indefinitely.

So, what's a person to do? Well, our recommendation would be to be cautious. These drugs are great for short periods of time. They control symptoms of heartburn quite well and have relatively few side effects. If a doctor recommends that you take a PPI for longer than 2 or 3 months, though, be prepared for rebound hyperacidity when you stop the medicine.[418]

Conclusions

Persistent symptoms of pain, burning, or pressure behind the breastbone should be investigated by a doctor to rule out a serious condition. For an occasional attack of indigestion, however, there are lots of things you need to consider. Before pulling out the heavy artillery of acid-suppressing drugs, there are many options to contemplate. Here is a quick snapshot:

- Avoid foods or drugs that might make the lower esophageal sphincter lazy and let gastric juice creep back into the esophagus. There are few good studies, but some possible culprits include chocolate, carbonated beverages, smoking, diazepam, and progesterone.

- Cut back on carbs. Although the data are preliminary, there is some suggestion that the typical high-carbohydrate American diet may be contributing to reflux.

- Keep your eyes on itopride. This prescription drug works differently than acid-suppressing drugs to relieve indigestion and heartburn. Its success in Japan and India and a fascinating report in the *New England Journal of Medicine* (February 23, 2006) have us looking forward to FDA approval.

- Saliva is the body's natural buffering agent and fire extinguisher for heartburn. Chewing gum or sucking on hard candy can help relieve symptoms.

- Chamomile or ginger tea also can wash acid out of the esophagus and back into the stomach where it belongs. These traditional remedies also may help calm an upset stomach.

- Home remedies such as sipping diluted apple cider vinegar or even swallowing yellow mustard may help. Each person is different, though, so trial and error will be the only way to find out if a home remedy will work for you.

- Baking soda remains a time-honored solution for occasional heartburn. Dissolve ½ teaspoon of powder in 4 ounces of water. For those on sodium-restricted diets because of congestive heart failure or high blood pressure, this is not an option.

• If you need an antacid, calcium carbonate remains one of the cheapest and most effective in the pharmacy. Tums Ultra contains 1,000 milligrams of calcium carbonate and is a cost-effective option.

• In our opinion, a sensible first choice for an OTC acid-suppressing drug is Pepcid Complete. It combines the immediate action of antacids (calcium carbonate and magnesium hydroxide) with the longer-acting H_2 antagonist famotidine. Short-term use should be safe.

• If you feel you must take a powerful acid-suppressing PPI, we would opt for Prilosec OTC. If you have great insurance coverage, you might save money if your doctor prescribes generic omeprazole instead. We think a little vitamin insurance is appropriate whenever acid-suppressing drugs are taken for any length of time (vitamin B_{12}, vitamin C, and vitamin E).

HEART DISEASE AND HIGH CHOLESTEROL

• Use olive oil in cooking and on salads	★★★★★
• Try limiting high-carb foods	
• Ask your MD about taking 160 milligrams of aspirin	★★★★★
• Consider taking fish oil	★★★★★
• Combine grape juice and Certo	★★★★★
• Drink pomegranate juice	★★★★★
• Nibble walnuts four or five times a week	★★★★★
• Treat yourself to a little dark chocolate	★★★
• Take niacin to lower cholesterol	★★★
• Consider taking magnesium to prevent atherosclerosis	★★★★
• Experiment with coenzyme Q_{10}	★★★
• Swallow psyllium three times a day	★★★
• Try red yeast rice	★★★
• Ask your doctor about statins	★★★★
• If statins cause trouble, ask about Zetia	★★★
• Ask about fibrate alternatives such as TriCor	★★★
• Ask about the bile acid binder WelChol	★★

Despite the billions of dollars spent each year on cholesterol-lowering drugs, heart disease remains our country's number one killer. More than 650,000 Americans—about one person every minute—die annually from a "coronary event."[419] More than 1 million people will have a heart attack this year, and 175,000 probably will not even realize that they suffered "silent" damage to the heart muscle.[420]

Although these stats may seem overwhelming, we are making some progress. Deaths from heart disease have been trending downward over the last 30 years.[421] That's the good news. The bad news is that even though the trend is in the right direction, you or someone you know is at great risk of dying of heart disease. According to the Centers for Disease Control and Prevention, one out of every three adults (71,300,000) has cardiovascular disease.[422]

So what can you do to avoid having a heart attack? If you watch the ads for cholesterol-lowering drugs like Lipitor (atorvastatin), Crestor (rosuvastatin), and Zocor (simvastatin), you would think that about the only thing that matters is getting your cholesterol under 200. For decades Americans have been told that cholesterol is the most important risk factor for heart disease. The cholesterol theory evolved from experiments carried out in the middle of the 20th century. Scientists found they could force rabbits to develop plaque in their arteries by feeding them butter and cheese. As a result of this research, fat was vilified, and most physicians forbade eggs because the yolks were high in cholesterol. Eating eggs, in fact, became tantamount to a sin. Needless to say, eating butter or steak was even worse.

All of these recommendations were presented as if they were chiseled in stone. The health gurus set them forth as facts rather than articles of faith. Millions of people gave up eggs and started eating high-carbohydrate breakfasts consisting of cereal, toast, or pancakes. They thought they were protecting themselves from heart disease. Now it turns out that most, if not all, of these dietary guidelines were built on a foundation of shifting sand.

Cholesterol Conundrum

The late Robert Atkins was ostracized when he challenged the low-fat, high-carb orthodoxy. Cardiologists condemned his high-protein weight-loss diet, which included eggs, bacon, and steak. They were sure cholesterol levels would skyrocket if people ate such sinful food.

When scientists actually did the research on healthy people, they could find no problem associated with people consuming cholesterol. The conclusion: "Analyses of several studies have also failed to find an association between the incidence of CHD [coronary heart disease] and egg consumption."[423] If anything, eating eggs converts more dangerous LDL cholesterol into a less hazardous form.[424,425]

Far more heretical than the discovery that eggs posed no problem for healthy people was the observation that an Atkins-type diet did not lead to hellfire and brimstone. Research published in the prestigious *Annals of Internal Medicine* reported that "over 24 weeks, a low-carbohydrate diet program led to greater weight loss, reduction in serum triglyceride level, and increase in HDL [good] cholesterol level compared with a low-fat diet."[426] For this particular study, participants were permitted unlimited amounts of animal foods (meat, fowl, fish, and shellfish), unlimited eggs, 4 ounces of hard cheese, 2 cups of salad vegetables (such as lettuce, spinach, or celery), and 1 cup of low-carbohydrate vegetables (such as broccoli, cauliflower, or squash) daily.[427]

Other studies have also demonstrated that a low-carbohydrate, high-protein, high-fat Atkins-type diet can have a beneficial impact on blood fats.[428,429,430] In one of the most astonishing experiments ever conducted, overweight patients with existing cardiovascular disease were switched from a diet that was low in saturated fats and cholesterol to a diet that was high in saturated fats and cholesterol and devoid of starches. They continued taking their statin medications with no change in dose.

Before the experiment, these patients followed their cardiologists' instructions to eat no more than two eggs a week and restrict red meat to less than three servings a week. During the 6-week experiment, they were to eat

> "We need to acknowledge that diverse healthy populations experience no risk in developing coronary heart disease by increasing their intake of cholesterol, but, in contrast, they may have multiple beneficial effects by the inclusion of eggs in their regular diet."[431]
>
> —M. L. Fernandez, *Current Opinion in Clinical Nutrition and Metabolic Care*, 2006

two to four eggs daily and half a pound of red meat at each meal. Such a study seems almost unethical, if not immoral. But surprisingly, this high-saturated-fat, no-starch diet led to decreases in body weight without increasing total cholesterol or bad LDL cholesterol. Triglycerides came down and, if anything, the overall lipid profile improved.[432]

> *Three years ago, my husband was up to 217 pounds. (He's 48 years old and 6 feet tall.) His cholesterol levels were off the charts, and his triglycerides were 942. His doctor tried him on several cholesterol-lowering medications. He could not tolerate the side effects, especially the memory loss.*
>
> *He then went on the Atkins diet and quickly dropped 20 to 25 pounds. To his doctor's amazement, his triglycerides dropped to 192, and his cholesterol is almost normal—without medication.*
>
> *Please keep your readers posted on further studies. I thought he was nuts to go on that diet until I saw the results. Now I follow some of its principles as well.*

The most telling study actually compared four popular diets: Atkins, Zone, Weight

Watchers, and Ornish. Conventional wisdom would predict that the low-fat Dean Ornish diet would beat every other diet hands down on the heart disease risk score. Au contraire. All of these diets were roughly comparable in helping people lose weight.[433] Many cardiologists were shocked to learn, however, that those following a high-protein, low-carbohydrate regimen ended up with a better score on heart disease risk factors than those following an Ornish-type low-fat, high-carbohydrate diet. That is because the higher-fat diets raised good HDL cholesterol more than the Ornish approach.

The final nail in the coffin of dietary dogma should have been driven by the Women's Health Initiative. This long-term research project cost more than $700 million and will likely never be repeated. Until this ambitious project, we relied mostly on observational studies: Ask people what they eat and see what happens to them. It is not a very good technique for actually proving whether something works or is dangerous. People have notoriously bad memories about what they really eat.

At the end of the 20th century, scientists decided to test their theories in a giant experiment. More than 48,000 women over 50 years old were recruited into a dietary intervention trial. Some (40 percent) of the women were instructed to reduce the amount of fat in their diet, replacing it with extra vegetables, fruits, and grains. The training took place in groups and individually, and the women made the suggested dietary changes. The other 60 per-

cent of the women were not asked to change the way they ate.

After approximately 8 years of follow-up and massive number crunching, the results are in, and they're disappointing. The researchers had expected that women who adopted the more virtuous low-fat, high-veggie diet would be protected from heart attacks, strokes, breast cancer, and colorectal cancer. But despite the large number of women participating, the differences in the results of the two groups were not statistically significant.[434]

For cardiovascular disease, the investigators found a trend favoring survival in women who ate the least amount of saturated fat and trans fatty acids (and the most vegetables). But a trend is hardly the kind of solid evidence policy makers need before they recommend major changes in a country's diet. These results were certainly not expected. The granola gurus were left scratching their heads, wondering what went wrong. They did their best to explain why the low-fat diet was a giant fizzle, but the answers were unsatisfying and could not counteract the loss of trust by the American public.

Cardiologists, internists, registered dietitians, and most other health professionals like to maintain that they follow "evidence-based medicine." In other words, science, not supposition, is their motto. But when data don't match dietary dogma, they frequently are ignored. That's what happened with MRFIT (the Multiple Risk Factor Intervention Trial). Until the Women's Health Initiative, MRFIT was the largest (nearly 13,000 men were recruited) and most expensive ($100 million was spent) study of lifestyle intervention.

In the early 1970s, these men were divided into two groups. One got "special intervention," which meant intensive counseling and follow-up to modify diet (by lowering saturated fat and cholesterol intake) and control blood pressure. The others got no special attention. After 6 years, there was no significant difference between the two groups of men in terms of heart attacks or deaths. The unexpected MRFIT findings matched those of the later Women's Health Initiative. This study sank without a trace. If the facts don't fit our preconceived notions, perhaps we need to reexamine our faith in the low-fat approach.

No one is suggesting that a high-calorie, high-fat diet of eggs and bacon, burgers and shakes, steaks and fries, and hot fudge sundaes is good for health. And we're not particularly fans of the high-protein Atkins approach. But the dietary changes that seemed so obviously beneficial in the early 1990s can no longer be treated as gospel.

Perhaps we should take a tip from the French. They have pretty much ignored our low-fat fanaticism. They continue to eat croissants, butter, brie, and chocolate mousse without a second thought. They get more exercise by walking and climbing stairs. They eat well, but not nearly as much as Americans. And they make meals social occasions to be savored with a glass of wine. Following their example of moderation might do us all some good.

Despite our national obsession with fighting fat, we weigh far more than the French, and our incidence of heart disease is much higher.

Types of Fat

By now we hope we have convinced you that eating fat or cholesterol does not necessarily raise your own cholesterol levels or even your risk of heart disease. There are exceptions, of course. Some people do react to dietary fat. For them, cutting back may be helpful. As with everything, though, you must pay attention to your body and monitor your lipid levels. The real issue is not how much fat you eat but what kind.

Walter Willett, MD, DrPH, MPH, is chair of the Department of Nutrition at the Harvard School of Public Health. Dr. Willett is arguably the most respected and knowledgeable nutrition expert and epidemiologist in the world. For a very long time he has tried to convince his colleagues and the public that the "fat is bad" belief is baloney. It has been an uphill struggle, but at last the tide is turning. His campaign against trans fats (hydrogenated vegetable oil) has led to labeling that will allow consumers to recognize and avoid this poison. Although trans fats have been removed from many margarines, you still will find them in lots of processed foods like crackers and cookies. They are also found at high levels in many fried fast foods.

The reason trans fats are so dangerous is that they are associated with an increased risk of heart disease. That may be because they are pro-inflammatory. So are many of the omega-6 fats (found in vegetable oils such as corn, safflower, and sunflower oil). Even though dietitians have been proclaiming that all cholesterol-free vegetable oils are heart healthy, we beg to differ. There is growing evidence that Americans consume way too much omega-6 and not nearly enough omega-3 fats (found in certain fish as well as walnuts and flaxseed). Because of this imbalance, we suggest you try to limit your intake of omega-6-rich vegetable oils.

Which fats are the superstars? Clearly, olive oil is one of the very best. It is high in monounsaturated fatty acids, and there are lots of data to support its positive health benefits.[435,436,437] Olive oil can be used to sauté almost anything. We use it not only for all the obvious vegetables like onions, garlic, tomatoes, and peppers, but also for scrambled eggs. Extra-virgin olive oil is our favorite because of its additional health benefits, such as prevent-

---

BREAD SPREAD

The best way to lubricate bread is with seasoned olive oil. The Italians really got this one right. If you feel compelled to use a spread, we recommend the new heart-healthy margarines that no longer have trans fats. They include Benecol, Promise, Smart Balance, and Take Control. Benecol and Take Control contain ingredients designed to lower cholesterol.

---

ing blood clots, improving the flexibility of blood vessels, and reducing the risk of certain cancers. It may have too strong a flavor for some, however. If you don't like it, look for a "light" olive oil that has a milder aroma and taste. Other healthy options include canola, almond, avocado, and walnut oils.

You won't want to use pure olive oil or walnut oil for stir-frying in a wok. Their "smoke point" is too low. For higher-temperature cooking, consider pure canola oil or combine half olive and half canola oil. If that seems a bother, look for "high heat" safflower or avocado oil. It should be higher in monounsaturated fat (oleic acid) than standard safflower oil.

A Contrarian Cholesterol Perspective

Most cardiologists believe that cholesterol is like golf: There's no such thing as too low a score. Anyone who questions that view is considered a menace to the public health. And the media have accepted the concept that cholesterol is evil without much question.

★ ★ ★ ★ ★ Olive Oil

Olive oil is the best source for monounsaturated fat. It lowers total cholesterol, bad LDL cholesterol, and blood pressure. It also has anti-inflammatory properties that should reduce the risk of atherosclerosis.

Cost: Highly variable depending on brand and quality. Can range from about $10 to $50 a liter and up.

It comes as a shock to a lot of people to learn that cholesterol is essential for good health. It is the basic building block for a number of crucial chemicals in the body, including vitamin D as well as sex hormones like testosterone and estrogen. Cholesterol also is found in cell membranes throughout the body and is an important component of the nervous system, especially the brain. Researchers have discovered that cholesterol is necessary for nerve cells to communicate. Without adequate cholesterol, the connections between neurons (synapses) fall apart.

> "Our data accord with previous findings of increased mortality in elderly people with low serum cholesterol, and show that long-term persistence of low cholesterol concentration actually increases the risk of death. Thus, the earlier that patients start to have lower cholesterol concentrations, the greater the risk of death."[440]
>
> —I. J. Schatz et al., *Lancet*, 2001

Scientists hypothesize that cholesterol helps strengthen the small arteries that feed the brain. Without it, they become more vulnerable to breakage under stress, which happens when blood pressure rises.[438] That might help explain research findings showing that very low cholesterol poses problems too.

Evidence comes from the Honolulu Heart Program.[439] Scientists at the University of Hawaii studied 3,500 Japanese-American men born between 1900 and 1919. The volunteers' total cholesterol levels were measured when they were middle-aged and again in the early 1990s, when they were elderly. Then the scientists kept tabs on who survived and who died.

To their surprise, the men with the lowest cholesterol levels had the highest risk of dying over the next several years. Those with cholesterol levels between 188 and 209 fared the best. Even men with elevated cholesterol, over 209, were less likely to die from any cause than were those with the lowest cholesterol readings. The investigators confessed their confusion: "We have been unable to explain our results. These data cast doubt on the scientific justification for lowering cholesterol to very low concentrations (less than 4.65 millimoles per liter) [less than 180 milligrams per deciliter] in elderly people."[441]

Some experts have tried to explain away the link between low cholesterol and higher mortality by suggesting that cholesterol drops when people come down with cancer or other life-threatening diseases. But the Honolulu researchers did not find excess cancer in the low-cholesterol group. Besides, many of these men had had low cholesterol 20 years earlier.

This isn't the first study to find a connection between low cholesterol and higher mortality. A report to the American Heart Association in 1999 showed that people with total cholesterol of less than 180 were twice as likely to suffer a bleeding stroke as those with cholesterol of more than 230. More than 15 years ago, Japanese researchers found that men with cholesterol under 178 and women with cholesterol under 190 were also at higher risk of brain hemorrhage.[442] In fact, people in Japan have traditionally experienced three times the risk of hemorrhagic stroke compared to Japanese people living in America. It is assumed that the lower-fat diet and lower cholesterol in Japan may be the most important difference.

Research has also shown that American women who eat very little meat or saturated fat may also be at higher risk for bleeding strokes, especially if they also have high blood pressure. For an investigation known as the Nurses' Health Study, researchers at Harvard University have been following more than 85,000 female nurses since 1980. Every 2 years the women answer questions about their diet, lifestyle, and health. The investigators found that the women who ate the least saturated fat and animal protein had the highest risk of bleeding stroke, twice as high as that of women who ate the most fat.[443]

One of the key investigators in the Nurses' Health Study is Dr. Willett of the Harvard School of Public Health. He told us that "in Japan, where cholesterol levels have been low, hemorrhagic stroke rates have been extremely high, so that total cardiovascular mortality has not been very different between the United States and Japan." In his opinion, "there is indeed some basis for real concern, even though it's not been absolutely proven that cholesterol levels can be driven down too low."[444]

Of course, none of this research means that people with high cholesterol can relax their guard. Too much of this blood fat is clearly dangerous and increases the risk of heart attack. But for people over age 70, or for women with high blood pressure, it may be counterproductive to lower cholesterol much below 200. Like body temperature or blood sugar level, cholesterol may need to stay in a middle range. Too little or too much can have negative health consequences.

Beyond Cholesterol: Other Risks

As we have said before in this book, when all you have is a hammer, everything looks like a nail. When it comes to heart disease, the nail is cholesterol. That's because the pharmaceutical industry has been extremely successful at creating hammers to lower this compound. At last count, Americans were spending more than $16 billion annually on statin-containing medications alone.[445]

STATIN-CONTAINING DRUGS

- Amlodipine/atorvastatin (Caduet)
- Atorvastatin (Lipitor)
- Ezetimibe/simvastatin (Vytorin)
- Fluvastatin (Lescol)
- Lovastatin (Mevacor)
- Pravastatin (Pravachol)
- Rosuvastatin (Crestor)
- Simvastatin (Zocor)

One prominent cardiologist believes that worldwide, at least 200 million people should be on statins.[446] Some physicians have jokingly suggested that it would simplify matters if we just added statins to the water supply or supplied "statin shakers" at every table the way we now have salt shakers.[447] This way people could sprinkle on a statin whenever they eat steak or eggs and not worry about cholesterol.

We're not knocking statins. They are extraordinarily effective at lowering bad LDL cholesterol, and they do prevent heart attacks and strokes and save lives. They also carry more risks than many physicians and patients have realized. (More about that shortly.) No, what really worries us about physicians' focus on cholesterol is that they may ignore other things that also contribute to heart disease. It's as if the conductor of a symphony orchestra were focusing only on the percussion section. Listening to a concert that featured just cymbals and drums would not be a very enjoyable experience.

In an editorial in the *New England Journal of Medicine*, Lori Mosca, MD, PhD, MPH, director of the preventive cardiology program at Columbia University Medical Center in New York City, states, "More than 20 years ago, 246 risk factors for coronary heart disease (CHD) had already been identified, and the number continues to grow."[448] Think about that. Physicians know of more than 240 risk factors for heart disease, yet most still single out only a couple of them: cholesterol and hypertension.

When is the last time a cardiologist asked you about your level of anxiety and depres-

OTHER RISK FACTORS FOR HEART DISEASE

- High level of C-reactive protein (CRP)
- Low level of HDL (good) cholesterol
- High level of LDL (bad) cholesterol
- High level of very low-density (VLDL) cholesterol
- High level of triglycerides
- Elevated level of lipoprotein (a), or Lp(a)
- High blood pressure
- Elevated homocysteine
- High uric acid level
- Insulin resistance
- Depression
- Stress and anxiety
- Anger and hostility
- Low level of physical activity
- Smoking
- Hormone Replacement Therapy (HRT)
- Marital strife
- Family (genetic) history of heart problems

sion, stress, or anger and hostility? How about your marital relationship or your support network? These are all key risk factors for heart disease.[449,450]

Cardiologists love numbers. Someone with a bad LDL cholesterol of 160 can lower that level to less than 100 with Lipitor within a few weeks. Stress, marital discord, and hostility are much more difficult to deal with, and progress is not so easily measured. And yet they may be just as important as a cholesterol number.

We used to hear that the so-called type A personality was a problem. Traditionally, these go-getters have been known for their impatience; they would have a hard time waiting in line, for example. But it turns out that hard-driving, multitasking, goal-oriented folks are not the most at risk. Rather, it seems that people with high levels of hostility may be more prone to heart disease.[452,453]

Researchers at the University of Utah report that marital strife is also a risk factor. They studied 150 couples between 2002 and 2005. If partners fought nastily, they were more likely to have significant signs of clogged coronary arteries.[454]

The lesson from all this research is clear: Heart disease is related to all sorts of things. While it is not practical to tackle 246 different risk factors, you can go after a few of the big ones. Some of our key recommendations won't surprise you. They include getting regular exercise and a good night's sleep, quitting smoking, managing anger and reducing hostility, controlling stress and depression, nurturing friendships, losing inches around the tummy if overweight, eating sensibly, and controlling cholesterol and other lipids.

Combating C-Reactive Protein

Sensible eating, exercise, and social support are all valuable, but sometimes we need more help than that against heart disease. Even having a great cholesterol level is no guarantee against heart attacks. According to renowned cardiologist Paul Ridker, MD, of Harvard Medical School, "Cholesterol screening is currently the gold standard for predicting heart attack risk, but nearly half of all heart attacks occur among men and women with normal cholesterol levels."[455]

We'll never forget the story of an athlete who was doing everything right but still suffered a heart attack. Even though his total cholesterol looked fabulous, his good HDL cholesterol was way too low. He also had a high level of lipoprotein (a), or Lp(a), a blood lipid that many physicians disregard because they don't have good drugs to lower it.

"*I'm a 44-year-old male and an active masters swimmer. I have always eaten a low-fat diet and have a total cholesterol of 160. For all intents and purposes, I'm the picture of health.*

However, I recently survived a heart attack caused by plaque and a blood clot blocking one coronary artery. Further testing showed that my HDL level is low (25) and my level of Lp(a) is very high (80). I've been told that these risk factors could help explain the recent heart attack."

Another reader shared a similar story about her good friend. Again, the numbers looked great. Many physicians would have given her a pat on the back and offered congratulations. Most cholesterol-lowering drugs couldn't produce such impressive results. And yet she suffered a heart attack. Perhaps both patients had high levels of C-reactive protein (CRP) and didn't realize that inflammation was silently attacking their arteries. CRP as a marker of inflammation may be even more important than cholesterol for alerting people to their risk of heart disease.

> ❝ *I thought you only got heart disease if you had high cholesterol. My friend, a woman 53 years old, had a heart attack even though her total cholesterol was 141 (HDL 49, triglycerides 124, and LDL 67). There's no heart disease in her family, she did not smoke, and she had low blood pressure. And yet she is scheduled for open-heart surgery because she has four blocked arteries.* ❞

CRP is a measure of general inflammation, which is now considered to be one of the most important underlying causes of heart disease. According to Dr. Ridker, "CRP has emerged as one of the most powerful predictors of cardiovascular disease."[456]

Do you know your CRP number? The test is affordable (usually $20 or less). If your number is above three, it is highly worrisome. If you fall between one and three, you are at moderate risk of heart disease. Ideally, your CRP level should be around one or less.

Because CRP is a measure of general inflammation within your body, there may be several ways to get the number down. A study from the Stanford School of Medicine demonstrated that people who score high on adherence to a Mediterranean diet (which emphasizes fruits, vegetables, beans, nuts, seeds, grains, fish, meat, monounsaturated oils, and alcohol) had a lower CRP level.[457] In addition, people who eat lots of fruit and/or take vitamin C supplements also have a lower CRP level, fewer signs of inflammation, and better blood vessel function.[458]

Statins have anti-inflammatory activity and can lower CRP levels. So can aspirin and fish

ANTI-INFLAMMATORY FOODS

- Wild salmon
- Bluefish
- Tuna
- Sardines
- Fresh or ground ginger
- Garlic
- Olive oil
- Broccoli
- Walnuts
- Almonds
- Pomegranates
- Strawberries
- Blueberries

oil.[459] Exercising regularly, controlling blood sugar, and drinking tea can lower CRP.[460] Even alcohol may be beneficial. Losing the love handles around the middle also can help lower CRP.

Heart Help

Aspirin

One of the simplest approaches to combating inflammation might be a cheap white pill. Never has one drug done so much for so many for so little. We're talking about aspirin, of course, the most versatile, miraculous, and inexpensive drug of all time. Even though inflation has affected the cost of aspirin just as it has the cost of everything else, it is still the best deal in the pharmacy. Over the last decade or so, aspirin has doubled or even tripled in cost—from half a penny a pill to about 1 or 2 cents per tablet. Yet you can still buy more than a year's worth of heart protection for $5. Compare that to prescription statins that can cost up to $3.50 per pill or the prescription blood thinner Plavix (clopidogrel), which can cost around $4 per pill.

By the way, a fascinating study published in the *New England Journal of Medicine* compared the effectiveness of low-dose aspirin (75 to 162 milligrams per day) to that of Plavix. More than 15,000 high-risk heart patients got either Plavix plus aspirin or aspirin alone. They were followed for more than 2 years. The conclusion: "Overall, clopidogrel [Plavix] plus aspirin was not significantly more effective than aspirin alone in reducing the rate of myocardial infarction [heart attack], stroke, or death from cardiovascular causes."[462]

Aspirin is more than 100 years old. On

★★★★★ **Aspirin**

Aspirin is the best deal in the pharmacy. It reduces the risk of heart attacks and thrombotic (clotting) strokes because of its anticlotting and anti-inflammatory actions.

Despite decades of research, the best dose of aspirin for heart attack and stroke prevention has been controversial. One leading expert concluded, "These [major] studies indicate that the most appropriate dose for the primary and secondary prevention of stroke and MI [myocardial infarction, or heart attack] is 160 milligrams/day."[461]

Downside: Damage to the stomach lining
Side effects: Indigestion, gastritis, and ulcers make this drug inappropriate for many. Bleeding or perforated ulcers can be life threatening. Some people are allergic to aspirin and must avoid it. Interactions with many other drugs are a potential problem. Anyone on long-term aspirin therapy must be under medical supervision.
Cost: Approximately $5 per year if purchased in economy-size packages

August 10, 1897, Bayer chemist Felix Hoffman created a stable form of acetylsalicylic acid. Little did he realize that the drug he hoped would ease his father's rheumatism would go on to save millions of lives by preventing heart attacks, strokes, and cancer. It seems to reduce the risk of developing malignancies of the colon, rectum, prostate, pancreas, lung, skin, ovary, and breast. In addition, it appears to lower the likelihood of coming down with Alzheimer's disease or diabetes.

Almost 30 billion aspirin tablets are swallowed annually. That represents 117 pills for every man, woman, and child. Such success did not come easily. Although aspirin was quickly recognized as the gold standard for relief of inflammation and pain, its other benefits seemed too good to be true.

Lawrence Craven, MD, was a general practitioner in Glendale, California. In 1948, when Aspergum was introduced, Dr. Craven started giving this aspirin-containing gum to his tonsillectomy patients so they could eat and sleep without pain. Some liked the Aspergum so much that they purchased additional packets and developed "serious postoperative hemorrhages which were difficult to control. The bleeding was sometimes so severe that hospitalization was necessary."[463]

Dr. Craven quickly realized that aspirin had a powerful anticoagulant effect. He could have dropped the matter and discouraged the use of aspirin. Instead he speculated that low-dose aspirin therapy might prevent blood clots in coronary arteries. By 1950, he was advising all of his male patients between ages 40 and 65 to start taking aspirin. In 1956, Dr. Craven wrote up his results: "Approximately 8,000 men have adopted a regime calling for from 5 to 10 grains [one to two tablets] of aspirin daily, with a surprising result. Not a single case of detectable coronary or cerebral thrombosis [heart attack or stroke] has occurred among patients who faithfully have adhered to this regime."[464]

Unfortunately, Dr. Craven's astounding observations were initially ignored by cardiologists. It took decades for the medical community to accept his results. Now physicians themselves often take low-dose aspirin to prevent heart attacks and strokes. And emergency rooms routinely give aspirin to patients they suspect may be experiencing a heart attack. If they don't administer aspirin, it is considered a major faux pas.

Over the last 50 years, evidence of aspirin's heart-protective effects has continued to accumulate. Two major reviews in prestigious medical journals (the *British Medical Journal* and *Annals of Internal Medicine*) analyzed the benefits and risks of aspirin. The British investigators reviewed nearly 300 clinical trials involving aspirin. Their American counterparts analyzed five major studies involving more than 50,000 patients. Both groups found that preventive aspirin therapy reduces the likelihood of heart attacks and strokes by one-fourth to one-third.[465, 466]

Yet millions of people who could benefit from this inexpensive, life-saving treatment are not taking it. The British scientists maintain that 40,000 additional lives could be saved every year if all those at risk were on low-dose aspirin. Men over 40 years of age; women who are past menopause; smokers; and those with diabetes, high blood pressure, clogged arteries, or angina should be considered susceptible to cardiovascular complications and therefore candidates for aspirin therapy.

Fish Oil

When we first started writing about the cardiovascular benefits of fish oil more than 2 decades ago, it was considered radical. Most cardiologists rejected the idea of fish oil supplements, though they were willing to encourage people to eat fish. Now, fish oil is a part of mainstream medicine, and cardiologists routinely recommend supplements. There is even a pharmaceutical-grade prescription fish oil product (Omacor) that has become quite popular among physicians.

At the time of this writing, there are more than 10,000 articles on fish oil in the National Library of Medicine database. More than 1,600 relate to cardiovascular issues. The evidence is in, and it is convincing. Fish oil dramatically lowers triglycerides by up to 45 percent (at doses of 4 grams daily). It can also raise good HDL cholesterol by up to 9 percent, something that is notoriously difficult to do with most prescription medications. The ratio of triglycerides to good HDL cholesterol (TG/HDL) is one of those numbers that we think is an excellent predictor of heart disease. The higher the ratio (four or above), the worse

---

★★★★★ Fish Oil

The omega-3 fatty acids (EPA and DHA) lower the risk of sudden cardiac death by 45 percent because they lower triglycerides and bad VLDL cholesterol, raise good HDL cholesterol, lower blood pressure, stabilize heart rhythm, and reduce the chance of blood clots. Fish oil together with a Mediterranean-type diet is a powerful aid in preventing cardiovascular disease.[467]

Recommended doses range from a total of 1 gram daily of EPA and DHA for people who are healthy to up to 4 grams total for those with high triglycerides or existing heart disease. Doctors may prescribe higher doses in some situations. Always take fish oil with food.

Downside: There is some concern that fish oil may interact with anticoagulant drugs like warfarin (Coumadin) to increase the risk for bleeding.
Side effects: An unpleasant aftertaste or even burping or indigestion. Purified fish oil may reduce this side effect and lower the risk of exposure to PCBs and other impurities.
Cost: Can range from as low as $3 a month when purchased in bulk (Kirkland Signature, Costco's brand, is United States Pharmacopeia verified) to more than $130 for prescription Omacor

---

things are, as it may indicate inflammation in the body and a prediabetic condition called *metabolic syndrome*. Ideally, the TG/HDL ratio should be like your CRP number: one or lower. Fish oil can help achieve this goal.

More important than the numbers, though, the omega-3 fatty acids in fish oil are powerful anti-inflammatory agents that retard the buildup of atherosclerotic plaque. They also discourage blood clot formation that might cause heart attacks or strokes. But wait, there's more. Fish oil can lower blood pressure, slow heart rate, stabilize the electrical activity of the heart and reduce the likelihood of serious heart rhythm abnormalities, and improve the flexibility of blood vessels.[468] In addition to these cardiovascular benefits, fish oil may be helpful against other chronic conditions like arthritis, Alzheimer's disease, depression, and asthma.

All in all, we cannot think of a more impressive dietary supplement than fish oil. In our enthusiasm for fish oil, however, do not think for a moment that we are abandoning fish. This should also be an important part of a heart-healthy diet. At least three servings of fish a week are recommended.

Nuts for Your Heart

For many years, people were told that nuts were not a good idea if they wanted to protect their heart. Dietitians worried that nuts were too high in fat. What was missing from the discussion was the fact that many nuts contain healthy fats that are actually good for the

★ ★ ★ ★ ★ **Walnuts**

Four to five servings (2 to 3 ounces each) a week can have a beneficial effect on blood lipids and lower the risk of coronary artery disease. In practical terms, that means about a handful of walnuts (8 to 16) on a regular basis.

Downside: Calories. Compensate for the additional calories by cutting back on sugar and other carbohydrates. Fortunately, a "nut diet" rarely causes weight gain.

Cost: In bulk, approximately $25 to $30 for a month's supply

heart. Walnuts are especially heart healthy, and there is a lot of research to prove it.

Several epidemiological studies have consistently demonstrated that people who eat nuts in general and walnuts in particular four or five times a week reduce their risk of coronary heart disease by 30 to 50 percent.[469,470,471] That's as impressive a response as you might expect from some cholesterol-lowering drugs.

In fact, eating walnuts has all kinds of positive effects on blood lipids. Total cholesterol, bad LDL cholesterol, and triglycerides all come down when you eat walnuts.[472] Good HDL cholesterol goes up.[473] More important, walnuts help block the oxidation of bad LDL cholesterol that leads to plaque buildup in coronary arteries.[474] A walnut-rich diet also makes blood vessels more flexible and improves circulation in people with high cholesterol levels.[475]

• • •

Q. *Eating walnuts nearly every day has brought my cholesterol down nicely. This experience makes me wonder: Why don't doctors prescribe natural remedies? The FDA should not object because items like walnuts are already safe for consumption. But my doctor was surprised when I told him how I have gotten my cholesterol under control.*

A. Natural remedies, such as specific foods, are not always the first things a doctor considers. Drug companies spend a lot of money promoting their products to physicians. There are no sales reps "detailing" walnuts to doctors for heart health.

The FDA now allows walnut packaging to carry a health claim based on research showing that 1½ ounces of walnuts daily (about ⅓ cup) can help lower LDL cholesterol.

• • •

Although walnuts have gotten most of the spotlight, other nuts are also good for the heart.[476, 477] We are especially fond of almonds because they are quite effective at lowering total cholesterol as well as LDL cholesterol and triglycerides. Canadian scientists found that a diversified diet containing almonds (approximately an ounce daily) was astonishingly effec-

tive. This "portfolio" diet was also rich in soluble fiber (including oats, barley, psyllium, and vegetables like okra and eggplant), cholesterol-lowering margarine, and soy-based milk and meat substitutes. People who stuck to the program were able to get their cholesterol down by an average of 30 percent, about as much as with the statin-type drug they also tested (lovastatin, or Mevacor).[478]

There is evidence that pecans, pistachios, and macadamia nuts produce heart-healthy lipid changes as well. Peanuts, which aren't really nuts at all but rather a legume, have been shown to lower triglycerides and raise magnesium, which is an essential mineral. Cashews are not nuts either. They are seeds from tropical trees. They are high in monounsaturated fat, which is part of a heart-healthy diet. Don't overdo, though, as they are also high in calories.

Alcohol

Americans have a moralistic streak that probably dates back to the Puritans. There is a sense that if it hurts or tastes bad, it must be good for you. That may be why generations of children were dosed with cod liver oil and had their skinned knees doused with alcohol. Those practices have faded, but people still have trouble imagining that their little vices might be healthy.

There is overwhelming evidence, however, that moderate alcohol consumption can protect the heart.[479, 480] The best study involved more than 38,000 male health professionals who were followed for 12 years. Men who had an alcoholic beverage 4 or 5 days a week reduced their risk of a heart attack by 30 to 35 percent compared to nondrinkers.[481] Contrary to popular belief, it didn't matter whether they were drinking beer, wine, or spirits. A drink is defined as 12 ounces of beer, 4 ounces of wine, or a shot of spirits (1½ ounces).

Most doctors are reluctant to tell patients they can have a glass of wine or a mug of beer with meals. Many worry that any patient who has a drink might be unable to stop after just one. And that is certainly a serious concern for alcoholics. But if a prescription medication were as effective as alcohol at preventing heart attacks, it would be a big bestseller.

Moderate alcohol consumption also appears to reduce the risk of ischemic (clotting) strokes.[482] Those same 38,000 male health professionals were followed for 14 years. The men who drank a glass or two of red wine three or four times a week lowered their risk of a stroke by more than 40 percent, but heavier drinkers actually increased their stroke risk.[483]

There is also evidence that people who drink moderately are somewhat protected against type 2 diabetes.[484] One final bonus: The Cardiovascular Health Study involving 5,888 older Americans in four communities has revealed that moderate alcohol consumption (one to six drinks per week) is associated with a lower likelihood of developing dementia.[485]

Of course, alcohol is not appropriate for everyone. Some people don't like it, while others can't tolerate the effects. Alcohol can inter-act with many medications and therefore would be inappropriate for millions. No one should start drinking for health reasons, and anyone with alcoholism in the family should avoid alcohol completely. There are, after all, many other ways to help the heart.

Grape Juice

Who would ever have guessed that a kid's drink, good old-fashioned purple grape juice, could have cardiovascular benefits? Then again, many of the same antioxidant flavonoids in red wine are found in grape juice. There has been impressive research suggesting that it can reduce bad cholesterol, prevent the oxidation of LDL cholesterol, lower blood pressure, help maintain the flexibility of blood vessels, improve bloodflow, and diminish the likelihood that platelets will clump together to form blood clots.[486, 487] There are even some data to suggest that the ingredients in grapes may enhance the immune system.

• • •

Q. *I've heard that red wine is good for the heart, but I don't dare drink alcohol. Would grape juice work as a substitute?*

A. Grape juice does seem to have intriguing benefits. Jane Freedman, MD, of Boston University School of Medicine, reported that Concord grape juice raised good HDL cholesterol and reduced inflammation when compared to a purple placebo beverage.[488] In previous research, Dr. Freedman and her colleagues had found that Concord grape juice helps keep blood platelets from clumping to form clots.

The anti-inflammatory effect of grape juice might help explain why some people find it eases arthritis pain: "After reading your article, my husband and I started to take grape juice and Certo. It works like magic! We each drink 8 ounces of grape juice containing 1 tablespoon of liquid Certo each day."

* * *

Some of our readers have become quite creative in trying various juice "tonics." The combination of apple cider vinegar, apple juice, and grape juice got some traction in the treatment of arthritis. Although there is no science to support this use, some of our readers have reported that this drink also lowers cholesterol.

> Last year my cholesterol was 284. I read your column about ½ cup apple cider vinegar mixed with 4 cups apple juice and 3 cups grape juice and began taking 6 ounces of this tonic every morning before breakfast.
>
> Slowly but surely, my cholesterol has dropped. Now it is down to 212. In addition, the arthritis pain in my knee is gone.

Apple Cider Vinegar

Apple cider vinegar all by itself may have some benefit. According to one reader, "I am 44

★★★★★ Grape Juice and Certo

You will find more information about Certo and grape juice in our discussion of arthritis (see page 87). Because Certo contains soluble fiber in the form of liquid plant pectin (used to make jams and jellies), we think this combination is a winner. It may do triple duty by relieving inflammation, increasing the flexibility of blood vessels, and lowering cholesterol.

We offer three different recipes for this remedy:
- 2 teaspoons Certo in 3 ounces grape juice (three times daily)
- 1 tablespoon Certo in 8 ounces grape juice (once daily)
- 1 packet Certo in 64 ounces grape juice (drink 6 to 8 ounces daily)

Researchers have used anywhere from two to three glasses of grape juice daily to achieve heart-healthy effects.

Downside: Grape juice contains too much sugar for many people with diabetes.

Cost: Approximately $3 for 64 ounces of grape juice and $2 for 3 ounces of Certo. This is enough for about a week.

years old with four grown children and four grandchildren. I take apple cider vinegar every day. My recent physical showed my HDL (good cholesterol) is 63 and my bad LDL cholesterol is 61. My husband was astonished, since before I started taking apple cider vinegar, my total cholesterol was 384. I also eat lots of garlic, drink green tea, and eat tons of vegetables." Anyone who tries this approach, though, should take no more than 1 teaspoon of vinegar in water and should rinse thoroughly afterward to protect the teeth. Dentists warn that acidic beverages can be tough on teeth.

Pomegranate Juice

If grape juice is too mundane for you, why not try something a bit more exotic? Pomegranates are an ancient fruit. Legend has it that the first pomegranate tree grew in the Garden of Eden. The ancient Chinese believed that pomegranates could offer longevity or even immortality. Pomegranates also played a key role in Greek mythology. According to one story, Hades, the lord of the underworld, kidnapped the beautiful maiden Persephone, daughter of the harvest goddess Demeter. Because Persephone ate a few pomegranate seeds before being rescued, she had to spend several months every year in the underworld with him. According to the myth, that's when the earth was forced to endure winter.

Modern stories about pomegranates are not quite as fanciful as the myth, but there is a lot of buzz about this exotic fruit. Like grapes, pomegranates are rich in antioxidants that can keep bad LDL cholesterol from oxidizing.[489] This degradation of LDL seems to be

---

★★★★★ Pomegranate Juice

This delicious fruit is also heart healthy. It lowers total and bad LDL cholesterol, assists in protecting arteries from plaque formation, and helps keep blood platelets from sticking together to form unwanted clots. Drinking 8 ounces daily improves bloodflow and oxygen delivery to the heart. Pomegranate juice also lowers blood pressure and may be beneficial against erectile dysfunction. There is also evidence to suggest that the anti-inflammatory properties of pomegranates may be helpful against arthritis and cancer.

Downside: Some preliminary evidence suggests that pomegranate juice might interact with some prescription drugs (including statins) in a manner similar to grapefruit juice. That could make these medications more likely to cause side effects. Too much juice may be constipating.

Cost: Pure pomegranate juice is pricey. A month's worth could run into hundreds of dollars unless you purchase pomegranate juice concentrate. Check out www.healingfruits.com for affordable products. A 1- to 2-month supply costs around $25.

an initial step in the development of athero-sclerosis.[490] A 3-year study in Israel discovered that patients who had thickening of their carotid arteries (in the neck) could reduce this complication by 30 percent with daily sup-plementation with pomegranate juice. Their blood pressure also went down.[491] Another study found that when hypertensive patients drank 2 ounces of pomegranate juice daily, their systolic blood pressure (the first number in a blood pressure reading) dropped by 8 points, on average.[492]

If that sounds impressive, the news just keeps getting better. Pomegranate juice, like aspirin and grape juice, can help keep blood platelets from clumping together to form unwanted clots. And a small study of diabetics with high cholesterol found that pomegranate juice concentrate lowered both total and bad LDL cholesterol.[493]

Another study, published in the *American Journal of Cardiology,* suggests that pomegran-ates may improve bloodflow to the heart. The researchers gave 45 patients with heart disease either 8 ounces of pomegranate juice or pla-cebo for 3 months. They then used a high-tech thallium scan to measure oxygen deficiency before and after exercise. Those patients who were drinking pomegranate juice had improved oxygen delivery, suggesting that pomegranates can have measurable heart-healthy effects.[494]

If our passion for pomegranates seems over the top, we're barely getting started. This fruit is so versatile that it reminds us of the old TV commercials for the Veg-O-Matic kitchen device that "slices and dices." There is evidence that pomegranate juice may help combat erec-tile dysfunction.[495] Investigators are also excited about the possibility that pomegranate com-pounds might prevent prostate cancer or slow its growth.[496,497] Other preliminary research suggests that pomegranate juice might help protect against skin and breast cancer.

Even arthritis may yield to the power of pomegranates. Scientists at Case Western Reserve University have reported that tissue cultures of human cartilage cells respond to pomegranate extract. Inflammation is reduced and the enzymes that break down cartilage become less active.[498]

Despite our great excitement about pome-granate juice, we do wish to offer a word of caution: Pomegranate juice appears to inter-fere with certain medications much as grape-fruit juice does.[499] At the time of this writing, this interaction has been demonstrated only in animals, so we don't know whether it poses a serious problem for humans. Until we know for sure, ask your physician and pharmacist to review your medications to see if there could be an interaction issue.

Grapefruit

Grapefruit has long had a reputation as a health food. Not only is it loaded with nutri-ents like vitamin C, potassium, and folic acid, it also has been reported to help people lose weight. For decades, dieters were convinced that grapefruit had special fat-burning power.

This idea was bolstered by advertisements like one for a diet plan in which a muscular construction worker pulled a grapefruit out of his lunch box with disdain, squeezed it, and tossed it away. Then he held up a little grapefruit pill and sang the praises of its grapefruit essence for weight loss.

One popular grapefruit diet has people either eating half a grapefruit or drinking 8 ounces of grapefruit juice three or four times daily. We haven't seen any studies showing that eating grapefruit will actually make anyone thinner, but new research does demonstrate that grapefruit can help lower cholesterol.

Scientists divided 57 volunteers into three groups of 19 people each. All of the subjects had undergone coronary bypass surgery, and all had high cholesterol and triglycerides. One group got a red grapefruit each day for a month; a second group got a white grapefruit daily. The control group got no grapefruit. At the end of the month, the total cholesterol levels of those who had eaten red grapefruit were 15 percent lower. The group that had eaten white grapefruit had lowered their total cholesterol by about half that much. Dangerous LDL cholesterol had also dropped, by 20 and 10 percent respectively, and triglycerides were lower as well.[500] Although grapefruit has ample dietary fiber, the scientists suspect that some other component of the fruit might be responsible for this fascinating effect.

As much as we love grapefruit, you do need to be somewhat cautious about using grapefruit for cholesterol control if you are also taking prescription medicines. Dozens of drugs are affected by grapefruit, especially cholesterol-lowering compounds like atorvastatin (Lipitor), lovastatin (Mevacor), and simvastatin (Zocor). For more information on this subject, see our Guide to Grapefruit Interactions at www.peoplespharmacy.com.

Chocolate

In his 1973 movie *Sleeper*, Woody Allen plays a character who ends up in a coma on life support due to a medical error. Two hundred years later, he wakes up to find that the conventional dogma on healthy living has been turned upside down. Woody's character is astonished to learn that wheat germ and brown rice, the ideal of 1970s health-food faddists, are considered terrible choices. Instead, hot fudge and steak are the new health foods.

Perhaps the most amazing thing about this "science fiction" is that it may be coming true. Scientists have found evidence that chocolate contains a number of compounds that can keep blood platelets from forming clots that may lead to heart attacks.

Some people find it hard to accept that chocolate could have health benefits. Yet the evidence keeps accumulating. Researchers have found that dark chocolate lowers blood pressure and helps improve the response to insulin.[501,508]

Researchers have also found that cocoa compounds improve the flexibility of blood vessels [502,503,504] and help keep blood platelets from clumping together to form clots.[505,506] Some

★★★ Chocolate

Dark chocolate is rich in cocoa flavonoids (plant-derived chemicals similar to those found in red wine and tea). These compounds can improve the flexibility of blood vessels, enhance insulin sensitivity, raise HDL cholesterol, lower blood pressure, and keep blood platelets from clumping together to form unwanted clots.

Downside: Calories. Compensate for the additional calories by cutting back on sugar and other carbohydrates.

Cost: Variable; approximately 30 cents for a day's supply (a small square of Ritter Sport Dark)

data indicate that dark chocolate may raise good HDL cholesterol and prevent the bad cholesterol from promoting atherosclerosis.[507]

The real question about any cholesterol-lowering tactic is, Will it prevent heart attacks? A long-term study from the Netherlands has good news in that regard for chocolate. For the study, researchers recruited 470 men over the age of 65. They were interviewed about their diet at the start of the study, then queried again 5 years and 10 years later. After 15 years of follow-up, the men who ate the most chocolate were only half as likely to have died of heart disease.[508] They also had slightly lower blood pressure. These fellows averaged about 10 grams of dark chocolate a day, a little less than you would get in a small square of Ghirardelli chocolate. That's far less than the

100 grams of dark chocolate that has been shown to lower blood pressure in double-blind trials.[509] So a little bit of dark chocolate every few days is a tasty, heart-healthy prescription.

• • •

Q. *How much chocolate should we eat per day to get maximum benefit and not gain weight?*

A. The minimum amount of cocoa needed to detect a cardiovascular benefit is about 4 grams. You can get that from a small, bite-size piece of dark chocolate (10 grams). To avoid the extra fat and sugar, you can always make your own cocoa. Look for a brand that is not "Dutch" or alkali-processed. Our favorites are Scharffen Berger and Valrhona.

• • •

Cinnamon

About 5 years ago, we heard from a reader that cinnamon might help lower blood sugar in someone with type 2 diabetes. That was news to us, but a little sleuthing did turn up some interesting animal cell research. Studies showed that cinnamon made cells more responsive to insulin, which theoretically would lead to better glucose control.[510,511] Since then we have heard from many readers that a little cinnamon does indeed help them keep their blood sugar in check. (To learn more about this effect, see the discussion of cinnamon in the section on diabetes on page 155.)

• • •

Q. *I have a history of high cholesterol dating at least to bypass surgery about 12 years ago. My cholesterol was running around 290.*

Several months ago I decided to try cinnamon, about a quarter teaspoon every morning. I usually put it on my oatmeal or in my coffee. Sometimes I use more because I like cinnamon.

After I started eating cinnamon, my cholesterol went down to 225. My next test was 4 months later and the reading was 175. Most recently, in June 2005, the reading was 122.

A. We are very impressed with your results. A study in rats showed that one ingredient in cinnamon, cinnamate, lowers cholesterol and triglyceride levels even better than the statin drug lovastatin by working through the same mechanism.[512]

Some readers who have tried taking cinnamon report that it can cause heartburn. We're glad you're not having any trouble with the amount you are taking. Anyone who uses this spice medicinally should monitor their blood sugar and be under medical supervision.

• • •

The cinnamon and blood sugar story was certainly interesting, but then a few years later we heard from a reader who discovered that cinnamon could help lower his bad LDL cholesterol while raising his good HDL cholesterol. Again we were astonished, but further investigation turned up a randomized, placebo-controlled trial published in *Diabetes Care*. The scientists found that cinnamon could help lower blood sugar, total cholesterol, bad LDL cholesterol, and triglycerides in type 2 diabetics.[513] Check with your doctor about adding cinnamon to your line-up of healthy foods that might work together with medical treatment to improve blood lipids.

Dietary Supplements

There are several dietary supplements that we think are important for maintaining heart health. Some of our old favorites, however, have not lived up to expectations. We had been big boosters of B vitamins because they lower homocysteine, a known risk factor for heart disease. We had hoped that taking vitamins B_6, B_{12}, and folic acid would lower the risk of heart attacks and strokes. To our disappointment, those hopes were dashed.

Studies published in the *New England Journal of Medicine* conclusively demonstrated that taking B vitamins did not protect high-risk patients from heart attacks or other "major vascular events." They may even pose a hazard in the relatively high doses used in these prevention trials. Such research demonstrates how critical it is to do these long-term trials in order to test any theory of heart attack prevention. Sometimes the data contradict our preconceived notions.

NIACIN

One B vitamin that does work to lower the risk of heart disease is niacin (vitamin B$_3$, or nicotinic acid). Doctors have prescribed this drug for more than 50 years. (At the doses required to produce results, niacin must be considered a medicine and its use should be supervised by a physician.) A landmark study published in 1986, the Coronary Drug Project, tracked heart attack victims for 15 years. Men who had been prescribed niacin had substantially fewer repeat heart attacks and 11 percent fewer deaths.[516] The benefit persisted for many years, even after they stopped taking the niacin.

Despite the fact that niacin has been prescribed for decades to improve lipid profiles, researchers still do not understand exactly how it works this magic. Niacin lowers bad LDL cholesterol by anywhere from 15 to 40 percent. Triglycerides also come down significantly.

★★★ Niacin

Niacin lowers the bad stuff and raises the good stuff. It diminishes heart attack risk at an affordable price. Decades of experience with this drug mean treatment holds few surprises.

Downside: Unpleasant side effects including flushing, tingling, and itching. Controlled-release products such as Bronson sustained-release niacin or prescription Niaspan may diminish this, but they require careful liver enzyme monitoring.

Other side effects: Nausea, diarrhea, fatigue, headache, dryness of the eyes and skin, and muscle problems

Cost: Variable; approximately $10 to $15 for a 2-month supply of Bronson Laboratories' over-the-counter 500-milligram niacin. Prescription Niaspan could cost up to $250 for a comparable amount.

Niacin is one of the few compounds that reduces Lp(a) and raises good HDL cholesterol by 10 to 20 percent.

Best of all, niacin is inexpensive. Compared to today's powerful prescription drugs, niacin is a steal. A 2-month supply can cost one-tenth as much as the same amount of a statin-type medication. Of course, at the doses that are required to lower cholesterol and reduce the risk of heart disease, medical supervision is essential. Liver function must be monitored periodically to detect any enzyme elevation that might signal damage. Doses that are prescribed range from 300 to 500 milligrams at the low end to up to 3,000 milligrams at the high end. Only a physician can determine the most appropriate dose and supervise safe treatment.

MAGNESIUM

Magnesium is a mineral that rarely gets the respect it deserves. Sodium has been in the spotlight for decades because we have been warned so frequently that too much salt is bad for us. (This notion is now under review. See our discussion of hypertension on page 292 for the latest update.) Physicians also focus on potassium, because having too little or too much can be life threatening. Many diuretics deplete the body of potassium. What is rarely mentioned is that magnesium is often in short supply in our diet, and the same diuretics that deplete the body of potassium may also deplete magnesium.

Magnesium plays a crucial role throughout the body. It helps control blood pressure, pre-

★★★★ Magnesium

This mineral can help improve the ratio of bad LDL cholesterol to good HDL cholesterol, reduce the oxidation of bad LDL cholesterol, diminish cellular inflammation, and lower the risk of atherosclerosis. It improves circulation to the coronary arteries and helps maintain a regular heart rhythm. The recommended dose of magnesium is 300 to 500 milligrams daily. Loose stools signal too much magnesium!

Downside: Dangerous for people with reduced kidney function or kidney disease.

Side effects: Diarrhea. Remember, milk of magnesia has been used to combat constipation for decades.

Cost: Variable; approximately $3 for a 3-month supply from Bronson Laboratories

vent migraine headaches, maintain bone strength in combination with calcium, improve bowel regularity, and—most important for this discussion—assist in keeping the heart healthy. The Honolulu Heart Program initially involved more than 8,000 men between 1965 and 1968. It examined lifestyle issues as well as diet and heart disease. A follow-up evaluation of 7,172 men after 15 years revealed that those with low magnesium levels in their blood had a substantially increased risk of heart disease and heart attacks. The investigators concluded that "the intake of dietary magnesium is associated with a reduced risk of CHD [coronary heart disease]."[517]

FOODS HIGH IN MAGNESIUM

- Almonds
- Cashews
- Halibut
- Oatmeal
- Peanuts
- Potatoes (baked)
- Soybeans
- Spinach

A different study of nearly 3,000 people was presented at the American Heart Association annual meeting in April 2005. It revealed that magnesium plays a crucial role in heart disease. Investigators found that those people who get the least magnesium are most likely to have clogged coronary arteries. Scientists believe that magnesium deficiency changes fat metabolism so that atherosclerosis becomes more likely.

Psyllium

We used to wonder why more physicians didn't recommend soluble fiber to patients with elevated cholesterol. Research carried out in the 1980s suggested that psyllium could lower total cholesterol by up to 15 percent and LDL cholesterol by as much as 20 percent.[518,519] That kind of improvement had us excited for years, since psyllium (the fiber in bulk laxatives like Metamucil and Fiberall) was inexpensive. Then we started digging deeper and discovered that the story is a lot more confusing.

More recent research suggests that psyllium does indeed lower cholesterol, but the effect is relatively modest. Several studies have shown that doses of about 10 grams of psyllium daily (equivalent to 3 tablespoons of Metamucil with sucrose) can lower total cholesterol by about 4 percent and bad LDL cholesterol by roughly 7 percent.[520,521] That's not nothing. But it is easy to understand why physicians would be far more impressed with statin-type drugs that lower cholesterol levels far more dramatically.

★★★ Psyllium

This soluble fiber may be quite helpful in helping lower total cholesterol and LDL cholesterol when it is part of a "portfolio" diet (see opposite page). If you are dedicated, such an approach may lower cholesterol almost as much as a statin-type medication.[522]

The "standard" dose of psyllium is 1 teaspoon (sugar-free) in 8 ounces of water three times a day before meals.

Downside: Not terribly tasty. If you don't drink a full 8 ounces of water, it could cause a digestive tract blockage.

Side effects: Digestive tract discomfort, including bloating, a feeling of fullness, and flatulence

Cost: Variable; Metamucil costs $8 to $10 for a month's supply in bulk.

Q. *My cholesterol has ranged from 240 to 300 for years. My doctor finds these numbers unacceptable and has insisted I take medication.*

First I was put on Lescol. My muscles hurt so much I could barely walk. Then I was put on Zocor. The muscle pain came back. The same pattern repeated with Lipitor. Is there any way to get my cholesterol down without one of these drugs?

A. A multifaceted approach to lowering cholesterol naturally can be successful. A study published in the *Journal of the American Medical Association* on July 23, 2003, showed that consuming a "dietary portfolio" of vegetarian foods lowered cholesterol nearly as well as the prescription drug lovastatin (Mevacor). The diet was rich in soluble fiber from oats, barley, psyllium, eggplant, and okra. It used soy substitutes instead of meat and milk and included almonds and cholesterol-lowering margarine (such as Take Control) every day.

• • •

Where psyllium shines is when it is included with a heart-healthy "portfolio" diet. Canadian researchers have found that combining cholesterol-lowering foods with psyllium can produce

---

ELEMENTS OF THE "PORTFOLIO" VEGETARIAN DIET

- Almonds (½ ounce, or 13 nuts)
- Barley
- Eggplant
- Margarine (like Take Control)
- Oats
- Okra
- Psyllium
- Soy meat analogues (burgers, dogs, deli slices)

---

impressive lipid changes after 1 month. For folks who followed the diet, LDL cholesterol came down almost 28.6 percent.[523] That was statistically comparable to the 30.9 percent reduction seen with added lovastatin (Mevacor). CRP, a marker for inflammation and an equally important risk factor for heart disease, came down 28.2 percent on the portfolio diet.

These results were fabulous, but the study was relatively short (1 month) and the subjects of the experiment received most of their food at the Clinical Nutrition and Risk Factor Modification Center at St. Michael's Hospital in Toronto. They ate a controlled, vegetarian diet that included lots of high-fiber vegetables, whole grains, special margarine, and almonds. A long-term follow-up trial "under real-world conditions" produced good results, though not quite as impressive as the 1-month study. After a year on the high-fiber, vegetarian program, about a third of the "motivated participants" had LDL cholesterol reductions of more than 20 percent, statistically comparable to their response with lovastatin.[524]

One especially novel concept is combining psyllium with a cholesterol-lowering drug. Researchers discovered that they could reduce the dose of simvastatin (Zocor) from 20 milligrams daily to 10 milligrams daily if they added 15 grams of Metamucil (about 4½ doses daily).[525] This could be a way to enhance the effectiveness of pricey prescription drugs and, by reducing the dose, minimize the risk of side effects.

Policosanol

Cuban researchers discovered many years ago that certain compounds found in sugarcane wax (long-chain alcohols collectively called policosanol) could lower both total cholesterol and bad LDL cholesterol and possibly even raise good HDL cholesterol. There have been more than a dozen randomized, double-blind, placebo-controlled clinical trials with Cuban policosanol. The results are surprisingly consistent with doses ranging between 5 and 20 milligrams daily. Total cholesterol comes down by between 13 and 23 percent, and LDL cholesterol is reduced by 20 to 26 percent.[526,527,528] What is even more impressive is that policosanol raises good HDL cholesterol by 10 percent or more. The problem is that much of this research was carried out by the same investigators and not confirmed by other scientists.

In a few comparative trials, policosanol was roughly on a par with statin-type medications like lovastatin, simvastatin, and pravastatin when it came to improving lipid levels.[529] When patients were given 2 grams of fish oil in capsules with 10 milligrams of policosanol

---

★ Policosanol

Several older studies conducted with Cuban policosanol have shown cholesterol-lowering power, but a newer, well-controlled study did not. Many scientists question whether US policosanol from beeswax or yams (which contain the same long-chain alcohols as sugarcane) is as effective as the patented Cuban product, which is now itself in question.

The standard dose ranges from 5 to 20 milligrams.

Downside: Effectiveness and quality control of US policosanol products have not been established. There could be an increased risk of bleeding when policosanol is combined with an anticoagulant like warfarin (Coumadin).

Side effects: Modest weight loss, digestive tract upset, headache, insomnia, and skin rash. Generally considered quite safe and very well tolerated.

Cost: US products of unproven efficacy and quality range from $5 to $20 for a month's supply.

---

daily, total cholesterol dropped by 15.3 percent, LDL cholesterol came down by 24.4 percent, triglycerides were reduced by 14.7 percent, and good HDL cholesterol went up by 15.5 percent.[530] Those are really terrific numbers. If a prescription drug were able to do all of those things, you would see commercials on the evening news and your doctor would prescribe it almost as frequently as a statin.

If only all of the research were consistent. A well-designed study at the University of Cologne in Germany found that policosanol from Cuba was no more effective than placebo at lowering LDL cholesterol, total cholesterol, or triglycerides or raising HDL cholesterol concentrations.[531] This suggests that policosanol is worthless when it comes to lowering cholesterol.

Despite these conflicting data, some people insist that policosanol has helped them improve their lipid profile. Until there is additional positive research, though, you should probably try some other approach to cholesterol control. If you forced us to make a policosanol recommendation, we would probably go with One-A-Day Cholesterol Plus from Bayer. The only reason is that Bayer is a major pharmaceutical company and presumably has high quality-control standards.

Red Yeast Rice

One of the first major policosanol products distributed in the United States was Cholestin, made by a company called Pharmanex. But before it contained policosanol, Cholestin contained red yeast rice. It's a tale of woe and intrigue—a story of Big Pharma and the FDA ganging up on a small herbal company.

Pharmanex discovered that Chinese researchers had found that red yeast rice could lower cholesterol and triglycerides. Nobody else was paying much attention to this kind of foreign research, so the company decided to do its own clinical trials. It published a randomized, double-blind study that was conducted at the UCLA School of Medicine.[532] The trial showed that red yeast rice was quite effective, lowering LDL cholesterol by 22 percent.

Red yeast rice contains several interesting compounds, one of which is lovastatin. This is the same chemical found in the first statin drug, Mevacor. When Merck discovered that Cholestin was being sold over the counter as a dietary supplement, the pharmaceutical giant complained to the FDA. The agency agreed that Pharmanex was selling an unapproved new drug, even though it has been used for hundreds of years in China to flavor and color meat and fish. Lengthy legal battles ultimately resulted in Pharmanex taking red yeast rice off the market and substituting policosanol in its Cholestin sold in the United States.

Despite the fact that the original company pulled the plug on a standardized, purified, and tested product, a number of other manufacturers have jumped into the game. The FDA has apparently turned a blind eye to the distribution of numerous red yeast rice products as dietary supplements. How safe and effective they are is hard to tell. Without the kind of research behind them that Pharmanex

★★★ Red Yeast Rice

The "standard" dose of 2,400 milligrams contains about 4 to 7 milligrams of lovastatin (much less than the 20 milligrams found in Mevacor). There are several statinlike compounds in this natural product, along with tannins and other phytochemicals. The mechanism by which red yeast rice lowers total cholesterol, LDL cholesterol, and triglycerides is probably more complex than just a "statin effect."

Downside: May interact with several prescription drugs that also interact with statins. Beware of combining it with certain antibiotics, antifungals, antidepressants, immune-suppressing medicine (cyclosporine), anticoagulants (warfarin), HIV/AIDS drugs, other cholesterol-lowering compounds, and grapefruit. Take it only under medical supervision! Monitor liver enzymes and creatine kinase levels.

Side effects: Elevated liver enzymes, flatulence, and heartburn. If muscle pain or weakness occurs, stop taking it immediately and consult a physician. Adverse events may be less common than with statin-type medications.

Cost: US products of unproven efficacy and quality range from $12 to $48 for a month's supply.

conducted, we are loath to endorse any particular brand of red yeast rice.

Before we could give a green light to any red yeast rice formulations, we would need to see new and expanded clinical trial evidence. Investigation has revealed that quality control may be lacking for many commercial red yeast rice products. [533, 534] The early Pharmanex data were intriguing, but it's time for someone to step up to the plate and give us new and better research. Nevertheless, we do hear from many readers that they have great success getting their cholesterol under control with this dietary supplement.

• • •

Q. *I am a 61-year-old retired physician. Over the past several years, my total cholesterol has crept up from 215 to 255 despite an almost vegetarian diet and daily exercise.*

I've never taken cholesterol-lowering drugs because my ratio of beneficial HDL cholesterol to total cholesterol has always been good. Four months ago I began taking red yeast rice at half the usual dose. My cholesterol fell to 192 and my LDL dropped from 166 to 118. Is it possible that a small amount of red yeast rice could be responsible for such a dramatic improvement?

A. Red yeast rice has been used in traditional Chinese cooking as far back as 800 AD. It is made by fermenting cooked rice with red yeast. During the Ming

Dynasty, healers used this flavoring to treat indigestion and cardiovascular problems ("blood circulation").

Your results are impressive. The few studies that have been done suggest that LDL cholesterol should go down by about 22 percent with the "usual" dose (2,400 milligrams daily). You were able to lower your LDL by almost 29 percent with a lower dose. Since there have not been good dosage standards, it is perfectly reasonable to start lower (1,200 mg) and see what happens.

Red yeast rice may affect the liver, so blood tests are advisable. Anyone who experiences muscle pain or weakness should stop taking it immediately and consult a physician.

● ● ●

Some people experience side effects even with this natural medicine. One reader wrote: "I cannot take conventional statin drugs. I've tried three different brands and got achy muscles from all of them. So I tried red yeast rice. Within a few weeks, I got the same muscle pain, although not quite as severe."

Statins

Statins are the most successful drugs in the history of the pharmaceutical industry. "Statin" is the shorthand name for a class of cholesterol-lowering drugs that includes atorvastatin (Lipitor), fluvastatin (Lescol), lovastatin (Mevacor), pravastatin (Pravachol), rosuvastatin (Crestor), and simvastatin (Zocor). At the time of this writing, annual worldwide sales of statins exceed $30 billion.[535] No other category of medicines even comes close to this astonishing sum. Worldwide, nearly 50 million people pop a statin-type drug each day.

The reason for the statins' popularity is that these drugs work extraordinarily well in reducing the creation of cholesterol. Cardiologists love them because statins bring LDL cholesterol levels down dramatically. Ads for Lipitor tell consumers, "Adding a cholesterol-lowering medication like Lipitor can lower your total cholesterol by 29 percent to 45 percent [and] your 'bad,' low-density (LDL) cholesterol by 39 percent to 60 percent (average effect depending on dose)." Those are impressive numbers. A study conducted by cardiologists at the Cleveland Clinic reported that high-dose Crestor treatment lowered LDL cholesterol 52 to 60 percent and reduced plaque buildup in coronary arteries by 9 percent.[536]

Anyone at moderately high risk for a heart attack (but without prior history of heart disease) is advised to get his or her LDL cholesterol below 100, and those at the highest risk are supposed to get their level below 70 mg/dl. Some cardiologists want the LDL level to be even lower. Such numbers can be achieved only by taking cholesterol-lowering drugs. According to the statin enthusiasts, at least 43 million Americans are now supposed to be on such medications. If you add in the number of diabetics who

★★★★ Statins

Statins dramatically lower total cholesterol and LDL cholesterol. They are only moderately effective at reducing triglycerides and raising good HDL cholesterol unless "intensive therapy" (a high dosage) is employed.

Downside: Muscle tenderness or pain may affect any part of the body, including the legs, back, arms, shoulders, and neck. At their worst, pain and weakness can be immobilizing. Any muscle symptoms require immediate medical attention, because they can be a sign of a life-threatening crisis (rhabdomyolysis). Memory and concentration problems and mood or personality changes have also been reported.

Coenzyme Q_{10} may help to counteract some statin side effects when it is taken in doses of 200 to 300 milligrams daily.

Some statins interact with other drugs, including amiodarone (Cordarone), certain antibiotics, antifungals, antidepressants, immune-suppressing medicine (cyclosporine), anticoagulants (warfarin, or Coumadin), HIV/AIDS drugs, and other cholesterol-lowering compounds, as well as grapefruit. Monitor liver enzymes and creatine kinase (CK) levels.

Side effects: Rare, but may include muscle pain, muscle weakness, joint pain, digestive tract upset, headache, peripheral neuropathy (pain, tingling, numbness in the extremities), cognitive problems, depression, rash, blood sugar changes, shortness of breath, pancreatitis, sexual difficulties, and elevated liver enzymes.

Cost: Variable. Can range from $66 for generic lovastatin to $125 for a month's supply of Lipitor. Add approximately $25 for coenzyme Q_{10} (200 to 300 milligrams daily).

take them, this number exceeds 50 million.

Statins are highly effective for middle-aged men with coronary heart disease. Men with bad total cholesterol to HDL ratios and multiple other cardiac risk factors may also benefit. At this writing, questions remain whether statins offer a significant benefit for women and those over the age of 70. A cost-benefit analysis suggests that even among middle-aged men, statins may be cost-effective only when the risk of a heart attack is 10 percent or more over 10 years.[537]

There is no doubt that statins save lives. Many people have reduced their risk of heart attack and stroke because of drugs like Crestor, Lipitor, Pravachol, and Zocor.[538] Although everyone has focused on the drugs' ability to lower cholesterol, that may not be the only mechanism through which they prevent heart disease and strokes. There is growing recognition that such medications also have anti-inflammatory activity.[539,540] They do lower CRP levels, one of the prime markers for inflammation.[541]

Some statins may have greater anti-inflammatory activity than others. This may account for Lipitor's edge in some clinical trials. We are not ready to recommend one statin over another, though. From a purely economic perspective, Zocor represents a very good deal. When this medicine lost its patent, Merck decided to price the brand name competitively with generic simvastatin. Consequently, you can have the assurance of a brand-name product that costs no more (and possibly less) than some generic competitors. Interestingly, when you compare aspirin with statins, they turn out to be roughly comparable in their effect on preventing a first heart attack.[542] A book review in the *New England Journal of Medicine* points out that "two fish meals a week are as effective as statins in preventing death among patients with cardiac disease."[543]

Regardless of how they work, we know that statin-type drugs are effective, which is why some cardiologists seem to want them in the water supply. Many patients are equally enthusiastic. One reason statins are so popular is that it allows them to "cheat." Regardless of what people eat, statins bring cholesterol levels down. Although physicians tell patients to cut back on saturated fat, it doesn't take some people long to figure out that they can have their cake and eat it too. Lots of folks resume eating burgers, fries, and hot fudge sundaes and still have great cholesterol levels. So patients appreciate drugs like Lipitor. If they can eat butter and Brie and still make the doctor happy with great lipid levels, what's not to love?

The Dark Side of Statins

Despite their incredible success, statins are not for everybody. Although most people do seem to tolerate these drugs very well, others experience serious or even life-threatening side effects. Just as penicillin is a lifesaver for many, others are allergic to this antibiotic and may die from anaphylactic shock if exposed to just one dose. Aspirin prevents heart attacks, but some people experience lethal bleeding ulcers. That's why it is so important for people to know the risks as well as the benefits of all the drugs they take, including statins.

> *"This summer my father committed suicide. After his death we became aware of the possibility that his death might have been related to a little-known side effect of a medication he took to lower his cholesterol.*
>
> *My father began taking Zocor 2 years ago. Prior to that he had never been depressed. I have since met a patient who can directly attribute the start of depression with beginning on Zocor and its end with stopping the drug. Depression is listed as a possible side effect of Zocor but only in the fine print of a full page of information."*

For more than a decade, readers of our newspaper column have been writing us about serious side effects caused by statins. At first we wondered whether these medications could really be responsible for so many debilitating reactions. For example, an extraordinary number of people told us that their pills were turning them into invalids. Severe muscle pain and weakness curtailed exercise or even everyday activities—despite normal lab tests. We also heard about problems such as depression, memory loss, nerve damage, and sexual dysfunction.

❝*I started taking Lipitor about 2 years ago and it was very effective in lowering my cholesterol level. As time went on, though, I became more and more inactive until I hardly had the strength to get up in the morning and bathe. I went from one resting place to another. My muscles just would not carry me very far.*

All the while I was complaining to my doctor, but he wouldn't listen. Finally I became so debilitated with awful joint pain that I quit the Lipitor. Since then I have been doctoring for the arthritis I never had before. I think Lipitor caused my profound weakness. Since I have gone off the drug, my energy level has increased a hundredfold. As soon as I can get rid of this joint pain I will be off and running. Lipitor ruined the quality of my life. It caused severe bouts of depression, short spells of memory loss, and was responsible for massive arthritis pain.❞

We tried to overlook these reports because the medical literature kept telling us that these medicines protect people from heart attacks and strokes. No one wants to discredit a miracle. Over time, our readers convinced us that something scary was happening. Gradually, the medical literature has caught up with our readers, but few physicians or patients yet realize the extent and severity of this hidden epidemic.

Most people don't recognize that seemingly unrelated symptoms can be drug-induced. Some side effects sneak up so slowly that a person may believe that he is suffering from age-related arthritis or Alzheimer's disease. Despite our best efforts to alert the FDA to these problems, the feds have turned a deaf ear to our concerns, much as the agency ignored early reports that the popular pain reliever Vioxx could cause heart attacks and strokes.

❝*My mother's doctors discovered that at age 74 her cholesterol had started to rise. They decided to put her on Lipitor. Since that time her life has changed in many ways. Before Lipitor she played golf on average two times a week. She has not played now in a year. She worked in her yard every day, now only once in a great while. She was walking 2 to 3 miles on the days she did not play golf. This she is still doing, only it is 1 mile. She would go to dinner with us almost every Friday night. She still does this only when we make her.*

Mother is 4 foot 11 inches tall and normally weighs 110 lbs. She has always been happy even though all her friends were passing away. Last week, she told me she wished she could die because of the pain she is in. She wakes up in the middle of the night in so much pain that she cannot go back to sleep. Her arthritis has flared up and that is what the doctor has told her is causing her pain. She has also developed diabetes. She is now taking so many drugs that I am not sure what all is wrong with her.❞

Physicians have become so enamored of statins that many deny that a patient's joint discomfort or muscle or nerve pain could be caused by such medications. Even when people become so crippled that they can no longer exercise or socialize with friends, they are sometimes admonished to stay on their statins. Given that remaining active and socializing are critical to maintaining heart health, not to mention the overall quality of life, this kind of cholesterol compulsiveness seems obsessive to us. If a person complains of memory loss or concentration problems, he may be laughed at or labeled a hypochondriac. Side effects associated with statins are routinely discounted.

Nerve damage is another potential complication of statin therapy that often goes unrecognized. Although there are reports in the medical literature documenting this reaction, many physicians seem unaware of it.[544] Tingling, numbness, prickling, burning, and pain, especially in the legs and feet, can come on so gradually that no one realizes they are related to a medication.

• • •

Q. *I have developed peripheral neuropathy in my legs over the last year. My feet are numb and my legs are weak. My doctor has eliminated causes like vitamin B$_{12}$ deficiency or diabetes but is at a loss to explain what's happening.*

I went to the Internet to look for answers and discovered that other people have reported similar symptoms while taking Lipitor. I have been taking this cholesterol drug for 2 years.

Could Lipitor be responsible for my neuropathy? My doctor says that you can't trust anything you find on the Internet.

A. An article in the journal *Neurology* (May 14, 2002) suggests that long-term use of statin-type cholesterol-lowering drugs may be associated with nerve damage.

• • •

Can cholesterol-lowering drugs affect memory? That is a question we have wrestled with for nearly 6 years. It started when we received a letter from a woman who complained that Lipitor affected her ability to verbalize thoughts and remember things.

" *Last fall my doctor prescribed Lipitor, and after several months I found I was having trouble remembering names and coming up with the right word. At dinner once I said, "Please pass the elephant" though I wanted the bread. I told my husband I thought I'd had a stroke.*

In January a friend came to visit. She was worried about her memory and couldn't think of her daughter's name on the telephone. She too was on Lipitor.

I asked my doctor to prescribe a different cholesterol medicine. Within a couple of weeks I was more mentally alert. But my friend (still on

Lipitor) was in worse shape and afraid she would lose her job. Her doctor said forgetfulness could not be due to the drug. She finally stopped taking Lipitor anyway and now is much sharper. "

We didn't know what to make of this story because we could find nothing in the medical literature connecting statin-type medicines like Lipitor to memory loss or poor word recall. Before long, however, letters started pouring in. One reader wrote:

" *Thank you. Validation at last! I have had enormous problems with concentration. I get confused and feel like there are big ugly holes burned in my memory. I am certain that Lipitor is causing my problems, but my doctor refuses to believe me and denies any connection.* "

Letters like these led us to suspect that some people develop cognitive problems on statins. We became alarmed when we received this story:

" *I am a retired family doctor and former astronaut. Two years ago at my annual astronaut physical at Johnson Space Center I was started on Lipitor. Six weeks later I experienced my first episode of total global amnesia lasting 6 hours. They couldn't find anything wrong with me so I suspected Lipitor and discontinued it.*

Other doctors and pharmacists were unaware of similar problems. Believing it must have been a coincidence, I restarted Lipitor a year later. After 6 weeks I landed in the ER with a 12-hour

episode of total global amnesia. I am more convinced than ever of a Lipitor relationship. "

The astronaut-physician is Duane Graveline, MD. In response to his experience, we heard from other readers who had suffered episodes of total global amnesia while taking Lipitor, Zocor, or similar drugs. Total global amnesia is a temporary but frightening loss of memory. Dr. Graveline forgot that he was a physician and an astronaut and didn't even recognize his wife. He has summarized his experiences in a book called *Statin Drugs: Side Effects and the Misguided War on Cholesterol* (available on the Web at www.spacedoc.net).

We heard of another disturbing statin reaction. Michael K. is a retired professor of business law and computer science. He was diagnosed with probable Alzheimer's disease that was progressing very rapidly. He went to his 50th college reunion with a sign around his neck that said, "I'm Mike. I have Alzheimer's disease." At his youngest daughter's wedding, he did not recognize people he had known for more than 20 years.

His decline made it clear that he would need long-term nursing care. But then he read our column about statins and memory problems. With his doctor's knowledge, he discontinued the Zocor he had been taking. Although it took many months, he gradually regained his memory and cognitive ability. He is back to reading three newspapers a day and is as sharp as a tack. A complete neurological workup showed no signs of Alzheimer's disease.

We suspect that such memory problems and episodes of amnesia are extremely rare. But with millions of people taking statins on a daily basis, even a relatively uncommon side effect can affect a large number of people. Judging from our mail bag, muscle pain is actually quite common. Many doctors disregard such symptoms because a blood test for muscle damage (creatine kinase, or CK) comes back normal. This is short-sighted, since many of our readers tell us that the pain gradually disappears (most of the time) when the medicine is discontinued. Whether coenzyme Q_{10} supplements can counteract these side effects remains to be determined.

66 *You have written about serious muscle and memory problems some people have when taking statins to lower cholesterol. Coenzyme Q_{10} might help reduce the muscle pain.*

I started taking this dietary supplement years ago. I had been on Lipitor for several months at that time and had severe pain in my arms. After taking CoQ$_{10}$ for a month, the pain disappeared and has not recurred. 99

No one should ever stop taking medicine on his or her own. Sudden discontinuation of a statin may lead to a rapid rise in both CRP and bad LDL cholesterol levels.[545] But if you are experiencing side effects that are interfering with the quality of your life, by all means discuss the situation with your physician. A surprising number of other options can get your cholesterol under control.

COENZYME Q_{10}

Most physicians have never heard of coenzyme Q_{10} (CoQ$_{10}$). When we mention it to cardiologists we frequently get a blank stare as if it is some sort of flaky dietary supplement. In truth, CoQ$_{10}$ is found in almost all of the cells in the body as well as in many foods, including spinach, broccoli, meat, and fish.

CoQ$_{10}$ is also known as *ubiquinone*, presumably because it is ubiquitous in tissue. The name is similar to *phylloquinone*, which is vitamin K. In reality, CoQ$_{10}$ acts very much like a vitamin, facilitating numerous biochemical reactions. It is also a powerful antioxidant. CoQ$_{10}$ might also be beneficial as an adjunct in the treatment of gum disease, angina, congestive heart failure,

★★★ Coenzyme Q_{10}

CoQ$_{10}$ is not an antidote to statins' side effects, but it may sometimes prevent or reduce symptoms of muscle pain and weakness associated with such drugs. The dose recommended by physicians we respect is 200 to 300 milligrams for patients on statins.

Downside: CoQ$_{10}$ may reduce the effectiveness of blood thinners like warfarin (Coumadin), but this interaction needs confirmation.
Side effects: Digestive tract upset, though it is rare
Cost: Variable; oil gelcaps (the best form) can cost $15 to $60 a month depending on brand and dose. Q-Gel and All-Q brands (solubilized CoQ$_{10}$) may be better absorbed than other formulations and require lower doses.

Parkinson's disease, high blood pressure, and certain irregular heart rhythms. This dietary supplement may be very helpful for patients taking statin-type cholesterol-lowering medication.

CoQ_{10} is critical for the energy factories of each cell—the mitochondria—to work efficiently. You want your mitochondria to be working optimally to supply your cells with energy. If CoQ_{10} is low, however, your cells have a harder time performing at their peak. Muscles in general, and the heart muscle in particular, may suffer if your CoQ_{10} level drops.

Stephen Sinatra, MD, a cardiologist, is a leading proponent of CoQ_{10} supplementation, especially for patients on statin-type cholesterol-lowering drugs like Crestor, Lipitor, and Zocor. These medications work by blocking an enzyme that is critical for the production of cholesterol. That same enzyme is essential for the manufacture of CoQ_{10}.

According to Dr. Sinatra, patients with heart disease or congestive heart failure "must be given supplemental doses of coenzyme Q_{10} to offset the depleting effects of cholesterol-lowering agents."[546] He recommends 90 to 150 milligrams of CoQ_{10} daily "as a preventive in cardiovascular or periodontal disease" and 180 to 360 milligrams daily "for the treatment of angina pectoris, cardiac arrhythmia, high blood pressure, and moderate gingival [gum] disease and for patients taking HMG-CoA reductase inhibitors (statin drugs)."[547]

Beatrice Golomb, MD, PhD, is an associate professor of medicine in residence in the Department of Medicine at the University of California at San Diego (UCSD). She is also a principal investigator of the UCSD Statin Study, which was undertaken to better understand how people react to this class of cholesterol-lowering drugs. Dr. Golomb has shared with us that some patients with low CoQ_{10} levels experience muscle pain or weakness. When they get 300 milligrams per day of CoQ_{10}, their symptoms may improve. She suggests that "coenzyme Q_{10} should be in gelcaps, in an oil or vitamin-E base to be absorbed."[548]

Other Drugs to Lower Cholesterol

Although statin-type drugs dominate do the cholesterol-lowering drug marketplace, many

★★★ Ezetimibe (Zetia)

Zetia has a modest effect on total cholesterol and LDL cholesterol.

Downside: While far less likely to interact with other medications than statins, Zetia should be used cautiously (if at all) by folks on cyclosporine. It may also interact with some other cholesterol-lowering drugs but poses no special problem for people taking statins. People also taking warfarin (Coumadin) should monitor their INR level carefully. INR is a blood test that indicates how quickly blood is clotting.

Side effects: Rare, but may include diarrhea, abdominal pain, sinusitis, back pain, arthritis, fatigue, cough, liver enzyme elevation, allergic reaction, and pancreatitis. We have heard from readers that both Zetia and statins may start turning white hair dark.

Cost: $80 to $90 for a month's supply

other drugs also do the job. One of the more popular these days is ezetimibe (Zetia). It works through a completely different mechanism than statins do. Rather than shutting down cholesterol synthesis, it blocks the absorption of cholesterol from the small intestine. In clinical trials, Zetia lowered total cholesterol by about 13 percent and LDL cholesterol by about 18 percent. When combined with a statin-type drug such as atorvastatin, lovastatin, or pravastatin, the results are much more impressive. In fact, there is a formulation on the market called Vytorin that combines simvastatin and ezetimibe in one pill. This dual-action medicine will lower total cholesterol by about 34 to 37 percent and LDL cholesterol by 46 to 50 percent.

Another category of medications that lowers cholesterol reasonably well is the fibrates. Gemfibrozil (Lopid) has been on the market for more than 25 years and is now available generically at $15 to $20 for a month's supply. That makes it one of the more cost-effective cholesterol-lowering drugs in the pharmacy. A newer compound called fenofibrate (TriCor) is also available. Both drugs are quite effective at lowering triglycerides, total cholesterol, and LDL cholesterol. They are also very good at turning small, dense particles of bad cholesterol into larger, less dangerous particles. As a bonus, fibrates raise good HDL cholesterol better than some other cholesterol-lowering drugs.

There is one other category of cholesterol medication. Although these drugs are not prescribed very often, they can lower cholesterol when other medicines are not appropriate. These drugs bind to bile acids, precursors to cholesterol. By preventing the reabsorption of cholesterol from the digestive tract, the body eliminates it more effectively. These drugs include cholestyramine (LoCholest, Questran), colestipol (Cholestid), and colesevelam (WelChol). These medications have a modest ability to lower total cholesterol and LDL cholesterol. They may actually raise triglyceride levels.

★★★ Gemfibrozil (Lopid) and Fenofibrate (TriCor)

Fibrates modify blood lipids in all the right directions. A long-term Finnish study showed that men taking gemfibrozil reduced their rate of heart attack by 34 percent.

Downside: Gallstone formation may be more likely on these fibrate-type medications. Can interact with the blood thinner warfarin (Coumadin). If this combination is required, dosage adjustments of warfarin may be necessary and very careful monitoring of INR levels is essential. INR is a blood test that indicates how quickly blood is clotting.

Side effects: Liver enzyme elevations (monitor carefully), nausea, vomiting, diarrhea, constipation, and stomach pain. Digestive tract discomfort may fade with time. If muscle pain occurs, a creatine kinase (CK) test is essential. Combining fibrates with statins may increase the risk of severe muscle problems (rhabdomyolysis).

Cost: Highly variable, ranging from $15 for generic gemfibrozil to $80 to $110 for a month's supply of TriCor.

Conclusions

Cholesterol is only one of more than 240 risk factors for heart disease. Focusing on this one element without addressing others is a little like trying to play a song with only one note. If we have learned anything about healthy lifestyles, it is that moderation in all things is the key to success. You will find a wonderful story in our appendix (page 467) from Laura Effel. It is titled "How I Lowered My LDL Cholesterol 44 Points in 5 Weeks without Drugs." Laura is our poster child for how sensible eating can make a difference for some people.

★ Bile Acid Binders

These drugs include cholestyramine, colestipol, and colesevelam. They lower total cholesterol by up to 20 percent and LDL cholesterol by around 15 percent. Triglycerides go up modestly.

Downside: These drugs are not for people with high triglycerides. Patients who have trouble swallowing should also avoid bile acid binders. Cholestyramine and colestipol may interfere with absorption of many other drugs and nutrients. Check with your pharmacist for compatibility and timing of dose.

Side effects: Digestive tract upset, including constipation, heartburn, and flatulence. Headache, rash, and fatigue have also been reported with cholestyramine.

- Cutting back on fat won't save your heart. Sugar and simple starches like potatoes, rice, and bread can raise triglycerides and other risk factors. A balanced diet of protein, low-starch vegetables, and monounsaturated fat such as olive oil is best for the heart.

- Don't smoke. If you do, quit. It may not be easy, but it will yield big dividends for your heart.

- Establish regular times for exercise and sleep and stick to them. Belly fat is a killer. Getting rid of your spare tire will save your life.

- Learn to manage your anger. Find ways to work out hostility that don't include dumping on or yelling at family members and friends. Supportive social relationships are good for the heart.

- Lower inflammation throughout your body by eating omega-3-rich fish and lots of other anti-inflammatory foods. Drink tea and sip wine in moderation. Measure CRP and keep your number around 1 or lower.

- Ask your doctor about taking 160 milligrams of aspirin daily. This is one of the cheapest and most effective heart insurance medications in the pharmacy. Beware of stomach ulcers and drug interactions, however.

- Try fish oil (up to 4 grams daily) to reduce inflammation and bring triglycerides under control. A great measure of heart health is the triglyceride/HDL ratio. It should ideally be around 1.

- Drink high-flavonoid beverages like purple grape juice, pomegranate juice, or a tonic of apple juice, grape juice, and apple cider vinegar. A glass of wine or beer three or four times a week can also be heart healthy.
- Eat a red grapefruit as often as possible. Daily consumption can lower both total cholesterol and dangerous LDL cholesterol. Beware of drug interactions, though.
- Nibble on nuts (such as walnuts, almonds, macadamia nuts, pecans, and pistachios) four or five times a week. They are part of a vegetarian dietary portfolio that includes oats, barley, psyllium, and vegetables high in soluble fiber (eggplant, okra) as well as soy-based substitutes for meat and milk and cholesterol-lowering margarine.
- A little bit of high-flavonoid dark chocolate can be good for the heart. Just 10 grams a day, on average, may be enough.
- Add some cinnamon to your food. As little as ¼ to ½ teaspoon a day may help bring down cholesterol and blood sugar levels. Results vary, so keep track of your progress.
- High-dose niacin can lower cholesterol, triglycerides, and Lp(a). It also raises beneficial HDL cholesterol. This vitamin therapy requires medical monitoring for liver enzymes and other potential problems.
- Magnesium may fight inflammation and improve cholesterol ratios as well. Many Americans don't get enough magnesium in their diet. Consider a supplement of 300 to 500 milligrams daily.
- Try coenzyme Q_{10}, especially if you take a cholesterol-lowering statin drug. They deplete the body of this nutrient that is crucial to the energy-making machinery inside each cell.
- Swallow a dose of psyllium three times a day to lower cholesterol effectively. Be sure to take it with adequate water. Psyllium seems to work best as part of the dietary portfolio.
- Experiment with policosanol if you want to lower your cholesterol without a prescription. Data on effectiveness are equivocal.
- Consider red yeast rice if your physician is unhappy about your cholesterol levels. Make sure the doctor monitors your liver enzymes and overall progress. Add coenzyme Q_{10} to reduce the risk of muscle problems.
- If your doctor prescribes a statin-type drug, ask for the lowest possible dose to start and monitor your progress. At the first sign of muscle pain or weakness, notify your physician immediately. Coenzyme Q_{10} may reduce the risk of some side effects.
- If you cannot tolerate statins and your doctor insists on better lipid control, ask about alternative medications. Zetia, TriCor, and Welchol all represent new options. Older generic possibilities include gemfibrozil and cholestyramine.

HIGH BLOOD PRESSURE

• Measure your blood pressure (Omron)	★★★★
• Monitor your stress level with a mood ring	★★★
• Take time-outs and relax (www.drmiller.com)	★★★★
• Learn to breathe (RESPeRATE)	★★
• Stay connected with friends and family	
• Follow the DASH diet	★★★★
• Lose weight (it's worth the effort!)	
• Drink tea and avoid coffee and soda	
• Try pomegranate juice	★★★★
• Drink Concord grape juice	★★★★
• Treat yourself to a little dark chocolate	★★★
• Maximize your minerals (magnesium!)	★★★★
• Beware of the beta-blocker blues	
• Avoid licorice and drugs that raise blood pressure	
• Ask your MD about chlorthalidone	★★★★
• Have an ACE up your sleeve	★★★★★

High blood pressure is a very big deal. According to the American Heart Association, it affects up to 65 million Americans (nearly one in three adults). The majority (more than 70 percent) are not controlling it adequately. For the most part, the experts are still trying to figure out what causes this common condition and why it becomes so widespread as people age.

If you were to reduce traditional medical wisdom on hypertension to its essence, it would probably come to these four points:

1. High blood pressure is bad! It contributes to atherosclerosis and leads to strokes, heart attacks, kidney damage, and dementia.

2. Low blood pressure is good.

3. Eat less salt.

4. Take your pills.

Wouldn't it be wonderful if it were that simple? Like so many things, though, blood pressure (BP) is complicated. For one thing, your blood pressure is not a single, solitary number that remains stable day in and day out. If you were to monitor your BP every few minutes throughout the day and night you would likely discover enormous variability. Over the course of 24 hours, readings could change by as much as 50 points.[549]

Some people may have relatively low blood

pressure in the morning when they first get up.[550] After drinking coffee and dealing with rush hour traffic, however, their BP may go up by 10 or more points.[551] A stressful interaction with a co-worker or family member can jack it up even higher.[552] Exercise (including sex) pushes up blood pressure dramatically, but after a strenuous workout, pressure often comes down below where it started. And blood pressure can vary while you are asleep, depending upon whether you are dreaming, sleeping peacefully, or snoring (with sleep apnea).[553]

Even the day of the week can affect your blood pressure. One study revealed that readings are substantially higher on Monday and Tuesday compared to Saturday and Sunday.[554] That's presumably because people relax on the weekends and are under a lot less stress at home than at work.

Then there's the whole issue of "white coat hypertension," so named because it is triggered by the presence of a health professional wearing a white coat. Some years ago Italian researchers demonstrated that when a doctor walked into a patient's room, systolic blood pressure (the first, or top, number of a blood pressure reading) went up an average of 27 points within 2 minutes.[555] This increase occurred in 47 out of 48 subjects regardless of whether they started with normal blood pressure or had a history of hypertension. Sitting

> "Although a large number of guidelines and recommendations describing how blood pressure [should be] measured are available, research shows that health care providers frequently do not comply with these guidelines. This leads to possible mistakes in the diagnosis and treatment of hypertension. Additionally, the guidelines are not always consistent with each other."[556]
> —S. T. Houweling et al., *Family Practice*, 2006

in a doctor's exam room in a goofy gown with your butt hanging out while you wait forever to see the doctor is not designed to put you at ease. The minute he knocks on the door and comes rushing in, you are likely to feel even more stressed out.

The point is that blood pressure is a constantly moving target. Relying on a single measurement in a doctor's office would be like looking at a still shot from a 90-minute movie and trying to decipher the plot. If you happened to catch a love scene, you might think the movie was romantic. If the actors were laughing, you might assume it was a comedy. In reality, though, you could not predict how the movie would play out based on a couple of quick snapshots. Likewise, trying to draw conclusions about someone's blood pressure based on a few readings in a doctor's office is virtually impossible.

Measuring Blood Pressure

Many physicians, nurses, and physician's assistants assume that they know how to take your blood pressure correctly. It is, after all, one of the primary tricks of the trade. In truth, there is tremendous variability in technique.[557] How your blood pressure is measured will affect the number recorded in your chart and, ultimately, whether you will receive a prescription.

European and American guidelines suggest that you be allowed to sit quietly for 5 minutes before any measurement is taken. Tight clothing should be removed from the upper arm. The health professional should measure your arm circumference and select the appropriate cuff to match your arm size. The cuff should be applied snugly to the bare arm about half an inch above the elbow crease. The arm should be resting comfortably on a desk, and the cuff should be at heart level. Your back should be supported. Sitting on the exam table to have your blood pressure taken could raise it by as much as 5 points.

You should never talk prior to or during measurements. Blood pressure should be measured twice in each arm with at least 15 seconds between readings. If there is a difference of greater than 5 points between readings, repeat measurements should be taken until this variability is below 5. The two numbers should then be averaged.

Even if everything is done correctly at the doctor's office or clinic, it is still only a snapshot of your 24-hour blood pressure. The only way to really know what is going on is to measure your own blood pressure on a regular basis under a variety of different circumstances. Many physicians now believe that even white coat hypertension may be a predictor of problems to come. Someone who has "normal" blood pressure at home and elevated readings in a doctor's office may react to other stressful situations (such as a demanding boss or a spat with a spouse) with bouts of high blood pressure. This might lead to true hypertension, with all its negative health consequences, down the road.

So, how would you begin to determine whether you have high blood pressure? If you even suspect you may be at risk, invest in a blood pressure monitor. If you have hypertension, this device is crucial for measuring your progress. We have looked at lots of machines over the last 3 decades and have found that those in the Omron line are as easy to use and as accurate as anything on the market. In past years *Consumer Reports* has given the Omron Automatic BPM with Intellisense its highest rating.[558] The ReliOn brand, available from Wal-Mart, is also manufactured by Omron, but is less expensive ($40 to $60). We prefer the old-fashioned arm cuff to a wrist device.

★★★★ Omron Digital Blood Pressure Monitor with IntelliSense

We like this device because it is so easy to use. The cuff wraps around the arm without requiring any assistance and fits people with medium to large arms (9 to 17 inches in circumference). This is important to get accurate readings. There is easy cuff storage and memory recall so you can monitor your progress over time.

Cost: Approximately $80 to $90

We think the arm cuff produces more reliable readings most of the time.

We encourage people with borderline or diagnosed hypertension to measure blood pressure regularly under a variety of conditions. Until you detect clear trends, we think it makes sense to monitor in the morning, in the middle of the day, and again in the evening. Keep a machine at work so you can check your blood pressure in stressful working conditions.

Once you have a pretty clear picture of what's going on, you can cut back to once a day or even a couple of times a week, as long as you change the time of day you take your measurement. Keep a diary of all your numbers so you can show them to your physician. If you want to really go high-tech, you can plug the values into your computer and use a program like Excel to plot out your readings in a graphical form. Your doctor will be blown away by your diligence. It will also make it easier for her to track your progress.

We cannot emphasize enough how critical it is to work closely with your physician to find a blood-pressure-lowering approach that controls hypertension and maintains your quality of life. It will take patience and persistence.

How High Is High? How Low to Go?

Just as cardiologists keep lowering the target levels for cholesterol, they are also reducing the goals for blood pressure. It used to be that many physicians didn't treat high blood pressure unless the systolic pressure (the upper number) stayed above 160 millimeters of mercury (mmHg) and the diastolic (the bottom number) was above 100 mmHg. These days many doctors define hypertension as anything over 140/90.[560] Some who would have us aim even lower have proposed a goal blood pres-

---

TIPS FOR BLOOD PRESSURE MONITORING

• Use the proper cuff size. If your arm is larger than 13 inches in circumference, you must use a larger cuff (just as your doctor must when taking your blood pressure!). Using a normal cuff if you have a large arm can lead to falsely elevated blood pressure readings.

• Maintain correct arm position. Rest your arm horizontally on a desk or the arm of a chair or couch. Your arm should be at roughly the same level as your heart and resting comfortably. If your arm is lower (like in your lap) your blood pressure reading may be falsely elevated.

• Do not talk! Doctors and nurses often try to put patients at ease by chatting them up while taking their blood pressure. A seemingly simple question like "How are the kids?" could trigger a dramatic jump in blood pressure. We don't know why, but talking while measuring blood pressure can increase a reading by more than 20 points.[559] Sit quietly and breathe deeply from the belly for 5 minutes before measuring blood pressure.

---

sure reading of 115/75.[561] To be perfectly candid, even the experts cannot decide precisely when it is necessary to treat. Different countries frequently have different guidelines.

Some data even suggest that very low blood pressure may have certain negative consequences. Although many physicians believe that there is no such thing as too low a cholesterol score or blood pressure reading (unless someone is really sick), that might not always be true. Older people may be more vulnerable to falls if they experience low blood pressure when they stand suddenly. (This can be caused by some blood pressure medications.) Dizziness is a frequent complaint when blood pressure drops dramatically.

Swedish researchers have reported that although elevated blood pressure in midlife is associated with Alzheimer's disease, so is a fall in blood pressure when people get older. In their study, elderly subjects who experienced a 15-point or greater decline in blood pressure had an elevated risk of Alzheimer's disease or dementia.[562]

● ● ●

Q. *My father has had trouble getting his blood pressure under control. His doctor has him on atenolol, reserpine, Accupril, Norvasc, and hydrochlorothiazide. Dad is terribly depressed and can barely drag himself out of bed. As a result, his doctor prescribed Lexapro. Isn't this too much medication?*

A. We are astonished physicians are still prescribing reserpine for hypertension. It is an old-fashioned medication. Reserpine is notorious for causing severe depression. Treating it with an antidepressant like Lexapro is not logical.

A meta-analysis of atenolol in the journal *Lancet* (November 6, 2004) "cast doubts on atenolol as a suitable drug for hypertensive patients." It may cause fatigue, dizziness, or depression in some patients, but such blood pressure medication should never be stopped suddenly!

Your father should discuss his symptoms with his doctor who should be able to control your dad's blood pressure without severe side effects like depression or fatigue.

● ● ●

The bottom line is that there is no bottom line for you. Hypertension guidelines are created for large populations or countries, but not for individuals. Remember, blood pressure is just one more risk factor for cardiovascular disease, like cholesterol, smoking, and diabetes. Granted, it is a key risk factor, but the point of treatment is not only to get your numbers down to some arbitrary ideal—the goal is to keep you as healthy as possible and prevent atherosclerosis that might lead to a heart attack, a stroke, or kidney damage.

Aggressive treatment may be called for in

some cases when there are many other risk factors like diabetes, overweight, high triglycerides, and coronary artery disease.[563] In other situations, a more modest approach may be appropriate.[564]

Lowering Blood Pressure without Drugs

Hundreds of medications lower blood pressure, but they all can cause side effects. In some cases the complications are extremely subtle, such as a loss of potassium. This serious situation can go undetected for years unless you get a blood test. If potassium levels go too low, an irregular heart rhythm may result or, in the worst case, cardiac arrest. Since there is no perfect pill to control hypertension, it only makes sense to try to manage things first with nondrug approaches.

Measuring Stress

Just as there are many factors that cause heart disease, so, too, there are many factors that raise blood pressure. Stress is an obvious culprit, yet it is frequently ignored.

For one study, researchers measured blood pressure changes in young adults while they played challenging video games. Thirteen years later, the study subjects underwent CT scans of their coronary arteries. Those who had reacted with elevations in their blood pressure during the psychological stress experiments had an increased risk of developing calcification of their coronary arteries more than a decade later.[565]

We have already established that daytime blood pressure is higher on weekdays than on weekends.[566] This is presumably because of work-related stress. We also know that the mere act of talking can increase blood pressure by 25 to 40 percent within 30 seconds.[567] The more emotional the content, the stronger the reaction is and the longer it lasts.[568,569] Interestingly, blood pressure medications such as diuretics, beta-blockers, and calcium channel blockers do not seem to block blood pressure increases caused by talking.[570]

Since it is not practical or healthy to retire to a cave, become a hermit, and stop talking, you may want to become sensitized to your reaction to stressful situations. Some people can literally "feel" their blood pressure going up when they are in an emotional or challenging environment. If you "listen" to your body, you will sense that an argument with a co-worker or a spouse can increase your blood pressure dramatically. You could measure your blood pressure with a digital monitor, but that's kind of hard to do in the middle of a stressful situation.

There's another unobtrusive way to monitor your internal stress level: Invest in a "mood" ring. It may look funny, but this kind of jewelry was quite popular in the late 1970s. It was supposed to reflect your emotions—from happy, romantic, and relaxed to nervous and stressed out.

In reality, the liquid crystals in the ring are sensitive to the surface temperature of your skin, which is a way of monitoring internal stress. Blood vessels constrict and temperature drops during stressful situations. Under normal conditions the average person should have a skin temperature of about 82°F and the ring should be calibrated to the color green. When you are really relaxed and feeling happy, your skin temperature should be a little higher and the ring should turn blue. If you are a little anxious and the capillaries in your skin start to constrict, the ring should turn amber. When you are stressed out, your hands may get cold and clammy and the ring should go to gray or black.

Cardiologists we know think this is a total waste of time. We'll let you be the judge.

★★★ Mood Ring

You can buy mood rings almost anywhere. Look for them on eBay, Amazon.com, or www.moodjewelry.com. Use Google to shop the Web for dozens of other options.

We love the Bio-Q Thermal Biofeedback and Stress Monitoring Ring because it provides a more sophisticated and elegant measure of skin temperature. For more information, visit www.futurehealth.org.

If a ring isn't your thing, you can buy a little liquid crystal "chip" that is smaller than a postage stamp. It sticks to your skin and changes color just like a ring.

Cost: From $1 to $5 and all the way up to about $25 for the Bio-Q. You can buy 100 Biofeedback Bio-Squares for about $15 from Amazon.com.

Use this biofeedback device to alert yourself to high-stress situations. Think of it as your body's thermometer. Just as you might check the outside temperature, you can use this to check your skin temperature. The more time you keep your mood ring showing green and dark blue, the calmer you are supposed to be.

If you see your ring changing to the wrong color, you will know that you need to calm down. Turn off the stress reaction by breathing deeply from the abdomen, taking an internal "time out," and exercising. Listening to a relaxation CD or calming music can help, too. Seek out friends and family members who make your hands warm. Avoid toxic people or situations that make your hands cold or turn your ring amber or black.

Your mood ring can be your guide. It may help you lower your blood pressure when coupled with a general stress-reduction and relaxation program.[571,572] One research team reported that about a fifth of the subjects in their biofeedback and relaxation study were able to lower their systolic blood pressure by 10 points, about as much as some medicines do.[573]

Breathe!

Some people have an incredibly hard time relaxing and breathing deeply. Most of us take breathing for granted. It's not something we think about. But how we breathe can influence our entire physiology. This concept is fundamental to yoga, a healing tradition that stretches back thousands of years. If you breathe shallowly from your chest, you probably take 16 to 20 breaths per minute, or up to 25,000 breaths per day. Deep, diaphragmatic breathing requires only six to eight breaths a minute, or a maximum of 12,000 breaths per day.

Most of us are too busy to take time out of our frantic schedules to sit quietly and breathe deeply. If yoga seems too exotic for you, there is now an alternative. It is called RESPeRATE. This dandy device combines high technology with an ancient healing tradition to teach you how to breathe deeply. It includes a small, computerized device, about the size of a thick paperback book or a portable CD player. There is also a chest strap that goes around your diaphragm, and a set of earphones.

At first you breathe normally as the sensor feeds a signal to the computer, which analyzes your breathing pattern. You then listen to melodious tones, which gradually prolong your exhalations. The goal is to slow your respiration to less than 10 breaths per minute.

Studies have demonstrated that slow breathing reduces blood pressure.[574,575] People who used the RESPeRATE device lowered their systolic blood pressure by around 5 points compared to control subjects who did not practice slow breathing.[576,577] The absolute reduction may be as much as 10 to 15 points in systolic blood pressure.

RESPeRATE is not a magic bullet; it won't take a blood pressure reading of 160/100 and normalize it to 120/80. But many people who want a nondrug approach to partial blood pressure control may see benefits if they use the device 15 minutes a day several times a week. Unfortunately, it is pricey. You should not consider it unless you are willing to devote a little time each day to deep breathing.

Social Interaction

When was the last time a doctor asked you whether you were lonely? It turns out that loneliness is linked to hypertension and may be a stronger risk factor for cardiovascular disease than more recognized things like salt, obesity, and lack of exercise. Physicians may feel more comfortable writing a prescription for a blood pressure medication, but they might also consider prescribing volunteer work or dance classes or a furry pet.

Older people around retirement age are most vulnerable to this effect. It is estimated that at least 9 million people over the age of 50 frequently feel lonely or cut off socially. Blood pressure could end up 30 points higher when people feel isolated.[578] When you are lonely, stressful events can become even more challenging.

Try to nurture friendships and social support networks. They may help you lower your blood pressure as well as reduce your need for medication.

Weight Loss, Diet, and Exercise

The safest, most effective ways to lower blood pressure are weight loss, exercise, and the DASH (Dietary Approaches to Stop Hypertension) diet.[579] Studies have shown that regular moderate exercise alone can bring down blood pressure by 2 to 3 mmHg or more. The DASH diet can reduce systolic blood pressure by 5.5 points in people with and without hypertension. People who are overweight and lose about 18 pounds can expect to lower their systolic blood pressure by 8.5 mmHg and their diastolic blood pressure by 6.5 mmHg.[580] These kinds of reductions are what you would expect from many blood pressure medications.

The benefits of diet, exercise, and weight loss are obvious. Even more important, they don't cause the side effects—sexual dysfunction, dizziness, forgetfulness, and depression—that drugs can. But losing weight is difficult. Trying to recommend one diet or

★★★★ DASH Diet

The DASH (Dietary Approaches to Stop Hypertension) diet was developed specifically to help lower high blood pressure. It has been studied extensively and proven effective.[581,582] People with hypertension (a reading higher than 140/90) showed reductions of 11.4 mmHg systolic and 5.5 mmHg diastolic, as much as you would see with blood pressure medicine. The key elements are daily intake of:

- 4 servings of fruits
- 4 servings of vegetables
- 7 to 11 servings of grains
- 2 to 3 servings of low-fat dairy foods
- Nuts, fish, and poultry
- Little red meat, sweets, and sugary drinks

Cost: $7 for the book *The DASH Diet for Hypertension,* which offers a detailed discussion of the diet. For a free overview on the Web, visit www.nhlbi.nih.gov/health/public/heart/hbp/dash/new_dash.pdf.

exercise program over another is foolhardy. Ultimately, you must pick the program that works best for you. Some people find the South Beach Diet suits their style. Others may prefer the Zone. They should all be beneficial, and some may be even more effective than the DASH diet.

Scientists at Johns Hopkins University tested three different diet plans. One was the DASH diet, which is rich in vegetables, fruits, and grains. It has clearly been shown to help lower blood pressure. Another plan substituted protein for some of the carbohydrates in the DASH diet. And in the third plan, monounsaturated fat, like that in olive oil, replaced calories from carbohydrates. According to the investigators' report in the *Journal of the American Medical Association,* the high-protein and monunsaturated fat diets lowered blood pressure and cholesterol even better than the higher-carb DASH diet.[583]

Losing weight, however you do it, should bring your blood pressure down.[584] The best diet is the one that you will stick with. That goes for exercise as well. And if all else fails, a diet pill may help. The medication we are most intrigued by is rimonobant (Acomplia). See page 411 for more details on this approach.

The Salt Wars: Man Bites Dog

People have been fighting over salt for hundreds, if not thousands, of years. In ancient times, it was a valuable commodity. Roman soldiers were even paid partly in salt (hence the word *salary,* derived from the Latin *salarium,* meaning *payment in salt*). But for the last 50 years doctors have been warning Americans to cut back on salt.

The modern-day salt wars are fought in the pages of medical journals. Although most Americans have been told repeatedly to avoid excess sodium because it will raise blood pressure, the data are not as clear as you might imagine for a belief that is so entrenched.

Even after 20,000 studies and decades of debate, scientists cannot agree about the dangers of salt. The current sodium guidelines are based primarily on salt restriction during relatively short-term clinical trials.[585] But in 2006, the second National Health and Nutrition Examination Survey (NHANES II)—which included more than 7,000 people and followed their progress for nearly 14 years—yielded one of the most bizarre results in modern medicine, a man-bites-dog story if ever there were one. People who ate *less* sodium were more likely to experience fatal heart attacks or strokes.[586]

The NHANES researchers suggested that there may be adverse consequences associated with low salt consumption. Having too little sodium in the system may affect the nervous system and blood pressure–controlling enzymes made in the kidneys and possibly increase insulin resistance (not good things). Some cardiologists are skeptical of these results and suspect that the information on salt intake may have been inaccurate.

No one is ready to suggest that people should overindulge in salt. But there is some concern that sodium restriction may not prolong life the way everyone expected. There is also a growing recognition that people differ in their salt sensitivity. Many folks do not experience a rise in blood pressure when exposed to sodium.[587] Others are so salt sensitive that it may increase their risk of heart attacks and strokes even if they do not have hypertension.[588,589]

There is no easy way to tell whether you are salt sensitive. It normally requires special testing in a research facility. But you could do your own crude experiment. Establish your baseline blood pressure for a few weeks while eating normally. Then cut back on salt for several weeks and measure your blood pressure a couple of times each day. Return to your normal eating behavior and measure your blood pressure again. After a few cycles like this, you may be able to tell whether your body is sensitive to salt.

Drink Tea and Avoid Coffee and Soda

For decades the link between coffee and high blood pressure has been confusing and controversial. Experts are almost as conflicted about coffee as they are about salt. One study showed that as little as 2 or 3 cups of coffee could raise blood pressure by 14 percent.[590] Other research, however, suggests that there is only a modest effect on blood pressure (a systolic increase of 1.22 mmHg and a diastolic increase of 0.5 mmHg).[591] A 33-year study of men who graduated from Johns Hopkins University School of Medicine uncovered a very

small increase in blood pressure among coffee drinkers who consumed about a cup a day.[592]

If coffee drinking produces such a modest increase in blood pressure, how could it possibly be dangerous? The answer to all the confusion may lie in our genes. It turns out that people are divided into two groups: slow caffeine metabolizers and rapid caffeine metabolizers. Until recently, researchers did not realize that many people rid their bodies of caffeine quite quickly, whereas for others, the effects linger for many hours. This may explain why one person can drink a cup or two of coffee with dinner and experience no jitteriness or insomnia, whereas another may have a cup of coffee at lunch and still be wired that evening.

A study has revealed that among coffee drinkers, slow caffeine metabolizers seem to be at substantially higher risk of heart attack than fast metabolizers.[593] The more coffee the slow metabolizers drank, the greater their danger. Since these variations have not been taken into account in prior studies, they may be the reason for the inconsistent findings about coffee and blood pressure. It is not possible to easily tell whether you are a rapid or slow caffeine metabolizer, so we encourage people with hypertension to err on the side of moderate caffeine consumption.

Coffee may not be that big a problem for women, but cola soft drinks (sugared or diet) may be. Researchers have been following more than 150,000 nurses for over a decade. They found that while women who drank coffee regularly were not at significant risk for developing hypertension, those who consumed colas were more likely to have higher blood pressure. The researchers speculate that it is probably not the caffeine, but rather something else in these soft drinks that may be predisposing women to hypertension.

Drinking tea (green and oolong) may actually protect against high blood pressure, at least in a Chinese population.[594] Researchers in Taiwan discovered that men and women who consumed at least ½ cup of tea daily decreased their risk of hypertension by almost 50 percent. If they drank up to 4 cups a day their likelihood of having high blood pressure was reduced by 65 percent.

Pomegranate Juice

Most cardiologists would agree that ACE inhibitors are about the most valuable blood pressure medications ever developed. These are drugs like benazepril (Lotensin), enalapril (Vasotec), lisinopril (Prinivil, Zestril), ramipril (Altace), and quinapril (Accupril). They block an enzyme called angiotensin-converting enzyme (thus the name ACE). Studies demonstrate significant blood pressure reduction and heart attack prevention with this class of medications. What most physicians don't realize, however, is that some foods can also inhibit this enzyme.

Pomegranate juice can reduce ACE activity by about 36 percent.[595] This may explain why drinking the juice regularly can help lower blood pressure. One study found that when hypertensive patients drank 2 ounces of pome-

★★★★ **Pomegranate Juice**

Small preliminary studies suggest that pomegranate juice may lower systolic blood pressure by almost as much as some medications. Pomegranate juice reduces total and bad LDL cholesterol and helps keep blood platelets from sticking together to form unwanted clots.

Downside: Drinking too much juice may be constipating.

Cost: Pure pomegranate juice is pricey. A month's worth could run into hundreds of dollars unless you purchase pomegranate juice concentrate. Check out www.healingfruits.com for affordable products. A 1- to 2-month supply costs around $25.

granate juice daily, their systolic blood pressure came down by an average of 8 points.[596]

Pomegranate juice has other heart-healthy benefits (see page 255 for more details). For one thing, pomegranate juice may improve bloodflow and oxygen delivery to the heart.[597] There are also data to suggest that pomegranates have antiplatelet activity, which could reduce the risk of blood clots. All in all, we think pomegranate juice has potential cardiovascular benefits that rival those of many drugs.

Purple Grape Juice

Pomegranate juice may not be the only beverage that inhibits angiotensin-converting enzyme. Japanese researchers have tested a red wine vinegar and grape juice drink called

★★★★ Concord Grape Juice

Purple grape juice has many cardiovascular benefits. It lowers cholesterol, improves the flexibility of blood vessels, reduces the likelihood that platelets will clump together to form clots, and lowers blood pressure.

The amount needed to accomplish an effect is unclear. One study found that about two glasses of juice daily produced a measurable blood pressure–lowering effect.

Downside: Grape juice has a lot of sugar and calories. This is not a good choice for diabetics or those on a low-carb diet.

Cost: $3 to $4 for 64 ounces. That is enough for about a week.

Budo-no-megumi. They found that it partially blocks this enzyme and activates another enzyme (nitric oxide synthase), which may account for its ability to dilate blood vessels and lower blood pressure.[598,599]

Since this drink does not appear to be available in the United States, you could experiment by mixing various proportions of red wine vinegar and grape juice to find a pleasing concoction. Check your blood pressure to see if you notice any benefit.

Even by itself, grape juice has health benefits. It can reduce bad cholesterol, prevent the oxidation of LDL cholesterol, help maintain the flexibility of blood vessels, improve bloodflow, and diminish the likelihood that platelets will clump together to form blood clots.[600,601] In one double-blind, placebo-controlled trial, Concord grape juice lowered systolic BP by 7.2 points, on average, and diastolic BP by 6.2 points, compared to 3.5 and 3.2 mmHg, respectively, for placebo.[602]

Chocolate

Don't laugh—chocolate really does have amazing health benefits. You've heard that red wine and green tea are loaded with beneficial antioxidant flavonoids. Well, it turns out that ounce for ounce, cocoa and chocolate have higher levels of these goodies. They also contain other compounds that are beneficial for the cardiovascular system. A study published in the *American Journal of Hypertension* demonstrated that 100 grams (3.5 ounces) of dark chocolate improved the flexibility, function, and diameter of arteries.[603]

Can chocolate really lower blood pressure? The Zutphen Elderly Study is a long-term research project that was started in 1985. Older

★★★ Chocolate

Dark chocolate improves blood vessel flexibility, lowers blood pressure, reduces insulin resistance and helps keep blood platelets from sticking together to form clots.

Downside: Calories. Compensate for the additional calories by cutting back on sugar and other carbohydrates or by drinking cocoa (not alkali or Dutch processed) without sugar.

Cost: Variable; approximately 30 cents for a day's supply (a small square of Ritter Sport Dark)

Dutch men (over the age of 65) were recruited and then followed every 5 years for 15 years. The investigators discovered that the men who ate the most chocolate were only half as likely to have died of heart disease.[604] They also had slightly reduced systolic blood pressure (3.7 mmHg lower). These fellows averaged about 10 grams (0.35 ounce) of dark chocolate a day. That's far less than the 100 grams of dark chocolate that has been shown to lower blood pressure in double-blind trials.[605]

Bottom line: A little chocolate is good for the soul and the blood pressure. If you are on a weight-reduction program, try cocoa (Scharffen Berger, Valrhona) instead.

> "The present study indicates that men with a usual daily cocoa intake of about 4.2 grams, which is equal to 10 grams of dark chocolate per day, had a lower systolic and diastolic blood pressure compared with men with a low cocoa intake. Although this amount is one tenth of the dose that is used in most intervention studies, it suggests that long-term daily intake of a small amount of cocoa may lower blood pressure."[606]
> —B. Buijsse et al., *Archives of Internal Medicine*, 2006

• • •

Q. *I've got a comment about the dark chocolate controversy: whether it is irresponsible to recommend chocolate for health benefits.*

I started eating Hershey's dark chocolate when it was on sale a few weeks ago. I enjoy about five of the little squares twice a day. Both my systolic and diastolic blood pressure numbers went down about 15 or 20 points each.

A. Chocolate will never substitute for blood pressure medicine, but there are some data to support your experience. Studies have demonstrated the modest blood pressure–lowering effects of cocoa and dark chocolate (*Hypertension*, August, 2005; *Archives of Internal Medicine*, February 27, 2006).

Your reaction to chocolate is much greater than average. The amount needed to affect blood pressure ranges from 10 grams (the size of one Ghirardelli chocolate square) to 100 grams (the size of a Ritter Sport bar).

• • •

Maximize Your Minerals

So much intellectual capital has been spent trying to convince people to avoid sodium that there hasn't been much left for encouraging people to consider the value of other minerals. Many physicians have been trained to be Doctor Don'ts: "Don't eat fat, don't eat eggs, don't eat salt." We're much more interested in do's than don'ts.

It turns out that calcium, magnesium, and potassium actually can lower blood pressure. The individual impact of each is relatively modest, but many well-conducted clinical trials have demonstrated that collectively, the three electrolytes have a measurable effect on blood pressure.[607,608,609]

Although all three are important, we tend to think of magnesium as the most magnificent mineral. For one thing, it may be lacking in the diet. For those on a blood pressure medicine containing a standard diuretic, there is a strong likelihood that their magnesium level (as well as potassium) will be low. That's because many water pills deplete the body of both potassium and magnesium.

Doctors frequently think of potassium and remind their patients to eat bananas and oranges to replenish this mineral if it is low. They may order a blood test to keep tabs on the potassium level. But magnesium often falls through the cracks. That is why it is so important to get adequate amounts of this mineral.

People with a low level of magnesium in their body may be at greater risk for metabolic syndrome, hypertension, diabetes, and atherosclerosis.[611,612] This is especially true for diabetics.[613] When the magnesium level is suboptimal, there are signs of inflammation, poor vascular function, and cardiovascular disease.[614,615] When people get extra magnesium from their diet or from supplements, their arteries function better, the heart pumps more regularly and effectively, blood pressure comes down, and the risk of heart disease is lower.[616,617,618]

Whenever possible, we prefer food sources of magnesium to dietary supplements. For those who are less interested in taking a supplement and would like to know which foods are highest in this essential mineral, please refer to our table of high-magnesium foods.

We don't want to slight potassium. As long as you are not taking a potassium-preserving diuretic or a blood pressure medication that allows the mineral to build up (such as an ACE inhibitor or an angiotensin receptor blocker),

---

★★★★ Magnesium

This mineral can help lower blood pressure, enhance arterial function, improve the ratio of bad LDL cholesterol to good HDL cholesterol, reduce the oxidation of LDL cholesterol, diminish cellular inflammation, and lower the risk of atherosclerosis. It improves circulation to the coronary arteries, helps maintain a regular heart rhythm, and improves exercise tolerance.[610] The recommended dose of magnesium is 300 to 500 milligrams daily. Loose stools signal too much magnesium.

Downside: Dangerous for people with reduced kidney function or kidney disease
Side effects: Diarrhea. Remember, milk of magnesia has been used to combat constipation for decades.
Cost: Variable; approximately $3 for a 3-month supply from Bronson Laboratories

FOODS THAT ARE HIGH IN MAGNESIUM*

Halibut, 3 ounces	90 milligrams
Almonds, 1 ounce	80 milligrams
Cashews, 1 ounce	75 milligrams
Soybeans, ½ cup	75 milligrams
Spinach, ½ cup	75 milligrams
Mixed nuts, 1 ounce	65 milligrams
Shredded wheat, 2 wafers	55 milligrams
Oatmeal, instant, 1 cup	55 milligrams
Baked potato, medium	50 milligrams
Peanuts, 1 ounce	50 milligrams
Black-eyed peas, ½ cup	45 milligrams
Yogurt, plain skim, 8 ounces	45 milligrams
Brown rice, ½ cup	40 milligrams
Lentils, ½ cup	35 milligrams
Avocado, ½ cup	35 milligrams
Banana, medium	30 milligrams

*Derived from data from the Office of Dietary Supplements of the National Institutes of Health.

you may want to consider eating your choice of the following potassium-rich foods: apricots, artichokes, asparagus, bananas, beets, bell peppers, blackstrap molasses, broccoli, brussels sprouts, buttermilk, cabbage, cantaloupe, carrots, cauliflower, chicken, fish, kidney beans, lentils, lima beans, nectarines, oatmeal, onions, oranges, peaches, plums, pomegranates, pork, potatoes, prunes, raisins, raspberries, spinach, squash, tomatoes, wheat germ, and yogurt.

Special Foods

We have heard for years that eating garlic or celery can lower blood pressure. The data on garlic are mixed, though. There have been nine meaningful studies to date. Six have demonstrated some benefit while the other three produced no reduction in blood pressure.[619] A meta-analysis of all the garlic research published in the *Archives of Internal Medicine* came to the following conclusion: "Trials suggest possible small short-term benefits of garlic on some lipid and antiplatelet factors, insignificant effects on blood pressure, and no effect on glucose levels."[620] We would not count on garlic to make a big difference in your blood pressure. On the other hand, cooking with garlic and using it in salad dressing can't hurt.

• • •

Q. *I've had high blood pressure since 1985 and have taken many drugs, including Vasotec, Maxzide, and others. All of them have side effects such as dry mouth or hair loss, and none has been effective at getting my lower number below 90.*

About 2 years ago, I heard about taking garlic for blood pressure. I take two pills a day. For over a year, my blood pressure has been around 135/80. I swear by garlic even though the doctors say it's not very effective.

A. Some preliminary research in animals and humans suggests that garlic may have a modest effect, especially on diastolic blood pressure (the lower number). Garlic cannot substitute for prescribed medication, however, and garlic supplements may interact with some prescription drugs to increase the risk of bleeding. Nevertheless, adding fresh garlic to food is certainly a reasonable approach.

• • •

Celery enthusiasts insist that if you eat eight ribs a day your blood pressure will come down. We have seen no solid research to support this concept. We happen to enjoy celery, however, and it probably can't hurt to do the experiment. Buy enough celery to last a couple of weeks and measure your blood pressure regularly. If it goes down, so much the better. Even if your blood pressure doesn't budge, you haven't lost anything. Celery has lots of healthy fiber.

Then there's the eggplant story. We got an astonishing letter from a reader and became quite interested. To our dismay, it looks like eggplant is a fizzle.

• • •

Q. *Have you ever heard of this remedy for high blood pressure?*

Wash but don't peel a medium eggplant. Dice it into 1-inch cubes.

Place the cubes in a glass gallon jug and cover the eggplant with distilled water. Put the jug in the fridge for 4

days. Drink 1 ounce of the water per day, taking your blood pressure daily.

After a week or so, the eggplant will begin to disintegrate; discard the cubes but keep drinking the ounce of water daily.

Be sure to check your blood pressure, as it may begin to drop dramatically.

Once your blood pressure is at a good level, you will need to experiment to determine how often to drink the eggplant water. It may be every other day or less often.

A. Your remedy is fascinating, but we were unable to confirm that it would lower blood pressure.

Eggplant is a popular vegetable in many parts of the world. It is also referred to as *aubergine, garden egg,* or *melanzana.* The peel contains anthocyanidins, compounds like those in blackberries or purple grapes, and the flesh is rich in soluble fiber, which may help lower cholesterol.

The Nurse's Health Study has been tracking tens of thousands of women for decades to see how diet and lifestyle affect health. Surprisingly, eggplant consumption was associated with higher blood pressure (*Hypertension,* May 1996). Based on this research, we wouldn't trade medicine for eggplant.

• • •

Researchers are looking into foods that may inhibit angiotensin-converting enzyme. Drugs that block this enzyme are some of the most successful blood pressure pills in the pharmacy. Scientists have found that ingredients in aged Gouda cheese may offer some promise. And Japanese investigators are looking at compounds in fermented milk products like kefir (available in health-food stores in the dairy section). It's still too early to recommend such foods for hypertension, but you could do your own experiment and see what happens.

Dietary Supplements

We would never suggest substituting an herb or a dietary supplement for a prescription blood pressure medicine. There's just not enough data to demonstrate clear effectiveness. That said, there are some data to support the possible effectiveness of coenzyme Q_{10} (CoQ_{10}).[621] As long as you check in with your physician to make sure he or she is on board with the program, it seems reasonable to add CoQ_{10} to your standard regimen and monitor your progress.

One other supplement has shown promise, especially for people with prehypertension (meaning those on the borderline of having high blood pressure). Researchers at the University of California at Davis gave a small group of such patients and some nonhypertensives either grape seed extract or placebo. Those taking the grape seed (150 or 300 milligrams daily) experienced an average drop of 12 points in their systolic BP and 8 points in their diastolic BP.[622] The investigators speculate that grape seed extract may work by dilating blood vessels.

Managing Your Medicines

Successful treatment of hypertension requires medical supervision. It is not a do-it-yourself project. The medicines you take should be adjusted to control your blood pressure and reduce your risk of having a heart attack or stroke. They should not make you miserable in the process. That's why good communication between patient and physician is essential for this project to be successful.

Avoiding Pitfalls

There are some things you should not be taking. For starters, avoid black licorice! It can completely screw up metabolism, deplete potassium, alter hormone levels—and cause a dramatic rise in blood pressure. And that can happen to folks with normal blood pressure. You can imagine what might happen to someone with hypertension.

● ● ●

Q. *I heard that licorice can lower a man's libido, so I thought I would see if it could help me. My husband has an overactive sex drive. He wants to make love every other day and I just can't get interested that often.*

He loves licorice, though, so I started buying licorice candy to see what would happen. Sure enough, his interest dropped off a bit.

Last week he came back from his physical worried because his blood pressure was high. It's never been a problem before, but the doctor wants to put him on medication. Now I'm afraid the licorice might be harming him.

A. If the candy contains real licorice, it could indeed affect your husband's libido as well as his blood pressure. A letter in the *New England Journal of Medicine* reported the results of a pilot study. Men who were given small amounts of licorice for a week ended up with substantially lower levels of testosterone.

In another study volunteers were given different doses of licorice for 2 to 4 weeks. The smallest dose (50 grams—equal to several jelly beans) produced a rise in blood pressure of almost 4 points. Those on the highest dose (200 grams—about the size of a candy bar) had their blood pressure go up by 14 points.

We suggest you eliminate the licorice from your husband's diet. Counseling might help you find a compromise that will satisfy both of you.

● ● ●

Pain relievers pose another problem. Millions of people pop nonprescription ibuprofen (Advil, Motrin IB) and naproxen (Aleve) day in and day out. That doesn't count the prescription NSAIDs (nonsteroidal anti-inflammatory drugs) like diclofenac (Voltaren), etodolac (Lodine), ketoprofen (Orudis), meloxicam (Mobic), nabumetone (Relafen), naproxen (Naprosyn), oxaprozin (Daypro), or piroxicam (Feldene). This entire class of medications can raise blood pressure. That's one of the reasons that the FDA has added stronger language about the cardiovascular risks associated with NSAIDs to the prescribing information for these drugs.

Unfortunately, most people tend to ignore these cautions. But trying to lower your blood pressure while taking an NSAID might be like running uphill while wearing cement overshoes. You won't make much progress.

● ● ●

Q. *I would like to alert you to a problem I encountered using Preparation H as a skin treatment. A long time ago I read something you wrote about this ointment being good for chafed skin, so for about a year I would rub it onto my genital area as needed—once every few weeks.*

I started to have frequent, frightening high blood pressure spikes of 255/140, which would come on suddenly and last several hours as my face turned red. (My usual reading is 150/75 with a low dose of Lotensin.) No one could pinpoint the cause, and it wasn't until many months had passed that I happened to read the tiny printed warning on the Preparation H box not to use it if you need blood pressure medication. That had been the cause of my numerous emergency events!

Neither my internist nor my pharmacist believed me at first, but when they looked up the ingredients they both agreed that I had uncovered something so important that they would tell all their older patients about it. You might want to warn people, too.

A. Thank you for alerting us to this issue. Preparation H used to contain shark liver oil and live yeast cell derivative (LYCD). Back then, we received many testimonials from people who found it helpful to speed wound healing, minimize wrinkles, and even repair scraped bark on trees.

When the FDA disallowed LYCD several years ago, the product was reformulated. Preparation H products now contain phenylephrine, a decongestant that constricts swollen blood vessels. When applied to delicate tissue such as the rectum (or the genitals), this ingredient may be absorbed into the bloodstream and might raise blood pressure.

The Preparation H label warns that you should ask a doctor before use if you have heart disease or high blood pressure or if you are presently taking a prescription drug for high blood pressure.

• • •

Hundreds of other medications should also be avoided if you have high blood pressure. Read the label on all over-the-counter medications and check with your physician to make sure any pills you may be taking for allergies aren't making your hypertension more difficult to treat.

Beware of the Beta-Blocker Blues

Beta-blockers are among the most commonly prescribed blood pressure medicines in the country. At last count, more than 115 million prescriptions were dispensed annually. If one were to assume that there are 30 pills per prescription, that would be 3,450,000,000 pills. While it is true that beta-blockers are prescribed for a variety of other conditions such as irregular heart rhythms, angina, and migraine headaches, high blood pressure has historically been the engine that pulls the beta-blocker train.

The reason they are so popular for treating hypertension is that they have been around for decades, so there is a familiarity factor. The first major beta-blocker was propranolol, which gained FDA approval in 1967 under the brand name Inderal. These days, atenolol (Tenormin, Tenoretic) and metoprolol (Lopressor, Toprol XL) dominate the beta-blocker marketplace. Between the two drugs,

> "We systematically analyzed all available outcome studies and found no evidence that beta-blocker based therapy, despite lowering blood pressure, reduced the risk of heart attacks or strokes. Despite the inefficacy of beta-blockers, the incidence of adverse effects is substantial. In the MRC [Medical Research Council] study, for every heart attack or stroke prevented, three patients withdrew from atenolol because of impotence, and another seven withdrew because of fatigue. Thus the risk/benefit ratio of beta-blockers is characterized by lack of efficacy and multiple adverse effects."[623]
>
> —F. H. Messerli et al., *American Journal of Hypertension*, 2003

more than 100 million prescriptions have been dispensed annually.

We suspect that one of the reasons beta-blockers are so popular with insurance companies and HMOs is that they are inexpensive. Since these drugs have been around so long, they are available generically and represent a big savings for the payers.

So what's a beta, and why would you want to block one anyway? What you're actually blocking when you take these drugs are beta receptors, which are found on cells all over your body—in your heart and your lungs and around the little muscles that surround blood vessels. When you block these receptors you make it harder for adrenaline (epinephrine) to stimulate the heart or other cells.

We like to think of beta-blockers as being a little like the governors on a school bus. To prevent the driver from going too fast, the engine has a device (a governor) that prevents it from exceeding a certain speed, no matter how hard you push the pedal to the metal. The same thing is true of beta-blockers. No matter how hard you exercise, you will never be able to rev your heart rate above a certain threshold. This action keeps the heart from overworking.

How good are beta-blockers in the fight against hypertension? Despite the fact that they have been enthusiastically prescribed for so long, there is a growing concern among cutting-edge cardiologists that beta-blockers in general and atenolol in particular are not that great for treating high blood pressure.[624] The cognoscenti of cardiology are saying that beta-blockers "should not remain first choice in the treatment of primary hypertension."[625,626] In fact, one group of physicians went so far as to write an article in the *American Journal of Hypertension* (October 2003) entitled "Beta-Blockers in Hypertension—The Emperor Has No Clothes."[627]

What is so astonishing is that some experts are now saying the evidence for beta-blockers' "effectiveness in the prevention of heart attacks and strokes in hypertension was always inadequate."[628] A review of the most important studies involving atenolol in the treatment of high blood pressure concluded that it did not reduce the risk of heart attacks or death any better than placebo or no treatment at all. In fact, there was an increased risk of stroke compared to other blood pressure drugs. The authors concluded that the results of their analysis "cast doubts on atenolol as a suitable drug for hypertensive patients."[629]

There is not only serious doubt about the effectiveness of beta-blockers like atenolol against hypertension, but also concern about their side effects. Such drugs can cause weight gain,[630] cholesterol elevation (not a good way to prevent heart disease), psychological depression (the "beta-blocker blues"), fatigue, stomach upset, insomnia, nightmares, confusion, memory problems, lethargy, cold hands and feet, shortness of breath, rash, hair loss, blurred vision, dizziness, joint pain, and sexual difficulties.

This seems a little reminiscent of the Vioxx scandal, except the media completely missed the significance of the research. And unlike Vioxx, which was only on the market for a couple of years, atenolol has been prescribed to tens of millions of hypertensive patients for decades.

• • •

Q. I believe I have been a victim of over-medication. My doctor put me on Inderal for high blood pressure and later changed the prescription to metoprolol and then to nadolol. I went through a living hell because I became severely depressed. When I complained of my depressed feelings and asked if the medication might be responsible, he brushed my concerns aside and prescribed an antidepressant. It made me anxious and gave me insomnia, so he added a tranquilizer.

Eventually I developed asthma and had to be taken off the beta-blockers. My energy came back, my mood improved, and I no longer needed the antidepressant and tranquilizer.

Now I'm taking Zestril and the only problem is a terrible cough that doesn't get better with cough medicine. Is this a side effect?

A. Beta-blocker heart medicines such as atenolol, metoprolol, nadolol, propranolol, and timolol are widely used because of their cardiovascular benefits: They reduce blood pressure and help normalize irregular heart rhythms. Some people complain of fatigue and depression while on such drugs. Patients with asthma generally must avoid beta-blockers. Weight gain can also be a problem with beta-blockers.

It often comes as a surprise that drugs for physical problems such as blood pressure pills can affect mood or personality. Zestril and other ACE inhibitors can sometimes cause a hard-to-kick cough.

• • •

No one should ever stop taking a beta-blocker suddenly! Doing so could cause rebound high blood pressure, a serious attack of angina, or even a heart attack. Anyone who contemplates discontinuing such medications must do so gradually and only under careful medical supervision.

Beta-blockers do play an absolutely crucial role in the treatment of other conditions such as coronary artery disease, irregular heart rhythms, and heart failure. They are especially valuable in preventing another heart attack after someone has already experienced one. But it is now pretty clear that these drugs should rarely be first choices in blood pressure treatment. They may be valuable when adequate control is not achieved with other classes of drugs, but you and your physician will need to find if the benefits outweigh the risks.

COMMON DIURETICS

- Bendroflumethiazide (Naturetin)

- Benzthiazide (Exna)

- Bumetanide (Bumex)

- Chlorothiazide (Diuril, Diachlor, Diurigen)

- Chlorthalidone (Hygroton)

- Ethacrynic acid (Edecrin)

- Furosemide (Lasix)

- Hydrochlorothiazide (Esidrix, HCTZ, HydroDIURIL, Oretic)

- Hydroflumethiazide (Diucardin)

- Indapamide (Lozol)

- Methyclothiazide (Aquatensen, Enduron)

- Polythiazide (Renese)

- Trichlormethiazide (Diurese, Metahydrin, Naqua)

Diuretics

The first real breakthrough in the treatment of high blood pressure occurred in 1958. That was when chlorothiazide was introduced. Before this "thiazide" diuretic was developed, physicians admonished patients to eliminate salt from their diets. It was one of their few treatment options and was only partially effective. Other available drugs like reserpine, which was derived from the *Rauwolfia serpentina* plant, often caused very serious side effects such as suicidal depression.

Although chlorothiazide and similar compounds started a revolution in blood pressure treatment, they eventually lost their luster. Newer medications like beta-blockers, calcium channel blockers, and ACE inhibitors seemed sexier and more powerful. Since diuretics were old and available generically, drug companies promoted the new, more expensive products. And physicians responded by prescribing Tenormin (atenolol) or Procardia (nifedipine). We now know that such drugs are not better and may even be worse than old-fashioned, unglamorous diuretics.

ALLHAT—the Antihypertensive and Lipid-Lowering Treatment to Prevent Heart Attack Trial—rocked the world of cardiology in 2002.[631] This government-sponsored study, which cost $120 million, tracked more than 40,000 subjects for years to determine the outcomes of various blood-pressure-lowering drugs. The scientists found that chlorthalidone, an inexpensive diuretic, was superior to some popular brand-name blood pressure pills.

★★★★ Chlorthalidone

Many physicians believe that all thiazide diuretics are created equal. Hydrochlorothiazide (Esidrix, HCTZ, HydroDIURIL, Oretic) is the most widely prescribed by far. Although it is unquestionably effective, we prefer chlorthalidone. For one thing, it was the thiazide diuretic used in the ALLHAT that proved so beneficial in reducing strokes and other cardiovascular events. For another, chlorthalidone remains in the body longer than other thiazides and may be more effective in controlling blood pressure, especially during the night.[632,633]

Downside: Increased urination, since this is part of the way the drug works. Sexual dysfunction may be more likely than with some other blood pressure meds.[634]

Side effects: Potassium and magnesium depletion, muscle cramps, gout, and increased blood sugar levels. Less common adverse reactions may include upset stomach, loss of appetite, diarrhea, dizziness, increased susceptibility to sunburn, rash, blurred vision, headaches, and blood disorders.

Cost: Approximately $4 to $6 per month when 100 pills are purchased from places such as Costco

The pharmaceutical industry had spent billions investigating and promoting products like Norvasc (amlodipine), Cardura (doxazosin), and Zestril and Prinivil (lisinopril). For FDA approval, drug companies need only prove that a medicine lowers blood pressure more effectively than placebo. They have little incentive to test medications head-to-head to determine how they compare in improving health.

That's what makes this government research so important. Instead of just looking at numbers on a blood pressure monitor, scientists determined whether people had suffered heart attacks, strokes, or heart failure or had died. Curt Furberg, MD, PhD, chair of the study's steering committee, shared his conclusions with us: "It's important to lower blood pressure, but it matters how you do it. The diuretics have

three advantages. They are unsurpassed in lowering blood pressure; they are superior in reducing the cardiovascular complications of hypertension; and they are 10 to 20 times cheaper than the newer branded drugs."[635]

Doctors were probably astonished to learn that in this trial the alpha-blocker Cardura (doxazosin) actually increased the likelihood of heart failure compared with diuretic treatment. That was also true of the calcium channel blocker Norvasc (amlodipine), which was responsible for a 38 percent increase in the risk of heart failure. Dr. Furberg estimates that with 7 million patients taking similar drugs, there would be 35,000 unnecessary heart failure events per year.

Of course no one should ever discontinue any blood pressure medication without care-

potassium. It is important to have blood tests regularly to measure both of these electrolytes and make sure they are maintained within normal limits. Allowing the level of magnesium or potassium to stay low has serious negative health consequences. Both minerals must be kept in proper balance. You will find a list of high-magnesium foods on page 293. For potassium sources, also see page 293.

To get around the loss of potassium caused by many thiazide-type diuretics, physicians have switched to potassium-preserving diuretics such as amiloride (Midamor), spironolactone (Aldactone), and triamterene (Dyrenium). They are prescribed alone or more commonly in combination with hydrochlorothiazide (Aldactazide, Dyazide, Maxzide, and Moduretic). Such drugs have some of the same adverse reactions and precautions that standard diuretics have.

Potassium-preserving diuretics pose a sig-

ful consultation with and supervision by a physician. And Norvasc and similar drugs do have an important role in some heart conditions. But ALLHAT suggested that not all blood pressure medicines are created equal.

As much as we value thiazide diuretics in general, and chlorthalidone in particular, these are not perfect blood pressure–lowering drugs. Although they are inexpensive and effective, they can cause several serious side effects. One potential complication of diuretic treatment is elevation of blood sugar levels, which can lead to an increased risk of diabetes. These drugs can also raise uric acid levels, which can cause excruciating bouts of gout.

The biggest complication, however, is depletion of the essential minerals magnesium and

ACE INHIBITORS

- Benazepril (Lotensin)
- Captopril (Capoten)
- Enalapril (Vasotec)
- Fosinopril (Monopril)
- Lisinopril (Prinivil, Zestril)
- Moexipril (Univasc)
- Perindopril (Aceon)
- Quinapril (Accupril)
- Ramipril (Altace)
- Trandolapril (Mavik)

nificant problem when combined with ACE inhibitors such as benazepril (Lotensin), captopril (Capoten), enalapril (Vasotec), fosinopril (Monopril), lisinopril (Prinivil, Zestril), quinapril (Accupril), and ramipril (Altace). Because the ACE inhibitors also help the body retain potassium, it is possible that one could end up with potassium overload. This is just as dangerous as too little potassium. Symptoms may include breathing difficulty, weakness, confusion, slow heart rate, and potentially life-threatening heart rhythm changes. Periodic blood tests are essential for a doctor to monitor the safe use of these medicines.

An ACE Up Your Sleeve

One of the most extraordinary advances in pharmaceutical research and blood pressure management evolved out of the jungles of Brazil. A Brazilian scientist noted that when people were bitten by the poisonous jararaca snake, they experienced a dramatic drop in blood pressure. By harnessing the power of the snake venom to lower blood pressure, pharmacologists were able to isolate chemicals that could be used as drugs.

These venom-derived compounds block an enzyme that converts a naturally occurring chemical called angiotensin I into a powerful

★★★★★ ACE Inhibitors

We think the ACE inhibitors are remarkable. They are very effective at controlling blood pressure and reducing the complications of cardiovascular disease. These drugs are usually well tolerated, resulting in less sexual dysfunction than some other blood pressure meds. We wish we could say one was better than another. Cardiologists we trust seem to lean toward the longer-acting perindopril (Aceon), ramipril (Altace), and trandolapril (Mavik), but without head-to-head trials it is hard to recommend one ACE inhibitor over another.

Downside: Some people are allergic to these drugs and may develop life-threatening swelling of the face, tongue, lips, and airways. At the first sign of an allergic reaction, get to the emergency room.

Cough is the other big complication. It is hard to control and may require an alternate type of high blood pressure treatment, such as an angiotensin receptor blocker.

Potassium levels may occasionally rise to dangerous levels. Monitor potassium carefully.

Always check with your physician and pharmacist about drug interactions. There are several, including potassium-sparing diuretics.

Side effects: A dry, hacking cough is the most common. Less common adverse reactions may include dizziness, weakness, rash, itching, stomach upset, headache, and elevated enzymes related to kidney function.

Cost: Approximately $10 to $15 per month for generic drugs like captopril or lisinopril and $45 to $60 per month for brand-name medications

vasoconstrictor called angiotensin II, which in turn raises blood pressure. The drugs are called angiotensin-converting enzyme (ACE) inhibitors. The first was captopril (Capoten), and it was followed by a wide range of other chemicals that have revolutionized the treatment of high blood pressure.

By all accounts, ACE inhibitors are now considered to be the best choices in the treatment of high blood pressure for many patients. They may also be beneficial in the treatment of congestive heart failure, kidney disease associated with diabetes, and secondary stroke prevention when they are combined with a diuretic. There is reason to believe that these drugs might reduce the risk of developing diabetes.[636]

Adding an ACE inhibitor to a thiazide diuretic may offset the loss of potassium and the risk of drug-induced diabetes. According to Dr. Furberg, this is a "combination made in heaven."[637]

• • •

Q. *Is coughing at night a side effect of any of the ACE inhibitors? I take Zestril, and I am having a terrible time with this cough. Even cough medicine with dextromethorphan doesn't quell it.*

A. As you have guessed, a persistent cough that does not respond to cough suppressants might be a reaction to blood pressure medicines like lisinopril (Prinivil, Zestril). Ask your doctor about an iron supplement (ferrous sulfate). One small study found that some patients taking such a supplement had a dramatic improvement in ACE-inhibitor cough (*Hypertension*, August 2001). Some people tough it out by sucking on hard candy. The cough may fade away after several weeks.

Another option is to take a different kind of blood pressure medicine. Another reader shared this: "For the past 2 years I had a chronic cough that was variously diagnosed as allergies, sinus, or acid reflux. I was taking lisinopril for my blood pressure. When I read that coughing could be a side effect, I checked with my doctor. He switched me to Cozaar. Within less than a week's time, the coughing subsided. I now sleep straight through the night without being wakened by coughs."

• • •

Angiotensin Receptor Blockers

There is an alternative to the ACE inhibitors. The angiotensin receptor blockers (ARBs) have a somewhat similar action, but since cough is an uncommon side effect, such drugs may substitute for ACE inhibitors in folks who cannot tolerate the latter drugs. The question that remains unanswered, however, is whether ARBs work as well as ACE inhibitors to prevent heart attacks. Some cardiologists are prescrib-

ANGIOTENSIN RECEPTOR BLOCKERS

- Candesartan (Atacand)
- Eprosartan (Teveten)
- Irbesartan (Avapro)
- Losartan (Cozaar)
- Losartan + hydrochlorothiazide (Hyzaar)
- Olmesartan (Benicar)
- Telmisartan (Micardis)
- Valsartan (Diovan)

ing lower doses of both ARBs and ACE inhibitors in combination to achieve better blood pressure control than either does alone.

Several years ago a controversial editorial appeared in the *British Medical Journal* entitled "Angiotensin Receptor Blockers and Myocardial Infarction [heart attack]: These Drugs May Increase Myocardial Infarction—and Patients May Need to Be Told."[638] The authors reviewed studies that showed that ARBs lowered blood pressure but actually seemed to increase the risk of heart attack. Needless to say, this commentary stirred up a hornet's nest of protest in the cardiology community.

Subsequent review and analysis have concluded that there is no difference between ACE inhibitors and ARBs. The authors of this later study reassure physicians and patients that all is well.[639] We would like to see more comprehensive trials looking at long-term meaningful outcomes (heart attacks and deaths) before we come to any final conclu-

sions about this controversy. If you have any concerns, please discuss this issue with your physician.

And this, dear reader, brings us back to the beginning. High blood pressure is a very serious condition. It is the most common risk factor for heart attacks, strokes, and other life-threatening cardiovascular conditions. Experts estimate that 50 million to 65 million Americans have hypertension and another 70 million have prehypertension (a systolic BP of 120 to 130 mmHg and a diastolic BP of 80 to 89 mmHg).[640] Chances are good that you belong in one group or the other.

Choosing the best treatment requires terrific communication between you and your health-care provider. You do not want to trade great blood pressure control for symptoms of dizziness, depression, fatigue, sexual dysfunction, or uncontrollable coughing. You do want to manage your blood pressure and still have a high quality of life.

Other Blood Pressure Meds

We have not listed all of the possible medications. For example, we have excluded calcium channel blockers and alpha blockers from our discussion because we have some concerns about their side effects. But there are situations where drugs like amlodipine (Norvasc), diltiazem (Cardizem), and verapamil (Calan, Covera-HS, Isoptin, Verelan) are clearly called for.

Another class of blood pressure–lowering

medications is called *aldosterone blockers*. Drugs like spironolactone (Aldactone) or eplerenone (Inspra) are intriguing and may offer some interesting advantages when traditional treatments are unsuccessful. Potassium levels must be monitored very closely, however. You and your physician need to work together to find the best treatment for you. It can be done!

Conclusions

- High blood pressure is common. The chances are very good that you or someone you love has this condition. It increases the risk of serious health problems like stroke, heart attack, dementia, and kidney disease.
- Measure your blood pressure properly. Purchase at least one digital device and plot your numbers in a diary or on a computer.
- Monitor your stress level. Purchase a mood ring or a Bio-Q Thermal Biofeedback and Stress Monitoring Ring. Take time-outs, exercise, and breathe deeply whenever you notice that you're stressing out.
- Never forget to make new friends but keep the old; one is silver and the other gold. Social support is crucial to good health!
- Lose weight and exercise. If you can do these two things, you may not need medication. Losing the belly and the love handles will do more to keep you healthy than almost anything else we can think of. The DASH diet, which is heavy on vegetables and fruits, can lower blood pressure by as much as some medications.

- Drink tea and avoid coffee and soft drinks. Drink some pomegranate or purple grape juice daily. Indulge in a little dark chocolate.
- Maximize your minerals: calcium, magnesium, and potassium. Get them from your diet if you can. You may need a magnesium supplement (300 to 500 milligrams daily) if you are taking a diuretic.
- Beware of the beta-blocker blues. Do not let your medicine cause fatigue, depression, or forgetfulness. Discuss the latest findings about beta-blockers for hypertension with your physician. *Do not stop* taking a beta-blocker suddenly! Check with your physician before stopping any medication.
- Diuretics are the first choice for most blood pressure regimens. Chlorthalidone is at the top of our list. It works well and is affordable. Potassium-sparing diuretics such as triamterene and hydrochlorothiazide (found in Dyazide and Maxzide) or spironolactone (Aldactone) may offer similar benefits without risking potassium depletion.
- The best ace up your sleeve is an ACE inhibitor. These drugs represent some of the best treatments modern medicine has to offer for high blood pressure.
- If you need additional antihypertensive treatment, work closely with your health-care professionals to find the approach that will best control your blood pressure without causing unacceptable side effects.

HYPERHIDROSIS

• Try Certain Dri (aluminum chloride)	★★★
• Experiment with MOM (milk of magnesia)	★★
• Give vinegar or baking soda a whirl	
• Try soaking your sweaty feet in tea	
• Ask about a prescription for Drysol	★★★★
• Look into iontophoresis	
• Consider Botox injections	★★

Why do we sweat? One important reason is to regulate body temperature. If we didn't have sweat glands in the skin all over our bodies, we'd need to stick out our tongues and pant like dogs to cool off in hot weather. Although that may be the function of sweating, plenty of people can tell you that's not all there is to it. They're the ones who perspire far more than is strictly necessary for cooling purposes. Almost all of us sweat when we are anxious as well.

Nearly 3 percent of adults sweat too much, a condition known as *hyperhidrosis*. Their armpits perspire and soak their shirt or blouse. Their hands sweat and make their handshakes slippery, or their feet sweat, contributing to the growth of odor-forming bacteria and fungi. Some people find perspiration dripping from their face even when they are not exerting themselves. It appears that their nervous system goes into overdrive, telling the eccrine glands in the skin that produce sweat to make more in response to emotion.[641]

Excessive perspiration can complicate life, but a surprising number of people don't discuss this issue with their doctor. That is a shame, because there are some effective treatments.

> *I have a problem with underarm perspiration. As a funeral director, I must wear a suit and tie, and in warm weather my coat gets soaked within 30 minutes. Some of my jackets have been ruined with perspiration stains, and I am distressed about my image.*

It's also important to discuss this issue with a physician so he or she can rule out any potentially serious medical conditions that might be causing excessive sweating. Infections (including tuberculosis and HIV), certain cancers, panic attacks, an overactive thyroid gland, menopause, Parkinson's disease, and a number of other conditions could be responsible.[642] There are also some medications that can trigger embarrassing perspiration. In most cases, though, damp armpits or sweaty feet are simply a consequence of sweat glands

> " *I suffered for years with sweaty feet and foot odor. I tried lots of over-the-counter foot products but none worked.*
>
> *One day I rubbed the bottoms of my feet and in between my toes with my underarm deodorant (Lady Mitchum Clear Gel) and it worked! Now I use it on my feet daily and have not had an odor problem since. Please let your readers know about this product, as it has made a tremendous difference in my life.* "

Another antiperspirant that is available without a prescription is Certain Dri. It is frequently effective even for people who perspire heavily. Certain Dri contains aluminum chloride, which is why it works well.

★★★ Certain Dri

This antiperspirant contains aluminum chloride and is available without a prescription. Like other aluminum chloride products, it should be applied to dry (not damp) armpits at bedtime. After the first few days, it should be applied only two or three times a week. Avoid broken skin. Information on sales outlets is available from 800-338-8079.

Side effects: May cause irritation or rash. Discontinue if this occurs.
Downside: Unresolved concerns about aluminum safety
Cost: $5 to $6 for a roll-on with 1.2 fluid ounces

being hypersensitive to the cues that normally stimulate perspiration.

Over-the-Counter Approaches

The first thing to try for damp armpits is a good strong antiperspirant. Nearly every antiperspirant contains aluminum. The stronger ones have higher concentrations. Some readers have reported success with a product called Mitchum antiperspirant. It contains aluminum zirconium tetrachlorohydrex 20 percent. It can be used on sweaty feet as well as on the underarms.

Home Remedies
MOM to the Rescue

• • •

Q. *I want to share a remedy I learned in Brazil. Just apply milk of magnesia to your armpits. It is the best underarm deodorant!*

A. What an unusual idea! Milk of magnesia (MOM) contains magnesium hydroxide, which acts as both an antacid and a laxative. We have never heard of applying it to the underarms, though. Perhaps it reduces the acidity of the skin to make odor-forming bacteria less welcome.

• • •

We don't know for certain how MOM would reduce underarm perspiration, though other people have also reported success with it. It may be able to inhibit odor by altering the environment for the bacteria that live on the skin and are responsible for the smell of sweat. We do know that MOM is safe. People have been swallowing milk of magnesia as a laxative for decades. The Phillips brand is probably the most famous. We also know that people frequently are low in magnesium. (See pages 261 and 292 for a discussion of this "magnificent mineral.") Other people have written to say they find milk of magnesia effective at stopping perspiration.

★★ Milk of Magnesia

Shake the bottle well before applying this product to the armpits with your fingers. It can be applied in either the evening or the morning, because it does not seem to stain clothing.

Side effects: Be alert for irritation or rash. Discontinue if this occurs.

Downside: No scientific studies support the use of MOM as an antiperspirant or deodorant. Proof of its effectiveness is purely anecdotal.

Cost: Approximately $6 for 12 fluid ounces

" *You expressed surprise that someone might use milk of magnesia as an underarm deodorant. I have been using milk of magnesia for several years. Despite my initial skepticism, I've found it to be a remarkably effective antiperspirant. I apply it directly from the bottle using my fingers.*

It is inexpensive (a bottle lasts months), goes on quickly and easily, has no odor, dries clear, does not stain clothing, and is completely effective in stopping odor and perspiration. It contains no aluminum. (Some people worry that aluminum contributes to Alzheimer's.) It contains no other harmful ingredients since it is made to be ingested. "

Vinegar and Baking Soda

If altering the pH of the skin helps control odor, it may explain why some people are enthusiastic about the use of plain vinegar as a deodorant. Others report good results with baking soda. Both of these kitchen remedies can change the balance of acid and base on the skin, which probably makes life less comfortable for odor-forming bacteria.

• • •

Q. *Thank you for writing about using vinegar and water on underarms. I have had a problem with underarm smell most of my life and have tried almost every product on the market. Nothing really stopped the odor.*

When I read about vinegar, I gave it a try. It has been a miracle. I can now go out in the heat, exercise, and go through the day without smelling at all. It is amazing and cheap.

A. Thanks for the testimonial. We heard this from another reader: "I had chemo treatment for breast cancer in 2002 and found that all antiperspirants caused redness and irritation. My doctor advised me not to use any deodorant, but that did not suit me. I tried plain white vinegar, and it worked so well I've kept it up ever since."

Dilute vinegar (half vinegar and half water) should be applied only to unbroken skin (not after shaving), or it will sting. If it causes any rash or another reaction, it should be discontinued immediately.

• • •

❝ *Several years ago I came across a tip from someone on a Web message board to use baking soda for excessive underarm sweating. For me it works like magic. I apply a dab the size of a dime just below the armpit. Any more than that and it may be irritating.*

I suffered for years prior to this. Deodorants and antiperspirants did nothing except cause white stains and stickiness. ❞

Tea Treatment for Hands and Feet

Many people with overactive sweat glands have a problem with excessive sweating on their hands and feet as well as under their arms. Some of the same products that work as underarm antiperspirants can be used for hands or feet.

❝ *My daughter has been plagued with hyperhidrosis since she was quite young. Every spring and summer she spends hours readying new sandals for wear. She lines the shoes with moleskin or some other absorbent material. Her feet perspire so much that if she does not take this precaution her feet slip right out of the shoes.* ❞

In some cases, tannic acid can be helpful in reducing the sweating of the palms of the hands and soles of the feet. One simple home remedy is to make a strong tea solution by steeping five tea bags in a quart of hot water for 15 minutes. Then soak the hands or feet in the solution for 30 minutes a day. The drawback of soaking hands in this tannin solution is that it stains the skin as well as acts as an astringent. It is inexpensive, however, and it works for some people. Clear tannic acid is available in some topical medications.

• • •

Q. *I read that some people use tannic acid to control excessive sweating of the palms. I currently use Drysol, but it's not completely effective.*

I know you can boil tea leaves to get a form of tannic acid, but it's a hassle and stains your palms brown. I'd like to try tannic acid but don't know what products to look for. Any information would be welcome, as this condition is embarrassing.

A. Commercial products with tannic acid include Ivy-Dry (10 percent) and Zilactin (7 percent).

• • •

No-Sweat Prescriptions

The two mainstays of prescription treatment for hyperhidrosis both contain aluminum chloride. The first thing a physician is likely to write down on the prescription pad is Drysol, which is 20 percent aluminum chloride hexahydrate. (A generic version is available.) The other prescription option is Xerac AC; it is a weaker concentration at 6.25 percent aluminum chloride hexahydrate.

The guidelines for using both of these prescription antiperspirants are the same as those for using Certain Dri: Apply it to unbroken, dry skin before bedtime (use a hair dryer to dry your armpits, if necessary); wash it off in the morning. This not only keeps the products from damaging clothing, it also improves their effectiveness by allowing them to penetrate and block the sweat ducts. Once perspiration is under control, reduce the frequency of application to once or twice a week, as needed, or even once every 2 or 3 weeks. If the doctor recommends "occlusion," apply the antiperspirant first, then cover the area with plastic wrap. Don't use tape to hold the plastic in place, though. Instead, wear a tight-fitting T-shirt.

Aluminum chloride hexahydrate 20 percent is said to offer excellent perspiration control for a majority of people. There are some concerns about the use of aluminum, however. Some research has linked excessive aluminum

★★★★ Drysol

This antiperspirant contains 20 percent aluminum chloride hexahydrate. It should be applied to dry (not damp) armpits at bedtime. Avoid broken skin. Once the amount of sweating is reduced, Drysol should be applied only as often as needed.

Side effects: May cause irritation, itching, or rash. Discontinue if this occurs.
Downside: Requires a prescription
Cost: $10 to $15 for a bottle (37.5 ml)

exposure to an increased risk of Alzheimer's disease.[644] Scientists don't know for certain that aluminum contributes to Alzheimer's disease, but they haven't determined that it does not, either.

In addition, a recent study suggests that aluminum salts may have estrogenic activity and can stimulate the growth of breast cancer cells in the laboratory.[645,646] There is no scientific consensus that aluminum-containing antiperspirants increase the risk of breast cancer. Dismissing the idea as completely wacko is no longer scientifically responsible, however.

> *I am 16 and have a problem with excessive sweating in my armpits. This has been going on since I was 12. I've used a variety of deodorants and antiperspirants.*
>
> *Certain Dri worked for a while, but my mom prefers natural approaches. She worries about aluminum exposure.*
>
> *I'm tired of soaking my shirts or uniform blouses and I'm always so embarrassed that someone will see the stains. Please help me find a natural, safe cure to stop my sweating.*

If there is any increased risk from aluminum-containing antiperspirants, it is probably small. It is understandable, however, that some people would prefer to limit their exposure.

> *Could you remind your readers about Drysol? This is a chemical treatment for underarm sweat. Apply as directed (two times over 2 nights, then as needed). I go about 4 to 6 days between treatments now.*
>
> *I am an extraordinarily heavy sweater, and the premium antiperspirants did not work. But after I asked my doctor for a referral to the Botox clinic for armpit shots, she prescribed Drysol. It works for me. I am dry, and it is a miracle of modern chemistry!*

Antiperspirants seem to be more effective for underarms than for sweaty hands and feet.[647] Hands and feet may need an aluminum chloride concentration as high as 30 to 40 percent.

A study of aluminum chloride in a salicylic acid gel base found that this worked well for a majority of the patients with sweaty feet and hands.[648] This prescription product needs to be compounded by a pharmacist, because it is not available commercially. Once the effect is achieved, the antiperspirant may need to be applied only once a week, or even as infrequently as once every 3 weeks.

Get a Charge

If aluminum chloride formulations are not effective for underarm sweating, the next step could be a process called *iontophoresis*, in which a device passes a mild electric current through the affected skin. Nobody seems to know exactly how it works, but the mild electric current, powered by a battery, disrupts the sweat glands somehow.

The Drionic device costs approximately $150. For underarms, it should be used for 20 minutes three times a week for 2 weeks. This may reduce sweating for up to 6 weeks. When excessive sweating resumes, the treatment can be repeated.

The Drionic device may be more effective for sweaty hands and feet than for armpits. After the initial course of 6 to 10 treatments, maintenance treatments are needed every week or two, or possibly only once a month. Possible side effects include burning, tingling, irritation, and drying of the skin. This is a prescription treatment that should be supervised by a physician.

Botox Injections

Botulinum toxin type A may be best known for its use in fighting wrinkles and keeping starlets (and others) from showing their age. It is also quite effective for controlling excess perspiration, and the FDA has approved it for this purpose. If you opt for this treatment, make sure that the dermatologist or plastic surgeon who administers the injections has had training and experience in this use of botulinum toxin (Botox). Each treatment requires multiple injections around the armpit and lasts for 6 to 8 months. When it wears off, another treatment is usually quite effective.[649] Each treatment may cost $500 or more. It makes sense to do some comparative shopping before determining which doctor will do your injections.

Surgery

Only a few people don't get an adequate response from any of the above treatments.

★★ Botox

Injections of botulinum toxin into the armpit disable the neurochemical messenger that triggers sweat glands. The injections are effective for the great majority of people with excessive sweating. They last for 6 to 8 months, then need to be repeated when the effect wears off. Botox injections can also be used for sweaty hands.

Side effects: Pain, itching, shoulder muscle soreness, allergic reactions, rash
Downside: Expensive; must be repeated every 6 months or so. Other areas (such as the face) may begin to sweat more heavily in compensation.
Cost: $500 or more per treatment

For them, surgery may be helpful. One option for hyperhidrosis that was not available in times past evolved from cosmetic surgery. Liposuction is usually used to remove excess fat, but it also can be employed to take some of the sweat glands from the armpits. Not many studies have been done on this approach, so thoroughly check out the plastic surgeon who will perform the procedure. It may take time, possibly as long as 6 or 8 months after the procedure, to get the full results.

There is a more drastic, last-resort surgery that has been studied more fully. It is known as *endoscopic thoracic sympathectomy*, or ETS for short. In this procedure, the surgeon severs the nerves that lead to the sweat glands of the hands or the armpits. Increased sweating of the face or other parts of the body following the surgery is a recognized side effect. There is also the possibility of surgical complications, so make sure the surgeon you choose has had a great deal of experience with this procedure. It is the most expensive way to deal with excessive sweating, but unlike the other treatments, it is permanent.

• • •

Q. I am in my forties and have had a problem with my hands and feet sweating excessively all my life. I've heard there is surgery to control this problem, but that seems extreme. Are there any other options?

A. Surgery can be effective, but it is expensive and requires general anesthesia. It is not recommended for sweaty feet because there would be a risk of sexual dysfunction as a complication of the surgery.

The FDA has approved Botox for use in treating excessive underarm sweating. Such injections have been used to control sweaty palms and feet.

It makes sense, though, to try topical aluminum chloride first. Available in products such as Drysol, it is far less costly and less invasive than surgery or injections and can be quite effective.

• • •

Conclusions

Excessive sweating, whether of the underarms, hands, or feet, can cause people a lot of anxiety and disruption in their lives. If you have this problem, make sure you tell your doctor about it and ask for help with it. There are treatments available, so you don't need to go on suffering.

- Begin with an over-the-counter antiperspirant such as Certain Dri. Apply it before bedtime so it has longer to work and won't ruin your clothes.
- If you want to avoid aluminum, experiment with milk of magnesia. It can be applied daily to armpits, hands, or feet, since it dries clear.
- Try white vinegar, straight or diluted, on armpits to control sweating and odor.
- Ask your doctor about a prescription for Drysol. Apply only to dry skin at bedtime and wash it off in the morning.
- If you don't get satisfactory results from aluminum chloride hexahydrate products, consider Botox injections every 6 to 8 months.
- Treat your sweaty hands or feet with electric current by using a prescription Drionic device.
- Soak your sweaty feet in a strong tea solution. Tannic acid is astringent and helps shut down sweat glands.
- Surgery (ETS) offers a permanent solution to hyperhidrosis, but it is also the riskiest and most expensive treatment.

HYPOTHYROIDISM

• Take levothyroxine (Synthroid, Levoxyl, Levothroid, Unithroid)	★★★★
• Experiment with Armour desiccated thyroid	★★★
• Supplement with selenium	★★★★
• Try zinc	★★★

Thyroid disease is one of the most common conditions in America, yet the cause remains mysterious. More than 20 million people suffer from a thyroid disorder; some of them don't even know it. They just feel awful. More than 80 million prescriptions are filled every year for thyroid hormones like levothyroxine (Synthroid, Levoxyl, Levothroid, Unithroid) and Armour desiccated thyroid. If we didn't know better, we would say there is an epidemic of hypothyroidism in America.

Nobody knows exactly what makes the thyroid gland stop working properly. In many cases of hypothyroidism (an underactive thyroid), the immune system attacks the thyroid gland and undermines its ability to produce thyroid hormone. Like diabetes, this may be considered an autoimmune disease. Environmental exposure to chemicals like perchlorate,[650,651] found in rocket fuel, and polychlorinated biphenyls (PCBs)[652,653] and polybrominated diphenyl ethers (PBDEs),[654] both used as flame retardants, may have an impact on the developing thyroid gland. Some of these are pervasive environmental contaminants, so it's plausible that they might be contributing to the prevalence of thyroid problems.

The thyroid gland is so small that it doesn't look particularly important. It is located in the neck and weighs just a few ounces, but it has an impact on the entire body. A healthy functioning thyroid gland normally puts out two hormones: triiodothyronine, or T_3, and thyroxine, known as T_4. (The numbers indicate how many atoms of iodine are part of the hormone molecule.) These hormones control how every cell in the body uses energy. They also affect a cell's response to growth hormone and other compounds, including estrogen and calcium. Because the thyroid regulates so many different activities, symptoms of thyroid problems may be vague and general. This can make diagnosis difficult.

What Is Hypothyroidism?

If the thyroid gland produces too little of the main thyroid hormone (thyroxine, or T_4), a person may become easily chilled, sometimes running a lower-than-normal body temperature. Although fatigue can have many causes, it is a common complaint of the hypothyroid person. Weight gain is also a tip-off, though again there are many other possible causes. The increased fluid retention that can occur with inadequate thyroid hormone levels contributes to weight gain, but so can the slow

SYMPTOMS OF UNDERACTIVE THYROID

- Apathy
- Fatigue
- Dry skin
- Weakness
- Constipation
- Hair loss
- Cold intolerance
- Swollen eyelids and puffiness under the eyes
- Decreased sweating
- Infertility
- Heavy menstruation
- Low libido
- Swollen hands or feet
- Brittle fingernails
- Slow pulse
- Anemia
- Elevated cholesterol
- Shortness of breath during exercise
- Hoarse voice
- Clumsiness
- Depression
- Mental slowness
- Carpal tunnel syndrome

metabolism, as well as the fatigue that makes it hard to exercise. Thyroid deficiency can sap muscle strength and lead to shortness of breath during exertion.

Dry skin, brittle fingernails, and coarse, sparse hair can be frustrating. Moisturizers or conditioners may help, but they can't fight the symptoms that result from too little thyroid hormone. When the outer third of the eyebrows is missing, it strongly suggests low thyroid function. Hair may fall out from other parts of the body as well as the scalp.

Doctors may use their little hammers to check for a slow Achilles reflex. They might ask a woman about her menstrual cycle. Heavy bleeding may be associated with inadequate thyroid hormone, and women sometimes have trouble getting pregnant when thyroid hormone is low. Although doctors don't usually ask about more subjective symptoms, problems such as depressed mood, difficulty concentrating, and clumsiness are common in people experiencing low thyroid function.

If the physician suspects hypothyroidism, he or she will order a blood test for thyroid-stimulating hormone (TSH). This is a chemical made by the pituitary gland (located in the brain) that sends a message to the thyroid to make more thyroxine hormone. That explains why a high level of TSH means that the thyroid gland isn't functioning properly. The brain is working extra hard to kick it into gear.

TSH (also called *thyrotropin*) controls the action of the thyroid gland the way a thermostat controls the activity of a furnace. When the gland is making too little thyroid hormone, the brain puts out more TSH to tell it to make more. If there is too much thyroid hormone in the bloodstream, the brain's output of TSH will drop, sometimes almost to nothing. As a result, the TSH level is a very good upside-down indicator of thyroid function: When you have too little thyroid hormone, TSH is high; if you have too much thyroid hormone, TSH is very low.

Should you be treated if your doctor discovers an abnormal TSH level but you have no other symptoms? This is controversial. People with subclinical hypothyroidism may become symptomatic, but they may also do well for years without treatment. Some experts believe that treatment to normalize TSH protects other body systems from the effects of hypothyroidism. Keep in mind that high cholesterol, for example, should be considered a symptom of hypothyroidism, but it may be overlooked.

If TSH is within the normal range but the person has symptoms suggesting that the thyroid gland is underactive, the doctor may order a TRH. This test utilizing thyrotropin-releasing hormone is a way of stimulating the pituitary gland to determine how it responds. If the pituitary gland mounts a large response to TRH, it suggests an underactive thyroid gland.

If there's a blood test, why worry about the symptoms? Won't the blood test tell the story? Usually it will, with appropriate interpretation. But the symptoms can help to determine if it even makes sense to do a blood test.

One publication on evidence-based medicine, *Bandolier*, reviewed a study in which symptoms were noted before patients underwent a thyroid function test. Out of 500 patients, 23 had five or more of the symptoms of thyroid problems. (The investigators looked at overactive as well as underactive thyroid.) Of those 23, 78 percent were diagnosed with a thyroid problem, compared to about 4 percent of the patients overall.[655] Anyone who has four or more of the symptoms of low thyroid function has grounds to ask the doctor for a blood test (a "thyroid panel").

TSH Controversy

Since the test that doctors rely on measures the level of TSH, it's important to understand what the value means. For years, doctors were told that a value of serum TSH between 0.5 and 5 microunits per milliliter (mcU/ml) represented normal thyroid function. Then in 2003, the American Association of Clinical Endocrinologists announced that physicians should consider treating any patients whose TSH fell outside a narrower range of 0.3 to 3 mcU/ml. More recently, some endocrinologists have called for narrowing the range even further—in particular, bringing the high end of "normal" down to 2.5.[656] Not all laboratories have kept up with these changes. Unless the physician has a specific interest in thyroid issues, she may not question the lab's characterization of a TSH level near 5 as within the normal range. But if other thyroid hormones (T_3 and T_4) are low, even low normal, it could indicate that the person is hypothyroid.

"For most of my life I was told my thyroid tests were "low normal" despite my freezing hands, feet, ears, and nose. I was also completely

exhausted every day. My cholesterol was 300 but that was considered acceptable back then.

Then the cholesterol cap was lowered to 200, but mine had gone up to 485. My daughter, a chiropractor, said unless I had a liver problem it had to be my thyroid. My doctor finally put me on Armour desiccated thyroid. I now feel happier, peppier, and more alert than I did in my twenties. Armour really gives me a great sense of well-being.

After several months on Armour, my cholesterol went down to around 160. That's where it's been for several years with no other treatment."

★★★★ **Synthroid**

Long the standard thyroid replacement hormone, Synthroid comes in a wide range of doses. Most doctors are comfortable prescribing it.

Side effects: Uncommon if the dose is properly adjusted. Too much Synthroid may produce palpitations, diarrhea, heat intolerance, insomnia, anxiety, and other symptoms of excess thyroxine.

Downside: Synthroid alone does not work for all hypothyroid people.

Cost: Approximately $12 to $20 for a month's supply

Treating Underactive Thyroid

To treat hypothyroidism, doctors generally prescribe synthetic levothyroxine hormone in pills such as Synthroid, Levoxyl, or Levothroid to supplement or replace the patient's inadequate supply. The dose may be started low and gradually increased until the TSH gets back down into the normal range. (That means a blood test is required 6 weeks after starting on a new dose to make sure it is working properly.)

Doctors used to think thyroid therapy had no side effects if the dose was appropriate. That may well be true. But getting the dose right can be trickier than it might seem. Scientists suspect that synthetic T_4, or levothyroxine, may increase the risk of osteoporosis, especially at higher than physiologic doses. This would be especially serious for older women, who are at the greatest risk of bone loss. Even at normal treatment doses, bone mineral density may drop after 48 weeks of thyroxine therapy.[657]

Synthroid is the brand of levothyroxine that has been around the longest, but the FDA has determined that other brands, including

NORMAL THYROID TEST VALUES

- Total serum T_4: 5–12 micrograms per deciliter (mcg/dl)

- Serum T_3: 80–180 nanograms per deciliter (ng/dl)

- T_3 resin uptake: 25–35 percent

- Thyroxine-binding globulin capacity: 15–25 mcg T_4/dl

Levoxyl and Levothroid, are equivalent to it in effectiveness. We suggest, though, that if you start using one brand, you should stick with it. Switching back and forth between brands every few months is probably unwise. Differences in formulation may lead to subtle differences in how well they are absorbed. In certain cases, that could result in undesirable changes in the amount of levothyroxine in your system.

If your doctor prescribes generic levothyroxine, you have little or no control over whether the pharmacy switches from one supplier to another without notifying you. So although this may be the least expensive alternative, it is not one we recommend.

● ● ●

Q. *The information I get with my Levoxyl prescription says I should wait 4 hours before consuming calcium. I don't have 4 hours in the morning. I take my thyroid pill when I get up, but within half an hour I have to be dressed, have breakfast, and get out the door to work. Usually breakfast is calcium-fortified orange juice, bran cereal with milk, and tea. Will this have an impact on the Levoxyl?*

A. The calcium in the fortified orange juice is likely to bind to the thyroid hormone and interfere with its absorption. If you switched to ordinary orange juice and took your calcium with dinner or at bedtime, you might absorb the Levoxyl more efficiently.

● ● ●

Levothyroxine is absorbed best if it is taken on an empty stomach, so doctors often recommend it be taken at least half an hour before breakfast. People with families and jobs often find this restriction inconvenient. They're lucky if they can get it together to swallow the thyroid pill before gulping a cup of coffee and grabbing a bowl of cereal while trying to get the kids ready for school.

It is particularly important not to take this thyroid hormone at the same time as or even within an hour of taking calcium or iron supplements. These minerals can prevent absorption of the hormone. The most important thing, though, is to be consistent in the way you take it. Once the proper dose has been determined, keep taking it in the same way so that is the dose you actually get. Remember that the dose you need may change over the years; that is why your doctor will want to repeat the thyroid panel periodically. Some people report that they feel better if the dose is adjusted seasonally, but this is something you and your physician should discuss.

There shouldn't be any obvious side effects of levothyroxine when the dose is adjusted carefully. For someone with heart problems, the dosage should be increased very gradually. If the level is too high, adverse reactions such as heart palpitations and a rapid heartbeat, insomnia, nervousness, and raised blood pressure may result. Other possible signs of overdose include headache, diarrhea, tremor, increased sweating, changes in appetite, weight loss, and reduced menstrual flow. Report such symptoms to your physician promptly, because continued overdosing may cause serious heart or nervous system complications

Symptoms of low thyroid activity, such as cold intolerance, fatigue, constipation, or hair loss are not side effects of levothyroxine but indications that the dose is not quite adequate, even if the numbers on the blood test look good. (We suggest you keep a record of your results, so you can watch for trends.) Be sure to let your doctor know how you are feeling.

Adding T_3

Despite the dogma that levothyroxine alone is the proper prescription for the hypothyroid patient, there is growing interest even among endocrinologists in the possible benefits of adding some T_3 to the therapeutic regimen. Many or possibly most hypothyroid patients do quite well on levothyroxine, once the proper dose is determined. But others just never feel quite right and still suffer from subtle or not-so-subtle symptoms.

Since the healthy thyroid produces both T_4 and small amounts of T_3, why do doctors so often insist on prescribing just levothyroxine? Here's the explanation: Even in a healthy person, the thyroid gland produces only a fraction of the T_3 that the body uses. Other tissues in the body normally convert T_4 to the more active T_3 as they need it, just by knocking off one of the iodine atoms. This works well for most people.

• • •

Q. *For several years I took Thyrolar for hypothyroidism. I had to change doctors because of a change in my insurance, and the new endocrinologist refused to prescribe Thyrolar. He said that the blood test results would not be accurate because this drug combines T_3 and T_4.*

He insisted on prescribing Synthroid. I am supposed to take it upon awaking and not eat or drink for 1 hour. I follow his advice, but in 3 years, I have gained 25 pounds, I am tired all the time, and I don't feel at all like my old self.

I have complained and had numerous blood tests but the results are always within the normal range. Those nice normal test results make my doctor feel good but I still feel lousy. Is it possible that the medication is getting into my bloodstream but I am not utilizing it properly?

A. There are individuals for whom levothyroxine just doesn't seem to do all it should. These people continue to experience symptoms even on doses of levothyroxine that should be adequate. Such patients occasionally say that their experience with Armour Thyroid is more satisfactory and wonder why the physician does not simply prescribe desiccated thyroid.

Because Armour Thyroid contains both T_3 and T_4, some endocrinologists are starting to prescribe it alone or in conjunction with levothyroxine for patients who may not be converting T_4 efficiently and who continue to experience symptoms. T_3 lasts a very short time in the body, though, so a single dose of Armour during the day might result in an initial surge of T_3 and then a drop in the level of this hormone later in the day.[658]

• • •

Other experts have found that adding a small amount of T_3 to patients' levothyroxine can alleviate the depression and mental cloudiness of low thyroid hormone better than T_4 alone. It is possible that some of these people are not capable of converting T_4 to T_3 efficiently.

In one study, researchers found the dose of levothyroxine that normalized TSH. Then, they replaced 50 micrograms of that dose with 12.5 micrograms of T_3, sold in this country under the brand name Cytomel.[659] Although these scientists reported benefits in mood and cognition on this combination therapy, it is still extremely controversial. Many endocrinologists remain unconvinced that it is worth trying.[660] In several studies, though, patients offered a combination regimen seem to prefer it to levothyroxine alone.[661]

" *I was diagnosed with a thyroid condition and put on Armour Thyroid at age 8. At 45, my TSH reading was too high and I was referred to a top-notch endocrinologist.*

★★★ Armour Desiccated Thyroid

This is the only "natural" treatment for hypothyroidism that is really worth considering. Herbs and seaweed are not recommended. Take note, Armour is not vegetarian.

Most endocrinologists shudder and twitch at the idea of using something so crude and old-fashioned. But there are patients who feel much better on Armour than on synthetic levothyroxine.

Side effects: Chest pain, increased pulse rate, palpitations, excessive sweating, diarrhea, heat intolerance, tremor, and anxiety. These are symptoms of excess thyroid hormone, suggesting that the dose may be too high. Contact the prescribing doctor promptly.

Downside: Derived from pork thyroid. Those who avoid pork for religious reasons need to avoid Armour. A majority of endocrinologists are opposed to prescribing it.

Cost: Approximately $8 to $15 per month

He was horrified that I had been taking dried animal thyroid and put me on Synthroid. He said the body makes T$_3$ (whatever that is) from it.

Within a month I had gained more than 10 pounds, had no energy, and felt so depressed I was nearly suicidal. The endocrinologist said these problems had nothing to do with the medicine, but I begged my family doctor to put me back on Armour. Within a week I felt normal again. It took a while to lose the weight, but I am convinced that natural thyroid actually saved my life."

There is considerable debate not only about whether T$_3$ should be added to the regimen at all, but also about how much T$_3$ is appropriate if it is used. One problem with the short time that T$_3$ stays active in the system is that it is difficult to maintain a steady dose, with either Armour desiccated thyroid or a T$_3$ preparation such as Cytomel. Cytomel, if used, may need to be given more than once a day. One thyroid expert, Ridha Arem, MD, prescribes a small amount divided into two or three daily doses.[662] Another thyroid specialist, Kenneth Blanchard, MD, uses a slow-release T$_3$ formulation that is compounded specifically for his practice.[663] Compounding can be tricky, however. One pharmacist who compounded a T$_3$ product was sued because the pills varied so widely in dose and some supplied a dangerously high level of this hormone.

As more doctors begin to treat patients based on how they feel (a *patient-centric* approach) instead of sticking to the test num-bers, they are likely to be more willing to experiment with new regimens. Some patients continue to suffer symptoms of low thyroid hormone despite TSH readings in the normal range. Too often such people are told, in essence, that their troubles are all in their head. It is very likely that psychological factors do contribute to problems such as lethargy in some instances. Both doctors and patients should keep in mind, however, that a thyroid imbalance can sometimes trigger psychological problems such as depression, anxiety, and feelings of low self-worth.

Foods and Supplements

It is simply a truism that a healthy lifestyle—one with enough sleep and exercise and a sensible diet (and, of course, no smoking)—is just as important for people with an underfunctioning thyroid as it is for everyone else. But when a person is diagnosed as hypothyroid, there is often a lot of free advice offered about what to take and what to avoid. It can be very confusing, so we will try to offer some clarification.

Iodine

People inclined to use natural treatments for their health problems are often advised to take iodine to straighten out a thyroid problem. There's some theoretical reason for this. Iodine is an essential element in thyroid hormones. The numbers (T$_3$, T$_4$) tell how many atoms of iodine are attached to the basic hormone. There are parts of the world where iodine deficiency is a real possibility. In regions where many people are iodine deficient, severe thyroid problems like goiters are not uncommon. The pregnant woman who is iodine deficient risks giving birth to a child whose brain has not developed properly—a *cretin*, to use the technical term. People living in such conditions might well benefit from iodine supplements.

This is just not relevant for most people in the United States, though, partly because iodine supplementation has been accomplished at the level of the general population. Iodized salt provided the answer to iodine deficiency more than a generation ago, and it is still so widely used that an American would have to be eating quite a bizarre diet to become iodine deficient.

Now, if a little is good, wouldn't more be helpful if the thyroid is not working well? Not necessarily. Most endocrinologists discourage people from taking iodine because it can be overdone. In that case, it would make matters worse instead of helping.[664] In fact, excessive iodine intake increases the risk of subclinical hypothyroidism.[665] But eating a little seafood from time to time would provide a bit of extra iodine in moderation, rather than excess.

Soy

There are foods that can tangle with the enzymes needed for thyroid hormones to work normally, and soy is one of them. (Others include many members of the cabbage family.) Some of the isoflavones, especially genistein and daidzein, that seem to make soy such a valuable food also inactivate thyroid peroxidase.[666] This enzyme is important for the production of the thyroid hormones T_3 and T_4.

Simply eating soy-based foods doesn't seem to produce thyroid problems all by itself. But iodine deficiency makes animals (and presumably humans) susceptible to clinical problems caused by soy isoflavones interfering with thyroid peroxidase.[667] A person who is already hypothyroid should probably be cautious about basing a diet on soy burgers, soy milk, soy hot dogs, soy shakes, and the like. And we are skeptical about the value of soy isoflavones in pill form for someone with an underactive thyroid. Dr. Arem suggests that those who are hypothyroid limit soy-based meals to no more than three per week.[668]

• • •

Q. *I was diagnosed with hypothyroidism in 1992 and started on 0.025 milligram of Synthroid a day. This was gradually increased to 0.075 milligram in 1999.*

Last month my blood test showed that my TSH (thyroid-stimulating hormone) was up to 5.0. (The normal range is 0.4 to 4.2.) The doctor increased my dose of Synthroid to 0.1 milligram. But I kept wondering why this had happened.

When I heard that foods could have an effect, I called the doctor. I had been eating the following thyroid-fighting foods every day:

1 cup raw broccoli or cauliflower
1 cup coleslaw or cooked cabbage

2 ½ cups soy milk

2 tablespoons of soy lecithin granules on my oatmeal

Handfuls of unsalted peanuts

Instead of filling the prescription for the higher dose of Synthroid, I kept taking the 0.075 milligram. But I stopped eating the thyroid-fighting foods and a recent TSH test was much better at 3.3.

A. Some foods that are capable of causing a goiter (an enlarged thyroid gland) when they are consumed in excess have recently become very popular for fighting cancer, heart disease, and other health problems. There is even a weight-loss regimen making its rounds on the Internet that is based on cabbage soup. Now, hypothyroid people have more trouble than most losing weight, so they might be especially tempted. But as with soy, it makes sense to consume these goitrogenic foods only in moderation (and primarily in cooked form).

• • •

Selenium

Selenium is an essential mineral that is part of the enzyme that converts T_4 to T_3. So, clearly, it is important to have enough selenium in your diet. The amount in your diet may vary widely depending on where you live—and whether you buy your vegetables and milk from local producers or from national or even international sources, as is increasingly common. The amount of selenium in the soil determines how much ends up in food.

Most of us have no way of evaluating whether our diet supplies adequate selenium. Foods rich in selenium aren't necessarily the most popular in the grocery: whole grains, organ meats, mushrooms, oatmeal, soybeans, wheat germ, and sunflower seeds. Big fish like tuna and halibut also supply selenium, though, and so does beef, unless the cattle were raised in a selenium-poor environment.[669]

FOODS THAT MAY INTERFERE WITH THYROID FUNCTION

- Broccoli
- Brussels sprouts
- Cabbage
- Cauliflower
- Millet
- Mustard greens
- Peanuts
- Pine nuts
- Radishes
- Rutabaga
- Soybeans
- Turnips

★★★★ Selenium

Check your multivitamin to see if it contains selenium. If it doesn't, or if you don't take a multivitamin, consider adding 50 to 100 micrograms of selenium a day.

Downside: Too much selenium is toxic. Don't worry about overdosing through food, but don't take a supplement if your diet is rich in fish or seafood, seaweed, mushrooms, and wheat germ.

Cost: Approximately $1 to $3 per month

Zinc

Like selenium, zinc is important for the proper functioning of the enzymes that make thyroid hormone. Also like selenium, it can be hard to tell if the diet contains enough zinc. It too is found in fish, whole grains, and sunflower seeds. If you are not confident about your diet, a supplement of 15 to 25 milligrams daily is sensible.[670]

★★★ Zinc

If you take a multivitamin, it probably contains zinc. Look for an amount of 15 to 25 milligrams per day. (If you take several supplements, add up the zinc in each one.)

Downside: Excess zinc can throw off the balance of copper in the body. Stick to less than 50 milligrams daily.

Cost: Approximately $1 to $4 per month

Conclusions

Untreated hypothyroidism can be a very serious condition, contributing to other problems like infertility, heart disease, and depression. Getting the proper diagnosis and treatment may take some negotiating. Remember, how you feel is an important criterion for how well your treatment is going, although the blood tests are also important.

- If you have four or five of the symptoms of low thyroid activity, ask your doctor to test your thyroid function.
- Keep track of your results, especially if you have been diagnosed with hypothyroidism. You will want to follow trends and see how your treatment affects the value of TSH, T_4, and T_3.
- Levothyroxine is the usual treatment. Especially in older people, the starting dose should be low and gradually increased until symptoms ease and the test results normalize.
- Some people do better on one levothyroxine formulation than on another. They are considered bioequivalent, so use the one that works for you. But don't switch back and forth between them, or between a brand name and generic. Differences in formulation can make a difference in the dose you need.
- If levothyroxine alone does not alleviate your symptoms, ask your doctor about a trial with a small amount of Armour desiccated thyroid or another source of T_3. You may need to reduce the dose

of levothyroxine slightly to compensate.

• T$_3$ (Cytomel) may need to be taken two or three times a day if it is added to the regimen. It does not last long in the body.

• Don't overdo on foods, especially soy, that interfere with thyroid peroxidase.

• Consider daily supplements of selenium (50 to 100 micrograms) and zinc (15 to 25 milligrams).

• For more information, consult Mary Shomon's book *Living Well with Hypothyroidism*.

INSOMNIA

• Avoid late-night TV, alcohol, and caffeine	
• Exercise during the day	
• Take a hot bath 1 hour before bedtime	
• Listen to soothing music or a relaxation CD	
• Seek cognitive behavioral sleep therapy	★★★
• Eat a high-carb snack before bedtime	
• Take magnesium before bedtime	★★★
• Scent your bedroom with lavender or jasmine	
• Try melatonin	★★
• Use acupressure	
• Consider valerian	★★★
• Ask your doctor about Ambien CR (zolpidem)	★★
• Check with your doctor about Lunesta (eszopiclone)	★★
• Inquire about Rozerem (ramelteon)	★★
• Ask your doctor about Sonata (zaleplon)	★★

Whoever coined the phrase "sleeping like a baby" must have been childless. No parent who has ever walked the floor for hours with a fussy infant or gotten up for numerous nighttime feedings would imagine that babies sleep well.

At the other end of the life span, sleep problems are just as common. Older people frequently have trouble getting to sleep. Another common complaint is that they wake up far too early. Some have to get up to visit the bathroom and then have difficulty falling back to sleep. Others find that they are wide-awake at 3:00 a.m. and toss and turn until morning. Up to half of all elderly people report trouble with insomnia.[671]

Babies and senior citizens are not the only ones who suffer. The number of people who have intermittent or chronic sleep problems is enormous, perhaps as many as 70 million.[672] That means that one in five of us is all too familiar with sleeplessness.[673]

Perhaps people slept better in past centuries. Back before Thomas Edison invented the electric lightbulb, even adults slept an average of 10 hours a night. But average sleep time has been dropping ever since. A poll in 2002 showed that the average American gets fewer than 7 hours of shut-eye on weeknights. And the deficit can't all be made up on weekends or holidays.

Think about a sleep debt as you would a financial debt. The more it grows, the harder it is to pay off. Eventually your body rebels. Chronic sleep deprivation is associated with high blood pressure, weight gain, diabetes, reduced immunity, daytime drowsiness, poor performance, traffic accidents, falls, memory problems, and cognitive impairment. But lying awake in bed worrying about these possible consequences won't help.

Inviting Sleep

Have you ever climbed into bed exhausted after a stressful day, only to discover that your brain won't slow down? The events of the day just keep replaying like an endless movie. Figuring out how to let go of those worries can be challenging. Watching the clock tick off the minutes or the hours just makes things worse. The later it gets, the more anxious you become, especially if you are concerned about being fresh the next day.

It's hardly any wonder that so many people get into the habit of reaching for a sleeping pill "just in case." They assume they will have difficulty falling asleep and pop a pill to prevent trouble. Of course, this leads to an endless cycle. Without the sleeping pill, they have rebound insomnia, which reinforces the fear of not being able to fall asleep, which triggers another round of pills. What else can you do to avoid tossing and turning for hours?

NIGHT LIGHT

Epidemiologists have found that too much light at night may increase a woman's risk of breast cancer.[674] Light suppresses the production of a natural brain hormone called melatonin. Blood levels of this hormone naturally rise at night. When you are exposed to a computer screen or bright light at night, the body cannot make enough melatonin. A low level of melatonin is associated with cancers of the prostate, lung, stomach, and breast.[675] To minimize disruption of melatonin, body-clock researcher William Hrushesky suggests the following sensible guidelines:

- Have a consistent bedtime.
- Darken your bedroom.
- Get regular exercise during the day.
- Abstain from alcohol before bed (it blocks melatonin).[676]

Cut Out Caffeine

Most people know that caffeine is a stimulant that can keep them awake. They avoid that evening cup of coffee, thinking that will solve the problem. But some people are so sensitive to the effects of caffeine that they should stay away from coffee, tea, and caffeinated soft drinks at any time in the afternoon. And don't assume that decaffeinated coffee is the solution to your insomnia problems. If heartburn is contributing to your nighttime sleep woes, the culprit could be decaf coffee, which can trigger acid reflux that may wake you up.

Beware Drugs That Can Keep You Awake

Caffeine is not the only drug that can interfere with a good night's sleep. A surprising number of prescription and over-the-counter medications can contribute to nightmares, insomnia, or disrupted sleep. Many of these drugs would not necessarily be expected to cause problems. Beta-blockers such as atenolol, metoprolol, and propranolol, which are prescribed for high blood pressure or heart trouble, may cause nightmares and insomnia. The osteoporosis medicine Actonel (risedronate) can interfere with sleep. So can many antidepressants, such as Effexor (venlafaxine), Prozac (fluoxetine), Wellbutrin (bupropion), Zoloft (sertraline), and others, and allergy medicines that contain decongestants such as phenylephrine and pseudoephedrine.

The list of drugs that can cause sleeplessness is so long that we cannot possibly include it in its entirety here. If you suspect that your medication may be interfering with restful sleep, discuss this issue with your pharmacist and your physician. There may be alternatives.

Forgo the Nightcap

And don't forget alcohol. An evening glass of wine or a nightcap may seem relaxing and even make you drowsy. But alcohol can affect melatonin levels and interfere with dreaming sleep. Waking too early is a common consequence of having an evening cocktail.[677] If you're having trouble sleeping, don't drink after dinner.

Exercise

Exercise is not only good for the heart and bones, it is also a great stress reliever. If you can take a brisk walk, play a couple of sets of tennis, or play a round of golf (without the golf cart), you will find that your level of anxiety will diminish. Do it in the afternoon and you may get some sun on your face. Bright light combined with exercise can relieve depression and insomnia.[678] The sun exposure can also affect melatonin levels that have an impact on sleep quality and could reduce the risk of breast cancer in women.[679]

Tai chi is an ancient Chinese exercise program. This gentle form of activity is actually quite beautiful to watch. Researchers at the Oregon Research Institute in Eugene recruited 118 men and women over 60 years old. Half were taught tai chi and the other half had a low-impact exercise session. The tai chi students reported that after 6 months, it took them less time to fall asleep (18 minutes less on average) and they slept longer (48 minutes longer).[680]

Timing is everything when it comes to exercise and sleep. If you exercise in the morning or early in the day, you should have less trouble sleeping. But if you exercise in the evening, just before bedtime, you're likely to have more trouble sleeping.[681]

Hot Bath

Another simple, inexpensive, and pleasant way to ward off insomnia is to take a hot bath. Here again, though, timing is critical. A hot bath or shower just before bedtime could be counterproductive. The trick is to schedule it about an hour before you plan to go to bed.[682] A hot bath raises the core body temperature. As it drops, the signal that goes to the brain is "sleepy time." Body temperature normally drops in the first part of a night's sleep, so pushing it up with a 30-minute soak, then allowing it to fall tricks the body into thinking it may already be asleep. Combined with a regular bedtime ritual, this can really help.

Winding Down

Turning off the internal dialogue is especially hard for some folks. "If only" is a dangerous game. People who replay the day's events, complaining to themselves that they should have done things differently, are destined to toss and turn. How can you stop obsessing? One way is to set aside time specifically for worrying much earlier in the day. It

sounds odd, but some people find that it helps.

Another way to quiet your mind at bedtime is to keep the television out of the bedroom. Not only will this make it easier to get to sleep, it might improve your love life. According to an Italian researcher, Serenella Salomoni, "If there's no television in the bedroom, the frequency (of sexual intercourse) doubles."[683] Satisfying sex can lead to deep relaxation and make it easier to fall asleep.

If your bedroom clock has a bright face that allows you to watch the minutes tick past, turn it away from the bed. Watching the time go by is a recipe for staying awake and increasing your anxiety about falling asleep.

Another way to relax is to listen to gentle music or guided imagery. Our favorites are by Emmett Miller, MD. Dr. Miller is one of the founding fathers of the mind-body movement. He is a poet, a philosopher, a musician, and a healing, caring physician. His voice is so soothing and reassuring that you will find yourself relaxing without even trying. To find out more about his CDs and tapes, visit www.drmiller. com or call 800-528-2737. Our Dr. Miller faves are *Easing into Sleep, Letting Go of Stress, 10-Minute Stress Manager, Healing Journey,* and *Rainbow Butterfly.*

Lest you think this is all touchy-feely New Age nonsense, we promise you that there is actual research to support these nondrug approaches. One study offered insomniacs a selection of soothing music to be played for 45 minutes at bedtime.[684] The participants selected the music they preferred and were instructed to relax in bed while listening to it. Measurements showed that they had less trouble getting to sleep, fell asleep more quickly, and had better sleep quality.

Another study compared progressive relaxation to anxiety management training for 9 weeks. Both groups of insomniacs benefited. They fell asleep faster and slept more soundly.[685] Such behavioral training can be a little pricey, which is why we like Dr. Miller's CDs.

Cognitive Behavioral Therapy

People who have persistent problems with insomnia may find it well worth their while to consult a counselor who offers cognitive behavioral therapy (CBT). A study compared this nondrug approach to a sleeping pill similar to Lunesta (eszopiclone) that is commonly used in Europe. Investigators found that CBT was more effective than either the placebo or the sleeping pill.[686] The intervention included

---

★★★ Cognitive Behavioral Therapy

In a study, learning about sleep hygiene, sleep restriction, and progressive relaxation and discussing fears about losing sleep worked better than a sleeping pill against insomnia.

Downside: It is difficult to find a trained counselor.

Cost: Approximately $125 to $140 per session. Six sessions should last a lifetime.

---

instruction on using the bedroom only for sex and sleeping, sticking to a regular schedule for rising and retiring, avoiding naps during the day, progressive relaxation, and discussion of beliefs and fears about sleep loss.

Bedtime Snacks

The cartoon character Dagwood Bumstead is famous for his giant sandwiches just before bed. The official recipe contains meatloaf, ham, bacon, sausage, fried egg, and lots of other goodies. We suspect that anyone who actually tries such a sandwich would have real trouble falling asleep. It's not just the possibility of heartburn, but also the protein that worries us. Although we are big fans of a low-carb approach for weight loss and blood sugar control, this principle does not hold in the evening. Protein can be energizing, which is the last thing you need before bed. Instead, we would recommend eating carbohydrates. According to Judith Wurtman, PhD, a research scientist at Massachusetts Institute of Technology, "If you eat carbohydrates when your internal clock wants you to sleep, the food will act like a sleeping pill."[687]

Relaxation foods include caramel-coated rice cakes, Cheerios with frozen fruit and honey, toasted waffles with maple syrup and half a banana, a handful of pretzels, graham crackers, fig bars, and a blueberry muffin. We would never recommend this dietary approach for someone with blood sugar problems (diabetes or prediabetes). And it obviously is not for someone who is trying to lose weight. But such high-carbohydrate foods can boost serotonin levels in the brain and make it easier for you to relax and fall asleep when you consume them 15 to 30 minutes before bedtime.

Magnesium

A simple mineral may be just the ticket for a good night's sleep. Magnesium is essential for good health, but often it is in short supply in the American diet. One reason many people are deficient is because of their medicine. Diuretics that deplete the body of potassium also can eliminate magnesium. Although physicians are usually good about monitoring the blood's potassium level, they may be less diligent when it comes to magnesium.

Several years ago, we began hearing from readers of our newspaper column that magnesium is helpful for insomniacs. With some searching, we discovered that there is at least a little scientific basis for this benefit.[688] Magnesium appears to be especially helpful for those who suffer from restless leg syndrome.[689] This

---

★★★ Magnesium

This mineral is helpful for bones, nerves, muscles, and brain function. The recommended dose ranges from 250 to 500 milligrams daily. If you develop loose stools, reduce the dose.

Side effects: Diarrhea
Downside: Not safe for people with poor kidney function
Cost: Approximately $2 to $3 per month

---

condition can make it hard to fall asleep or can awaken you once you are sleeping sweetly.

• • •

Q. *I have suffered from episodes of insomnia for years. Cutting down on caffeine didn't work. Over-the-counter sleep aids such as Benadryl made me groggy the next day. Even prescription drugs like Ambien didn't help.*

Then a friend suggested I try taking magnesium at bedtime. I started taking magnesium (250 milligrams) at night. Magnesium has helped my insomnia more than anything else I've ever tried.

A. Magnesium is essential for good health. This mineral plays a role in more than 300 biochemical reactions in the body and is crucial for the proper functioning of nerves, muscles, bones, and blood vessels.

Magnesium is used in some laxatives (milk of magnesia) and antacids (Maalox, Mylanta, etc.). This nutrient may also be helpful in preventing osteoporosis and migraines and alleviating premenstrual symptoms. We've not heard of magnesium being used to treat insomnia, however. We'd be interested to learn if anyone else finds this mineral helpful against insomnia.

• • •

In response, we heard from several readers. Some found that they could eliminate over-the-counter sleeping pills after starting magnesium supplements. One reported, "I started taking Citracal Plus with Magnesium at bedtime. Ever since, I've been sleeping like a baby (a lazy one, mind you, not the colicky kind)." But here is a cautionary tale. Timing is everything:

● ● ●

Q. *You asked if anyone has had success taking magnesium for insomnia. Years ago I was visiting my sister, who urged my husband and me to start taking magnesium in addition to vitamins. We took the first dose the morning we left for home.*

We usually split the driving. I drive in the evening, when I am most alert, and my husband drives in the daytime while I drowse. That trip neither of us could keep our eyes open. We nearly pulled into a rest stop to sleep, but somehow we managed to get home.

I told my sister, who responded, "Sleepiness is a side effect. We take magnesium at night." I've used it for insomnia ever since.

A. You've confirmed what some other readers noted: Magnesium makes them sleepy. Magnesium can cause diarrhea, usually at doses above 350 milligrams daily. People with kidney problems must avoid magnesium, because it could be harmful.

● ● ●

Sleepy-Time Smells

Smelling yourself to sleep seems like a pretty strange concept. We have to admit that aromatherapy for insomnia seemed like a stretch to us, too. Most people are used to swallowing medicine, not smelling it. Nevertheless, scientific research supports the idea that soothing smells may be relaxing and actually enhance sleep.[690] Lavender and jasmine are the two scents that seem to promote sleep. Sleep researchers at Wesleyan University in Middletown, Connecticut, found that lavender increased deep sleep in both men and women, and they concluded that lavender aroma has sedative and sleep-promoting activity.[691]

Some people put a sachet under their pillow. Others spray the pillowcase with scented water.

> *Several friends and I have discovered a wonderful natural way to help insomnia. It is called "lavender and vanilla pillow mist." It can be purchased at the bath shops found in a shopping mall.*
>
> *When I first heard a friend tell me that she had been using sleeping pills for several years, and then did not need them once she discovered the lavender pillow mist, I originally thought it*

was all in her head. But I gave it a try and found it most relaxing.

You just spray a little on the corners of your pillow, where your face will be. It even seemed to help my stopped-up nose!

To brag a little more, I sprayed some on my dog's pillow, and she slept about an hour longer in the morning. I have been told that the Egyptians have used lavender for relaxing for more than 500 years. Perhaps this will help those who are having insomnia and want a natural way to go to sleep."

Those who don't find lavender appealing may want to consider jasmine instead. Researchers at Wheeling Jesuit University compared sleeping environments infused with jasmine, lavender, and no smell at all. Twenty subjects were tested for 3 nights each and then given mental function tests. Those who slept under the influence of jasmine woke up more refreshed and alert. They scored better on the tests by responding more quickly and accurately. Lavender also seemed to help, but not as much as jasmine.[692] Scientists have found that both jasmine and lavender odors have measurable effects on nerve activity, mood, and heart rate.[693] A caller to our national radio show also reported that the scent of eucalyptus helped her sleep.

Breaking the Vicious Pill Cycle

It may be difficult for people with chronic sleep problems to break out of the medication merry-go-round. Anyone who has relied on sleeping pills like diazepam (Valium), lorazepam (Ativan), or temazepam (Restoril) will discover that stopping suddenly may lead to several sleepless nights. Often, this sets in motion a vicious cycle in which the insomniac reverts to the medication just to get a little sleep but finds once again that when he or she stops the medicine, rebound insomnia kicks in.

It is not likely that natural sleep aids will be able to counteract this effect. Instead, you may need to discuss such a drug dependency problem with your physician to develop a withdrawal strategy. It may take several weeks (or longer) to wean yourself off a traditional sleeping pill habit. Once "clean," though, it may be possible to substitute an herb or a dietary supplement to get a decent night's sleep without creating another vicious circle of rebound insomnia.

Melatonin

Because melatonin is a natural chemical created in the brain and is essential for normal sleep, it seems logical that taking melatonin in a pill would be helpful for insomnia. Many people believe that melatonin is a wonderful natural sleep aid. Unfortunately, the studies that have been done have produced mixed results. One careful review of clinical trials concluded, "There is evidence to suggest that melatonin is not effective in treating most primary sleep disorders with short-term use (4 weeks or less)."[694]

People taking melatonin did fall asleep more quickly—11 minutes on the average—

★★ Melatonin

Taken 30 minutes before bedtime, melatonin may help a person get to sleep faster and improve sleep quality. The dose is controversial. As little as ⅓ milligram (300 micrograms) may be optimal (this dosage is available from Nature's Bounty). Most supplements provide 3 milligrams, which is probably too much.

Side effects: Tiredness, dizziness, headache. Don't mix with warfarin (Coumadin).
Downside: Finding 0.3-milligram doses is hard. You may have to split a 1-milligram tablet three ways.
Cost: Approximately $2 to $3 for a month's supply

not enough to write home about. The authors concluded that melatonin appears to be safe, at least in the short term. Another meta-analysis of 17 sleep studies reached a different conclusion. Those investigators found that melatonin reduced the amount of time it took for people to fall asleep and increased the amount of time they spent sleeping.[695]

The one condition for which melatonin appeared to work well is "delayed sleep phase insomnia." People with this problem go to bed very late (perhaps 3:00 or 4:00 a.m.) and get up late (around 10:30 a.m. or later), have trouble going to sleep at a normal time, and experience morning grogginess.[696] Taking 5 milligrams of melatonin 3 to 4 hours before bedtime allowed such people to go to sleep more easily around midnight.

Acupressure

We never considered acupressure a viable sleep aid until we received a most unorthodox home remedy from one of our readers. He suggested taping a dried bean to the inside of the wrist between the two tendons. He measured three finger-widths from the crease of the wrist. The point he described is known in traditional acupuncture as the Inner Gate. Pressing on it is supposed to relieve anxiety, slow the heart rate, and promote sleep.

> **I read in your column about an acupressure point on the inner arm to aid sleep. You suggested taping a kidney bean between the two tendons, three finger-widths from the wrist.**
>
> **My husband and I tried it, and it's been amazing! The tape was uncomfortable on our skin, so we're using plastic "marbles" (for arranging flowers in vases) instead of a kidney bean, and we secure it with an elastic band. It has improved our sleep tremendously, and we wanted to thank you.**

Other ingenious readers devised wristlets with buttons to exert pressure on the proper point. Apparently, though, the acupressure point our reader described is not the only one that could be used. A commercial product, 1st Choice Sleep Band, from the makers of Acuband, exerts pressure at a spot on the heart meridian (Ht7). The manufacturer claims that wearing the bands on both wrists promotes restful sleep (for more information, go to www.acuband.com).

There is relatively little research to support acupressure for treating insomnia. Not surprisingly, most of what there is has been done in places where people are familiar with the concepts behind acupuncture and acupressure. A Korean study found that acupuncture of the ear assisted elderly people in getting to sleep.[697] A Taiwanese study found that acupressure improved the quality of sleep in older people.[698]

Herbal Solutions

Compared to pharmaceuticals, herbs get no respect. Physicians think they are wimpy at best and ineffective and dangerous at worst. This is despite the fact that the sleeping pills they have prescribed for decades carry substantial risks of their own. More about sleeping pill problems in a moment, though. The question is whether it would even be worth trying an herbal approach to insomnia.

Valerian (VALERIANA OFFICINALIS)

Do you remember the story of the Pied Piper of Hamlin? He used music to rid the town of a rat infestation. Some herbal experts suggest that he may have used valerian as well. It was popular in medieval times to flavor soups and stews. Because dried valerian root smells like sweaty socks or stinky cheese, presumably the aroma would be appealing to rats. Some even suggest he could have given valerian to the town's children to quell their fears before playing his pipe for them. That would have made it easier for him to lure them away after the town

> ### ★★★ Valerian
>
> Taken 30 minutes to 2 hours before bedtime for at least 2 weeks, valerian can help a person get to sleep faster. It may also improve sleep quality. The dose is 300 to 600 milligrams daily. For tea, use 2 to 3 grams of dried root and steep for 10 to 15 minutes.
>
> **Side effects:** Digestive upset, rare headache. Don't mix with prescription sedatives such as barbiturates or benzodiazepines.
> **Downside:** Smells bad; quality variable
> **Cost:** Approximately $8 to $12 for a month's supply

fathers refused to pay him what they owed him for ridding the town of rats.

Regardless of whether this legend has any basis in fact, the herb has long been used as a mild sedative. A number of small trials suggest that valerian reduces the amount of time it takes a person to fall asleep and may improve the quality of sleep.[699] In one 6-week study, standardized valerian extract proved just as effective for mild insomnia as the prescription sedative oxazepam (Serax). Do not expect valerian to work instant magic. Unlike traditional sleeping pills, it appears that valerian is more effective when taken nightly for at least 2 weeks.

The biggest advantage of this herbal approach over antihistamines like diphenhydramine (Benadryl or Tylenol PM) and prescription sleeping pills like temazepam (Restoril) is that valerian does not affect coordination or make you woozy.[700] This is critical if you wake up in the middle of the night to go to the bathroom. Anyone who is a little unsteady could fall if taking standard sleeping pills.

OTHER SLEEPY-TIME HERBS

Other herbs that people have used to treat insomnia include hops, chamomile, lemon balm, passionflower, St. John's wort, kava, and fennel seeds. There are, unfortunately, few large, randomized, controlled studies to verify the effectiveness of any of these natural products.[701] Kava works, but concerns have been raised that it might cause liver toxicity. This may have to do with how the kava is manufactured, but until this issue is resolved, we cannot recommend the long-term use of this herb.

Chamomile tea is what Mrs. Rabbit gave Peter to ease his tummyache and help him get to sleep after his mischief in Farmer MacGregor's garden. (In one of her other books, Beatrix Potter suggests that lettuce can make little rabbits sleepy, though she doesn't find it affects her that way.) Chamomile has traditionally been suggested to be a very gentle sedative, but there is hardly any evidence that it would have an effect in insomnia. On the other hand, a cup of chamomile tea might settle the stomach and be a nice way to calm down before climbing into bed.

Sleeping Pills

Like Rip Van Winkle, the sleeping pill business is waking up after a long period of hibernation. During the 1990s, sleeping pills fell out of favor. Triazolam (Halcion) was extremely popular after coming on the market in 1983. Here was a sleeping pill that worked quickly to put people to sleep and would not leave a morning hangover like its predecessors (Dalmane, Restoril, or Valium). Since the drug was rapidly eliminated from the body, it was believed to have no measurable effect the following day. Halcion quickly became the market leader.

Then odd reports started cropping up. Scientists taking Halcion to prevent jet lag while traveling to international conferences noted bizarre lapses in memory concerning events that happened the following day. These people appeared normal to friends and relatives while they were giving speeches, recovering lost luggage, and sightseeing the day after taking Halcion. But sometimes they later could not remember having done any of those things. It was as if a piece of their memory had been erased, like words from a blackboard. There were also reports of depression associated with Halcion use and even some suggestions that it was linked to violent and aggressive behavior.

With all the bad press, Halcion in particular and sleeping pills in general fell into disfavor. A lot of insomniacs worried about drug dependency, morning grogginess, and memory lapses. Instead, they chose to toss and turn rather than rely on benzodiazepines like estazolam, flurazepam, quazepam, temazepam, and triazolam.

Then along came zolpidem (Ambien) in 1993. It gradually captured the sleeping pill market. Eventually zaleplon (Sonata) showed up, but the real competition didn't arrive until 2005 in the form of eszopiclone (Lunesta) and ramelteon (Rozerem). Sleeping pills were aggressively marketed directly to consumers. The Lunesta commercial featured a beautiful green Luna moth gently fluttering through a bedroom. But just because the ads are alluring doesn't mean a prescription is the best approach.

An in-depth analysis indicated that for the elderly, at least, some sleep medications are more likely to hurt than help.[702] The medications may help some older individuals fall asleep more quickly. But the overview found that, for the most part, sleeping pills have only a modest effect.

The prospect of dangerous side effects is especially troubling. Older people taking a sleeping pill were nearly five times more likely to become confused or forgetful as those tak-ing an inactive placebo.[703] Dizziness that might lead to a fall and daytime drowsiness that could lead to an accident were also significantly more common. These risks should lead an older insomniac to ask lots of questions about possible problems if his physician offers a prescription. The authors of the review suggested that cognitive behavioral therapy or other nondrug treatment might be preferable for some elderly people with sleeping difficulties.[704]

As is so often the case, there are few head-to-head clinical trials comparing the effectiveness or safety of the newer sleep aids.[705] As a result, ranking them requires a certain amount of guesswork and judgment. Here is our overview.

Ambien and Ambien CR (Zolpidem)

Until Lunesta arrived, Ambien dominated the sleeping pill landscape. Before it lost its patent, the manufacturer came up with a controlled-release (CR), long-acting formulation.

★★ Ambien CR (Zolpidem)

Zolpidem helps people fall asleep and stay asleep. For reasons that are somewhat mysterious, the FDA has limited use to about 2 weeks at a time. Insurance companies often won't pay for more than 15 pills a month. Dependency is uncommon, but some people do report rebound insomnia when they stop suddenly.

Side effects: Headache, dizziness, next-day drowsiness, fatigue, difficulty with coordination, and nightmares

Downside: Possible memory difficulties. Sudden discontinuation can lead to worse insomnia during the first night or two. Other symptoms of withdrawal may include anxiety and agitation. Do not take Ambien with an SSRI-type (Prozac, Zoloft, etc.) antidepressant.

Cost: Approximately $100 for 1 month (30 pills)

The pill is coated with two layers; the first dissolves immediately to help people fall asleep quickly, while the second dissolves more slowly to help people stay asleep. Studies suggest that Ambien CR helps people fall asleep more quickly (by about 10 minutes) and reduces nighttime awakenings. The immediate-release zolpidem was not associated with much morning sedation and did not seem to affect driving performance. The newer sustained-release product may cause some next-day grogginess. This might make driving more dangerous. When Ambien CR is stopped suddenly, it may produce rebound insomnia.[706]

Lunesta (Eszopiclone)

What makes Lunesta unique is the special status the FDA has granted this medication. Instead of the usual short-term restriction associated with other prescription sleeping pills, the agency gave the manufacturer permission to market Lunesta for long-term use. Since most people with insomnia suffer for more than a few nights at a time, this labeling is likely to propel Lunesta to becoming the most successful sleeping pill in the United States. Whether it deserves this marketing edge remains to be seen. Lunesta works in a manner similar to that of Ambien and Sonata, but it has a longer-lasting effect.

One study suggested that Lunesta could be used for up to 6 months without losing its effectiveness or leading to dependence. Nevertheless, the FDA classifies it as a Schedule IV controlled substance, which means "limited

---

★★ Lunesta (Eszopiclone)

Eszopiclone helps people fall asleep and stay asleep. It probably lasts a little longer than Ambien but likely is comparable to Ambien CR. Because the manufacturer submitted a 6-month study, Lunesta is approved for long-term use.

Side effects: Unpleasant taste, headache, next-day drowsiness, dizziness, dry mouth, next-day memory impairment (anterograde amnesia), difficulty with coordination

Downside: Possible memory difficulties. Sudden discontinuation can lead to worse insomnia during the first night or two. Lunesta can be very dangerous if taken in combination with alcohol or other sedatives. Avoid itraconazole (Sporanox), clarithromycin (Biaxin), and ritonavir (Norvir).

Cost: Approximately $100 to $110 for 1 month (30 pills)

---

dependence liability." When Lunesta is stopped, rebound insomnia is a distinct possibility.

Rozerem (Ramelteon)

This is the first truly unique sleeping pill to come to market in years. It targets melatonin receptors to help people fall asleep. Unlike all other prescription sleeping pills, Rozerem is not classified as a "controlled substance." That means there are no restrictions on the length of time it can be used and no fears about abuse or dependency.

On the surface, it might seem as if Rozerem

★★ Rozerem (Ramelteon)

Ramelteon helps people fall asleep. It works differently from all other sleeping pills and poses no risk of dependency. Take it 30 minutes before retiring and not with a high-fat meal.

Side effects: Next-day drowsiness, dizziness, nausea, fatigue, and headache
Downside: Not safe for people with liver problems. Avoid fluvoxamine (Luvox), fluconazole (Diflucan), and ketoconazole (Nizoral). Safety during pregnancy has not been determined.
Cost: Approximately $80 to $85 for 1 month (30 pills)

represents a wonderful new solution to insomnia. Unfortunately, we are not overly impressed with its effectiveness. In clinical trials, it reduced the amount of time it took people to fall asleep by 8 to 16 minutes.[707] That may be helpful for some, but Rozerem did not reduce nighttime awakenings or help people get back to sleep once they had awakened. In addition, there is one side effect that bothers us. The manufacturer reports that this compound lowers testosterone levels and increases a hormone called prolactin. This change in hormone balance may be associated with reduced libido, infertility, and osteoporosis.

Sonata (Zaleplon)

Sonata is a very short-acting sleeping pill that works in a manner similar to that of Ambien and Lunesta. Because its effects wear off quickly, it can be used when someone wakes up in the middle of the night and cannot get back to sleep. The only caution, though, is that you need at least 4 more hours of sleeping time for the effects to wear off. If you wake up at 5:00 a.m., take a Sonata, and then expect to be able to hit the ground running at 7:00 a.m., you could be in trouble. If Sonata is taken at bedtime, it is less likely than other sleeping pills to cause morning hangover or affect driving ability the next day. The downside to this short effect is that some people may wake up early in the morning because the drug's effect has worn off.

For people who wake up too early in the morning, there is another trick to try. Bright light exposure in the evening may help them

★★ Sonata (Zaleplon)

Zaleplon is a good choice for people who wake up in the middle of the night and cannot easily fall asleep again. At least 4 hours of sleep time are needed. Do not take after a fatty (heavy) meal because the food will delay absorption.

Side effects: Headache, stomachache, dry mouth, constipation, back pain, and occasional next-day drowsiness
Downside: Sonata's very short effect may mean that the drug wears off during the night and results in early morning awakening. People with liver problems should avoid Sonata.
Cost: Approximately $100 per month

reset their body clock so that they can sleep through the night.[708] Those who cannot fall asleep until the wee hours may benefit from bright light in the morning.[709]

Diphenhydramine

This antihistamine, the active ingredient in Benadryl, is notorious for causing drowsiness. During the daytime, this side effect is a real liability if you want to drive or do anything that requires alertness. But at bedtime, drowsiness might be a good thing. There are many over-the-counter sleeping pills that contain diphenhydramine (Nytol, Simply Sleep, Sominex, Unisom Sleepgels, etc.). The manufacturers of nighttime pain relievers like Alka-Seltzer PM, Exedrin PM, and Tylenol PM have been successful at getting consumers to buy into the need for a combination analgesic and sleep aid.

• • •

Q. *Several years ago I developed severe dry eyes. About a year later, my husband developed the same condition. The only common denominator our doctors could find is that we were both taking Tylenol PM to sleep at night.*

The ingredient that helps one sleep in that product is an antihistamine, which can be drying. Your readers should be told.

A. Diphenhydramine, which puts the *PM* in Tylenol PM and many other night-time pain relievers, can dry out mucous membranes. Sensitive individuals could notice a dry mouth. This is the first time we have heard that this anti-histamine may also cause dry eyes.

• • •

The main problem with diphenhydramine as a sleep aid is that some people experience next-day grogginess. As a result, driving performance may be impaired. In addition, some people may experience dry mouth or difficulty with urination. The sleep-inducing effect can wear off after a few days.[710] Older people may be especially vulnerable to side effects such as cognitive impairment.

Conclusions

Getting a good night's sleep is crucial for good health. We never cease to be amazed that health-conscious people who exercise, eat carefully, and take their vitamins often skimp on sleep. We hope you will make getting adequate sleep an important health priority. If you can find a psychologist who specializes in cognitive behavioral therapy for sleep disorders, this approach may be the safest and produce the longest-lasting benefits.[711]

Here is an overview of our other recommendations.

• Practice good sleep hygiene. Try to go to bed at the same time each night. Avoid alcohol and caffeine. Keep the bedroom dark, and do not watch TV in the bedroom.

• Exercise during the day (not in the evening) and take a hot bath about an hour before bedtime.

• A high-carb snack before bedtime may raise serotonin levels, helping you fall asleep. Relax with soothing music or a relaxation CD.

• Cognitive behavioral therapy is one of the most cost-effective approaches to insomnia. Finding a practitioner with experience will be your biggest challenge.

• Try magnesium supplements before bed.

As long as your kidneys are healthy, 250 to 500 milligrams may help. If you develop diarrhea, reduce the dose.

• Aromatherapy may be helpful. The scents of jasmine or lavender can be relaxing and facilitate sleep.

• If a nondrug herbal approach appeals to you, valerian is our first choice. We would recommend a standardized extract of 300 to 600 milligrams before bed. Several days to 2 weeks may be needed to see results.

• If a sleeping pill is your last resort, we suggest zolpidem. Because it is available as a generic, it will be the most cost-effective.

LEG CRAMPS

• Place a bar of soap under the bottom bedsheet	★★★★
• Eat a teaspoonful of yellow mustard	★★★
• Sip an ounce of pickle juice	★★★
• Try ¼ teaspoon of baking soda in water	
• Pinch your upper lip between your thumb and forefinger	
• Stretch calf and foot muscles before bed	
• Drink 8 ounces of low-sodium V8 vegetable juice	
• Take 300 to 500 milligrams of magnesium	★★★★
• Try 4 ounces of Pedialyte electrolyte solution	★★★★
• Take a B-complex vitamin	★★★
• Ask your doctor about quinine	★★

Imagine this: You're sleeping peacefully, with not a care in the world. Then, like a bolt of lightning, you are wide awake and in excruciating pain. A muscle in your leg is contracting so strongly that it wakes you out of a sound sleep. To ease the pain, you need the muscle to relax. But coaxing a muscle to let go can be tricky. If such sudden nighttime leg pains occur frequently, they can wreak havoc with your rest. And that can have negative consequences for your overall health.

> "When I get severe leg cramps, my calf muscle becomes hard as a rock. The pain is so severe that I panic until I can stop it. It's rather like being asleep and getting woken up with a hammer blow to the thumb.
>
> I tried massaging my calf. That didn't work. The pain doesn't quit until I can flex my calf muscle. During a leg cramp, my foot is in a position as if I had on high heels. Forcing the foot into a more normal position by pushing the toes and heel onto the floor usually stops the pain. This hurts, but it works.
>
> Every time I have gotten this kind of cramp it was because I was dehydrated. Any sports trainer will tell you that cramps are a sign of dehydration."

Although dehydration may lead to mineral imbalances that could contribute to muscle spasms, doctors don't always know why some people develop nighttime leg cramps. They often don't have good treatments, either. Many physicians prescribe quinine, a natural medicine derived from the bark of the cinchona tree. It has been used for centuries to treat fevers, especially those due to malaria. While this drug can be effective against leg cramps, there are a number of potentially serious side effects associated with quinine. They include ringing in the ears, rash, and, rarely, liver damage or life-threatening anemia.

Consequently, it makes sense to try home remedies or dietary supplements first to see if they work. That's true even though some of the home remedies may seem a little strange. What works like a charm for one person may be totally worthless for someone else. This is truly a case of trial and error.

Soap under the Sheets

One of the strangest home remedies we have ever encountered requires nothing fancier than a bar of soap. When we first heard about this approach, we assumed it had to be a placebo effect. That's because we have no scientific explanation for why it would work. Because it defies logic, we almost wrote it off as too weird. But so many of our readers have shared their successes with us that we can no longer ignore one of the cheapest and easiest ways to prevent leg cramps.

How someone came up with the idea to put a bar of soap under the bottom sheet is a mys-

---

★★★★ Soap

Any soap except Dove or Dial should work. Inexpensive, without side effects, and amazingly effective, according to many readers. Place a bar under the bottom sheet near your legs.

Cost: Approximately 70 cents for a bar that should last up to 6 weeks

---

tery. Whoever came up with the idea, however, was a creative genius and now has a lot of devoted followers. Basically, the instructions are to take an ordinary bar of soap, unwrap it, and stick it under the bottom (fitted) sheet about where your calves would be. The cheaper the soap, the better it seems to work. Folks tell us that even a small bar of hotel soap works just fine. Every so often, someone will report that she had concluded that the soap had stopped working until she discovered that it had fallen out of the bed. The bar does need to be replaced from time to time, perhaps every month or 6 weeks. And we have been told that it may take from a few days to a week for the full effect to take hold.

> *I read that a bar of soap under the bottom sheet near the bottom of the bed might help prevent leg cramps at night and decided to give it a try. I have been plagued with terrible leg cramps several times a night for months. None of the many remedies I've tried helped—until the soap.*
>
> *It is hard to believe that a simple bar of soap could possibly make a difference, but it did. Not a single cramp in over a week. I was desperate for a good night's sleep and finally got it. One bonus: There are no side effects!*

> *My physician husband was having severe leg cramps at night, and when he'd wake with one, I would wake up as well. He tried tonic water and quinine, but they didn't help.*
>
> *Under cover of darkness, so he wouldn't see, I placed a soap bar under the sheets on his side.*

> *He's had no more cramps since then. It was 2 nights before he even noticed the soap.*

> *I used one of your ridiculous remedies (the soap under the bedsheet) to stop nighttime leg cramps. Sufferers of leg cramps will try anything. I didn't tell my friends about trying this dumb suggestion. But what do you know, it worked!*

By the way, while you are messing with your sheets, make sure that the top sheet is not tucked tight. A military-style bed with sheets so tight that a quarter will bounce off them may contribute to foot or leg cramps by pulling the foot into an awkward position. Even your average hotel bed can be improved by loosening the top sheet.

Mustard

Soap might not prevent all leg cramps. An inexpensive option for relieving the pain quickly is to swallow a teaspoon of mustard—the cheap yellow kind, not a fancy French or German variety. Again, we have no idea how someone discovered this astonishing remedy.

We cannot tell you why yellow mustard seems to work so well for so many people. Presumably, the turmeric added for coloring and flavoring plays a role. The active ingredient in turmeric is curcumin, which has been shown to have anti-inflammatory properties. How it could work so fast mystifies us.

Most people who have tried this remedy report that they get quick relief, but some complain that mustard in the middle of the night,

★★★ Mustard

Eating cheap yellow mustard may soothe the pain of leg cramps. A teaspoonful or the amount in a self-serve packet should be enough.

Downside: It might cause heartburn.

Cost: Approximately $1 for a 9-ounce jar that will last for weeks. You can get little packets of yellow mustard for free at fast-food restaurants.

with no sandwich, is unpalatable or, worse, gives them heartburn. Be sure to wash it down with water if this is a problem. Other folks have found that the packets of mustard distributed in fast-food restaurants are easy to keep on the nightstand and deliver just the right dose.

Clearly, the mustard remedy for leg cramps has been around for a very long time. Many readers tell us it works great for either daytime or nighttime cramps. What is so astonishing is that people report such quick results. That makes no sense pharmacologically. If this were a druglike effect, the active ingredient or ingredients in mustard would have to be absorbed from the digestive tract, circulate through the bloodstream, and eventually relax the muscle causing the cramp. That could take anywhere from 15 to 30 minutes.

"My mother has leg cramps almost every night. Because of your reports on yellow mustard, I got a huge supply of individually wrapped mustard packets. She keeps them on her nightstand and in her purse. When a leg cramp starts, she takes the mustard and the cramps disappear immediately.

She got a cramp recently in a doctor's office. Since she had used all her packets up, I asked the nurse to get some mustard from the break room. She'd never heard of the remedy but was impressed when the cramps went away. The turmeric in the mustard is the lifesaver."

Not everyone agrees that mustard is marvelous. One reader reported that "a spoonful of mustard did *not* do anything to alleviate my cramp, but it kept me up the rest of the night with indigestion. My esophagus burned all night long. What a terrible remedy." Interestingly, some folks tell us that yellow mustard actually relieves their heartburn, proving once again that everyone is different!

Pickle Juice

Another odd remedy for leg cramps is a sip or two of pickle juice. A former pro football player who played with the San Francisco 49ers and the Dallas Cowboys wrote to tell us that yellow mustard is not his favorite remedy for leg cramps. And if anyone should know about leg cramps, it is someone who had to run around the football field at maximum exertion in the Dallas heat. He praised prescription quinine but also said that by far the best home remedy for leg cramps is a jigger of pickle juice (about an ounce).

This remedy may be especially popular in his home state of Texas, where an entrepreneur sells Pickle Juice Sport. He claims the electro-

About an ounce of dill pickle juice, with no seeds or spices, may quell cramps.

Downside: Pickle juice is high in sodium and so is not appropriate for those on a salt-restricted diet.
Cost: Approximately 10 cents an ounce from a pickle jar. A 16-ounce bottle of Pickle Juice Sport sells for $1.50.

lytes in this drink help reverse leg cramps. (His Web site, for those who are interested, is www.goldenpicklejuice.com.) Most people just use the liquid from a jar of pickles.

With pickle juice, as with mustard, those who experience relief do so very quickly. Who knows what mechanism is at work? Perhaps the pickle juice replenishes minerals, especially sodium, that are lost during exertion. Aside from having too much sodium for those who need to watch their salt intake, though, there is no downside.

> *My favorite remedy for leg cramps is pickle juice. When my youngest son was in school, the track coach used to get the leftover pickle juice after the band boosters had sold all the dill pickles in a jar. He kept it to give to an athlete when he cramped. I use it myself (when I can find it) during long bike rides."*

Baking Soda

Athletes often complain of leg cramps after vigorous exercise. Pickle juice may restore the sodium lost in sweat. Another remedy that may work on the same principle is baking soda, a time-honored remedy for indigestion. The dose for treating cramps is about half as much as that for treating indigestion, according to one reader:

> *A neighbor of mine has a remedy that I find very helpful. He was an avid skier in his younger days and advocates taking $\frac{1}{4}$ teaspoon of baking soda in a glass of water after a day on skis or doing other strenuous activities. He claims the soda neutralizes the lactic acid that forms in muscle upon heavy exercise.*

Lip Pinch

One of the more unusual approaches to leg cramps is a home remedy that many people find helpful. The idea is to pinch the upper lip, hard, for several seconds until the cramp lets up. We have never been successful with this approach, but many readers are enthusiastic about it.

> *For 15 years I suffered agonizing leg cramps, usually at night. I couldn't sleep and would almost panic at the thought of having one. I found relief with quinine, but this drug had some unpleasant side effects, mainly ringing in the ears.*
>
> *Then one day I read an article about a coach who would tell his players to pinch the upper lip right beneath the nose when they had leg cramps. The cramps would ease. I thought it sounded odd but decided to try it. When the*

cramps started, I pinched my upper lip, and the cramps gradually went away. I did this every time the cramps started for several months, then finally they quit altogether. "

Preventing Symptoms with Exercise

Anyone who suffers recurrent leg cramps will be anxious to prevent them. Many people are aware that strenuous exercise during the day may trigger nighttime cramps. But so can inactivity. Reader Ruth Mannich of Oxford, North Carolina, teaches exercises to seniors and offered the following instructions for stretching before bed.

Calf Stretch: Stand close behind a sturdy chair or other stable support. With your feet about hip-width apart, hold on to the chair back. Shift your weight to your left leg. Move your right foot about 12 inches back, placing your toes on the floor and elevating your heel. Keep your left knee over your left ankle (left knee will bend) as you slowly ease your right heel down and up (no faster than 1 second moving down and 1 second moving up) about 15 times. Repeat with your left calf. For a static stretch, hold the heel down for 15 seconds at a time rather than moving it.

Hamstring Stretch (back of thigh): Sit on a chair with a footstool in front of you. Place your left foot flat on the floor and your right heel on the footstool so that the right leg is fully extended and your toes point to the ceiling. Flex your right foot, drawing the toes back toward your body. With your back straight and your right knee "soft," not locked, bend from the hips and reach toward your right toes. Take a full second to reach toward your toes and a full second to return to the starting point. Repeat about 15 times. Repeat with your left hamstring. For a static stretch, reach toward your toes as far as is comfortable and without pain. Hold for 15 seconds; repeat three more times on each leg.

Active Quadriceps and Shin Stretch (front of thigh and shin): Hold on to a chair or table for support. Stand erect without leaning forward. Bending one leg at the knee, curl your heel behind you toward your buttocks. Take 1 second to curl your leg behind and 1 second to return your leg to the straight position. Repeat about 15 times on each leg.

Static Quadriceps and Shin Stretch: Stand close behind a sturdy chair that allows you to stand tall without leaning forward. Place a second chair with a seat that is no higher than your knee about a foot behind you. Bend your right leg at the knee and place the top of your right foot on the seat of the chair behind you. Your right knee should be directly under or slightly behind your hip. Gently press the top of your right foot down against the chair to stretch the entire front of the leg. The knee of the supporting leg should have a slight bend in it. Hold for four sets of 15 seconds, or a total of 1 minute. Repeat with left leg.

Other exercises may also be useful in helping to stretch muscles that tend to cramp. Some people use a stair step to stretch the back of the leg. Stand close to the edge of the step with the ball of one of your feet and drop your heel below the level of the step to stretch out the leg.

> *I am often bothered with foot cramps that are annoying and uncomfortable at night and during dance class. A physical therapist friend suggested a small rubber ball, about the size of a tennis ball. I put it on the floor and roll each foot on it firmly, especially the arch and ball of the foot, to prevent the cramps.*

Minerals

Over the years our readers have offered us dozens of suggestions for preventing nighttime leg cramps. Many of them involve minerals. Some people swear by potassium. Others are enthusiastic about calcium. Another contingent insists that magnesium is the magic mineral. There's no way to predict which mineral (or combination) will work best for you, so experiment until you find the right approach.

Before you start popping pills, though, why not start with food? Eight ounces of low-sodium V8 vegetable juice provide 840 milligrams of potassium at only 50 calories.

> *For many years I was plagued with severe muscle cramps, usually in the middle of the night. Several months ago one of your readers suggested low-sodium V8 juice, noting that it has more potassium and fewer calories than bananas.*
>
> *I decided to try it and began drinking 8 ounces daily. In 4 months I have not had a single muscle cramp. Quite a relief, to say the least!*

> *I heartily recommend it to anyone who has nighttime leg cramps.*

Other foods that are rich in potassium include vegetables such as artichokes, asparagus, beets, bell peppers, broccoli, cabbage, cauliflower, chard, mushrooms, spinach, squash, and tomatoes. A banana has about 400 milligrams of potassium, and so does a medium-size sweet potato. Other fruits packed with potassium include apricots, blackberries, cantaloupe and other melons, nectarines, oranges, peaches, plums, pomegranates, raspberries, and strawberries. Fish is generally rich in potassium, and many flavorings, such as ginger, onions, paprika, parsley, and red pepper, also contribute potassium to the diet. So do chicken and pork. Don't forget molasses, especially blackstrap molasses, which has about 500 milligrams in a tablespoon. The Food and Nutrition Board of the Institute of Medicine has determined that for adults, 4,700 milligrams of potassium a day is adequate.[712]

A word of warning: Potassium can interact with many prescription drugs, particularly blood pressure medications. Quite a few of these medications could boost the potassium level dangerously if a person on one of these drugs also took a potassium pill or used a potassium chloride salt substitute. Older people and those with reduced kidney function might be especially vulnerable. Too much potassium can lead to cardiac arrest, so be wary if you are taking any of the following: benazepril (Lotensin), captopril (Capoten), enalapril (Vasotec), fosinopril (Monopril), lisinopril (Prinivil, Zestril), losartan (Cozaar), moexipril (Univasc), quinapril (Accupril), spironolactone (Aldactone), ramipril (Altace), triamterene/hydrochlorothiazide (Dyazide, Maxzide), trandolapril (Mavik), or valsartan (Diovan).

Magnesium is another mineral that is frequently overlooked and in short supply in the diet. People on diuretics may be especially low in this crucial nutrient. Not only is magnesium essential for normal muscular contraction, it also plays a crucial role in heart health, blood pressure control, and hundreds of enzymatic reactions in the body. It also helps reduce the risk of kidney stone formation.

People have been using magnesium for decades (as milk of magnesia) to counteract constipation. The normal dose ranges between 300 and 500 milligrams daily. One study demonstrated moderate effectiveness in battling nighttime leg cramps at 300 milligrams.[713] Pregnant women are especially vulnerable to leg cramps. Another study concluded that

---

★★★★ Magnesium

This essential mineral may help with cramps and many other problems as well. Usual dose: 300 to 500 milligrams at bedtime—some people report it is gently sedating.

Downside: May cause diarrhea. Not for those with kidney failure.
Cost: Approximately $4 for 100 pills, or about a 3-month supply

---

"magnesium supplementation seems to be a valuable therapeutic tool in the treatment of pregnancy-related leg cramps."[714] Be aware that too much can cause diarrhea, and people with kidney problems should take magnesium only under medical supervision.

Some people are equally enthusiastic about calcium for preventing leg cramps. The research that has been done on this remedy has been equivocal. In one study, pregnant women with nighttime leg cramps were given calcium supplements or vitamin C as a "control." Since there is no evidence that vitamin C can reduce leg cramps, it seemed that the difference between the two groups would be readily apparent if calcium worked well. Both groups did equally well, however, suggesting that calcium really didn't make much difference.[715] A systematic review of the research on calcium for nocturnal leg cramps concluded that the evidence for its effectiveness is weak, at least in pregnant women. The reviewers found more support for supplemental magnesium.[716]

One way to get extra minerals is with a special pediatric formulation called Pedialyte. It was developed to "quickly replace fluids and electrolytes lost during diarrhea and vomiting to help prevent dehydration in infants and children." Pediatricians frequently recommend this ready-to-use liquid for sick children instead of juice or other beverages. Ingredients include water, dextrose, potassium citrate, sodium chloride, sodium citrate, and citric acid. Pedialyte is sold in drugstores and supermarkets in the baby section. One athlete

★★★★ Pedialyte

This rehydration solution for babies and children provides a balance of electrolytes that may help adults avoid muscle cramps. Drinking about 4 ounces after exercising should help.

Downside: Somewhat expensive
Cost: Approximately $8 for a liter, or about $1 per "dose"

offered an amazing testimonial for its benefits against leg cramps.

> *I have experienced a fair amount of cramping in my legs at night after I play tennis. The cramps occur more during the hot summer months when I perspire more.*
>
> *I tried a lot of the sports drinks, but they didn't seem to help with the cramping. Someone suggested that I either eat bananas or drink tomato juice. Unfortunately for me, I don't like either food.*
>
> *I was told that the cramping was due to a loss of potassium in the body. An assistant tennis pro suggested I try drinking the infant solution called Pedialyte. I thought that was a crazy idea, but I tried it because I didn't like waking at midnight with a leg cramp. To my surprise, the Pedialyte has worked like a charm and has eliminated my cramping.*
>
> *Pedialyte has one other unexpected benefit. I usually play singles tennis, and I am usually pretty worn out after I play. Like a lot of people my age, my middle-aged body is usually pretty darn sore after playing, particularly the next day.*

> *Like everyone else, I take Motrin for sore muscles. The Pedialyte has substantially reduced the soreness that I experience, and I don't need to take Motrin the next day.*

B Vitamins

B vitamins have become the superheroes of nutrients. Not only do compounds like folic acid, B_6, and B_{12} have cardiovascular benefits, folic acid and niacin may help reduce the risk of Alzheimer's disease. One study from Taipei offers evidence that a B-complex vitamin formulation can reduce nighttime leg cramps. "After 3 months, 86 percent of the patients taking vitamin B had prominent remission of leg cramps, whereas those taking placebo had no significant difference from baseline,"[717] reported the study's authors. This study used a formulation that is not available in the United States. It contained vitamins B_1 (50 milligrams), B_2 (5 milligrams), B_6 (30 milligrams), and B_{12} (250 micrograms).[718]

★★★ B Vitamins

A combination of B vitamins may reduce nighttime leg cramps. Keep the dose of vitamin B_6 below 100 milligrams per day to avoid nerve damage from long-term use.

Downside: The B-complex formulas available are not specifically designed to prevent leg cramps.
Cost: Approximately $11 for 100 tablets, or a 3-month supply

> ❝My husband has suffered horrible leg cramps at night all his life. He would writhe in pain.
>
> I read that B vitamins might help. He now takes multiple B-100s every day and has no leg cramps.
>
> We found a "dose-response curve." With B-50s, he'd still have cramps, but they were less severe. With B-75s, he wouldn't have cramps, just twinges in his legs. At the 100 level, he has not even a twinge.❞

A B-complex with 100 milligrams of vitamin B_6 may be too much. We worry that regular consumption of this nutrient may lead to nerve damage. Anyone who contemplates taking more than 50 milligrams of vitamin B_6 should be under medical supervision.

Quinine

If you tell your physician that you suffer from frequent leg cramps at night, you may be offered a prescription for quinine. This botanical medicine (derived from the bark of a South American tree) has been used against malaria since a monk sent a sample to Spain in 1633. (At that time, the diagnosis was probably "fever" or "the ague" rather than malaria.)

Doctors began using quinine against leg cramps in 1940. Despite this long history, there is still some controversy over whether its effectiveness outweighs the risks of side effects.[719] In the 1990s, the FDA determined that the possibility of a susceptible individual experiencing a life-threatening blood reaction (idiopathic thrombocytopenic purpura, or ITP) was just too great to allow the drug to be sold without a pre-

---

★★ Quinine

This traditional prescription for leg cramps is probably effective. One or two glasses of tonic water may contain enough quinine to help some people avoid nighttime cramps.

Downside: Tinnitus (ringing in ears), rash, changes in color vision, headache, nausea, diarrhea, liver damage, low blood sugar, life-threatening anemia (ITP), vomiting, and trouble breathing are possible reactions.
Cost: Approximately $65 in the United States for 100 pills or $33 from a Canadian pharmacy

---

scription. One reader reported that a single glass of tonic water (which contains quinine) put her in the hospital with an almost fatal anemia.

It is hard to predict ahead of time whether a person might react to quinine by developing severe anemia. Pregnant women should stay completely clear of quinine (even though they may suffer leg cramps) because it could cause birth defects and induce premature labor. Other side effects from quinine, whether ingested in pills or in tonic water, include ringing in the ears, rash, changes in color vision, headache, nausea, diarrhea, liver damage, low blood sugar, life-threatening anemia (ITP), vomiting, and trouble breathing. Anyone experiencing such symptoms should get medical attention promptly.

The amount of quinine in tonic water may vary from one brand to another. Some brands contain as much as 80 milligrams in a quart of tonic. The dose that proved effective in preventing muscle cramps in one placebo-controlled study was 400 milligrams.[720] That suggests that a person would have to drink more than a gallon to get an effect, but many readers report that they notice a benefit from one or two glasses of tonic. Doctors may prescribe a dose of 260 to 300 milligrams; older people should generally start with a lower dose.

> *I used to take quinine, but then it became unavailable over the counter. My doctor recommended that I drink a glass of Schweppes Tonic Water. It has enough quinine that it might help.*
>
> *I tried it and it works. I have recommended this to others bothered with cramps after exercising, and they have been pleased.*

One word of caution is probably unnecessary. Even though some people are accustomed to putting gin in their tonic water, the alcohol does nothing to prevent leg cramps. If it is taken shortly before bedtime, alcohol can disrupt sleep—the last thing a sufferer wants.

Conclusions

Health care professionals generally consider leg cramps more of a nuisance than a serious health problem. Nonetheless, anyone who suffers from nighttime leg cramps knows that they can disrupt sleep, and that can eventually have consequences for health as well as mood. Finding the remedy that suits you best may require some trial and error. Don't be afraid of the home remedies: They may seem silly, but since the only prescription treatment,

quinine, can have such serious adverse effects, we think they are worth considering.

> *I had terrible leg cramps, and nothing helped. Then my husband got some liquid calcium, and that worked immediately. I have not had another leg cramp.*
>
> *He decided to try mustard for leg cramps, but he still had leg cramps and really did not savor the mustard. He decided to try turmeric, an ingredient in mustard. He took ½ teaspoon at bedtime and ½ teaspoon at breakfast. BINGO! This worked great. Not only did it cure his leg cramps, but it also eased the pain in his hip and feet.*
>
> *He recommended I try it for my awful foot problems. It felt like an ice pick was stuck in the ball of my foot. As soon as I started taking the turmeric, I had no more pain. I can now wear my lovely high-heeled shoes on Sunday without suffering.*

• Tuck a bar of ordinary soap under the bottom sheet when you make the bed. It should be near your legs, and may need to be replaced every 6 weeks or so. We don't know why it would prevent leg cramps, but many readers report success—and we know of no side effects.
• Swallow a teaspoonful of yellow mustard—the inexpensive kind sometimes dispensed in individual packets. We think it may be the turmeric in the mustard that helps. This remedy can work very quickly, though some readers have reported heartburn as a result.
• Sip about an ounce of pickle juice. Some pickles may contain turmeric, so perhaps

that explains why this helps some people fight off muscle cramps so quickly. Or, it may provide some missing minerals. Pickle juice is high in sodium, so this home remedy is not for anyone on a low-sodium diet.

• Baking soda, ¼ teaspoon in 8 ounces of water, is reputed to fight painful leg cramps quickly. Baking soda contains sodium, so it is not for anyone on a low-salt regimen.

• Pinch your upper lip firmly between your thumb and forefinger until the cramp eases. This may have the effect of providing a distracting pain that is under your control. Many readers claim it is helpful, although we have not been impressed.

• Stretch leg muscles for several minutes before bedtime.

• Consume plenty of potassium-rich vegetables, especially low-sodium V8 juice. Increasing potassium intake seems to help prevent leg cramps.

• Take a supplement of 300 to 500 milligrams of magnesium a day. Reduce the dose if this gives you diarrhea. Avoid magnesium if you have kidney disease.

• Try 4 ounces of Pedialyte after vigorous exercise to replenish minerals and prevent muscle cramps.

• Consider B-complex vitamins to prevent cramps. Keep the dose of vitamin B_6 under 100 milligrams per day to avoid nerve damage.

• Ask your doctor about quinine. It is available by prescription (or at low doses in some brands of tonic water). Severe side effects are uncommon but may be life-threatening, especially a blood disorder called ITP.

MENOPAUSE

• Turn the thermostat down to reduce hot flashes	
• Use the lowest-dose estrogen and progesterone therapy for the shortest time possible	★★
• Try Remifemin for hot flashes	★★★
• Eat tofu or tempeh or drink soy shakes	★★
• Ask your doctor about Paxil (paroxetine) or Effexor (venlafaxine) for hot flashes	★★
• Inquire about Neurontin (gabapentin) for hot flashes	★
• Apply olive oil topically for vaginal dryness	★★★
• Squeeze vitamin E out of a capsule as a sexual lubricant	★★
• Experience slippery sex with Sylk	★★★★
• Experiment with aloe vera gel	
• Get a prescription for Estring (estradiol)	★★★

Decades ago, menopause used to be referred to in whispers as The Change. The mystery surrounding the event gave it a sinister aura. Now, though, more than 5,000 women enter menopause every day in the United States.[721] That's because the baby-boom generation is aging. We are not a bashful bunch, and female boomers have brought menopause out in the open. Women refer to hot flashes, somewhat jokingly, as power surges. But few women relish them. Most would like some way to ease this symptom, even if it is the consequence of a perfectly natural biological process.

We ought to begin with some explanation of menopause. Most people know this refers to the time when a woman's ovaries stop making the hormones that support the ripening and release of eggs. It is a gradual process that may be spread out over years, perhaps even a decade, and is properly referred to as *perimenopause*. Menopause itself is technically just one point in time: the day when an entire year has passed since the end of a woman's last menstrual cycle.[722] The average age on this day is 51 years, but women may be as young as 40 or as old as 58 and still be within the normal range for menopause.

Just as the timing of this change in ovarian function differs from one woman to another, so do the timing and intensity of menopausal symptoms (yes, we should be calling them *perimenopausal symptoms*). Some women barely notice a hot flash or two. We've even spoken with women who had "cold flashes" rather than hot flashes. Others are distressed by intense heat waves that may plague them daily for years. Most fall between those extremes but would still welcome some respite from the sweating, the flushing, and the distracting feeling that they might spontaneously combust. (Not to worry—that has never happened!)

> **"***I hope you can recommend something for my wife, who feels like she is about to burst into flames. Her doctor suggested Premarin, but she refuses to take it because she is worried about the increased risk of breast cancer. What other options are there?***"**

If it is any comfort, this period of discomfort lasts about 4 years, on average. That means, though, that some women zip through it much more quickly, whereas others take longer, sometimes much longer, to get through to relief.

The Hormone Controversy

For years, women suffering from hot flashes and other menopausal discomforts were told that their doctors had the magic solution: Just take hormones to replace the ones their ovaries were no longer making. Hormone replacement therapy, or HRT, has had its ups and downs over the decades, beginning with Premarin's approval in 1942. Since then, more than 30 billion doses of this hormone distilled from pregnant mares' urine have been dispensed.

When doctors discovered that women taking Premarin were at greater risk of developing cancer of the uterine lining, this prescription went out of vogue for a while. But then researchers found that adding progestin, a synthetic form of progesterone (usually prescribed under the brand name Provera), could reduce this risk. In the 1990s, Premarin became the most prescribed pill in history. Besides easing hot flashes, night sweats, and other menopausal problems, HRT was supposed to save women's lives by reducing their risk of heart disease, colon cancer, osteoporosis, and other serious health threats.

These days, though, the story has changed, and a lot of menopausal women are feeling confused and betrayed. For years, they were told that they were suffering from an estrogen deficiency syndrome. Replacing the hormones their bodies no longer made was supposed to ease menopausal symptoms. Women who resisted a prescription for HRT were sometimes treated as difficult cases. Some were told that though HRT might raise the risk of breast cancer, it was a much less significant concern than heart disease, which HRT might protect against.

> *After I was operated on for breast cancer, I was told that I could no longer take estrogen, because my tumor was, 'estrogen-dependent.' My primary physician actually had the gall to tell me: 'The benefits of estrogen far outweigh the threat of breast cancer, and besides, we can cure breast cancer.'*

Women have a right to be furious. The hormone hype that lasted for several decades represents one of the biggest scams in modern medicine. Millions of women were guinea pigs in an uncontrolled experiment. Physicians who pride themselves on practicing "evidence-based medicine" prescribed drugs that were unsupported by data. Many women who expressed their fears to their physicians were told in no uncertain terms that the benefits of HRT outweighed the risks.

When the National Institutes of Health announced a huge, long-term study of hormone replacement therapy, advocates of HRT were thrilled. They anticipated that the best available science would support their convictions that HRT had many health benefits, far beyond simply easing hot flashes. Thousands of women were recruited to the study and randomly assigned to take either Prempro or a look-alike placebo pill.

When the results of this study—called the Women's Health Initiative (WHI)—were announced in 2002, many physicians were surprised and women were shocked to learn that instead of protecting women from heart disease and cardiovascular complications, HRT actually increased their risk. A few doctors had anticipated that the study might show an increased risk of breast cancer. As early as 1995, the Nurses' Health Study, which followed more than 100,000 women, had confirmed that estrogen replacement therapy significantly increased the risk of breast cancer in postmenopausal women and demonstrated that progestin did not diminish that risk.[723] If anything, the data suggested that adding progestin could increase the risk.[724]

Although there had been hints from previous research that estrogen, with or without progesterone, might increase a woman's risk of breast cancer, such concerns were mostly downplayed. Opinion leaders reminded physicians that the leading cause of death in postmenopausal women is heart disease. (Breast cancer comes in second.) Some eminent gynecologists opined that if breast cancer was a risk, it was a minimal one, associated only with long-term HRT use. Such cancers were thought to be "good" cancers in that they were "early" cancers, easily detected and treated and not associated with increased mortality.

Further results from the WHI gave the lie to that claim. The investigators found that women taking combined HRT (Prempro) were more likely to be diagnosed with breast cancer than those on placebo and were more likely to have invasive, more advanced cancers. They concluded, "These results suggest estrogen plus progestin may stimulate breast cancer growth and hinder breast cancer diagnosis."[725]

As a result of these new findings, doctors may also be feeling betrayed. They too were sold a bill of goods that did not turn out to be as advertised. It is now clear to all that HRT is not a panacea for the miseries of menopause. But what remains unclear is exactly how women should cope with hot flashes, night sweats, sleep disruption, and vaginal dryness. Finding out that estrogen doesn't really prevent heart disease still leaves women with plenty of options for reducing their risk of heart trouble. And there are other possible treatments for osteoporosis, another condition for which women were given long-term estrogen treatment. But what can be done for those annoying, sometimes debilitating hot flashes?

Alleviating Hot Flashes

Certain simple lifestyle adjustments might be all that some women need to make hot flashes tolerable. First, turn down the thermostat. This seems too simple to work, but many menopausal women are less uncomfortable when the temperature is cooler.[726] Second, dress in layers that can be easily removed. This is simple common sense. Third, follow the Southern belles' example and keep a fan and a nice cool (nonalcoholic) drink handy. Fourth, keep exercising. Or if you are not already walking, swimming, or dancing, start. It's not a miracle, but women who exercise regularly seem to have fewer hot flashes or find them less bothersome. Besides, exercise eases depression and anxiety and is beneficial for the heart and the bones as well.

Hormone Replacement Therapy

When it comes to taming hot flashes, estrogen is undeniably the gold standard. Estrogen, either alone or in combination with progestin, clearly reduces the frequency and severity of hot flashes by about 75 percent.[727] This is significantly better than placebo, although women with hot flashes are susceptible to the placebo benefit.

In most studies of HRT or herbal alternatives, women taking the placebo had nearly 60 percent fewer hot flashes per week at the end of the studies, on average, than at the beginning.[728] Women on HRT, either estrogen alone or estrogen together with progesterone, also seem to have less trouble with night sweats that awaken them and disturb their sleep. There's little evidence that herbal treatments have much effect on menopausal sleep problems, which many women find extremely disturbing.

If it weren't for the WHI, doctors would still be prescribing Prempro (a combination of Premarin and Provera) to virtually every menopausal woman who would take it. And they would still be encouraging women to keep taking it long after menopausal symptoms faded away, as a general-purpose "health and beauty aid."

The characteristics of the women who were willing to use HRT before the WHI results were available probably accounted for many of the benefits seen with HRT in earlier, observational studies. Women were told that HRT was good for their health, so those who chose to take it were more likely to be the health-conscious, careful eaters, regular exercisers, nonsmokers, and occasional drinkers. Their healthy behaviors, rather than the HRT per se, are now believed to be responsible for their lower rates of heart attack, stroke, and many other problems.

★★ Estrogen and Progesterone

Hormone replacement therapy reduces hot flashes significantly for most women. Women who still have a uterus need to take progesterone along with estrogen to protect themselves from endometrial cancer.

The risks of this therapy rise significantly at 5 years of use. For most women, intense hot flashes last less than 5 years. Ask for the lowest possible dose, and increase the dose only if that does not adequately relieve the hot flashes and night sweats. Hot flashes may return if HRT is stopped abruptly, so gradually tapering off it may be more successful. Transdermal estrogen (Climara, Estraderm) may be less likely to trigger nausea, but there haven't been good head-to-head comparisons.

Side effects: Breast tenderness, nausea, gallbladder problems, migraine headaches, intolerance to contact lenses, elevated blood sugar. If progesterone is given only 1 week a month, vaginal bleeding resembling a menstrual period is common.

Downside: HRT increases the risks of breast cancer and blood clots that could trigger heart attacks and strokes. These risks increase over time. HRT should be used only as long as it is needed for perimenopausal symptoms.

Cost: Approximately $40 to $75 per month for brand-name HRT; generic is available for $12 to $20 per month

The WHI put the issue of HRT and heart attack prevention to the test with more than 16,000 postmenopausal women. Unfortunately, HRT did not pass. Women who had never undergone hysterectomy were randomized to Prempro or placebo, but the study was stopped early when it appeared that the women taking HRT were at greater risk than those on placebo.[729] Although Prempro had been expected to protect women from heart attacks and strokes, the results showed that women taking this HRT were nearly 30 percent more likely to develop coronary heart disease and twice as likely to come down with a pulmonary embolism, a dangerous blood clot in the lung.[730]

None of this has much bearing, though, on the use of hormones to treat hot flashes. The risks are primarily for women who take Prempro or other forms of estrogen and progesterone for extended periods of time. The most recent recommendations, based on subanalyses of the WHI data, suggest that women just entering menopause (ages 50 to 54 in particular) may be more resistant to the dangers of estrogen and might even get some protection from heart attacks by taking it.[731] Short-term use (for a few months up to a couple of years) to get through the worst of the hot flashes doesn't seem to pose an excessive risk for most women. Those who have previously had dangerous blood clots or breast cancer or who have a strong family history of breast cancer should probably avoid estrogen even in the short term, however.

● ● ●

Q. *I took hormones for 4 years and then discontinued them for a year. Now I have started again, at the urging of my doctor. While I was not taking hormones, I had hot flashes, night sweats, and vaginal dryness.*

I stopped taking hormones because the progesterone component made me irritable and depressed. (I was taking Premarin and Provera.) My doctor put me on Estrace and Prometrium this time, but I still feel prickly and sad.

I'm convinced progesterone is the problem, so I wonder if I can take the estrogen alone. I recently read that estrogen has heart benefits.

A. The hormone controversy has heated up again. A study showed that women between the ages of 50 and 59 taking estrogen alone were not at increased risk of heart attacks (*Archives of Internal Medicine*, February 13, 2006). These women had previously undergone hysterectomies, so they did not need progesterone.

Estrogen alone is not safe for a woman who still has her uterus since it increases the risk of endometrial cancer. Progestins like Provera protect against this kind of cancer. When added to estrogen, however, they may increase the risk of heart attacks and strokes and possibly breast cancer as well. For some women, progesterone lowers libido and leads to depression.

● ● ●

Doctors have followed the practice of prescribing progestin along with postmenopausal estrogen for many years, since research determined that estrogen alone increased the risk of cancer of the lining of the uterus (the endometrium). Endometrial cancer is not an issue for women with no uterus, and in the WHI study, these women were randomized to Premarin (estrogen alone) or placebo. This works just fine for hot flashes. Don't count on it to provide any cardiac benefits, though. Overall, women in the WHI study were not protected from heart attack or stroke by HRT whether they took Prempro or Premarin alone.[732]

Some critics of the WHI have objected to the use of Premarin or Prempro and suggested that other forms of postmenopausal estrogen replacement therapy would be preferable. There aren't studies to prove or disprove that idea. Epidemiologists at Group Health Cooperative, a big health maintenance organization in Washington, compared rates of heart attack and stroke among women taking Premarin and those taking another form of estrogen such as Estratab or Menest. They found a hint that the other forms of estrogen might be somewhat less likely to trigger a heart attack or stroke, but these data need to be confirmed.[733]

Bioidentical Hormones

● ● ●

Q. *I am a family physician. Back when we were prescribing HRT regularly, I used to offer women the option of plant-based estrogens instead of synthetic hormones. Since we learned the results of the Women's Health Initiative (WHI), though, I've viewed all estrogens as carrying similar risk until proven otherwise.*

There are practitioners who are saying that bioidentical hormones are safer. They encourage women to use them as an alternative for treating menopausal symptoms. Is there any research that shows that the risks are lower for plant-based HRT than for synthetic?

A. There is no comparable study of plant-based estrogens, and there is not likely to be one. The WHI was a very large and expensive study funded by the National Institutes of Health. Women were randomly assigned to receive Prempro or placebo. The results showed that postmenopausal hormones increased the risk of breast cancer, heart attack, and stroke.

Women's health expert Susan Love, MD, responded to a question like yours: "I think that it is very unlikely that bioidentical hormones, as they're called, will be any safer than Prempro."

● ● ●

The American College of Obstetricians and Gynecologists (ACOG) came out with a very strong caution about bioidentical hormones in 2005. Michele Curtis, MD, is associate professor of obstetrics and gynecology at Houston's University of Texas Medical School. On behalf of ACOG she said, "There are a growing number of women who are seeking therapy with bioidentical hormones, but there is a lot of misinformation about the assertion that these are plant-derived and therefore more closely mimic the estrogen that is in a woman's body. . . . These are hormones. They act just like estrogens that are commercially produced."[734]

The obstetricians and gynecologists of ACOG are concerned that plant-based hormones are unregulated and, as a result, women may not be informed about risks. In addition, lack of oversight may mean that it is hard to guarantee quality. Many of these products are made in small compounding pharmacies that act like micro–drug companies but escape the kind of regular FDA inspections one might expect a bigger manufacturer to undergo. When the FDA did check on samples from 12 compounding pharmacies, ACOG reports that "34 percent of them failed one or more standard quality tests."[735]

Progesterone

Many women are intrigued by the possibility that a progesterone cream derived from plant sources can be applied to the skin to relieve hot flashes naturally. Although wild yam can be used as a raw material for the manufacture of progesterone-like compounds, the human body can't convert wild yam to progesterone. A controlled study suggests that a cream containing wild yam extract is not much better at reducing hot flashes than a placebo.[736] Other creams formulated to contain progesterone can provide a dose comparable to taking progesterone by mouth.[737] Progesterone pills or long-lasting injections such as Depo-Provera can ease hot flashes, but questions remain about the long-term safety of this hormone for postmenopausal women.[738]

• • •

Q. *A nasty divorce has left me feeling slightly depressed, despite the relief of being out of a bad marriage. At times my heart races and then I break out in a sweat. I don't know if these episodes are just anxiety or if they are hot flashes, since I am menopausal.*

I am reluctant to take estrogen because I've heard about negative effects. I'd rather use a more natural approach. Would a progesterone cream be safe?

A. Many women experience hot flashes much as you have described them, with an accelerated heart rate, a vaguely anxious feeling, sweating, and feeling too warm. Progesterone cream may help reduce hot flashes. Women's health expert Susan Love, MD, points out, however, that high levels of progesterone are not natural after menopause. She worries that potential side effects might arise with long-term progesterone use. In addition, progesterone has been linked to depression.

• • •

Black Cohosh

One of the most popular herbal supplements used to alleviate hot flashes is black cohosh. This plant is native to North America and was used by Native Americans for a range of medicinal purposes. The botanical name has been changed in recent years, so some references refer to this plant as *Cimicifuga racemosa* whereas others use the current term, *Actaea racemosa*. The famous 19th-century patent medicine promoted for "women's problems," Lydia E. Pinkham's Vegetable Compound, contained black cohosh as a prominent ingredient.

★★★ Remifemin

This standardized extract of black cohosh is consistent and widely available. The recommended dose is 40 to 80 milligrams per day.

Side effects: Digestive upset
Downside: Not to be taken during pregnancy; monitor for liver toxicity
Cost: Approximately $15 to $30 per month

A standardized extract of black cohosh called Remifemin has been studied in Europe and found to effectively reduce hot flashes.[739] Physicians who scoff at herbal remedies appreciate that this research was published in a highly respected peer-reviewed journal, *Obstetrics and Gynecology* (May 2005). In one trial, Remifemin was compared to a low-dose transdermal estrogen preparation.[740] The treatments were equally effective in reducing hot flashes, and neither one was associated with serious side effects.[741]

Most reviews suggest that the side effects of black cohosh are infrequent and generally mild—mostly digestive upset with some headache or dizziness reported.[742] Just the same, we think that women should discuss this supplement with their doctor. Although recent studies of black cohosh have monitored liver enzymes and found no changes, there are reports of liver toxicity among women taking black cohosh.[743] Women who have had hepatitis or other liver problems might want to consider a different approach. For most healthy women, 6 months or so of black cohosh may be worth trying, and it seems fairly safe.[744] Unfortunately, black cohosh does not relieve hot flashes that result from breast cancer treatment with tamoxifen.

The Soy Solution

One of the other popular approaches to managing hot flashes is soy. Isoflavones such as genistein and daidzein are phytoestrogens, estrogen-like compounds derived from plants.

★★ Soy

The results of studies on soy have been inconsistent. Soy may be consumed as shakes, bars, or more traditional soy foods such as tofu or tempeh. Women who have more hot flashes may derive more benefit.

Side effects: Unpalatable taste, digestive distress
Downside: Not advised for women being treated for breast cancer; excess soy may interfere with the production of thyroid hormone
Cost: Approximately $15 to $50 per month

Even though they are far weaker than the estrogen a woman's own ovaries make before menopause, it seems logical to use these compounds to ease hot flashes. Studies from cultures like Japan, where women consume soy products such as tofu and tempeh as part of their normal diet, suggest that hot flashes and other menopausal symptoms may be less common there.[745]

Despite the epidemiological promise, research on soy against hot flashes has been disappointing overall.[746,747] One review of many trials, however, found that women who began the studies with frequent hot flashes got more relief from soy foods or isoflavone supplementation than did women who rarely had hot flashes.[748] A different systematic review delivered a less-than-ringing endorsement of the effectiveness of soy preparations against hot flashes, but the authors did conclude that the risks appear to be low.[749] As the authors of one

pilot study concluded, a soy extract (they were testing Phytosoya) appears to reduce hot flashes and night sweats and is probably worth a try if women don't want to take standard HRT.[750]

Red Clover

Another source of isoflavones that is marketed for perimenopausal women is red clover (*Trifolium pratense*). Although this plant is native to North America, its extracts are sold by an Australian firm as Promensil and Rimostil. Most of the research on red clover isoflavones has been funded by the manufacturer Novogen. Nonetheless, the results vary. One small Dutch study found a significant effect, with Promensil reducing hot flashes by 44 percent more than placebo.[751] But a larger, multicenter trial in the United States found no clinically significant effect on hot flashes with either Promensil or Rimostil.[752]

On the bright side, though, very few women dropped out of the study, and no side effects were significantly more common among those taking red clover extracts than among those on placebo. Analyzing the data for subgroups uncovered a trend toward heavier women getting more benefit from Promensil.[753] Overall, however, red clover does not seem very impressive.

Vitamin E

The North American Menopause Society suggests taking vitamin E along with keeping cool, exercising, not smoking, eating soy isoflavones, and taking black cohosh as inexpensive, probably helpful nonprescription measures to alleviate hot flashes. Quite a few women have heard that vitamin E can be helpful for this symptom, and some have passed the advice along to their friends.

• • •

Q. *I'm 53 and haven't had a period for a year. I have no problems other than hot sweats.*

I recently started taking 400 IU of vitamin E each day and, much to my amazement, it really works. Is there anything I should know about this vitamin?

A. **Many women tell us that vitamin E can be helpful for hot flashes. Don't count on it to protect you against cancer, though. Smokers should probably not take vitamin E supplements, because there is some fear it may actually increase their risk of lung cancer. For others, moderate doses of vitamin E seem safe for short periods of time.**

• • •

Unfortunately, there appears to be very little research on the effectiveness of vitamin E. Some of the buzz may have come from a study done more than 50 years ago.[754] Usually we would like to see more recent research to back up a recommendation, but little seems to have been done. Nonetheless, the North American

Menopause Society considers vitamin E, like black cohosh and isoflavones, safe enough to be worth a try.

Vitamin E has performed poorly in several recent studies of cancer prevention, and women who are at particularly high risk of lung cancer—smokers, for example—should probably avoid taking large doses of vitamin E without other antioxidant nutrients. But healthy women planning to take vitamin E for a year or two to ease hot flashes probably will not notice any unpleasant effects. The best product is a combination of natural tocopherols. As with other products, start with the lowest dose available and gradually increase it to find the lowest dose that helps with your symptoms.

It is disappointing that vitamin E has received so little scientific attention over the years. That hasn't stopped women from trying it, though. Of course, we frequently hear about other interesting nutritional supplements that have worked for a few women but have no scientific evidence to support or refute their effectiveness. If they are otherwise safe, we see no harm in experimenting.

❝ *I can't help but wonder why most doctors do not treat hot flashes and night sweats with bioflavonoids. As a retired registered nurse, I have found that daily use of bioflavonoids will relieve both the hot flashes and the night sweats. It saves the worry of cancer threats from hormones and is much less expensive. I use Citrus Bioflavonoid Complex, 1,000 milligrams, providing 35 percent hesperidin, 350 milligrams. [Hesperidin is a compound found in citrus fruits that has anti-inflammatory activity.]*

At one time, I was hesitant to suggest this to my daughter-in-law because she had been successfully treated for breast cancer. When we were visiting and she was showing the lack of sleep from hot flashes and night sweats, I finally bought bioflavonoids for her. She often thanks me for the relief that it has given."

Nonhormonal Therapies

For years, women have worried about the possibility that estrogen and progesterone could increase their risk of breast cancer. Women who have already been treated for breast cancer can't take these hormones safely. As a result, and in light of the negative results from the WHI research, physicians have been looking for other ways to alleviate hot flashes. One approach that seems to help is an antidepressant in the selective serotonin reuptake inhibitor (SSRI) family.

PAXIL

Some doctors now prescribe antidepressants like Paxil (paroxetine) to help women deal with hot flashes. A recent study found that Paxil was significantly better than placebo in reducing the number of hot flashes and easing their intensity.[755] Low-dose Paxil (10 milligrams per day) was also better than placebo in preventing nighttime awakening, presumably due to night sweats. Women in this study did not have to be depressed to get benefit. That also seems to be the case

---

★★ Paxil (paroxetine)

Paroxetine eases hot flashes due to menopause or associated with breast cancer drugs such as tamoxifen. The effect on hot flashes is independent of its antidepressant activity. Women found a lower dose easier to tolerate.

Side effects: Nausea, digestive problems, weakness, sleep disturbances, dizziness, nervousness, sexual difficulties, hypertension, weight gain

Downside: Paxil can be hard to stop taking. You may need your doctor to switch you to a longer-acting drug such as Prozac and then decrease the dose gradually over several weeks or months.

Cost: Approximately $75 to $90 per month

---

for drugs such as Effexor (venlafaxine).[756]

Such medications are not without their own drawbacks, though. They can cause sweating, nausea, dry mouth, constipation, insomnia, jitteriness, and sexual problems such as difficulty achieving orgasm. Both Paxil and Effexor also can be difficult to discontinue. Stopping suddenly can lead to odd and distressing symptoms such as dizziness, sensations similar to electric shock, and a peculiar feeling that has been described as "brain sloshing" or "head in a blender." If antidepressants are taken for hot flashes, they should be taken at the lowest dose that works for the shortest time needed, just like hormone replacement therapy. And, also like HRT, they may need to be tapered off gradually.

• • •

Q. *I have been having hot flashes, night sweats, mood swings, and other change-of-life problems for more than a year. I had hoped these problems would eventually go away, but so far they haven't.*

My doctor wants me to consider Premarin, but I worry about side effects, especially breast cancer. It runs in my family.

The other drug my doctor has suggested is Zoloft. But I am not depressed and don't want to deal with side effects from that drug either. Do you have information on natural alternatives that might help me withstand hot flashes, night sweats, and interrupted sleep?

A. Black cohosh extract has been recommended for hot flashes. A double-blind study published in *Obstetrics and Gynecology* (May 2005) showed that the standardized product Remifemin was significantly more effective than placebo.

Another reader shared her experience with a different herb: "I have been using St. John's wort since discontinuing hormone replacement therapy. It has relieved many symptoms, including sleeplessness, stress, and fits of temper."

• • •

NEURONTIN

Another approach that may help some women who are suffering with hot flashes is an anticonvulsant drug called Neurontin (gabapentin). Pilot studies show that 900 milligrams daily of Neurontin reduces both the frequency and intensity of hot flashes, and that it works better than placebo.[757] Because Neurontin, like the SSRI antidepressants, does not have any estrogenic activity, it may be especially helpful for women who have had breast cancer and must avoid HRT. This medicine has been associated with some potentially serious adverse reactions, such as a reduction in white blood cells that could leave a woman susceptible to infection. We recommend having a thorough discussion of its likely benefits and risks

> ### ★ Neurontin (gabapentin)
>
> Gabapentin eases hot flashes due to menopause or associated with breast cancer drugs such as tamoxifen. The effect on hot flashes is not related to its anticonvulsant effects.
>
> **Side effects**: Drowsiness, dizziness, problems with balance, fatigue, swelling of the feet, nausea or vomiting, depression, reduction in white blood cells
>
> **Downside**: Neurontin should not be discontinued suddenly. You should ask your doctor for help in reducing the dose gradually over several weeks or months.
>
> **Cost**: Approximately $60 to $150 per month, depending on whether you get a brand-name or generic product

with the prescribing doctor. This is good advice for any medication, of course, but especially for one being used for an "off-label" condition like this.

Relieving Vaginal Dryness

Hot flashes may be the most obvious symptom of menopause, but for many women, vaginal dryness is just as troublesome. And despite our culture's greater acceptance of public discussion of sexual issues such as erectile dysfunction, for example, vaginal dryness is often too personal and too embarrassing to bring up. When the WHI highlighted the potential dangers of long-term use of oral estrogen, millions of women stopped their HRT and then searched high and low for a personal lubricant that would be safe and effective.

● ● ●

Q. *I know this is a sensitive issue, but it affects a lot of women. Vaginal dryness is ruining our sex lives. I had breast cancer, so hormones are out. I'm embarrassed to ask my doctor about this.*

My husband works long hours, and our opportunities for intimacy are unpredictable. Is there any natural lubricant I could use just at that time?

A. Readers have suggested olive, almond, and vitamin E oils. Some people are allergic to topical vitamin E,

though, and it can cause a nasty rash. In addition, using any oil in combination with latex condoms may weaken them. One woman breaks a leaf off her aloe vera plant and uses the slippery gel that oozes out.

● ● ●

For some women, this problem is an issue only for sexual relations, but others find that dryness is uncomfortable throughout the day. Oral HRT generally relieves this symptom along with hot flashes, but just as sudden sweats may return when HRT is stopped, so can vaginal dryness.

Olive Oil

No studies have identified diets, exercises, or other lifestyle approaches that work for vaginal dryness. We have heard from many women who have found remedies that work for them, however. One of the simplest is olive oil. Other women have found that almond oil has a more pleasant aroma and that it still helps with everyday moisturizing.

❝ *I would like to suggest a natural lubricant that is not greasy but is good for your body. It is pure olive oil. (It can be edible, too.) I have been using olive oil for this purpose for a couple of years. When my doctor did a pelvic exam, he thought I was taking hormones although I am not. I think olive oil has natural compounds to keep women youthful.* ❞

There is, unfortunately, no research to show whether any kind of oil applied topically will moisturize vaginal tissues. Our reader got a lot of other people interested in using olive oil for this purpose, though, and some of them contacted us to tell us that it helped. We really don't know of any hazard to this one except for people who are allergic to olive oil. It doesn't take very much, so use the best-quality extra-virgin olive oil you can find, or substitute almond oil or another vegetable oil if you prefer.

Vitamin E

The underground popularity of vitamin E capsules taken orally for hot flashes has apparently inspired some women to try this dietary supplement "off-label." We don't think any vitamin manufacturer envisioned women using the contents of a vitamin E capsule for personal lubrication, but some are enthusiastic about it. They prick the capsule and squeeze out the oil for application by hand. Others use the capsule as a vaginal suppository. We caution, though, that some people are sensitive to vitamin E and might develop a rash. In addition, using any oil in combination with latex condoms may weaken them.

Improbable Lubricants

Whoever said "necessity is the mother of invention" must be smiling at the ingenuity of women who have taken common, inexpensive cleansers or moisturizers and tried them to combat vaginal dryness. But some household products have been especially popular. Some years ago, we heard from a couple in their seventies who were using Corn Huskers Lotion, an old-fashioned hand lotion, as a sexual lubricant. Other readers were interested in their experience and tried the product out.

• • •

Q. *I suffered for years from vaginal dryness and tried a lot of treatments for it. Then I read about using Corn Huskers Lotion. The results have been incredible! The lotion is inexpensive and works better than a progesterone cream my doctor prescribed.*

A. We've heard from others who have found that this old-fashioned hand moisturizer can be helpful for vaginal dryness. Some of the ingredients are identical to those in pricier personal lubricants.

• • •

Corn Huskers Lotion contains glycerin, guar gum, and methylparaben, as well as a few other ingredients. It is not dissimilar to K-Y Jelly (glycerin, hydroxymethylcellulose, methylparaben), Astroglide (glycerin, propylene glycol, parabens), or Replens (glycerin, mineral oil, methylparaben). All of these drugstore products are designed specifically as vaginal lubricants. Although they are a bit pricier, such products are certainly worth a try. Corn Huskers is promoted as an oil-free hand treatment lotion. The manufacturer makes no claims regarding this "off-label" use.

Do keep in mind that mineral oil, as found in Replens, could compromise latex condoms.

We have also heard from many readers who sing the praises of an old-time facial cleanser for this purpose.

• • •

Q. *My husband and I have used Albolene as a sexual lubricant since the early 1970s. I'm not sure how we heard about it, but it's great: odorless, tasteless, slick, but not messy.*

It comes in a white tub you can keep by the bed without embarrassment. A 12-ounce jar costs about $11, but a little goes a long way. We've purchased five jars in 27 years of marriage. I haven't seen this anywhere else and wanted to share our secret.

A. Thanks for the tip. Finding a sexual lubricant that suits both partners can be challenging.

Albolene is a moisturizing cleanser that contains mineral oil, petrolatum, paraffin, ceresin, and beta-carotene. It should not be used with condoms or a diaphragm since petroleum jelly degrades latex.

• • •

Albolene is certainly cost-effective. Although it is solid in its container, a small amount applied to the skin soon liquefies and becomes slippery. One drawback, though, is the mineral oil and petrolatum base. These petroleum products will destroy latex, so they must not be used with barrier contraceptives such as condoms or a diaphragm. (The postmenopausal woman may not need to worry about contraception, but many perimenopausal women still need to be vigilant.) Albolene is available in pharmacies and online; for more information, you can contact the manufacturer, Numark Laboratories, at 800-338-8079.

> " I've been using a product from New Zealand named Sylk for over a year now and find it does a great job in lubricating and relieving pain associated with vaginal dryness during relations. "

Quite a few people these days are reluctant to introduce petroleum-based products into their bodies, and they also worry about the effect of such products on latex condoms. Many of them have been pleased to learn about Sylk, a natural lubricant from New Zealand. It contains kiwifruit vine extract and, more importantly, does not contain petroleum products. As a result, it is safe to use with barrier contraceptives. Sylk is not available in most drugstores, but it can be ordered by telephone at 602-957-7955 or on the Web at www.sylkusa.com.

People have devised a number of other clever ways to use natural products as lubricants. Some people have found that the gel from an aloe plant is ideal. It certainly is inex-

★★★★ Sylk

This natural personal lubricant contains kiwifruit vine extract, citrus seed extract as a preservative, and vegetable glycerine. It is water-based, so it can be used with condoms. It is not sticky.

Side effects: None known
Downside: Effectiveness has not been scientifically tested.
Cost: One bottle costs $22 to $23 and lasts 3 to 4 months.

pensive! A few drugstore lubricants contain aloe as one of the ingredients, so presumably this is usually well tolerated.

• • •

Q. *My husband and I can't use K-Y Jelly or any other brand of lubricant we have tried. They make me itch and burn.*

We have found, though, that the slimy gel that oozes from an aloe leaf when you break off a piece is a very good lubricant. I hope this will add to your uses of aloe vera and help another couple.

A. This is a most unusual sexual lubricant. Aloe vera gel has been used for centuries to help burns heal and ease skin irritation.

Others who would like to try this should test the gel on the inside of the elbow first. If there is no allergic reaction, the slippery texture should make it a surprisingly effective sexual lubricant.

• • •

Hormonal Approaches

For decades, when women complained of vaginal dryness as a symptom of menopause, doctors prescribed estrogen, often as a vaginal cream. Most of the time when a vaginal cream or tablet was prescribed, the doctor would point out that it would have local effects and would not be absorbed into the bloodstream. Although vaginal estrogen creams can often help alleviate dryness, the dogma that the estrogen in the cream stays put and doesn't get into the rest of the body is bogus. The delicate tissue of the vagina is quite efficient at absorbing estrogen and passing it into the bloodstream.[758]

• • •

Q. *I have been reluctant to take estrogen because I worry about possible side effects, in particular breast cancer. The worst thing about menopause has been the lack of vaginal lubrication, which makes sex very uncomfortable.*

My doctor prescribed a vaginal estrogen cream for this problem. He has assured me that it is locally acting with negligible absorption.

It certainly has helped the vaginal dryness, but my hot flashes have also dropped off considerably. Is this cream getting from the vagina to the rest of my body to control the hot flashes? And if so, what about the risk of breast cancer?

A. Estrogen is easily absorbed from the vaginal lining. In fact, one study of Premarin and Estrace creams published in the *Journal of the American Medical Association* (December 14, 1979) found that "estrogen vaginal cream preparations, as widely used in clinical practice for their local effects on the vaginal mucosa, actually result in sustained high estrogen levels in the systemic circulation."

We suggest that you discuss your risk factors for breast cancer with your physician. If oral estrogen is inappropriate for you, a cream formulation is not likely to be much safer.

• • •

There are certainly times when a vaginal cream or tablet is appropriate. When other approaches aren't effective, an estrogen cream often will help. As with oral estrogen, the idea is to use the lowest effective dose for the shortest possible period of time. Frequently the prescription cream will be dispensed with an applicator. Ask the doctor if you should fill the applicator or use less cream than that. It may be possible to apply just a small dab on the tip of your finger and get adequate relief with less overall exposure to estrogen. Topically applied estradiol (a form of estrogen) is available as Estrace cream and Vagifem vaginal tablets.

• • •

Q. *A couple of years ago vaginal dryness was causing me a lot of discomfort. I am prone to blood clots, so I can't take oral estrogen.*

My doctor prescribed Estring, an estradiol vaginal ring that is inserted every 3 months. It has only 2 milligrams of estrogen and has solved my problem. Please tell others about this approach.

A. Estring has been available in Sweden since 1993 and in the United States since 1996. The 2-milligram dose of estrogen is very low, especially since it is released gradually over 3 months. This approach may solve the problem of vaginal dryness with fewer side effects than oral estrogens.

• • •

There is one more way to apply estrogen topically to the vaginal tissues—with a vaginal ring. This silicone ring is inserted into the vagina, where it releases estradiol at a low but steady rate for 3 months. Like other forms of estrogen, it's not appropriate for women who

★★★ Estring

Estring is a vaginal silicone ring that contains estradiol that is released at a steady, low rate over 3 months, which minimizes fussing. It is placed in the vagina, usually so that it is comfortable or almost unnoticeable.

Side effects: Stomachache, nausea, vaginal discharge, headache, insomnia
Downside: Must pay for 3 months' treatment up front
Cost: $100 to $150 for a 3-month ring

have or have had breast cancer. Because the dose at any given time is lower than if a woman were taking estrogen orally, it might be used even by women who are nervous about using estrogen.

Conclusions

Although menopause is a natural process, hot flashes and night sweats can be bothersome. Vaginal dryness also may be uncomfortable. The ideal treatment for these symptoms should be used at the lowest effective dose for the shortest possible period of time, since most symptoms will eventually fade away on their own.

Here is an overview of our recommendations.

• Keep cool by turning down the thermostat and wearing layers that can be easily removed if you start to sweat. A tall, cool (nonalcoholic) drink is less likely to trigger a hot flash than a steaming cup of coffee.

- Keep exercising to minimize your hot flashes and help you sleep. Then follow up with relaxation and deep breathing.
- Try Remifemin. Black cohosh can help with hot flashes if they are not too extreme.
- Eat moderate amounts of soy products with isoflavones. They may help reduce hot flashes.
- Take vitamin E capsules. Up to 400 IU daily should be safe and might help.
- If nothing else helps with the hot flashes, try hormone replacement therapy at the lowest effective dose for the shortest possible time. Transdermal estrogen might be worth considering.
- An antidepressant such as Paxil (paroxetine), Effexor (venlafaxine), or Prozac (fluoxetine) may calm hot flashes even if you are not depressed. Don't take any of these drugs for longer than you need them; you may need help getting off them.
- The antiseizure drug Neurontin (gabapentin) may ease hot flashes and does not have the same risks as hormone replacement therapy. Do not stop this drug suddenly, though, since that could trigger withdrawal symptoms.
- Vaginal dryness may respond to olive oil, almond oil, or the oil from inside a vitamin E capsule.
- Corn Huskers Lotion or Albolene offers slippery lubrication for sexual relations.
- For more natural lubricants, try the gel from a broken aloe vera leaf or Sylk, which has kiwifruit extract.
- Estring is the most convenient form of vaginal estrogen. The need for Estring should be reevaluated every 3 or 6 months so you won't use it for longer than necessary.

NAIL FUNGUS

• Soak your nails in a solution of one-third vinegar to two-thirds water	★★★★
• Prepare a cornmeal suspension and soak nails for an hour a week	★★★
• Apply Listerine to infected nails daily	★★★
• Coat the nails with Vicks VapoRub	★★★★
• Soak the nails in tea tree or vitamin E oil	
• Try Pau d'Arco tea soaks	
• Ask your MD about a prescription for urea paste 40 percent to remove the infected nail	★★★
• Apply prescription Penlac (ciclopirox)	
• Consider the pros and cons of Lamisil (terbinafine) and Sporanox (itraconazole)	

Over the last several years, nail fungus has garnered public attention completely out of proportion with its seriousness. The medical term, *onychomycosis* (oh-nick-o-my-CO-sis), is long and scary, but it just means fungal infection of the nail. Perhaps so many people are curious about this topic because nail fungus is very common. In addition, the development of new antifungal drugs that can treat (dare we say *cure?*) nail fungus has encouraged the pharmaceutical industry to advertise in magazines, in newspapers, and on television. The popularity of sexy sandals as footwear may also have contributed to the interest in treating nail fungus.

For diabetics, nail fungus is a medical issue. They need to be extremely vigilant about foot care and attend promptly even to things that may seem minor. For the rest of us, though, thick, yellow toenails that are crumbly or hard to cut are more of a nuisance than a serious health concern. They look ugly, and if they get very thick, they may be uncomfortable as well. Sometimes they split, which can be quite painful.

In our opinion, though, it would be a mistake to put your life on the line to clear up your funny-looking nails. That's why we have collected so many home remedies for this problem. They probably won't work for everyone, but they shouldn't be very risky, either.

● ● ●

Q. *My husband took Lamisil to treat toenail fungus. The drug worked but was ultimately responsible for his death.*

The fine print for this prescription drug noted that it might cause neutropenia. For my husband, it did. This led to MDS (myelodysplastic syndrome), which was followed thereafter by AML (acute myeloid leukemia) and his subsequent death.

He had suffered with periodic flare-ups of toenail fungus and athlete's foot for most of his life. Neither condition was life threatening. The Lamisil was!

Even though serious side effects mentioned in prescription drug labels may affect only 1 percent of users, anyone could be in that 1 percent. People should ask themselves if it is worth taking that chance!

A. We are so sorry to hear of your husband's tragic death. In rare cases, Lamisil may trigger serious blood disorders such as neutropenia, a lack of white blood cells. This drug can also damage the liver; there have been deaths associated with this problem. This is a high price to pay to cure toenail fungus.

Patients must always take into account not only common side effects but also the possibility of rare but deadly adverse reactions.

● ● ●

Home Remedies

It's hard to say just where nail fungus comes from and why some people appear to be more susceptible than others. Occasionally readers report that they first noticed nail fungus after going for a manicure or a pedicure. Presumably, it is possible to pass the organism that causes nail fungus from one person to another, and surely from one nail to another. To minimize that likelihood, we suggest that any tools such as scissors or clippers that have been used on a nail that might be infected be soaked in rubbing alcohol for 15 minutes before being used on an uninfected nail.

We think home remedies are the place to start for treating nail fungus, whether it affects the toenails or fingernails. (This does not apply to people with diabetes, who should seek medical care for this problem.) Needless to say, some doctors are not fond of the idea of using home remedies for nail fungus.

Some time ago, we heard from a podiatrist who was very unhappy with our recommendations. "Home remedies hardly ever work," he wrote. "The unproven treatments you mentioned are little more than urban legends. In 23 years of practice, I have never seen even one patient who responded favorably to Vicks VapoRub, dilute vinegar soaks, or vitamin E oil. Don't make me waste time dispelling these myths." He recommended that people take FDA-approved prescription drugs like Lamisil, Penlac, or Sporanox instead.

We certainly heard from readers who disagreed with him. One person who had success treating nail fungus with vinegar soaks expressed this opinion: "If a treatment is relatively harmless, as this is, and there's even a chance it can work, I believe doctors should encourage alternative methods instead of high-priced medicines laden with potential side effects."

A pharmacist also weighed in with some information on the effectiveness of the prescription medications:

> *I would like to point out some facts about the FDA-approved drugs the podiatrist prefers (Lamisil, Penlac, Sporanox). Does this doctor know that Penlac's success rate for a complete cure, according to the manufacturer's prescribing information, is only 5.5 to 8.5 percent after 48 weeks? When using Sporanox, the percentage of overall success rises to a dizzying 35 percent.*
>
> *Also, does he know the costs of these medications? A bottle of Penlac costs $72.99. To reach 48 weeks of treatment once a day to a single affected nail, I conservatively estimate that the patient will need six bottles of the lacquer (one bottle approximately every other month). So Penlac will cost the patient, without insurance, $437.94 to reach an outstanding 8.5 percent cure rate.*
>
> *For Sporanox, one pulse-pak costs $255.99. This is a 14-day supply. The manufacturer recommends 12 weeks of treatment, bringing the patient cost, without insurance, to $1,535.94! No wonder people are looking for alternatives to these medications.*

Oral medicines such as Sporanox can occasionally trigger serious reactions as well. No wonder some people are willing to spend time and effort—but not much money—trying a low-risk home remedy.

> *I assumed toenail fungus was a fact of life for me. It had spread to five or six toenails when I finally saw a dermatologist. The prescribed treatment was costly, and after it began, the dermatologist told me the odds of reinfection after treatment were about 50 percent.*
>
> *I had a nightmare reaction to the pills a week later. I was in remote Finland, of all unlikely places, when I developed hives and severe itching. After 24 hours of nonstop, nonsleep itching, I got through to my doctor and was told to stop taking the pills.*
>
> *When I got home, I decided to try the vinegar treatment. I applied a drop of distilled white vinegar to my toenails with a cotton swab each time I got out of the shower. As the nails grew out, the fungus was completely gone, along with slight traces of athlete's foot.*
>
> *Cost: under $2.00 over 9 months.*
>
> *Side effects: none.*
>
> *Effectiveness: 100 percent (or 200 percent if you include the athlete's foot).*

★★★★ Vinegar

Use two parts of water to one part vinegar for a soaking solution. It does not seem to matter whether you use white vinegar or apple cider vinegar, so we suggest the cheaper white vinegar.

Downside: Your toes may smell of vinegar.
Cost: $1.60 to $2 for 64 fluid ounces—enough for at least four treatments, and possibly eight

Vinegar

One of our favorite home remedies is a vinegar soak. It is surely one of the cheapest remedies for nail fungus. People who sit still to read, use the computer, or watch television could soak the foot with the affected toenails or hand with the affected fingernails in a solution of one part white vinegar to two parts water. Vinegar is acidic, and acid makes the environment inhospitable to nail fungus. Because it is a home remedy, there is no "prescribed" method. Some people have had success soaking for an hour each week, all at one go; others soak once a day; and still others use the technique of daubing undiluted vinegar on the affected nail with a cotton swab every day. Persistence is needed with any home remedy. Nails grow slowly, especially toenails, and you need to give them time to grow out healthy and fungus free.

Cornmeal

Another natural fungus fighter may be cornmeal. We first learned of this approach from a public radio listener: "Put about an inch of cornmeal in a plastic dishpan. Pour in hot water, stir it so the cornmeal gets dissolved, and when it is cool enough not to hurt, soak your feet for an hour. If you do this regularly, it will get rid of the fungus."

> *When examining me my doctor noticed that I had nail fungus affecting toes on each foot. He recommended that I make a batter by mixing corn-*

★★★ Cornmeal

A footbath of cornmeal mush is neither expensive nor dangerous, and it takes just 1 hour a week. Put about an inch of cornmeal in a shallow pan and add enough hot water to dissolve it. Let it cool to a comfortable temperature and soak your tootsies for an hour.

Downside: This treatment could be somewhat messy. Don't spill it on the carpet!

Cost: $2 to $4 for 5 pounds of cornmeal—enough for at least five treatments, and probably more

meal and water in a shallow pan, let it sit for an hour, and then soak my feet for an hour. He told me to do this once a week for a month. I did the cornmeal therapy for 3 weeks and the fungus was gone. I don't know why it works, but it's cheap, harmless, and it worked for me."

We haven't found any scientific support for cornmeal as a nail fungus treatment, and fewer people have written us regarding their success with cornmeal than with vinegar, but some have used it to eliminate their nail fungus.

Cornmeal does seem to be a popular home remedy in the garden, though. Gardeners claim that working some cornmeal into the soil around a rose bush will discourage black spot disease, a fungus that affects roses.

Vitamin E

We are always impressed by our readers' ingenuity. We would never have thought of putting vitamin E oil on fungus-infected toenails, for example. We can't think of a good reason why vitamin E in particular would be useful against fungus, and yet a number of people have tried this approach with some success.

"*I keep reading about treatments for toenail fungus so I thought I would pass on my solution. When I had this problem several years ago, I used a simple approach. I kept my toenail soaked with vitamin E oil and the fungus disappeared completely. I can't recall exactly how long it took but it wasn't too long.*"

As we understand the vitamin E tactic, a capsule that you would take as a vitamin—any dose will do—is pierced with a needle or a pin. Then the contents are squirted out all around the edge of the nail and particularly under the nail, between it and the skin. The key here, as with most nail fungus treatments, is patience and persistence.

Listerine

The old-fashioned mouthwash Listerine is one of America's favorite all-purpose home remedies. (The other is Vicks VapoRub; more about it in just a bit.) Amber-colored original flavor Listerine contains a mixture of herbal extracts that can fight fungal nasties from dandruff to jock itch. Some people have also reported having good success with soaking infected nails in Listerine.

Q. *I cured my toenail fungus using a fifty-fifty mixture of vinegar and Listerine. I kept the mixture in a quart jar with a screw-on lid and used a clean paintbrush to apply the liquid to the affected toes morning and night. I wore socks to protect the bedsheets at night.*

The fungus took about 3 months to clear up. It is slow growing but is also slow to cure. I hope this helps someone else.

A. You combined a couple of favorite remedies. Many people have reported success with soaking infected nails in one part vinegar to two parts water. Others got good results soaking their toes in Listerine. Such remedies won't work for everyone and take several months to produce results.

• • •

We have no studies at all examining the effectiveness of Listerine original mouthwash against nail fungus, but it is relatively inexpensive and should not be harmful. Perhaps someday we'll get reports from a scientifically minded reader who treats one nail with Listerine and the other with vinegar to see if there is a difference in how well they work. For now, all we can counsel is patience with either approach.

Vicks VapoRub

Another ever-popular old-time product that has found its way into many a home remedy is Vicks VapoRub. Like Listerine, Vicks contains thymol, eucalyptol, and menthol, along with other herbal oils (camphor, cedarleaf oil, nutmeg oil, and turpentine oil) that may fight fungus.

Pharmacist Lunsford Richardson of Greensboro, North Carolina, had other purposes in mind when he developed this aromatic salve around the turn of the 20th century. It was sold to treat coughs, congestion, colds, and croup and became extremely popular during the deadly 1918 flu season.

A foot-care nurse in Richmond, Massachusetts, alerted us to the potential of using Vicks to treat nail fungus. Many years ago, when

Jane Kelley, RN, first told us about using a dilute vinegar soak for nail fungus, she also mentioned that she'd heard about applying Vicks to the affected nails and the cuticle around them twice daily. If Vicks is used, it must be applied consistently, every day, until the infection clears. This may take 6 months or even longer.

We think we were the first to bring this remedy to the attention of the American public. Subsequently, we have seen it written up in the *Wall Street Journal* and *Consumer Reports*.[760]

"*People have conjectured why Vicks seems to be beneficial against nail fungus. There is a compound in Vicks—thymol—that is now listed as an inactive ingredient.*

When I was a premed student at UCLA in 1951, I met a mycologist (an expert on fungus). During World War II he devised a preparation to treat fungal infections that were common among the troops in the North African campaign. It was an ointment that relied heavily on thymol as the most effective antifungal agent and reeked of thyme.

Vicks contains three active ingredients and 22 considered inactive. One or more of these might help thymol penetrate the tissues. I suspect that a pure preparation of diluted thymol, without other ingredients except a solvent, would be a good antifungal nail treatment."

> "Applying Vicks VapoRub to fungus-infected toenails can clear up the notoriously hard-to-treat condition. Michigan State University clinicians found that applying the product daily to the infected nail cleared the condition in 32 of 85 patients, though it took anywhere from 5 to 16 months. While the study had notable weaknesses, it nevertheless suggests that VapoRub's efficacy may at least rival that of more costly, prescription topical medication."[759]
> —*Consumer Reports*, 2006

Vicks VapoRub certainly does not work for everyone. But we have heard from a great many people who have tried it and gotten a positive response. Some could see the results within a few weeks; others needed to keep applying it for months. Even prescription

★★★★ Vicks VapoRub

This ointment contains herbal oils such as camphor, menthol, thymol, eucalyptol, cedarleaf, nutmeg, and turpentine. Some of these have antifungal activity, and they may work synergistically. Apply Vicks VapoRub all around and under the affected nail or nails once or twice a day. Putting it on right after a shower or bath seems to help. If you apply it at night, wear socks to bed to protect the sheets. It may take 6 months to see results.

Side effects: Allergic rash is possible. In addition, we heard from a few people whose fungus-infected nails came off with this treatment. This might increase the effectiveness of the remedy, but it could be painful.

Downside: Inconvenience

Cost: Approximately $12 for 6 ounces. You could probably treat several toenails twice daily for 6 months with this much Vicks.

drugs take quite a while to clear toenail fungus, however, because the toenails grow so slowly. The infected nail must grow out completely and be replaced by uninvolved nail.

" *I had nail fungus for a long time. Medicines recommended by my doctor didn't work. Then I read about using Vicks VapoRub. I applied it to the nail every day for about 5 months and now the fungus has disappeared. I've been cured.* "

Tea Tree Oil

Tea tree oil comes from an Australian tree, melaleuca. It has long been used to treat skin problems, particularly fungal infections. You don't need to go to Australia to get it, though. It is marketed widely in stores and on the Internet in the United States. Applying tea tree oil to the infected nails daily can overcome some cases of nail fungus. Some people do develop allergic rashes in response to tea tree oil, however, so be alert for any itching or redness.

• • •

Q. *Some years ago I was diagnosed with a fungal infection on one toenail. The intense throbbing pain made it difficult to wear a shoe.*

My podiatrist said the only way to treat the toenail was to remove it. I had several more months of pain while the toe healed.

After the surgery I was alarmed when *another toe showed signs of fungus. I asked about a natural treatment at the health-food store and was told to try tea tree oil.*

I applied it liberally several times that day. Within 10 hours, the pain had diminished. I continued using tea tree oil on the nail daily for a few months. The base of the nail grew in pink and healthy.

I am angry that my podiatrist chose to operate on my toenail rather than recommend a natural, pain-free treatment.

A. Tea tree oil (derived from the Australian melaleuca tree) has antifungal activity. It has long been used to combat skin and nail problems. Your podiatrist may not know about this herbal product, however.

• • •

Pau d'Arco Tea

The lure of the exotic can be seen not only in tea tree oil but also in Pau d'Arco, also called *taheebo*. This product is the inner bark of a South American tree that has been used medicinally by the natives of Brazil, Argentina, and Paraguay. It contains at least one compound with antifungal activity. Some readers report that using an infusion of Pau d'Arco to soak toenails, much as one would use vinegar or Listerine, can help clear the infection.

Oregano Oil

Oregano oil doesn't come from a tropical rain forest, but it is hardly a common household staple. Nonetheless, some people have used it topically for fighting athlete's foot, and others have reported success in using it against nail fungus. Like Listerine and Vicks VapoRub, oregano oil contains thymol. It also contains carvacrol. These two herbal oils together seem to have some antifungal action. Some people are allergic to oregano oil. Anyone who has experienced a reaction to basil, sage, lavender, marjoram, or mint probably should steer clear of oregano oil.

66 *Can you stand another toenail fungus cure? I have found one that works for me, and I have tried them all, including prescription Lamisil pills.*

I read somewhere that oil of oregano will kill anything, so I tried putting a drop down between the nail and the skin every day. Slowly but surely the toenail is growing out normally! I hope someone else can benefit from this as well. 99

Lemon

Some years ago, we heard from a reader who maintained that sleeping with a lemon attached to the toe for 3 nights running would clear up toenail fungus. Only a few others have tried this and reported back to us. It did not work for at least one person, though it seemed to help another.

• • •

Q. *Many people write to you about toenail fungus, but you have never mentioned a remedy I learned from an elderly lady in South Carolina. This remedy requires three fresh lemons. At night cut a hole in the top of one and scoop out a hollow just large enough for the toe.*

My mother had a great toenail so thick and hard that she could hardly wear a shoe on that foot. I used duct tape to hold the lemon on Mother's foot, and put a sandwich bag over it to protect the bed. Do this for 3 nights in a row. The toenail becomes so soft that it can be peeled right off, and the new nail that grows in is normal. It worked for my mother!

A. We have been collecting nail fungus remedies for years, but this is the most unusual. Fungus doesn't thrive in an acidic environment, which may be why dilute vinegar soaks are so effective. The citric acid in the lemon may work in a similar manner.

Prolonged exposure to pure lemon might be irritating for some people, so we suggest that anyone who wants to try such an approach test it first. Removing a toenail should be done only with medical supervision, because there is a risk of infection.

• • •

Prescription Treatments

Unlike home remedies, prescription medications for nail fungus have been scientifically tested and have performed better than placebo. That is the criterion applied by the FDA before approving any prescription product. Don't expect too much from these medicines, though: They don't work for everyone, even though they might be more effective than home remedies. Before beginning a prescription medicine for nail fungus, make sure you understand the risks.

Urea Paste

One treatment for toenail fungus is to remove the nail surgically and then treat the underlying skin with an antifungal cream while the nail grows back without fungus. Many people are understandably reluctant to undergo surgery for nail fungus. Infection is always a risk. We hate it when the cure is worse than the condition it's intended for.

Dermatologists have studied a different approach that is far less traumatic. Urea paste at a 40 percent concentration will dissolve infected nail and leave healthy nail alone. It is essential to work together with the prescribing physician, however, as removing a nail is not a trivial issue. Please do not do this at home by yourself.

• • •

Q. *I have ugly, thick, yellow toenails that are hard to clip. My doctor says they are infected with fungus but he doesn't want to prescribe Sporanox because it could interact with other medicine.*

I have tried home remedies, including Vicks VapoRub, and none has worked. The podiatrist wants to remove the nails surgically. I know you have written about urea paste to dissolve away the infected nail. Where do I get it and how do I use it?

A. Surgical removal of nails can be painful and there is a risk of infection. Stanford dermatologist Eugene Farber, MD, discovered the urea treatment many years ago while traveling in Russia.[761] Urea (40 percent) is available only by prescription (Ureacin-40, Carmol 40, Gordon's Urea 40). Your doctor should supervise the treatment.

• • •

★★★ Urea Paste

The high-strength 40 percent urea paste that dissolves infected nails is available only by prescription. Its use should be supervised by a physician who is familiar with the treatment.

Side effects: Irritation, itching, or burning
Downside: Many doctors are not familiar with this approach.
Cost: Approximately $75 for an 85-gram tube

Penlac

A lot of people are reluctant to take an oral antifungal drug. Some worry about side effects; others are concerned about potential interactions with other drugs they take. Both are valid concerns.

One manufacturer came up with a topical prescription antifungal medicine that is applied like nail polish. Penlac (ciclopirox) was approved by the FDA for the treatment of mild to moderate nail fungus. Like most of the home remedies we've already discussed, Penlac requires a lot of persistence. It needs to be applied to the affected nail, including between the nail and the skin, every day. It can cause redness or irritation, and it may take up to 6 months to produce results.

When people use Penlac, they need to see a health-care professional on a regular basis to have any unattached, infected nail removed so it won't continue to spread the infection. We have no way of comparing Penlac's effectiveness to that of other treatments. Presumably it is as good as most of the untested home remedies, but it is not really too astonishing. About 12 percent of the patients treated with Penlac in clinical trials were able to clear their toenails of fungus. One of the biggest differences between Penlac and a home remedy is the cost. A little bottle (6.6 milliliters) costs $130 or more.

Sporanox or Lamisil

The heavy artillery for treating nail fungus is an oral antifungal medication. If it is crucial to eliminate the infection, the physician will prescribe a drug such as itraconazole (Sporanox) or terbinafine (Lamisil). (You may have seen magazine or television ads for Lamisil that feature a cartoon character, Digger the Dermatophyte.)

In a long-term head-to-head study, patients with toenail fungus were given either terbinafine or itraconazole according to the recommended dosing procedure for 3 to 4 months.[762] At the end of that time, 46 percent of the people who had taken Lamisil and 13 percent of those who had taken Sporanox had no detectable fungus in their nails. The follow-up extended for another 4 years or so. The investigators (some of whom worked for the maker of Lamisil) found that relapse rates were significantly higher among those who had taken Sporanox.

An analysis of cost-effectiveness found that terbinafine is the most cost-effective treatment a doctor can prescribe.[763] Penlac was judged to be at least three times more expensive than the others, considering cost per cure. This analysis did not take any of the home remedies into account. If there were scientific data on them, they might well demonstrate low effectiveness, but because they are cheap, their cost-effectiveness might compare well to some of the standard treatments.

Another advantage of home remedies is the low likelihood of serious side effects. Lamisil is considered fairly safe, even for children and the elderly.[764] Nonetheless, some people taking Lamisil have developed liver failure.[765] People who already have liver problems should not be given this drug. Other people taking Lamisil have come down with a very serious skin reaction, so anyone who develops a rash should get in touch with the doctor promptly. People who have lupus could get worse while taking Lamisil, so it's generally not recommended for them.

As we mentioned at the beginning of this discussion, Lamisil occasionally can lower white blood cell counts to dangerous levels. Usually, the count comes back up once the person stops the drug. This drug may interact with other prescription medicines, including antidepressants, beta-blockers, and certain other medications that regulate the heart's rhythm. By now, we hope we have convinced you to stay in very close touch with the doctor who prescribes Lamisil for your toenail fungus. It'll probably run you more than $800 for the 12 weeks of treatment, but because it works so well, it is quite cost-effective.

Conclusions

Nail fungus, particularly toenail fungus, is usually more of a nuisance than a serious medical problem. (For diabetics, however, nail fungus or any other foot problem qualifies as serious and requires medical care.) As a result, we feel comfortable in recommending that most people try home remedies first. We don't have any data on how well they work, but the testimonials we have received indicate that they do work for some people. In addition, they are inexpensive and don't cause dangerous interactions or reactions.

A person who needs a higher likelihood of cure may need a prescription for Lamisil. It is the most cost-effective of the prescription nail fungus drugs. Even so, it does not work for everyone, and it is not always appropriate. Some people may be taking other medicines that could interact with Lamisil. Others may be at risk of liver problems or complications such as lupus. Most of the time, nail fungus is a problem you can live with; some of the rare side effects could be deadly.

- Toenails grow slowly. It takes a year to a year and a half for them to grow out completely, so be very patient and persistent.
- After cutting fungus-infected nails, soak the clippers or scissors you used in alcohol for 15 to 20 minutes so you don't spread the infection.
- Soak your feet in a footbath of one part vinegar to two parts water for 20 minutes a day.
- Mix cornmeal with hot water, allow it to cool to a comfortable temperature, and soak the affected nails for 1 hour once a week for at least a month.
- Squeeze vitamin E oil or tea tree oil around the cuticle and under the nail once or twice a day.
- Soak the feet in original Listerine or apply it daily to the affected nails.
- Smear Vicks VapoRub around and under the nail every day.
- Brew an infusion of Pau d'Arco for soaking the affected nails every day.
- Stick your toe in a lemon overnight to soften the infected nail for removal.

- If the nail needs to come off, ask your doctor about prescribing urea paste (40 percent).

- Lamisil is the most effective prescription pill for fighting nail fungus.

OSTEOPOROSIS

• Exercise regularly to keep bones strong	★★★★★
• Take vitamin D along with your calcium supplements	★★★★
• Experiment with Menostar (estradiol) instead of hormone replacement therapy	★★
• Consider Evista (raloxifene) to reduce risks of spinal fracture and breast cancer	★★★★
• Ask your doctor about the benefits and risks of Fosamax (alendronate)	★★★
• Make Miacalcin (calcitonin) an option if back pain from fractures is an issue	★★

We tend to think of our bones as hard and unchanging, like the bones we find on our dinner plate. But actually, they are living tissues that undergo constant change and renewal, just like our other organs. Cells called *osteoclasts* break bone down, and cells called *osteoblasts* build it back up, just as if you were remodeling your house a room at a time. The osteoblasts build up living tissue and reinforce it with minerals like calcium, magnesium, boron, and manganese.

Normally, these two processes—resorption and formation of bone—are closely linked so that bone stays strong. Quite a few factors can upset the balance, though. If the osteoclasts race far ahead of the osteoblasts, bone density can drop and eventually the bones are not strong enough. A minor fall can result in a broken hip, which can be catastrophic for an older person.

Osteoporosis, a condition of weakened bone, is responsible for 1.5 million fractures each year, including 300,000 hip fractures.[766] The National Institutes of Health (NIH) estimates that 10 million Americans currently have osteoporosis. Two million of them are men. While osteoporosis is thought of as a women's issue, it is not limited to women.

There's no shortage of controversy surrounding osteoporosis. Perhaps the first issue is just how many people should be concerned about it. According to the NIH, 34 million people have low bone density. Add that to the 10 million who have been diagnosed with osteoporosis, and you come up with 44 million Americans for whom "osteoporosis is a major public health threat."[767] That's more than half of the population over 50 years of age.

Lumping those 34 million who have low bone density together with those who have

The availability of bone density screening is a two-edged sword in this respect. On the one hand, it is helpful for those who are truly at risk to find out before they break a hip or develop debilitating back pain from vertebral fractures. Unfortunately, many of those being screened are not those who need it most. An analysis of nearly 44,000 women on Medicare found that the oldest women, ages 81 to 85, were only half as likely to be screened as women ages 66 to 70.[770] The older women, however, are far more likely to have reduced bone density, even osteoporosis, putting them at risk of a fracture.

Increasingly, middle-aged women are being screened for bone density. The scoring system is a bit complicated, since it is based on standard deviations below the bone density of a young

IS IT CELIAC DISEASE?

Anyone can break a bone by falling off a horse or out of a tree. But some people break bones without even trying. If you have experienced fractures for no logical reason, you and your doctor may want to figure out why your bones are not as strong as they should be.

One possible explanation is celiac disease. It should be investigated in young people with low bone density measurements. Celiac disease is due to gluten intolerance. If it is not diagnosed and a gluten-free diet is not followed, the resulting damage to the small intestine can interfere with proper absorption of the nutrients needed to build bone.

already been diagnosed with osteoporosis certainly makes for a larger potential market for the drugs that have been developed to prevent or treat bone loss. Some public health researchers have criticized this tactic by calling it "disease-mongering."[768] Instead of characterizing osteoporosis or low bone density as a risk factor for fracture, calling it a disease implies that it requires treatment.[769] The critics claim that this tactic mobilizes fear (and helps sell drugs) rather than promoting understanding and positive action.

person at peak bone mass. Most of us don't have the grounding in statistics to make much sense of "standard deviations," so if the doctor does not explain carefully what the numbers mean, women often end up confused and alarmed. Critics point out that defining osteoporosis as bone density that is 2.5 standard deviations (T score –2.5) below the mean for a young person practically guarantees that approximately 30 percent of postmenopausal women will be diagnosed with this condition, whether they are truly at risk for osteoporosis or not.[771,772]

Reducing the Risk of Fracture with Nondrug Approaches

Although osteoporosis treatment now includes many more options than it did just 10 years ago, each drug that is prescribed for weakened bones has some drawbacks. That's why it makes sense to start with nondrug approaches and see how far they will take you. If you begin early enough, you may be able to slow bone loss and prevent a fracture. But even if you already have osteoporosis, these tactics may be a good addition to pharmacological treatment to make it more effective.

Exercise

Your doctor may not be accustomed to prescribing a walk around the block, but getting more exercise should be just what the doctor orders. In so many cases nowadays we must go out of our way to work up a sweat. Few of us do manual labor to earn a living; walking to our jobs or just to the store is almost as rare, espe-

cially in many suburbs. So instead of incorporating physical movement into everyday life, we need to find time—and funds—to go "work out" somewhere. This may be too inconvenient for many people.

It has become clear that our bodies adapt to the demands we make of them. Weight-bearing exercise like walking, running, or mowing the lawn encourages bones to grow stronger. Sitting in front of a computer screen, sadly, does nothing to stress our bones in a healthy way. In fact, differences in traditional patterns of activity may explain why women usually have less bone mass than men, even as young, healthy adults. In the past, boys were expected and encouraged to be active by playing sports and helping

★★★★★ Exercise

Moving your bones helps strengthen them. Doing something enjoyable on a regular basis—walking, gardening, dancing, or another weight-bearing activity—acts to delay bone loss as well as strengthen muscles, benefit cardiovascular health, improve mood, and reduce the risk of dementia. Exercise alone may not be enough to reverse bone loss, but it can improve the effectiveness of other treatments.[773]

Side effects: Sore muscles
Downside: If the exercise program is overly ambitious or too dangerous, a person with reduced bone density may experience injuries, including fracture.
Cost: Too variable to estimate

with strenuous chores. Girls, by and large, were not. Although these differences are diminishing among today's children, physical activity has been declining across the board.

A lifetime of activity is ideal for the strength of the skeleton, but it may never be too late to benefit from more exercise. Anyone who has already experienced fractures from osteoporosis should check first with his or her physician, but appropriate weight training or walking may be helpful even for those who are quite elderly or a bit debilitated. The exercise program should be carefully designed, of course, so that it does not put the person at a higher risk for fracture from a fall or injury.

The Calcium Craze

Calcium supplements are the first thing most people think of for preventing or treating osteoporosis. Although an adequate calcium intake is necessary to maintain strong bones, just taking calcium doesn't seem to help very much once bone density has begun to decline. Calcium supplementation can make a difference in young people, whose bones are still developing. But in postmenopausal women, the evidence is murky. Some studies have shown that 500 to 1,000 milligrams of calcium a day together with 700 to 800 IU of vitamin D can reduce the number of fractures (though this benefit does not extend to the spine).[776,777,778]

The results of the Women's Health Initiative on this issue were less encouraging. The study was very large, involving more than 36,000 postmenopausal women. Though supplements of 1,000 milligrams of calcium and 400 IU of vitamin D_3 daily improved the density of bone in the hip, it did not reduce the number of hip fractures.[779] Scientists have tried to explain the disappointing results: The

---

★★★★ Calcium and Vitamin D

Calcium is important for preventing and treating osteoporosis—but by itself it isn't enough. Taken together with adequate vitamin D, it may help reduce the risk of falling as well as improve bone mineral density.[774]

Most of the experts who do research on osteoporosis agree that a calcium-rich diet (or a supplement of around 1,000 milligrams daily) and 15 to 20 minutes of sun exposure 3 or 4 days a week (or a supplement of 800 to 1,000 IU of vitamin D_3, also known as cholecalciferol) are a sensible approach. Take no more than 500 or 600 milligrams of calcium at a time for better absorption.

Calcium also works with dietary protein to benefit the skeleton.[775] Make sure you are getting enough protein.

Side effects: Gas, intestinal bloating, constipation
Downside: Too much calcium increases the risk of kidney stones.
Cost: $6 to $10 per month for a supplement that contains both nutrients

---

women were not in the oldest age category at highest risk for fracture; the women on placebo pills could take calcium on the side if they chose to; many of the women in the active supplement group did not take their calcium and vitamin D_3 every day.

In addition, 400 IU of vitamin D_3 just may not be enough. An analysis of a number of studies concluded that it takes at least 700 IU of vitamin D_3 a day to make a difference in fracture risk.[781] Lower dosages simply aren't effective.

Human skin can make vitamin D when it is exposed to sunlight, but older people are often careful not to go out in the sunshine without their sunscreen. Aging skin is less efficient at making vitamin D, so a health-conscious older person may actually be making very little of it. If this is true for you, a supplement may be advisable.

We weren't as surprised as others may have been at the lackluster results seen with calcium supplements in the Women's Health Initiative. Walter Willett, MD, DrPH, MPH, the Frederick J. Stare Professor of Nutrition and Epidemiology and chair of the department of nutrition at the Harvard School of Public Health, had told us years earlier that calcium is not the whole story. Women in Scandinavia have the highest calcium intake in the world, but they also have the highest rates of osteoporosis. Women in some parts of Africa get very little calcium in their diets yet rarely have trou-

CALCIUM-RICH FOODS[782]

FOOD	SERVING SIZE	CALCIUM (MG)
Milk, skim	1 c	302
Yogurt, low-fat	1 c	300
Gruyere cheese	1 oz	287
Swiss cheese	1 oz	272
Figs, dried	10 figs	269
Tofu	½ c	258
Calcium-fortified orange juice	6 oz	200
Mozzarella cheese	1 oz	183
Collards, cooked	½ c	179
Blackstrap molasses	1 Tbsp	172
Cottage cheese	1 c	126
Sardines	2 sardines	92
Parmesan cheese	1 Tbsp	69
Kale, cooked	½ c	47
Broccoli, cooked	½ c	36

ble with fractures as they age. Sun exposure is one obvious difference that might account for women having relatively low levels of vitamin D in Scandinavia.

Clearly, other factors are at work here. That doesn't mean you should cut down on calcium. But don't count on it to do the job alone.

If you do choose a calcium supplement, keep in mind that calcium citrate may be taken with or without food, but calcium carbonate is absorbed best if taken at mealtime.[783] Many sources recommend taking 300 to 500 milligrams of magnesium with the calcium supplement.

Drugs to Treat Osteoporosis

Calcium supplements may be necessary but not sufficient against bone loss. Joel Finkelstein, MD, of Massachusetts General Hospital, has suggested that supplements of calcium plus vitamin D should be thought of as the ante for a poker game: It's the bare minimum if you are going to play.[784] Most of the drug treatments for osteoporosis work best if a person gets adequate amounts of these nutrients as well.

Low-Dose Estrogen (Menostar)

Women used to be told that once they reached menopause, they needed to take hormone replacement therapy to keep their bones strong. The idea was that they would be on estrogen (plus progesterone, unless they had undergone a hysterectomy) for decades and that this would prevent osteoporosis and the resulting fractures.

The findings of the WHI threw the wisdom of that simple approach into question. Although hormone replacement therapy (HRT) did cut the risk of hip fracture by more than 30 percent, it increased the risk of coronary heart disease, stroke, and breast cancer.[785] After these findings were released, many women decided that they were more concerned about heart attacks and strokes than broken bones. So they stopped taking their HRT.

Since then, clinicians have been trying to find a way to get the benefits of HRT without all the risks. One way to do that is with an estrogen-receptor modulator such as Evista (see page 389). Another way might be with a different form of estrogen. In 2004, the FDA approved a low-dose estrogen patch to prevent osteoporosis. This transdermal patch, called Menostar, releases 14 micrograms of estrogen as (17-beta)-estradiol a day. This form of estrogen is different from the mixture found in Premarin or Prempro but the same as that found in some other estrogen pills for postmenopausal women. Estrogen is absorbed well through the skin, so the dosage delivered in a skin patch can be a lot lower than the dosage in a pill. This dose is quite a bit lower than those of other commonly prescribed estrogen patches used to treat menopausal symptoms.[786]

Menostar is not for treating menopausal symptoms such as hot flashes or vaginal dryness. It is not for use by women who already have osteoporosis with vertebral fractures. But for women whose bone mineral density is low or who are at risk for developing osteoporosis, Menostar might be one way to try to get the bone benefits of estrogen while sidestepping the cardiovascular risks.

The research done on Menostar indicates that it is not likely to cause problems in the uterus, even though there is no progesterone in the regimen to protect the uterine lining.[787] It does increase bone mineral density, particularly in the spine, better than placebo.[788] There are not enough data to indicate whether women using Menostar are less susceptible to fractures, either of the spine or of the hip.

The bottom line on Menostar is that women who choose to use it at this time should recognize that in some respects they are experimenting. There are still some important facts about its potential long-term benefits and risks that need to be clarified.

Raloxifene (Evista)

Raloxifene (Evista) was specifically designed to be as much like estrogen as possible in its effects on bone and unlike estrogen in many other ways. The researchers who developed this selective estrogen receptor modulator, or SERM, were hoping that it would strengthen bone and prevent fractures as hormone replacement therapy seems to, but that it would not increase the risk of uterine or breast cancer as HRT does. They were largely successful in their efforts. This medication does reduce the risk of fractures in the spine, although it does not seem to have much impact on hip fractures.[789]

Because any osteoporosis drug must be taken for many years, a study considered the safety of raloxifene over a period of 8 years and found that it did not increase the risk of heart attack, stroke, uterine cancer, or ovarian cancer.[790] Like HRT, raloxifene increases the risk of blood clots forming in the veins. In fact, this drug increases the risk of fatal strokes as well as dangerous blood clots.[791] As a result, doctors and patients need to weigh its benefits—reducing the risk of spinal fractures and of invasive breast cancer—against the possibility of a blood clot or a stroke.

In the spring of 2006, scientists announced that Evista had performed well in the STAR

★★ Menostar

Menostar is a relatively new ultra-low-dose transdermal estrogen patch. It can increase bone mineral density and has been approved for preventing osteoporosis in postmenopausal women. Menostar comes as a patch applied to the belly. Each one lasts a week.

Side effects: Redness or irritation under the patch. Estrogen has a number of side effects, such as blood clots, stroke, increased risk of breast or endometrial cancer, and gallstones. It is not clear to what degree Menostar will cause estrogenic side effects.

Downside: No evidence that Menostar will prevent fractures; no long-term data on cardiovascular safety

Cost: About $50 a month

★★★★ Raloxifene (Evista)

This pill strengthens bone and is especially effective at preventing fractures in the spine. It is approved both for preventing and for treating osteoporosis. In addition, raloxifene can reduce the risk of invasive breast cancer in high-risk (postmenopausal) women by approximately 50 percent.

Side effects: Blood clots, vaginal dryness, hot flashes, joint pain, leg cramps
Downside: Raloxifene does not appear to have a significant effect on hip fractures. In addition, it does not reduce the risk of noninvasive breast cancer.
Cost: Approximately $75 for a month

trial, the Study of Tamoxifen and Raloxifene for preventing breast cancer. The women who had volunteered for this National Cancer Institute–sponsored study were at increased risk of developing breast cancer. Both drugs reduced their likelihood of a breast cancer diagnosis by about 50 percent. Women who took raloxifene were less likely to experience blood clots, cataracts, or uterine cancer than those given tamoxifen.

The investigators concluded that women who had already taken tamoxifen for 5 years following treatment for breast cancer would get no further benefit from taking raloxifene. Women who had not taken tamoxifen but were at high risk of breast cancer could get two benefits—breast cancer prevention and osteoporosis treatment—in one pill if they took raloxifene instead.

Actonel, Boniva, and Fosamax

All three of these osteoporosis drugs fall into the category called *bisphosphonates*. Alendronate (Fosamax), ibandronate (Boniva), and risedronate (Actonel) work by slowing down bone resorption. They zip to places where bone remodeling is going on and mess with the osteoclasts so that these bone-wreckers work more slowly. Usually, that is enough to give the osteoblasts a chance to catch up a bit on bone formation.

Fosamax was the first bisphosphonate to be developed and approved by the FDA for treating osteoporosis. It has been available for more than 10 years in this country. Women who have taken it for that long have continued to increase their bone mineral density. Although it was originally prescribed as a once-daily pill, the inconvenience of getting up early enough to take it an hour before breakfast or even coffee and juice, as advised, cut down on its popularity. Taking Fosamax with anything other than plain tap water reduces the amount that is absorbed and lessens its effectiveness. Changing the regimen so that it is taken only once a week, and only half an hour before breakfast, has made it easier for women to follow the doctor's orders.

The effectiveness of all of the bisphosphonate medicines is clearest in people who are at highest risk: those who already have osteoporosis, particularly those who have experienced one or more fractures. The bisphosphonates are not hormones and don't work through the same mechanisms as hormones. As a result, presumably they would be equally effective for men and women with osteoporosis.

Many of the studies that have been done on the bisphosphonates involved only women. Among a group of women who'd already had one vertebral fracture, Fosamax cut the number of hip fractures in half.[792] A head-to-head trial of Fosamax against Actonel showed that Fosamax had a slight edge. Subjects taking once-a-week Fosamax had higher bone mineral density scores and were less likely to have lost bone than subjects taking once-a-week Actonel.[793]

A 3-year study of more than 9,000 women with osteoporosis found that Actonel reduced hip fractures significantly, from 3.2 percent in the placebo group to 1.9 percent in the Actonel group.[794] This study found no significant benefit among women who did not actually have osteoporosis but were included because of their age or other risk factors. Boniva, which is given just once a month rather than once a week, can increase bone mineral density. In a study that included nearly 3,000 women with at least one vertebral fracture, Boniva significantly reduced the number of new vertebral fractures.[796] It did not reduce the rate of hip fractures or fractures elsewhere besides the spine, however.

A few complications of bisphosphonates that are especially worrisome have been getting significant attention lately. Some people taking Actonel or Fosamax have developed osteonecrosis of the jaw, a condition in which part of the jawbone dies. This seems to be an uncommon side effect, but it is frightening

★★★ Alendronate (Fosamax)

Alendronate works by slowing bone resorption. It is commonly given once a week. It must be taken with 8 ounces of plain tap water, not mineral water, at least 30 minutes before eating or drinking anything else. The patient must remain standing or sitting during that time to keep the pill from lodging in the throat, where it can cause damage.

Side effects: Digestive disturbances, including heartburn, esophageal irritation or inflammation that can become severe, stomachache, and diarrhea; severe bone, joint, and muscle pain; osteonecrosis of the jaw, a rare but serious complication following tooth extraction, root canal, and other significant dental procedures; inflammation of the eye, resulting in blurred vision, eye pain, conjunctivitis, uveitis, or scleritis

Downside: Although alendronate has been around for more than 10 years, some of the more worrisome side effects are just now coming to light. No one knows how this drug will affect bone in the long term. Could the increased mineralization of bone end up making bones more brittle instead of stronger? As yet, there are no good answers to this question.[795]

Cost: Approximately $77 per month, a little more than Actonel ($72) and Boniva ($74)

because there is no good treatment for it. Most of the cases reported so far have occurred after tooth extraction or some other major dental procedure. There is no indication that Boniva would be exempt from this issue.

If you are taking any of these drugs for osteoporosis, be sure to tell your dentist and your endodontist about it. We don't know yet if discontinuing the medication for some months before a dental intervention would reduce the risk of this unusual adverse reaction.

Two other concerns that have come up with the bisphosphonates are severe joint, bone, or muscle pain, and eye inflammation. The eye inflammation may affect vision. In one case, the only way to control it was to discontinue the medication.[797] Be sure to discuss your osteoporosis medication with your eye doctor, particularly if you notice any problems with your vision.

The joint or muscle pain required narcotic pain relievers in some cases. The confirmation that it was related to the osteoporosis drug came when drug treatment was stopped and the pain went away—but when the drug was restarted, the pain returned.[798]

Teriparatide (Forteo)

Currently, there is no other osteoporosis drug like teriparatide (Forteo). It is a genetically engineered copy of the active part of parathyroid hormone. This hormone, which is produced by a gland in the neck right next to the thyroid, governs the body's utilization of minerals such as calcium. Like most of the human endocrine glands, it operates on a feedback system and shuts down when it senses there is enough calcium in circulation. If it senses too little, it stimulates bone breakdown to liberate calcium.

If the hormone stimulates bone breakdown, how can it help treat osteoporosis? Forteo—which is given by injection—is active for only a short time, reaching maximum concentration after about 30 minutes and disappearing completely within about 3 or 4 hours.[799] When the hormone is administered in this kind of short pulse, the body responds by building bone. Forteo is the only osteoporosis drug currently in use that stimulates bone formation.

Studies have shown that Forteo can increase bone mineral density in the spine and the hip. It also reduces fractures in the spine and elsewhere. It performs significantly better than placebo in men as well as women. In a small head-to-head trial against Fosamax, Forteo increased the bone mineral density of the spine by about twice as much and reduced fractures in places other than the spine significantly more than Fosamax did.[800]

The FDA has approved Forteo to treat osteoporosis in men and women. It sounds great, but of course there are drawbacks. Side effects with Forteo are mostly mild: nausea, dizziness, headache, and leg cramps. It is given by injection, so redness and swelling may rarely occur at the injection site. A patient just starting on Forteo may experience "orthostatic hypotension," or dizziness if she stands up suddenly. Fortunately, this side effect usually goes away within a couple of hours.

The big worry with Forteo involves its long-term use. Studies in rats have shown that this drug increases the rate of a bone cancer called osteosarcoma. This may have factored in to the FDA's decision to limit use of Forteo to 2 years. The medication is so new that no one has a good handle on what the long-term effects will be, but so far no cases of osteosarcoma have been reported in humans using the drug.[801]

Another disadvantage of Forteo is that it must be injected every day. It comes in a self-injectable "pen," and the shot is administered in the thigh or belly. Each pen lasts for a month and needs to be kept in the refrigerator.

In comparison to other treatments for osteoporosis, Forteo is extremely expensive. A single month's treatment can cost $750 to $800. Given all these negatives, we think Forteo might best be reserved for people whose risk for adverse events with other osteoporosis treatments is too high.

Calcitonin (Miacalcin)

Another hormone that may be prescribed to treat osteoporosis is calcitonin. It, too, is made by the thyroid gland. It binds to osteoclasts and slows down their bone munching. It also helps regulate the action of vitamin D and works together with parathyroid hormone to control the balance of calcium and phosphorus within the body.

Salmon calcitonin can be given either as an injection or in a nasal spray. It can reduce fractures of the vertebrae significantly more than

---

★★ Calcitonin (Miacalcin)

Calcitonin is given not to prevent but to treat osteoporosis. In women who already have at least one fractured vertebra, Miacalcin is significantly better than placebo at preventing additional spinal fractures. Some studies suggest that it helps alleviate back pain by stimulating production of beta-endorphins, the body's natural opiates.

Side effects: Nausea and vomiting, flushing, redness or soreness at the injection site, rash, reduced appetite, severe allergic reaction; runny nose and nosebleed may occur with the nasal spray

Downside: Expensive. It does not appear to have a substantial effect on preventing hip fractures.

Cost: Nasal spray, $95 per bottle; injection, $45 for 2 milliliters (a 4-day supply)

---

placebo. Some scientists have suggested that it may relieve back pain, which is frequently a serious problem for women whose osteoporosis has caused numerous fractures of the vertebrae. There is no solid consensus on this issue, however. [802,803]

Conclusions

When it comes to preventing broken hips and painful spinal fractures, there is no single treatment that stands head and shoulders above the rest. Each has benefits and disadvantages. People at risk for osteoporosis will need to think about the issues that might affect their treatment and their ability to stick with the program.

Even when the primary goal is prevention by getting adequate calcium and vitamin D together with exercise (and we strongly encourage that for everyone who can do it), the studies show that nutritional supplements are effective only if people actually take them all the time. Surprise! So consider whether you will take a pill or an injection every day, or if you're better off with once-a-week or even once-a-month therapy.

Consider combining Evista or Menostar with one of the bisphosphonate medicines, such as Actonel or Fosamax. Some research shows that combining these treatments can increase bone density more than either one alone.[804] We don't know whether the combination also reduces the risk of fractures synergistically. There are, of course, costs associated with taking more than one drug. But if the therapy you are using does not seem to be working adequately, this option might be worth discussing with your doctor. There isn't any advantage in combining Forteo with other medicines.

There are a couple of other treatments to watch for, although they are not currently available in the United States. A new hormone replacement therapy called Angeliq has been introduced in Europe. It contains a lower dose of estrogen (1 milligram per day of estradiol) along with a different type of progestin called drospirenone.[805] We can't tell at this point whether it would be safer than the usual HRT or how effective it might be at preventing fractures. Another new drug is called Preos. Like Forteo, it is based on parathyroid hormone.[806] Not enough information is available at this time to tell if it would offer any significant advantages.

• A lifetime of healthy living, with plenty of physical activity and adequate intake of calcium and vitamin D, is the best osteoporosis preventive. It's (almost) never too late to start. But if you already have had fractures, check with your doctor before you begin a new exercise program! You don't want to make things worse.

• Bone density screening can be a useful tool for determining who may need treatment for osteoporosis. It is underutilized for those most at risk, women of more than 80 years of age.

• Don't bother with calcium supplements alone. Make sure they are paired with adequate vitamin D. Your skin can manufacture its own D with roughly 15 minutes of sun exposure three or four days a week. If you shun the sun, you should be getting a minimum of 700 IU of vitamin D_3 a day; 1,000 IU daily might be even better, but don't go overboard because vitamin D can be toxic at very high doses.

• Evista can do double duty, reducing the risk of both osteoporosis fractures and breast cancer. If you are concerned about both issues, discuss this possibility with your doctor.

• The bisphosphonates are fairly similar in

side effects and efficacy, though alendronate (Fosamax) may have an edge. Consider one of these medicines unless you have had problems with your esophagus (such as bleeding or trouble swallowing) or expect to need dental surgery.

• Forteo builds bone, but its long-term benefits and risks are unknown. As a daily injection, it is less convenient and more expensive than most other treatments.

• Miacalcin might be a good choice for a person who already has osteoporosis and vertebral fractures. It may ease back pain as well as increase spinal bone density.

• Menostar offers an alternative for women. This ultra-low-dose estrogen patch can increase bone mineral density and may not cause the harm associated with conventional HRT.

TINNITUS

• Test drive a hearing aid/masking device	★★★
• Take melatonin at bedtime	★★
• Ask your doctor about misoprostol (Cytotec)	★

Can you imagine anything more annoying than hearing a mosquito buzzing around your head and not being able to catch it? A dentist's drill might be a close match. Now imagine what it would be like to have crickets chirping in your ear 24 hours a day, 7 days a week.

Experts estimate that more than 30 million Americans hear a constant noise in their ears.[807] Roughly one in eight men between the ages of 65 and 74 experiences some form of tinnitus (pronounced *TIN-a-tus* or *tin-EYE-tus*).[808] Women and children are not spared the unwanted sound effects, which some describe as hissing, humming, chirping, whooshing, whistling, squeaking, or roaring.

Many tinnitus sufferers hear a high-pitched ringing, while others say it sounds more like steam escaping. Others complain of radio static or an electronic whine inside their head. One person described it this way: "I have an ocean between my ears every day, 24-7." Whatever the sound, it never lets up—but nobody else can hear it, either.

❝ *My husband has a constant buzz in his ears and also hears a sound he likens to a dishwasher running. This particular sound bothers him most when he goes to bed or wakes up at night, and it wakes him frequently. The doctor says lots of people have tinnitus and the problem isn't serious, but it has my husband on the ropes.* "

According to the medical establishment, "Many patients with tinnitus believe that they have a serious medical problem. This is rarely the case."[809] We beg to differ. People with tinnitus look normal, but the affliction can be as crippling as arthritis. Some individuals are so distressed by the sounds they hear that they become severely depressed and contemplate suicide. A study has found that even moderate tinnitus can interfere with cognitive ability, making it harder to focus and achieve peak performance while working on demanding tasks.[810]

Tinnitus can be caused by many things, including very loud noises. More than 15 years ago, Joe was preparing to cohost a radio show when a student engineer made an error and created a feedback loop through Joe's headphones (the kind of screech you sometimes hear through speakers in an auditorium). The sound was so loud and so close to his ears that from that day to this, Joe has heard a ringing and hissing sound. Some days the noise is so overpowering that it is hard for him to concentrate. For people who cannot imagine what you are going through, it is difficult to describe how disconcerting it is to have a fieldful of crickets inside your head all the time.

We fear that millions of teenagers and young adults may be setting themselves up for tinnitus and other forms of hearing loss by exposing themselves to high volume levels while listening to iPods and other music devices. There are so many loud noises in our environment that the cumulative effect can damage our ears and increase our risk of tinnitus. We're talking about everyday things in our lives like blenders, vacuum cleaners, motorcycles, leaf blowers, and lawn mowers. All of them are loud and can contribute to hearing problems.

● ● ●

Q. *I have just developed a hissing sound in my ears. The onset was very rapid!*

The doctor diagnosed it as tinnitus but would give me no reason for the problem. He said there wasn't anything I could do. I've noticed some days it is less disturbing than others, but some nights it awakens me because it has become so loud.

I was drinking large quantities of tonic water, which contains quinine, when this started. Do you have any suggestions to help me?

A. Stop the tonic water! Quinine gives tonic its distinctive bitter flavor, but it can cause tinnitus, especially at high doses. Hopefully the hissing sound will gradually go away once the quinine is out of your system.

● ● ●

Drugs are another common cause of tinnitus. An amazing number of prescription and over-the-counter medications can cause ringing in the ears. Aspirin is one of the most common culprits, but many other arthritis drugs can also contribute to the problem. If you suspect that a medicine is causing ringing, hissing, or whooshing, please discuss this with your physician promptly.

Drug-Induced Tinnitus

• • •

Q. *I am desperate to find some way to alleviate my arthritis pain without experiencing unbearable tinnitus. I have taken aspirin for some time, and it has been quite effective. If a joint flares up, I increase the dose for a few days. Then I heard your radio show where you mentioned that aspirin can contribute to tinnitus.*

The noises in my head had been getting worse. I was resigned to this, but after listening to your program I stopped the aspirin. The result for my ears was dramatic! But then the joint pain came back. I feel I am walking a very thin line between arthritis and tinnitus.

A. Sadly, you are caught between a rock and a hard place. Aspirin and other arthritis drugs (nonsteroidal anti-inflammatory drugs, or NSAIDs, like naproxen and ibuprofen) can cause ringing in the ears. Some people are

DRUGS THAT CAN CAUSE TINNITUS*	
GENERIC	**BRAND NAME**
Aspirin	Alka Seltzer, Ascriptin, Bayer
Bleomycin	Blenoxane
Bumetanide	Bumex
Bupropion	Wellbutrin SR and XL
Cetirizine	Zyrtec
Chloroquine	Aralen
Cisplatin	Platinol
Diclofenac	Cataflam, Voltaren
Erythromycin	E-Mycin, Ery-Tab, Eryc
Furosemide	Lasix
Ibuprofen	Advil, Motrin
Meloxicam	Mobic
Methotrexate	Rheumatrex
Nabumetone	Relafen
Naproxen	Aleve, Anaprox, Naprosyn
Quinine	Quinamm, Quinerva, QM-260
Risedronate	Actonel
Tetracycline	Sumycin
Valproic acid	Depakene
Vancomycin	Vancocin
Vincristine	Oncovir

*This is just a partial list. Hundreds of drugs can contribute to tinnitus.

susceptible to even low doses. You may need to investigate other options for arthritis pain. (See page 78 for some nondrug approaches.)

• • •

In addition to sound-induced injury (like Joe experienced) and drugs, many other things can cause tinnitus. Impacted earwax is probably the most benign and easiest to correct. Some other contributors include head injury, multiple sclerosis, hypertension, infections (otitis media, Lyme disease), and tumors (acoustic neuroma). That's why it is important to be seen by a specialist (an otorhinolaryngologist, or ear, nose, and throat doctor) to rule out any treatable condition. Sometimes there is no obvious reason for the ringing or whooshing.

> *A few months ago I suddenly developed a case of tinnitus in my left ear. It sounds like the high-pitched noise the computer makes when logging onto the Internet. I am 36 years old and in extremely good health. I have not experienced any head trauma and am not exposed to loud noises.*
>
> *I had an MRI to rule out a brain tumor. Neither my family physician nor an ear, nose, and throat doctor could find anything wrong with me and they have not suggested any remedies. I currently just barely manage it with white noise (a fan) at night.*

Treatments for Tinnitus

When everything else has been ruled out and you are left with ringing in the ears, what can be done? First and foremost, do not expose yourself to noise pollution. Chances are good you already have some hearing loss. Be cautious around all appliances (blenders and vacuum cleaners, for example) and power tools. When flying, take along hearing protectors (you can buy earplugs that fit in your ears unobtrusively) to block out some of the jet engine sounds at airports or on loud commuter airplanes. Do the same when attending concerts or sports events. Protect your ears from any further damage.

The official word from the medical establishment is that "most treatments [for tinnitus] are unsuccessful."[811] A review of 69 randomized clinical trials published in 1999 concluded that there was no proof that any therapy provides long-term improvement.[812] Investigators have experimented with powerful medications that control irregular heart rhythms (intravenous lidocaine, and oral flecainide and tocainide), but the results were disappointing and the side effects scary. Antianxiety agents (benzodiazepines) such as alprazolam (Xanax) may help ease the psychological impact of tinnitus, but when the drug is discontinued, the problem can return with a vengeance. The antidepressant nortriptyline has shown more promise than many other approaches, but the benefits still are not overwhelming.[813] Acupuncture, biofeedback, hypnosis, and "tinnitus retraining therapy" have all been disappointing and do not make the ringing go away.

Most physicians will say that the primary goal of treatment for tinnitus is "management." Usually this means things like masking devices. In its crudest and cheapest form, a

★★★ Hearing Aid/Masking Device

High-tech hearing aids that combine frequency-specific amplification and masking in one device may be worth consideration. Some folks report both improved hearing and reduced tinnitus with such equipment. Sometimes the tinnitus relief lasts for some time after the device is turned off or removed.[814]

Downside: These special hearing aids are pricey, costing several thousand dollars. Insurance is not likely to cover the cost. They require professional fitting. Do not expect them to solve the problem, but they may make it more tolerable.

Cost: Approximately $1,000 to $3,000 per ear. Try to work out a "test drive" to make sure they work well and adequately relieve your tinnitus discomfort. Another option: Lease with an option to buy. If they do not solve your problem, you can at least give them back when the lease is up.

masking device is an FM radio tuned so that you do not get a signal, just static. The theory is that this "white noise" will mask the sound of the tinnitus. Some people find this helpful, whereas others report that it just intensifies the annoying sounds.

There are also white noise generators or masking devices that can be "tuned" to an individual's general noise frequency. There are also sophisticated new hearing aids that both amplify sound in the hearing range that is impaired and use a masking signal that is adjusted to the specific range of the patient.

"" *My husband has suffered for years from tinnitus and hearing loss (due to his time in Vietnam). He recently found great relief with the new technology in hearing aids. Since getting his hearing aids, the ringing, buzzing, etc., has completely gone away and his hearing is now very acute.*

Many folks have tried hearing aids in the past without success. I know my husband did. He said they just made the ringing louder! He is thrilled with this new technology. I believe this might help many who haven't tried the devices. ""

No one should buy these pricey instruments unless they actually work. That means you should be able to either test the device for a short while or lease it for somewhat longer before shelling out thousands of dollars to purchase it.

Ginkgo Biloba

There has been some interesting research on this ancient Chinese herbal medicine. From the more than 100 clinical trials that have been published, there seems to be a reasonable amount of data suggesting that standardized ginkgo extracts (Ginkgold, Ginkoba, and Ginkai) improve circulation throughout the body, in general, and may modestly improve symptoms of dementia.[815] A 1999 review of clinical studies of ginkgo concluded that "overall, the results of these trials are favorable to ginkgo biloba as a treatment for tinnitus, but a firm conclusion about efficacy is not possible . . . the body of evidence is small."[816]

Since then, there have been two studies that have not found ginkgo to be any better than placebo for relieving symptoms of tinnitus.[817,818] At this time it would be fair to say that the evidence is mixed at best and probably not very promising. On the other hand, ginkgo does seem to improve circulation and may be worth a try. Do not expect any miracles, though.

Adding a little zinc to the mix (50 milligrams) might be worth consideration since a small study suggested that this mineral produced some modest clinical improvement.[819]

★★ Melatonin

Melatonin is natural, safe, and not very expensive. Although there is some controversy about its effectiveness for insomnia, two preliminary studies suggest that it may help people with tinnitus and sleeping problems associated with ear ringing. The dose that has been tested is 3 milligrams.

Downside: The data are not yet strong enough to elicit a ringing endorsement.
Cost: Approximately $2 to $4 per month when purchased in bulk

---

If after several weeks there is no improvement, we would give up on this approach.

Melatonin

One of the least studied but most promising new approaches for the treatment of tinnitus may be melatonin. This natural compound is inexpensive and safe. Melatonin is a hormone that is made primarily by the pineal gland in the brain in response to darkness. During the daytime, the blood level is low, but at night melatonin climbs until it reaches its peak between 2:00 and 4:00 a.m. It is crucial for regulating sleep and wake cycles.

Some extraordinary claims have been made for melatonin. Some proponents say that it can reverse aging, improve immune function, reduce the risk of cancer, control blood pressure, and lower cholesterol. The best-known use of melatonin is as a sleep aid. An extensive review of the existing studies published in the Cochrane Database concluded, "Melatonin is remarkably effective in preventing or reducing jet lag, and occasional short-term use appears to be safe. It should be recommended to adult travelers flying across five or more time zones, particularly in an easterly direction, and especially if they have experienced jet lag on previous journeys."[820]

Despite this good news, two reviews of melatonin's use for easing insomnia were less glowing. They concluded that melatonin does not work for sleep disorders.[821,822] Nevertheless, a small preliminary study carried out by the Ear Research Foundation in Sarasota,

Florida, in 1998 revealed that a dose of 3 milligrams of melatonin was helpful for patients with tinnitus that interfered with their sleep.[823] Following up on this research, investigators at Washington University in St. Louis also found that a dose of 3 milligrams was beneficial for people with tinnitus: "In summary, our study demonstrates that melatonin use is associated with improvement of tinnitus and sleep."[824] Although the research to date is preliminary, melatonin seems to be worth a try because of its safety and affordability.

Misoprostol (Cytotec)

Sometimes doctors teach old drugs new tricks. That might be the case with misoprostol (Cytotec), a medication approved more than a decade ago to help prevent stomach ulcers. It was hoped that Cytotec would be especially beneficial for people taking aspirin or other NSAIDs like ibuprofen or naproxen. This medication has become controversial in recent years because some obstetricians have used it to induce labor. Others have combined misoprostol with mifepristone to induce abortion.

An entirely different use for misoprostol is treating tinnitus. We first stumbled across a pilot study that was published in 1993 in the *Archives of Otolaryngology—Head & Neck Surgery*.[826] One of the most prestigious ear clinics in the world (House Ear Institute in Los Angeles) enrolled 24 subjects. These volunteers

---

★ Misoprostol (Cytotec)

This prescription medication has FDA approval for the prevention of stomach ulcers. An "off-label" use may ultimately turn out to be for tinnitus. Preliminary studies have found that misoprostol may help roughly one-third to two-thirds of tinnitus sufferers, with those who experienced a sudden onset of tinnitus or who had a history of acoustic trauma getting the most benefit. The dose used by the researchers was "200 micrograms per day for the first week, increased by 200 micrograms every 5 days" to reach a maintenance dose of 800 micrograms per day. This latter amount is also the dosage commonly used in gastroenterology."[825]

Downside: Very expensive! Misoprostol must never be taken by a woman who is pregnant or might become pregnant. It can induce premature labor and cause other serious complications. Patients with heart or inflammatory bowel problems should also avoid misoprostol.

Side effects: Common adverse reactions include abdominal pain, indigestion, diarrhea, nausea, vomiting, flatulence, constipation, headache, and menstrual changes. Rare but potentially serious side effects include allergic reaction, irregular heart rhythm, heart attack, high blood pressure, low blood pressure, breathing difficulty, and blood clots.

Cost: Approximately $160 to $300 for a 2-month supply (depending on whether you purchase from a Canadian or US pharmacy)

were given either misoprostol or placebo. Not surprisingly, the placebo did not work. Misoprostol, on the other hand, provided improvement for eight (33 percent) of the subjects. According to the investigators, "Responders reported improvement in tinnitus severity, sleep, and concentration."[827]

More than a decade later, Turkish investigators noted that 13 of 28 patients (46 percent) who were given misoprostol reported a decline in the volume of their tinnitus, compared to only 2 of 14 subjects (14 percent) in the control group.[828] A follow-up study found that 18 of 28 patients "showed improvement in tinnitus loudness, representing an improvement rate of 64 percent."[829] These are all small studies, and larger, more comprehensive, and longer follow-up research is required to prove that misoprostol represents a true advance in the treatment of tinnitus.

Conclusions

Compared to heart disease, diabetes, and cancer, tinnitus seems like a trivial complaint. But ask anyone who suffers from it and you will discover that it can have devastating consequences on the person's quality of life. The constant ringing or hissing not only affects concentration, it also can interfere with sleep. Many people with tinnitus are depressed, and some even contemplate suicide. There is no cure and no perfect treatment. Nevertheless, there are some options worth considering.

- Avoid loud noise, including common household appliances like blenders, hair dryers, vacuum cleaners, and power tools. Concerts, sporting events, and airports call for ear protection. Noise can make tinnitus worse.

- Beware of prescription medicines and over-the-counter remedies that can trigger tinnitus or make it worse. Even the quinine in tonic water can be a problem for some people.

- Some people benefit from antianxiety agents like alprazolam (Xanax) or antidepressants such as nortriptyline. These drugs are not without side effects, however.

- Seek professional advice about new technology that combines a hearing aid with a masking device. This equipment may help improve hearing and reduce the ringing. Try to negotiate for a trial period to test the hearing aid so you can make sure you are satisfied before shelling out thousands of dollars to purchase it.

- Give ginkgo biloba a try. Although the research is not very supportive, ginkgo may help and it is relatively inexpensive. Make sure that it won't interact with any other medicine you are taking.

- Consider melatonin. This natural compound appears to be quite safe and may help tinnitus sufferers get some much-needed sleep.

- If all else fails, your physician might prescribe misoprostol. A few small studies have found it useful for about one-third to two-thirds of tinnitus patients. Its price and side effects are daunting, however.

WEIGHT LOSS

• Find a diet plan that fits your style	
• Keep a dietary diary	★★★★★
• Eat a high-protein breakfast	
• Use a pedometer to reach 10,000 steps	★★★★★
• Try Alli (orlistat) for an OTC weight loss crutch	★★
• Ask your doctor about Acomplia (rimonabant)	★★★★

By now you are probably sick and tired of hearing about the obesity epidemic in America. You already know that bigger is *not* better and that a large waist size increases the risk of diabetes, high blood pressure, and heart disease. But shedding pounds—and keeping them off—is one of the great challenges of modern life.

It's not that there is any shortage of advice. There are dozens of diet programs and probably hundreds of diet books available to help you shed pounds, preferably painlessly. Effortless weight loss seems to be the perennial American dream. Some of the diets keep popping up like perennials, as well.

One of them, misleadingly titled "the new mayo clinic diet," has been circulating on the Internet for a decade. Even then, it was a resuscitation of the "old" mayo clinic diet that had been passed from person to person since the 1960s. The actual Mayo Clinic has disavowed this diet in any of its incarnations, but that doesn't stop enthusiasts from claiming that you can achieve weight loss of 50 pounds in 2 months by following the plan. People are instructed to breakfast upon eggs, bacon, and grapefruit. Lunch consists of salad, meat, and the ubiquitous grapefruit. For dinner, the dieter has (you guessed it) half a grapefruit plus as much meat as he or she wants and a green or red vegetable cooked in butter. People are encouraged to eat until they are full.

The sad and simple truth is that there are no shortcuts to the shape you want. Taking off pounds requires taking in less energy than you are using up. This equation has two parts: how much you eat and how much you exercise. Changing either part calls for more effort than many of us can muster in an environment that encourages us to eat more and exercise less. No doubt that's why new diets have such appeal, even though they are often a familiar approach recycled with a new twist.

There are so many diet plans out there that we can't possibly tell you about each one. Instead, we will stick to some general guidelines that may help you figure out the best approach for you. This is an arena in which one size does not fit all and, sadly enough, there is no magic bullet. Getting weight under control can be quite a challenge, but it is also a great opportunity to improve your health.

Dietary Approaches

There is no question that diet is crucial to weight loss. You may not want, or even need, to count calories. But even if you take a diet pill, you can't lose weight without paying attention to what you eat. Dietitians are fond of pointing out that losing weight is a simple matter of using up fewer calories than you take in. "Simple" it may be, but it isn't easy, as too many of us know! For best results, of course, you need to work on both sides of the equation.

Pick a Plan

Which diet is best for weight loss? That is a difficult question to answer. Most of the popular diets have not been subjected to rigorous study. Even when they have been studied, few of them have gone head-to-head with others to determine the better or best one.

Scientists at Tufts University did undertake a comparison of four popular diets under "real world" conditions. They enrolled people in the trial and then assigned them randomly to the low-carbohydrate Atkins diet, the low-fat Ornish diet, the Weight Watchers diet plan, or the Zone diet. Although there were some interesting differences in the blood fats at the end of the study, in terms of weight loss, the programs were about the same.[830] People on the more extreme diets—the low-carb Atkins and the low-fat Ornish—lost a bit more weight than those on the more moderate diets. But more people dropped out of those diet groups as well, perhaps because the more extreme diets are harder to follow.

The main trick is to figure out what diet plan you prefer. We don't mean "what you like to eat"; if you use a diet that focuses heavily on what you like to eat, it will be far too easy to eat too much. No, you need to ask yourself what you are willing to eat. If going without a single piece of cheese for a year will be a major deprivation, you might not want to adopt a super-low-fat approach. If your Italian soul can't survive without pasta, an ultra-low-carb approach is probably out. But don't fret too much. Either diet will work, if you stick with it. And so will a lot of the more moderate diet approaches. The social reinforcement built into the Weight Watchers plan can be very helpful for some people; it drives others nuts.

A meta-analysis of diet studies shows that both low-carbohydrate and low-fat diets are about equally effective for weight loss.[831] The question is, Do you need to raise good HDL cholesterol and lower triglycerides as well? If so, choose a low-carb diet. But if you really need to get your total cholesterol and your bad LDL cholesterol under control, the low-fat diet is a better way to go.

We have a friend who has managed to lose and keep off about 30 pounds over the years. This weight loss has brought his total cholesterol down so well that he does not need a cholesterol-lowering drug. This surprised his doctor, who assumed that he would require a prescription for Lipitor (atorvastatin) or Zocor (simvastatin) sooner or later.

What impresses us is his persistence. He is always very careful about what he eats. We asked him how he manages to keep it up day after day, and he said he makes it like a game with himself. He actually shifts back and forth between a low-carb pattern and a low-fat pattern, which helps him prevent boredom. But on any given day, he decides which diet he is following and challenges himself to see how closely he can adhere to it. We don't know if he gives himself points or has a reward system set up. But playing the game of eating right has a lot of rewards built into it, not the least of which is weight control.

If you like the idea of a game, then we have a wonderful "diet" book to recommend: *Eat, Drink, and Weigh Less,* by the fabulous vegetarian cookbook author Mollie Katzen and the respected nutrition researcher Walter C. Willett, MD, DrPH, MPH. They devised a numeric concept, the body score, that makes it easy to measure how well you are eating and challenge yourself to do even better.[832]

Write It Down

Aside from getting you to focus more on low-calorie, high-nutrient vegetables and fruits, calculating your body score brings another tool into play: the dietary diary. Even if you do nothing else in your weight loss efforts, do this. Get yourself a portable notebook. It can be as nice as you like, or as inexpensive as a little flip pad. But it does need to be small, because you should take it with you everywhere you go and write down everything you eat. Not just the menus of your meals, though that is necessary and can be fun. You must also note every tidbit, every nut, every chocolate chip that you eat between meals.

And don't forget to write down what you drink as well. Some of us get a lot of calories

★★★★★ Dietary Diary

No matter which diet you plan to follow, this allows you to track your progress. The simple act of writing it down can help you become more aware of what you are eating. You learn to ask yourself, Do I really want this?

In addition, you can analyze the information in your dietary diary to see what circumstances conspire against your sticking to your plan. Try to figure out other ways to deal with problems like having to rush from appointment to appointment and therefore missing lunch, then discovering that you are starving before dinner and gobbling down a bag of tortilla chips with nacho cheese sauce.

Downside: Inconvenience. But if you stick with it, writing down what you eat and what else is happening can be a great way to reinforce your diet.

Cost: It's up to you. You could spend as little as 69 cents on a small notebook or as much as $30 on an elegant bound diary.

from sweetened beverages like soft drinks, fruit drinks, or sweet teas. In fact, this makes up 21 percent of our national calorie consumption.[833] Switching to water most of the time could make a substantial difference in energy intake for some people.

Eat Breakfast

It might seem like a good idea to save on calories—and time—by skipping breakfast. You've got enough trouble just trying to get dressed, pull together everything you'll need for the day, and get out the door. If you're a parent, you may need to do all of that for your children, as well! It's not easy. But going without breakfast, or grabbing just a cup of coffee and a piece of toast, is a bad idea. A study that has looked at people who have successfully lost weight and kept it off found that most of them make breakfast an important meal, or at least a reliable one.[834]

There are probably some breakfast choices that might be worse for dieters than no breakfast at all. Coffee and a Danish pastry come to mind; so do orange juice and a big stack of pancakes dripping with butter and maple syrup. Foods like this are high in sugar and refined flour that are quickly absorbed and push blood sugar and insulin up rapidly. (This can be quantified in scientific terms as the glycemic index of a food, which compares the food's effect on blood glucose to that of table sugar.) The result, though, may be that your blood sugar level will crash in 2 or 3 hours, resulting in fatigue and maybe even hunger. Instead of these high-glycemic-index treats that will send

blood sugar and insulin on a roller-coaster ride—first way up, then down, way down—you want a meal that will carry you through until lunchtime. That way you have a better chance of resisting the midmorning siren call of cookies or pastry. Breakfast is especially important for children, who pay better attention in school with a little nutrition under their belts.

We like a light scramble made of mostly egg whites plus a whole egg. If that's too much trouble, how about low-fat cottage cheese with some vegetables? Our quickest breakfast, a smoothie, still has a fair bit of protein in it: a frozen banana (peel it before you put it in the freezer!), a couple of scoops of powdered whey protein, a few teaspoons of powdered egg white, a cup or so of frozen fruit or berries, and about ¾ cup of yogurt and just enough fruit juice to get the blender to work. With the juice, you don't need any sweetener; the whey and egg white are good protein, much better than yogurt alone; and the berries offer all kinds of nutrients as well as fiber. Anyway, the point here is that you should find a breakfast that fits your tastes and lifestyle and satisfies you so you won't need a snack before lunch.

Keep Moving

As we pointed out earlier, even the most rigorous diet is only half of the story. The other half is increasing your energy expenditure through physical activity. It needs to be tailored to your lifestyle just as carefully as your meal plan.

The majority of Americans just don't use their muscles very much. If there were games or sports you enjoyed when you were younger, think about whether you might find the time to dust off the rust and go back to playing tennis, say, or dancing. Choosing something you love means you'll want to do it frequently, and that is more important than the type of exercise. Gardening, swimming, martial arts, yoga, bicycling, or anything else that gets you moving is fair game. There is definitely some activity that will help you use your muscles; it is up to you to figure out what it is and go for it.

If you can't think of anything else, consider walking. It's cheap and readily available, and it's good exercise. All you need is a pair of decent

shoes and about 20 minutes to spare. If you have been very sedentary, you don't even want to start with 20 minutes. Begin with 5 minutes and gradually work your way up to longer walks. To give yourself something of an extra challenge, get a step-counting pedometer. Then strive for 10,000 steps a day. Write down your step count every night in your dietary diary. When you can get to 10,000 steps reliably, day after day, set yourself a new challenge.

Herbal Disappointment

Dozens of dietary supplements are promoted as weight loss aids, but the science supporting most of them is lacking. Even when a study is done, the difference between those who took the product and those who took placebo is generally quite modest, possibly just a few pounds over several months. So if someone tries to sell you an all-natural supplement from somewhere exotic—whether it's the Amazon, Outer Mongolia, or the North Pole—be suspicious. If you are told that the agent will turn on your fat burners or turbocharge your metabolism, double your skepticism. People have been selling herbal diet pills for more than 30 years. If they really worked, we'd all be as thin as we'd like to be. In most cases, the only thing that will lose weight is your wallet.

The track record for herbal diet pills is frankly rather discouraging. For quite a while, ephedra (*Ephedra sinica*) was promoted as a natural weight loss aid. Companies producing ephedra products made a lot of money until, eventually, the FDA reviewed all the reports of

---

★★★★★ **Pedometer**

This gadget is a favorite at our house. It's small and lightweight, so you can set it to 0, clip it on your belt, and wear it all day long just to see how many steps you take. Of course, if you have a favorite walking or running course, you can measure the distance in miles or kilometers by wearing the pedometer while you traverse it. The goal of taking 10,000 steps a day is definitely doable, but it provides a good challenge. Public health folks offer it as a starting point.

Downside: It can be tricky to figure out the best place to wear this gadget to get an accurate count. Setting the pedometer so it measures your stride is not as hard as programming a VCR, but it can be a challenge.

Cost: Approximately $25 to $30. You can spend more, but you don't need to.

problems with this herb. The agency determined that ephedra was associated with a number of strokes, heart attacks, and other serious complications and called for its removal from the market. Aside from being overweight, some of the people who suffered life-threatening or even fatal side effects were otherwise in good health. This stimulant might have helped people shed pounds in the short term, but it was not safe enough to be used for the long haul.

Ephedra has stimulant properties, which probably account both for its ability to promote some weight loss and for its potential to trigger a dangerous reaction. A couple of other natural products with stimulant activity have been suggested for use in weight loss. Green tea[835] and yerba maté[836] have been considered for this purpose, though the research so far is not impressive. Both contain caffeine, along with other compounds that might be relevant.

Another purported stimulant, *Garcinia cambogia* (hydroxycitric acid), has also been included in a number of herbal weight loss preparations. A 3-month randomized controlled diet did not demonstrate any weight loss benefit beyond that of placebo.[837]

• • •

Q. *What is hoodia? I keep getting e-mail messages that this is a wonderful way to lose weight. Does it work? Is it safe?*

A. Hoodia is a cactus that grows in the Kalahari Desert in southern Africa. It is being promoted as a marvelous weight loss agent, but there is very little clinical research to support the claims.

One small, unpublished study (18 obese patients) demonstrated some benefit, but we would need to see far more evidence before recommending this plant product. Questions have been raised about the quality control used in manufacturing hoodia products, and long-term safety has not been established.

• • •

Nonprescription Help

One of the reasons that ephedra became so popular was that there were only a few other choices available without a prescription. The most popular over-the-counter (OTC) weight loss ingredient was a decongestant called phenylpropanolamine, or PPA for short. In its heyday during the 1970s and 1980s, Dexatrim was one of the most popular brands.

PPA was not as safe as most dieters assumed, however. As early as 1980, British researchers had raised a red flag. When they gave PPA to healthy young medical students, they noted side effects such as an alarming elevation in blood pressure along with dizziness, heart palpitations, headache, insomnia, anxiety, and restlessness. By 1990, doctors in the United States had reported 142 bad reactions to PPA, including bleeding stroke, seizure, and even death. But it

★★ Orlistat (Alli)

This weight loss medication is also available by prescription under the name Xenical. It appears to be one of the few weight loss drugs considered safe for long-term use. Orlistat is intended to be used in conjunction with a reduced-calorie, reduced-fat diet. The drug prevents the absorption of fat from the gastrointestinal tract. Nearly twice as many people on orlistat manage to lose 15 percent of their body weight in a year as people on diet restrictions alone.

Side effects: Most of the side effects are gastrointestinal. Because orlistat prevents the absorption of fat, fat is retained in the intestines. This may result in stomachache, diarrhea, nausea, flatulence, rectal discharge, and fecal incontinence. Headache is also a possible side effect.

Downside: The drug may interfere with the absorption of fat-soluble vitamins. Take a multivitamin either 2 hours prior to or 2 hours after taking Alli.

Cost: Approximately $50 to $60 per month

took the FDA 10 years to make a move. It requested a study of PPA's safety, particularly with respect to bleeding stroke. Yale investigators found that women who took PPA for the first time in a cough or cold remedy tripled their risk of a stroke. Those using the drug as an appetite suppressant appeared to be at 16 times the stroke risk of a woman not taking the drug.[838]

Given these data, FDA staffers estimated that PPA might be responsible for 200 to 500 strokes in people under the age of 50 each year. Extrapolating over all the years it was on the market, PPA could have accounted for as many as 10,000 strokes in people who otherwise would not have been vulnerable to that problem. The agency announced in 2000 that OTC weight loss products would need to be reformulated without PPA. This meant that most dieters could no longer rely on a pill to help them. Ephedra had been taken off the market because it was too

dangerous. And PPA was removed as well, also because it was not safe enough.

With the approval of orlistat (available by prescription as Xenical) to go over the counter under the name Alli, people finally have a tested do-it-yourself option. The company has chosen the name Alli to imply that it will work best if allied with a full program of dietary and behavior modification approaches. The FDA appears confident that this drug does not pose significant safety issues.

Orlistat is a compound that prevents the absorption of fat. It can help people lose weight, but there are some drawbacks. For one thing, there's the underwear risk: spotting with oily stool. There also may be increased flatulence, sometimes with discharge. Orlistat doesn't take you off the hook for eating carefully: The 5- to 6-pound weight loss advantage over placebo occurs only when people eat a reduced-calorie, low-fat diet. Unfortunately, once people stop the medication, they often gain back the weight they lost.

Perhaps Alli would be best used as a "jump start" by someone who's having a hard time pulling together the pieces of a diet plan. Few people will want to take it year after year, although it does appear to be cost-effective.[839]

Prescription Weight-Loss Drugs

The history of prescription diet pills in the United States is full of woe and intrigue. Starting in the 1950s, millions of overweight Americans were prescribed amphetamines to help them shed a few extra pounds. Such stimulants were supposed to be taken for only a few months at a time, but they were extremely seductive. Many respectable housewives became dependent on "speed." This made physicians a bit more cautious about prescribing such medications to help people lose weight.

During the 1990s doctors began to combine two diet pills that had been around for decades. The combination of fenfluramine and phentermine ("fen-phen") seemed to work better than either drug alone. The only trouble was, the combination led to heart valve complications. At about the same time, a new appetite suppressant, dexfenfluramine (Redux), was approved. It, too, was associated with heart problems and a potentially life-threatening condition called pulmonary hypertension.

In 1997, the FDA asked the manufacturer to withdraw Redux from the market, although it had been approved only the year before. Fenfluramine was also taken off the market. The fen-phen fiasco was certainly a spectacular disaster. Quite a number of people were left with damaged hearts just because they took drugs to help them lose weight.

Despite this uninspired track record, many people can hardly wait for the FDA to approve a new diet pill. The claims being made about rimonabant (Acomplia) are extraordinary. It is easy to understand why some people might be eager to try it, even if others are skeptical.

The manufacturer, Sanofi-Aventis, is being especially careful to downplay the cosmetic weight-reducing potential of Acomplia. Instead, they are highlighting other benefits, such as the improvement of lipid profiles. In three large clinical trials, Acomplia resulted in promising metabolic improvements.[840,841,842] Good HDL cholesterol rose and bad triglycerides dropped. Insulin efficiency improved and blood sugar levels came down. The positive changes were twice what researchers would have anticipated from weight loss alone. Such metabolic effects may be especially beneficial for people with type 2 diabetes.

What really has millions of people excited, though, is Acomplia's ability to lower weight. After 1 year on the drug, subjects lost approximately 15 pounds, significantly more than those on placebo. In the world of diet pills, such a loss is impressive.

The buzz surrounding Acomplia is enormous. Weight loss and improvements in blood glucose, blood pressure, and lipids are certainly much needed. In addition, investigators

★★★★ Rimonabant (Acomplia)

Acomplia is different from other prescription diet pills because it works on an entirely new mechanism. It blocks brain CB(1) (cannabinoid 1) receptors that respond to natural marijuana-like compounds. It is more effective than any other medication for weight loss, helping people lose more than 15 pounds over the course of a year.

Acomplia also has beneficial effects on good HDL cholesterol, triglycerides, insulin efficiency, blood sugar level, and blood pressure.

Side effects: Nausea, diarrhea, dizziness, headache, sore throat or flu, anxiety, insomnia, and depression. Most of these were mild and transient, although the depression does give us pause.

Downside: We don't have much information on the long-term effects of this new medicine.

are studying whether Acomplia may help people quit smoking. There is even some hope that the compound may help people deal effectively with other drug dependencies, including the most prevalent one, alcohol.[843]

Whether Acomplia lives up to such high expectations remains to be seen. It could take years to assess whether the drug is really safe enough for long-term use.

Conclusions

Losing excess weight is notoriously difficult, but it can have a profound effect on health. Dropping pounds can help lower blood pressure and get cholesterol under control, as well as alleviating the strain on arthritic joints. Weight loss is probably approached best as a long-term change in lifestyle rather than a short-term goal. If Weight Watchers or a similar program that offers social support appeals to you, by all means try it out. Here are some other suggestions that may help.

- Find a diet plan that appeals to you. The only program that will work is one that you can stick with long-term.
- Keep a dietary diary. Write down every single morsel that you stick in your mouth and when. Most of the weight loss gurus that we have consulted over the last few decades emphasize that this one behavior is essential for lasting success.
- Eat a high-protein breakfast. No more bagels and butter. Skip the orange juice and coffee. A low-glycemic-index meal will carry you through to lunch.
- Find an exercise you like. Get a pedometer and strive for 10,000 steps a day. Plot your progress in your dietary diary or on a computer.
- If you need a pharmacological boost, consider Alli (orlistat). This fat blocker may help you lose a few pounds, though the side effects might be embarrassing. Don't forget to take your vitamins if you take this drug.
- If all else fails, Acomplia (rimonabant) may provide the help you need to lose weight, improve your cardiometabolic risk factors, and quit smoking. Check with your doctor about the benefits and risks of this prescription drug.

REFERENCES

Acne

[1] Cordain, L., et al. "Acne Vulgaris: A Disease of Western Civilization." *Arch. Dermatol.* 2002;138:1584–1590.

[2] Cordain, L., et al. "Origins and Evolution of the Western Diet: Health Implications for the 21st Century." *Am. J. Clin. Nutr.* 2005;81:341–354.

[3] Thiboutot, D. M., and Strauss, J. S. "Diet and Acne Revisited." *Arch. Dermatol.* 2002;138:1591–1592.

[4] Treloar, V. "Diet and Acne Redux." *Arch. Dermatol.* 2003;139:941.

[5] Bershad, S. "The Unwelcome Return of the Acne Diet." *Arch. Dermatol.* 2003;139:940–941.

[6] Wolf, R., et al. "Acne and Diet." *Clin. Dermatol.* 2004;22:387–393.

[7] Adebamowo, C. A., et al. "High School Dietary Dairy Intake and Teenage Acne." *J. Am. Acad. Dermatol.* 2005;52:207–214.

[8] Wait, M., ed. *1,801 Home Remedies: Trustworthy Treatments for Everyday Health Problems.* Pleasantville, NY: Reader's Digest, 2004. p. 31.

[9] Bassett, I. B., et al. "A Comparative Study of Tea Tree Oil versus Benzoyl Peroxide in the Treatment of Acne." *Med. J. Aust.* 1990;153:455–458.

[10] Dreno, B., et al. "Erythromycin-Resistance of Cutaneous Bacterial Flora in Acne." Eur. J. Dermatol. 2001;11:549–553.

[11] Shalita, A. R., et al. "Topical Nicotinamide Compared with Clindamycin Gel in the Treatment of Inflammatory Acne Vulgaris." *Int. J. Dermatol.* 1995;34:434–437.

[12] Tanno, O., et al. "Nicotinamide Increases Biosynthesis of Ceramides as Well as Other Stratum Corneum Lipids to Improve the Epidermal Permeability Barrier." *Br. J. Dermatol.* 2000;143:524–531.

[13] Bissett, D. "Topical Niacinamide and Barrier Enhancement." *Cutis* 2002;70:S8–S12.

[14] Garner, S. E., et al. "Minocycline for Acne Vulgaris: Efficacy and Safety." *Cochrane Database Syst. Rev.* 2003;(1):CD002086.

[15] Margolis, D. J., et al. "Antibiotic Treatment of Acne May Be Associated with Upper Respiratory Tract Infections." *Arch. Dermatol.* 2005;141:1132–1136.

[16] Thiboutot, D. M., et al. "Adapalene Gel, 0.1%, as Maintenance Therapy for Acne Vulgaris." *Arch. Dermatol.* 2006;142:597–602.

[17] Leyden, J., et al. "Comparison of Tazarotene and Minocycline Maintenance Therapies in Acne Vulgaris: A Multicenter, Double-blind, Randomized, Parallel-Group Study." *Arch. Dermatol.* 2006;142:605–612.

[18] Panzer, C., et al. "Impact of Oral Contraceptives on Sex Hormone–Binding Globulin and Androgen Levels: A Retrospective Study in Women with Sexual Dysfunction." *J. Sex. Med.* 2006;3:104–113.

Allergies

[19] Bender, B. G. "Cognitive Effects of Allergic Rhinitis and Its Treatment." *Immunol. Allergy Clin. North Am.* 2005;25:301–312.

[20] Ibid.

[21] Ramaekers, J. G., and Vermeeren, A. "All Antihistamines Cross Blood-Brain Barrier." *BMJ* 2000; 321:572.

[22] Verster, J. C., and Volkerts, E. R. "Antihistamines and Driving Ability: Evidence from On-the-Road Driving Studies During Normal Traffic." *Ann. Allergy Asthma Immunol.* 2004:92:292–303.

[23] Thomas, K. "Distracted Drivers Risky Behind Wheel." *Associated Press*, April 21, 2006.

[24] American Academy of Allergy, Asthma and Immunology. *The Allergy Report: Science Based Findings on the Diagnosis & Treatment of Allergic Disorders*, 1996–2001.

[25] "New Concerns about Ionizing Air Cleaners." *Consumer Reports* May 5, 2005.

[26] "Ratings: Whole-House Cleaners CR Quick Recommendations." *Consumer Reports* October 2005.

[27] McDonald, E., et al. "Effect of Air Filtration Systems on Asthma: A Systematic Review of Randomized Trials." *Chest* 2002;122:1509–1510.

[28] Wood, R. A., et al. "A Placebo-Controlled Trial of a HEPA Air Cleaner in the Treatment of Cat Allergy." *Am. J. Respir. Crit. Care Med.* 1998;158:115–120.

[29] Green, R., et al. "The Effect of Air Filtration on Airborne Dog Allergen." *Allergy* 1999;54:484–488.

[30] Bernstein, J. A., et al. "A Pilot Study to Investigate the Effects of Combined Dehumidification and HEPA Filtration on Dew Point and Airborne Mold Spore Counts in Day Care Centers." *Indoor Air* 2005;15:402–407.

[31] Terreehorst, I., et al. "Evaluation of Impermeable Covers for Bedding in Patients with Allergic Rhinitis." *N. Engl. J. Med.* 2003;349:237–246.

[32] Woodcock, A., et al. "Control of Exposure to Mite Allergen and Allergen-Impermeable Bed Covers for Adults with Asthma." *N. Engl. J. Med.* 2003;349:225–236.

[33] Dharmage, S., et al. "Encasement of Bedding Does Not Improve Asthma in Atopic Adult Asthmatics." *Int. Arch. Allergy Immunol.* 2006;139:132–138.

[34] "Vacuums: New Choices, New Problems." *Consumer Reports* March 2006.

[35] Bucca, C., et al. "Effect of Vitamin C on Histamine Bronchial Responsiveness of Patients with Allergic Rhinitis." *Ann. Allergy* 1990;65:311–314.

[36] Johnston, C. S. "The Antihistamine Action of Ascorbic Acid." *Subcell. Biochem.* 1996;25:189–213.

[37] Anderson, R. "The Immunostimulatory, Antiinflammatory and Anti-Allergic Properties of Ascorbate." *Adv. Nutr. Res.* 1984;6:19–45.

[38] Bucca, op. cit.

[39] Thornhill, S. M., and Kelly, A. M. "Natural Treatment of Perennial Allergic Rhinitis." *Altern. Med. Rev.* 2000;5:448–454.

[40] Mittman, P. "Randomized, Double Blind Study of Freeze Dried *Urtica dioica* in the Treatment of Allergic Rhinitis." *Planta Med.* 1990;56:44–47.

[41] Melmon, K. L., et al. "Autocoids as Modulators of the Inflammatory and Immune Response." *Am. J. Med.* 1981;71:100–106.

[42] Bent, S., et al. "Saw Palmetto for Benign Prostate Hyperplasia." *N. Engl. J. Med.* 2006;354:632–634.

[43] Schapowal, A., et al. "Randomised Controlled Trial of Butterbur and Cetirizine for Treating Seasonal Allergic Rhinitis." *BMJ* 2002;324:1–4.

[44] Otsuka, H., et al. "Histochemical and Functional Characteristics of Metachromatic Cells in the Nasal Epithelium in Allergic Rhinitis: Studies of Nasal Scrapings and Their Dispersed Cells." *J. Allergy Clin. Immunol.* 1995;96:528–536.

[45] Taussig, S. "The Mechanism of the Physiological Action of Bromelain." *Med. Hypothesis* 1980;6:99–104.

[46] Busse, W. W., et al. "Flavonoid Modulation of Human Neutrophil Function." *J. Allergy Clin. Immunol.* 1984;73:801–809.

[47] Conboy-Ellis, K. "Management of Seasonal Allergic Rhinitis: Comparative Efficacy of the Newer-Generation Prescription Antihistamines." *J. Am. Acad. Nurse Pract.* 2005;17:295–301.

[48] Bender, op. cit.

[49] Bender, B. G., et al. "Sedation and Performance Impairment of Diphenhydramine and Second-Generation Antihistamines: A Meta-Analysis." *J. Allergy Clin. Immunol.* 2003;111:770–776.

[50] Bender, op. cit., 2005.

[51] Weller, J. M., et al. "Effects of Fexofenadine, Diphenhydramine, and Alcohol on Driving Performance: A Randomized, Placeo-Controlled Trial in the Iowa Driving Simulator." *Ann. Intern. Med.* 2000;132: 354–363.

[52] Vermeeren, A., and O'Hanlon, J. "Fexofenadine's Effects, Alone and With Alcohol, on Actual Driving and Psychomotor Performance." *J. Allergy Clin. Immunol.* 1998;101:306–311.

[53] "Drugs for Allergic Disorders." *Treatment Guidelines from the Medical Letter.* 2003;1:93–100.

[54] Bender, op. cit.

[55] Prenner, B. M., and Schenkel, E. "Allergic Rhinitis: Treatment Based on Patient Profiles." *Am. J. Med.* 2006;119:230–237.

[56] Mucha, S. M., et al. "Comparison of Montelukast and Pseudoephedrine in the Treatment of Allergic Rhinitis." *Arch. Otolaryngol. Head Neck Surg.* 2006;132:164–172.

Arthritis

[57] Lethbridge–Cejku, M., et al. "Summary Health Statistics for U.S. Adults: National Health Interview Survey 2002." *Vital Health Stat.* 2004;10(222); 1–151.

[58] Bolen, J., et al. "Racial/Ethnic Differences in the Prevalence and Impact of Doctor-Diagnosed Arthritis: United States, 2002." *MMWR* 2005;54;119–123.

[59] Lethbridge–Cejku. op. cit.

[60] Bjordal, J. M., et al. "Non-Steroidal Anti-Inflammatory Drugs, Including Cyclo-Oxygenase-2 Inhibitors, in Osteoarthritic Knee Pain: Meta-Analysis of Randomised Placebo Controlled Trials." *BMJ* 2004;December 4;329(7478):1317. Epub. 2004 Nov. 23.

[61] Huskisson, E. C., et al. "Effects of Anti-Inflammatory Drugs on the Progression of Osteoarthritis of the Knee." *J. Rheumatol.* 1995;22:1941–1946.

[62] Rashad, S., et al. "Effect of Non-Steroidal Anti-Inflammatory Drugs on the Course of Osteoarthritis." *Lancet* 1989;2:519–521.

[63] Vignon, E., et al. "Effects of Naproxen (Naprosyne) on the Metabolism of Arthrotic Cartilage in Man in Vivo." *Rev. Rhum. Mal. Osteoartic.* 1991;58:11S–15S.

[64] Reijman, M., et al. "Is There an Association Between the Use of Different Types of Nonsteroidal Anti-Inflammatory Drugs and Radiologic Progression of Osteoarthritis." *Arthritis & Rheumatism* 2005;52:3137–3142.

[65] Wilcox, C. M., et al. "Patterns of Use and Public Perception of Over-the-Counter Pain Relievers: Focus on Nonsteroidal Anti-Inflammatory Drugs." *J. Rheumatol.* 2005;32:2218–2224.

[66] Ibid.

[67] Ibid.

[68] Laine, L. "Proton Pump Inhibitor Co-Therapy with Nonsteroidal Anti-Inflammatory Drugs: Nice or Necessary?" *Rev. Gastroenterol. Disord.* 2004;Suppl. 4:S33–S41.

[69] Singh, G., and Triadafilopoulus, G. "Epidemiology of NSAID-Induced GI complications." *J. Rheumatol.* 1999;26:Suppl. 26:18–24.

[70] Wolfe, M. M., et al. "Gastrointestinal Toxicity of Nonsteroidal Anti-Inflammatory Drugs." *N. Engl. J. Med.* 1999;340:1888–1899.

[71] Wolfe, M. M., op. cit.

[72] Graham, D. Y., et al. "Visible Small-Intestinal Mucosal Injury in Chronic NSAID Users." *Clin. Gastroenterol. Hepatol.* 2005;3:55–59.

[73] Qureshi, W. A., Personal Communication, February 12, 2005.

[74] Bombardier, C., et al. "Comparison of Upper Gastrointestinal Toxicity of Rofecoxib and Naproxen in Patients with Rheumatoid Arthritis." *N. Engl. J. Med.* 2000;343:1520–1528.

[75] Topol, E. J. "Failing the Public Health: Rofecoxib, Merck, and the FDA." *N. Engl. J. Med.* 2004;351:1707–1709.

[76] Goozner, M. "What Went Wrong? FDA veteran David Graham speaks out on the drug safety dilemma." *AARP Bulletin*, February 2005.

[77] Topol, E. "Arthritis Medicines and Cardiovascular Events: 'House of Coxibs.'" *JAMA* 2005;293:366–368.

[78] Mamdani, M., et al. "Gastrointestinal Bleeding After the Introduction of COX 2 Inhibitors: Ecological Study." *BMJ* 2004;328:1415–1416.

[79] Hippisley-Cox, J., et al. "Risk of Adverse Gastrointestinal Outcomes in Patients Taking Cyclo-Oxygenase-2 Inhibitors or Conventional Non-Steroidal Anti-Inflammatory Drugs: Population Based Nested Case-Control Analysis." BMJ 2005;331:1310–1316.

[80] FDA Public Health Advisory, "FDA Announces Important Changes and Additional Warnings for COX-2 Selective and Non-Selective Non-Steroidal Anti-Inflammatory Drugs (NSAIDs)." April 7, 2005.

[81] Chan, F. K. L., et al. "Celecoxib versus Diclofenac and Omeprazole in Reducing the Risk of Recurrent Ulcer Bleeding in Patients with Arthritis." *N. Engl. J. Med.* 2002;347:2104–2110.

[82] Maillard, M., and Burnier, M. "Comparative Cardiovascular Safety of Traditional Nonsteroidal Anti-Inflammatory Drugs." *Expert Opin. Drug Saf.* 2006;5:83–94.

[83] Reijman, op. cit.

[84] Rogriguez, L. A. Garcia, and Gonzalez-Perez, A. "Long-Term Use of Traditional Non-Steroidal Anti-Inflammatory Drugs and the Risk of Myocardial Infarction in the General Population." *BMC Med.* 2005;3(1):17 [Epub ahead of print].

[85] Gislason, G. H., et al. "Risk of Death or Reinfarction Associated with the Use of Selective Cyclooxygenase-2 Inhibitors and Nonselective Nonsteroidal Antiinflammatory Drugs After Acute Myocardial Infarction." *Circulation* 2006;113:2906–2913.

[86] Hochman, J. S., and Shah, N. R. "What Price Pain Relief?" *Circulation* 2006;113:2868–2870.

[87] Helin-Salmivaara, A., et al. "NSAID Use and the Risk of Hospitalization for First Myocardial Infarction in the General Population: A Nationwide Case-Control Study from Finland." *Eur. Heart J.* 2006;27:1657-1663.

[88] Patrono, C., et al. "Low-Dose Aspirin for the Prevention of Atherothrombosis." *N. Engl. J. Med.* 2005:353:2373–2383.

[89] Maillard, op. cit.

[90] Lanas, A., and Ferrandez, A. "Treatment and Prevention of Aspirin-Induced Gastroduodenal Ulcers and Gastrointestinal Bleeding." *Expert Opinion Drugs Saf.* 2002;1:245–252.

[91] Patrano, op. cit.

[92] Laine, op. cit.

[93] Moore, R. A., et al. "Quantitative Systematic Review of Topical Applied Non-Steroidal Anti-Inflammatory Drugs." *BMJ* 1998;316:333–338.

[94] Mason, L., et al. "Topical NSAIDs for Acute Pain: A Meta-Analysis." *BMC Fam. Pract.* 2004;5:10.

[95] Mason, L., et al. "Topical NSAIDs for Chronic Musculoskeletal Pain: Systematic Review and Meta-Analysis." *BMC Musculoskelet. Disord.* 2004;5:28.

[96] Lin, J., et al. "Efficacy of Topical Non-Steroidal Anti-Inflammatory Drugs in the Treatment of Osteoarthritis: Meta-Analysis of Randomised Controlled Trials." *BMJ* 2004;329:324.

[97] Baer, P. A., et al. "Treatment of Osteoarthritis of the Knee with a Topical Diclofenac Solution: A Randomised Controlled, 6-Week Trial." *BMC Musculoskelet. Disord.* 2005;6:44.

[98] Arthur, A. M., et al. "Effect of a Topical Diclofenac Solution for Relieving Symptoms of Primary Osteoarthritis of the Knee: A Randomized Controlled Trial." *CMAJ* 2004;171:333–338.

[99] Roth, S. H., and Shainhouse, Z. "Efficacy and Safety of a Topical Diclofenac Solution (Pennsaid) in the Treatment of Primary Osteoarthritis of the Knee: A Randomized, Double-Blind, Vehicle-Controlled Clinical Trial." *Arch. Intern. Med.* 2004;164:2017–2023.

[100] Niethard, F. U., et al. "Efficacy of Topical Diclofenac Diethylamine Gel in Osteoarthritis of the Knee." *J. Rheumatol.* 2005;32:2384–2392.

[101] Tugwell, P. S., et al. "Equivalence Study of a Topical Diclofenac Solution (Pennsaid) Compared with Oral Diclofenac in Symptomatic Treatment of Osteoarthritis of the Knee: A Randomized Controlled Trial." *J. Rheumatol.* 2004; 31:2002–2212.

[102] "Beating Arthritis with the Right Food Choices." *Tufts Univ. Health Nutr. Letter* 2002;20(3):4.

[103] Jordan, J. Communication on *The People's Pharmacy* radio show, November 19, 2005.

[104] Jordan, J. "Study Links Low Selenium Levels with Higher Risk of Osteoarthritis." News Release, University of North Carolina at Chapel Hill, November 14, 2005, No. 570.

[105] Sokoloff, L. "The History of Kashin-Beck Disease." *N. Y. State J. Med.* 1989;89:343–351.

[106] Jordon, J., et al. "Low Selenium Levels Are Associated with Increased Risk for Osteoarthritis of the Knee." Research presented at the American College of Rheumatology Annual Scientific Meeting, November 15, 2005.

[107] Ryan-Harshman, M., and Aldoori, W. "The Relevance of Selenium to Immunity, Cancer and Infectious/Inflammatory Diseases." *Can. J. Diet. Pract. Res.* 2005;66:98–102.

[108] Rayman, M. P. "Selenium in Cancer Prevention: A Review of the Evidence and Mechanism of Action." *Proc. Nutr. Soc.* 2005;64:527–542.

[109] Pattison, D. J., et al. "Dietary Beta-Cryptoxanthin and Inflammatory Polyarthritis: Results from a Population-Based Prospective Study." *Am. J. Clin. Nutr.* 2005;82:451–455.

[110] Holick, M. F. "Sunlight and Vitamin D for Bone Health and Prevention of Autoimmune Diseases, Cancers, and Cardiovascular Disease." *Am. J. Clin. Nutr.* 2004;80(6 Suppl.):1678S–1688S.

[111] Bischoff-Ferrari, H. A. et al. "Fracture Prevention with Vitamin D Supplementation: A Meta-Analysis of Randomized Controlled Trials." *JAMA* 2005;293:2257–2264.

[112] McAlindon, T. E., et al. "Relation of Dietary Intake and Serum Levels of Vitamin D to Progression of Osteo-arthritis of the Knee among Participants in the Framingham Study." *Ann. Int. Med.* 1996;125: 353–359.

[113] Ibid.

[114] Drosos, A. A., et al. "Epidemiology of Adult Rheumatoid Arthritis in Northwest Greece 1987–1995." *J. Rheumatol.* 1997;24:2129–2133.

[115] Shapiro, J. A., et al. "Diet and Rheumatoid Arthritis in Women: A Possible Protective Effect of Fish Consumption." *Epidemiology* 1996;7:256–263.

[116] Skoldstam, L., et al. "An Experimental Study of a Mediterranean Diet Intervention for Patients with Rheumatoid Arthritis." *Ann. Rheum. Dis.* 2003;62:208–214.

[117] Hagfors, L., et al. "Fat Intake and Composition of Fatty Acids in Serum Phospholipids in a Randomized, Controlled, Mediterranean Dietary Intervention Study on Patients with Rheumatoid Arthritis." *Nutr. Metab.* 2005;2:26.

[118] Goggs, R., et al. "Nutraceutical Therapies for Degenerative Joint Diseases: A Critical Review." *Crit. Rev. Food Sci. Nutr.* 2005;45:145–164.

[119] Melhus, H., et al. "Excessive Dietary Intake of Vitamin A Is Associated with Reduced Bone Mineral Density and Increased Risk for Hip Fracture." *Ann. Int. Med.* 1998;129:770–778.

[120] Sears, B. *The Anti-Inflammation Zone: Reversing the Silent Epidemic That's Destroying Our Health.* New York: Regan Books, 2005, p. 80.

[121] Goggs, op cit.

[122] Halpern, G. M. "Anti-Inflammatory Effects of a Stabilized Lipid Extract of *Perna canaliculus* (Lyprinol)." *Allerg. Immunol. (Paris)* 2000;32:272–278.

[123] Bui, L. M., and Bierer, T. L. "Influence of Green Lipped Mussels (*Perna canaliculus*) in Alleviating Signs of Arthritis in Dogs." *Vet. Ther.* 2003;4:397–407.

[124] Halpern, G. M. *The Inflammation Revolution: A Natural Solution for Arthritis, Asthma & Other Inflammatory Disorders.* Garden City Park, NY: Square One, 2005, p. 103.

[125] Freedman, J. E., et al. "Select Flavonoids and Whole Juice from Purple Grapes Inhibit Platelet Function and Enhance Nitric Oxide Release." *Circulation* 2001;103:2792–2798.

[126] USDA Database for the Proanthocyanidin Content of Selected Foods, Prepared by the Nutrient Data Laboratory, August 2004.

[127] Albers, A. R. "The Antiinflammatory Effects of Purple Grape Juice Consumption in Subjects with Stable Coronary Artery Disease." *Arterioscler. Thromb. Vasc. Biol.* 2004;24:e179–e180.

[128] Folts, J. D. "Potential Health Benefits from the Flavonoids in Grape Products on Vascular Disease." *Adv. Exp. Med. Biol.* 2002;505:95–111.

[129] Aviram, M., et al. "Pomegranate Juice Consumption Reduces Oxidative Stress, Atherogenic Modifications to LDL, and Platelet Aggregation: Studies in Humans and in Atherosclerotic Apolipoprotein E-deficient Mice." *Am. J. Clin. Nutr.* 2000;71:1062–1076.

[130] Azadozoi, K. M., et al. "Oxidative Stress in Arteriogenic Erectile Dysfunction: Prophylactic Role of Antioxidants." *J. Urol.* 2005;174:386–393.

[131] Ahmed, S., et al. "*Punica granatum L.* Extract Inhibits IL-1beta-induced Expression of Matrix Metalloproteinases by Inhibiting the Activation of MAP Kinases and NF-kappaB in Human Chondrocytes in Vitro. *J. Nutr.* 2005;135:2096–2102.

[132] Haqqi, T. Communication on *The People's Pharmacy* radio show #559, September 17, 2005.

[133] Jacob, R. A., et al. "Consumption of Cherries Lowers Plasma Urate in Healthy Women." *J. Nutr.* 2003; 133:1826–1829.

[134] Blau, L. W. "Cherry Diet Control for Gout and Arthritis." *Tex. Rep. Biol. Med.* 1950;8:309–311.

[135] Shakibaei, M., et al. "Curcumin Protects Human Chondrocytes from IL-11beta-Induced Inhibition of Collage Type II and Beta1-Integrin Expression and Activation of Caspase-2: An Immunomorphological Study." *Ann. Anat.* 2005;187:487–497.

[136] Chainani-Wu, N. "Safety and Anti-Inflammatory Activity of Curcumin: A Component of Tumeric (*Curcuma longa*). *J. Alt. Comp. Med.* 2003;9:161–168.

[137] Reichling, J., et al. "Dietary Support with Boswellia Resin in Canine Inflammatory Joint and Spinal Disease." *Schweiz. Arch. Tierheilkd.* 2004;146:71–79.

[138] Kimmatkar, N., et al. "Efficacy and Tolerability of *Boswellia serrata* Extract in Treatment of Osteoarthritis of Knee: A Randomized Double Blind Placebo Controlled Trial." *Phytomedicine* 2003; 10:3–7.

[139] Badria, F., et al. "Boswellia-Curcumin Preparation for Treating Knee Osteoarthritis." *Alt. Comp. Ther.* 2002;December:341–348.

[140] Altman, R. D., and Marcussen, K. C. "Marcussen "Effects of a Ginger Extract on Knee Pain in Patients with Osteoarthritis." *Arthritis Rheum.* 2001; 44:2531–2538.

[141] Randall, C., et al. "Randomized Controlled Trial of Nettle Sting for Treatment of Base-of-Thumb Pain." *J. Roy. Soc. Med.* 2000; 93:305–309

[142] Mason, L. "Systematic Review of Topical Capsaicin for the Treatment of Chronic Pain." *BMJ* 2004; 328:991–996.

[143] McAlindon, T. E., et al. "Glucosamine and Chondroitin for Treatment of Osteoarthritis: A Systematic Quality Assessment and Meta-analysis." *JAMA* 2000;283:1469–1475.

[144] Richy, F., et al. "Structural and Symptomatic Efficacy of Glucosamine and Chondroitin in Knee Osteoarthritis: A Comprehensive Meta-Analysis." *Arch. Intern. Med.* 2003;163:1514–1522.

[145] Clegg, D. O. GAIT Results Presented at the American College of Rheumatology Annual Scientific Meeting in San Diego, California, November 15, 2005.

[146] "The GAIT Trial: Good News for Osteoarthritis Sufferers." Council for Responsible Nutrition Fact Sheet.

[147] Kim, L. S., et al. "Efficacy of Methylsulfonylmethane (MSM) in Osteoarthritis Pain of the Knee: A Pilot Clinical Trial." *Osteoarthritis Cartilage* 2006; 14:286–294.

[148] Sokken, K. L., et al. "Safety and Efficacy of S-Adenosylmethionine (SAMe) for Osteoarthritis: A Meta-Analysis." *J. Fam. Pract.* 2002;51:425–430.

[149] Berman, B. M., et al. "Effectiveness of Acupuncture as Adjunctive Therapy in Osteoarthritis of the Knee." *Ann. Intern. Med.* 2004;141:901–910.

[150] Ibid.

[151] Vas, J., et al. "Acupuncture as a Complementary Therapy to the Pharmacological Treatment of Osteoarthritis of the Knee: Randomised Controlled Trial." *BMJ* 2004;329:1216–1221.

[152] Witt, C., et al. "Acupuncture in Patients with Osteoarthritis of the Knee: A Randomised Trial." *Lancet* 2005;366:136–143.

[153] Harlow, T., et al. "Randomised Controlled Trial of Magnetic Bracelets for Relieving Pain in Osteoarthritis of the Hip and Knee." *BMJ* 2004;329:1450–1454.

[154] Wolsko, P. M, et al. "Double-Blind Placebo-Controlled Trial of Static Magnets for the Treatment of Osteoarthritis of the Knee: Results of a Pilot Study." *Altern. Ther. Health Med.* 2004;10:36–43.

Constipation

[155] American College of Gastroenterology Chronic Constipation Task Force. "Evidence-Based Position Statement on the Management of Chronic Constipation in North America." *Am. J. Gastroent.* 2005;100:S1–S22.

[156] Ibid.

[157] Ibid.

[158] Brandt, L. J., et al. "Systematic Review on the Management of Chronic Constipation in North America." *Am. J. Gastroenterol.* 2005;100:S15.

[159] Massey, L. K., et al. "Ascorbate Increases Human Oxaluria and Kidney Stone Risk." *J. Nutr.* 2005; 135:1673–1677.

Cough

[160] Saketkhoo, K., et al. "Effects of Drinking Hot Water, Cold Water, and Chicken Soup on Nasal Mucus Velocity and Nasal Airflow Resistance." *Chest* 1978;74:409–410.

[161] Eccles, R. "Mechanism of the Placebo Effect of Sweet Cough Syrups." *Respir. Physiol. Neurobiol.* 2006; 152:340–348.

[162] Usmani, O., et al. "Theobromine Inhibits Sensory Nerve Activation and Cough." *FASEB J.* 2005;19: 231–233.

[163] Albers, A. R., et al. "The Antiinflammatory Effects of Purple Grape Juice Consumption in Subjects with Stable Coronary Artery Disease." *Arterioscler. Thromb. Vasc. Biol.* 2004;24:e179–e180.

[164] Paul, I. M., et al. "Effect of Dextromethorphan, Diphenhydramine, and Placebo on Nocturnal Cough and Sleep Quality for Coughing Children and Their Parents." *Pediatrics* 2004;114:e85–e90.

[165] Paul, I. Personal communication, July 24, 2004.

Dandruff

[166] DeAngelis, Y. M., et al. "Three Etiologic Facets of Dandruff and Seborrheic Dermatitis: *Malassezia* Fungi, Sebaceous Lipids, and Individual Sensitivity." *J. Investig. Dermatol. Symp. Proc.* 2005;10:295–297.

[167] Ro, B. I., and Dawson, T. L. "The Role of Sebaceous Gland Activity and Scalp Microfloral Metabolism in the Etiology of Seborrheic Dermatitis and Dandruff." *J. Investig. Dermatol. Symp. Proc.* 2005;10:194–197.

[168] Bisset, N. G, ed. and trans. *Herbal Drugs and Phytopharmaceuticals: A Handbook for Practice on a Scientific Basis.* Boca Raton, FL: CRC Press, 1994, pp. 428–429, 440–441.

[169] Ody, P. *Healing with Herbs: Simple Treatments for More Than 100 Common Ailments.* Pownal, VT: Storey Books, 1999, p. 145.

[170] Ody, op. cit.

[171] Gupta, A. K., et al. "Role of Antifungal Agents in the Treatment of Seborrheic Dermatitis." *Am. J. Clin. Dermatol.* 2004;5:17–22.

[172] DeAngelis, et al., op. cit.

[173] Gupta, A. K., et al., op. cit.

[174] Gupta, A. K., and Nicol, K. A. "Ciclopirox 1% Shampoo for the Treatment of Seborrheic Dermatitis." *Int. J. Dermatol.* 2006;45:66–69.

Depression

[175] Kessler, R. C., et al. "Lifetime Prevalence and Age-of-Onset Distributions of DSM-IV Disorders in the National Comorbidity Survey Replication." *Arch. Gen. Psychiatry* 2005;62:593–602.

[176] Maugh II, T. "A Varied Assault on Depression Yields Gains." *Los Angeles Times*, March 23, 2006.

[177] Teicher, M. H., et al. "Emergence of Intense Suicidal Preoccupations During Fluoxetine Treatment." *Am. J. Psychiatry* 1990;147:207–210.

[178] Glenmullen, J. *The Antidepressant Solution: A Step-by-Step Guide to Safely Overcoming Antidepressant Withdrawal, Dependence, and "Addiction."* New York: Free Press, 2005.

[179] Vedantam, S. "Against Depression, a Sugar Pill is Hard to Beat." *Washington Post*, May 7, 2002, p. A01.

[180] Khan, A., and Schwartz, K. "Study Designs and Outcomes in Antidepressant Clinical Trials." *Essent. Psychopharmacol.* 2005;6:221–226.

[181] Moncrieff, J., and Kirsch, I. "Efficacy of Antidepressants in Adults." *BMJ* 2005;331:155–159.

[182] Rubinow, D. R. "Treatment Strategies After SSRI Failure—Good News and Bad News." *N. Engl. J. Med.* 2006;354:1305–1307.

[183] Vedantam, S. "Drugs Cure Depression in Half of Patients." *Washington Post*, March 23, 2006, p. A01.

[184] Rush, A. J., et al. "Bupropion-SR, Sertraline, or Venlafaxine-XR After Failure of SSRIs for Depression." *N. Engl. J. Med.* 2006;354:1231–1242.

[185] Trivedi, M. H., et al. "Medication Augmentation After the Failure of SSRIs for Depression." *N. Engl. J. Med.* 2006;354:1243–1252.

[186] "Drugs for Psychiatric Disorders." *Treatment Guidelines from the Medical Letter* 2003;1:69–76.

[187] Mathews, A. W. "Reading Fine Print, Insurers Question Studies of Drugs." *Wall Street Journal*, August 24, 2005, p. A-1.

[188] Mann, J. J. "The Medical Management of Depression." *N. Engl. J. Med.* 2005;353:1819–1834.

[189] Ebmeier, K. P., et al. "Recent Developments and Current Controversies in Depression." *Lancet* 2006;366:933–940.

[190] DeRubeis, R. J., et al. "Cognitive Therapy vs Medications in the Treatment of Moderate to Severe Depression." *Arch. Gen. Psychiatry* 2005;62:409–416.

[191] Hollon, S. D., et al. "Prevention of Relapse Following Cognitive Therapy vs Medications in Moderate to Severe Depression." *Arch. Gen. Psychiatry* 2005;62:417–422.

[192] Penedo, F. J., and Dahn, J. R. "Exercise and Well-Being: A Review of Mental and Physical Health Benefits Associated with Physical Activity." *Curr. Opin. Psychiatry* 2005;18:189–193.

[193] Warburton, D. E., et al. "Health Benefits of Physical Activity: The Evidence." *CMAJ* 2006;174:801–809.

[194] Dunn, A. L., et al. "Exercise Treatment for Depression: Efficacy and Dose Response." *Am. J. Prev. Med.* 2005;28:1–8.

[195] Lang, L. H. "Study Shows Light Therapy to Effectively Treat Mood Disorders, Including SAD." Press release, University of North Carolina School of Medicine, April 4, 2005.

[196] Golden, R. N., et al. "The Efficacy of Light Therapy in the Treatment of Mood Disorders: A Review and Meta-Analysis of the Evidence." *Am. J. Psychiatry* 2005;162:656–662.

[197] Benedetti, F., et al. "Morning Light Treatment Hastens the Antidepressant Effect of Citalopram: A Placebo-Controlled Trial." *J. Clin. Psychiatry* 2003;64:648–653.

[198] Leppamaki, S., et al. "Drop-Out and Mood Improvement: A Randomized Controlled Trial with Light Exposure and Physical Exercise." *BMC Psychiatry* 2004;4:22–33.

[199] Peet, M., and Stokes, C. "Omega-3 Fatty Acids in the Treatment of Psychiatric Disorders." *Drugs* 2005; 65:1051–1059.

[200] Linde, K., et al. "St. John's Wort for Depression (Review)." *Cochrane Database Syst. Rev.* 2005, April 18; (2):CD000448.

Diabetes

[201] The Diabetes Control and Complications Trial. "Intensive Diabetes Treatment and Cardiovascular Disease in Patients with Type 1 Diabetes." *N. Engl. J. Med.* 2005;353:2643–2653.

[202] Kleinfield, N. R. "Diabetes and Its Awful Toll Quietly Emerge as a Crisis." *New York Times,* January 9, 2006.

[203] Elliott, S. S., et al. "Fructose, Weight Gain, and the Insulin Resistance Syndrome." *Am. J. Clin. Nutr.* 2002;76:911–922.

[204] Alonso-Magdalena, P., et al. "The Estrogenic Effect of Bisphenol A Disrupts Pancreatic ß-Cells Function *In Vivo* and Induces Insulin Resistance." *Environ. Health Perspect.* 2006;114:106–112.

[205] Wen, C. P., et al. "Increased Mortality Risks of Pre-Diabetes (Impaired Fasting Glucose) in Taiwan." *Diabetes Care* 2005;28:2756–2761.

[206] "Solving Metabolic Syndrome's Addition Problem." *Tufts University Health & Nutrition Letter,* November 2005.

[207] Norris, S. L., et al. "Long-Term Effectiveness of Weight-Loss Interventions in Adults with Pre-Diabetes: A Review." *Am. J. Prev. Med.* 2005;28:126–139.

[208] Schulze, M. B., et al. "Dietary Pattern, Inflammation, and Incidence of Type 2 Diabetes in Women." *Am. J. Clin. Nutr.* 2005;82:675–684.

[209] Bernstein, R. K. *Dr. Bernstein's Diabetes Solution.* Boston: Little, Brown and Company, 2003. pp. 79–88.

[210] Yancy, W. S., et al. "A Low-Carbohydrate, Ketogenic Diet to Treat Type 2 Diabetes." *Nutr. Metab. (Lond.)* 2005;2:34.

[211] Nielsen, J. V., and Joensson, E. "Low-Carbohydrate Diet in Type 2 Diabetes. Stable Improvement of Bodyweight and Glycemic Control during 22 Months Follow-Up." *Nutr. Metab. (Lond.)* 2006;3:22 [doi:10.1186/1743-7075-3-22].

[212] Nielsen, J. V., et al. "A Low-Carbohydrate Diet May Prevent End-Stage Renal Failure in Type 2 Diabetes. A Case Report." *Nutr. Metab. (Lond.)* 2006;3:23 [doi:10.1186/1743-7075-3-23].

[213] Grassi, D., et al. "Cocoa Reduces Blood Pressure and Insulin Resistance and Improves Endothelium-Dependent Vasodilation in Hypertensives." *Hypertension* 2005;46:398–405.

[214] Nielsen and Joensson, op. cit.

[215] Van Dam, R. M., and Hu, F. B. "Coffee Consumption and Risk of Type 2 Diabetes: A Systematic Review." *JAMA* 2005;294:97–104.

[216] Lee, S., et al. "Caffeine Ingestion Is Associated with Reductions in Glucose Uptake Independent of Obesity and Type 2 Diabetes before and after Exercise Training." *Diabetes Care* 2005;28:566–572.

[217] Shearer, J., et al. "Quinides of Roasted Coffee Enhance Insulin Action in Conscious Rats." *J. Nutr.* 2003;133:3529–3532.

[218] Orchard, T. J., et al. "The Effect of Metformin and Intensive Lifestyle Intervention on the Metabolic Syndrome: The Diabetes Prevention Program Randomized Trial." *Ann. Int. Med.* 2005;142:611–619.

[219] Herman, W. H., et al. "The Cost-Effectiveness of Lifestyle Modification or Metformin in Preventing Type 2 Diabetes in Adults with Impaired Glucose Tolerance." *Ann. Int. Med.* 2005;142:323–332.

[220] Orchard, et al., ibid.

[221] Herman, et al., ibid.

[222] Hu, F., et al. "Walking Compared with Vigorous Physical Activity and Risk of Type 2 Diabetes in Women: A Prospective Study." *JAMA* 1999;282:1433–1439.

[223] Moore, H., et al. "Dietary Advice for Treatment of Type 2 Diabetes Mellitus in Adults." *The Cochrane Database of Systematic Reviews* (issue 4) 2005. *The Cochrane Library* [online at http://www.cochrane.org/reviews/en/ab004097.html.]

[224] Krucoff, C., and Krucoff, M. *Healing Moves: How to Cure, Relieve, and Prevent Common Ailments with Exercise.* Cranston, RI: The Writers' Collective, 2004.

[225] Mathieu, C., et al. "Vitamin D and Diabetes." *Diabetologia* 2005;48:1247–1257.

[226] Harris, S., et al. "Vitamin D Insufficiency and Hyperparathyroidism in a Low Income, Multiracial, Elderly Population." *J. Clin. Endocrinol. Metab.* 2000;85:4125–4130.

[227] Mathieu, C., et al. "Vitamin D and Diabetes." *Diabetologia* 2005;48:1247–1257.

[228] Tangpricha, V., et al. "Vitamin D Insufficiency among Free-Living Healthy Young Adults." *Am. J. Med.* 2002;112:659–662.

[229] Holick, M. F. "Sunlight and Vitamin D for Bone Health and Prevention of Autoimmune Diseases, Cancers, and Cardiovascular Disease." *Am. J. Clin. Nutr.* 2004;80(6 Suppl.):1678S–1688S.

[230] Stuebe, A. M., et al. "Duration of Lactation and Incidence of Type 2 Diabetes." *JAMA* 2005;294:2601–2610.

[231] Bergenstal, R. M., and Gavin III, J. R. "The Role of Self-Monitoring of Blood Glucose in the Care of People with Diabetes: Report of a Global Consensus Conference." *Am. J. Med.* 2005;118:1S–6S.

[232] Edelman, S. V. *Taking Control of Your Diabetes.* Caddo, OK: Professional Communications, Inc., 2000. p. 27.

[233] "SMBG in Type 2 Diabetes." *Bandolier* (148) 2006;13:3–4.

[234] Tisdale, James E., and Douglas A. Miller *Drug-Induced Diseases: Prevention Detection, and Management.* Bethesda, MD: American Society of Health-System Pharmacists, 2005. Pp365–372

[235] *Physicians' Desk Reference Companion Guide.* Montvale, NJ: Thomson PDR, 2005.

[236] Broadhurst, C. L., et al. "Insulin-like Biological Activity of Culinary and Medicinal Plant Aqueous Extracts in Vitro." *J. Agric. Food Chem.* 2000;48:849–852.

[237] Kim, S. H., et al. "Antidiabetic Effect of Cinnamon Extract on Blood Glucose in db/db Mice." *J. Ethnopharmacol.* 2005;October 3 [Epub ahead of print].

[238] Verspohl, E. J., et al. "Antidiabetic Effect of *Cinnamomum cassia* and *Cinnamomum zeylanicum* in Vivo and in Vitro." *Phytother. Res.* 2005;19:203–206.

[239] Ostman, E., et al. "Vinegar Supplementation Lowers Glucose and Insulin Responses and Increases Satiety after a Bread Meal in Healthy Subjects." *Eur. J. Clin. Nutr.* 2005;59:983–988.

[240] Sugiyama, M., et al. "Glycemic Index of Single and Mixed Meal Foods among Common Japanese Foods with White Rice as a Reference Food." *Eur. J. Clin. Nutr.* 2003;57:743–752.

[241] Johnston, C. S., and Buller, A. J. "Vinegar and Peanut Products as Complementary Foods to Reduce Postprandial Glycemia." *J. Am. Diet. Assoc.* 2005;105:1939–1942.

[242] Hosoda, K., et al. "Antihyperglycemic Effect of Oolong Tea in Type 2 Diabetes." *Diabetes Care* 2003; 26:1714–1718.

[243] Liu, J. P., et al. "Chinese Herbal Medicines for Type 2 Diabetes Mellitus." *The Cochrane Library*, 2005.

[244] Huang, K. C. *The Pharmacology of Chinese Herbs*, 2nd ed. Boca Raton, FL: CRC Press, 1999.

[245] Duke, J. A. *Handbook of Medicinal Herbs*. Boca Raton, FL: CRC Press, 1985, pp. 315–316.

[246] Hendler, S. S., and Rorvik, D., chief editors. *PDR for Nutritional Supplements*, 1st ed. Montvale, NJ: Medical Economics, 2001, pp. 96–99.

[247] Rabinovitz, H., et al. "Effect of Chromium Supplementation on Blood Glucose and Lipid Levels in Type 2 Diabetes Mellitus Elderly Patients." *Int. J. Vitam. Nutr. Res.* 2004;74:178–182.

[248] Anderson, R. A., et al. "Elevated Intakes of Supplemental Chromium Improve Glucose and Insulin Variables in Individuals with Type 2 Diabetes." *Diabetes* 1997;46:1786–1791.

[249] Shane-McWhorter, L. "Biological Complementary Therapies: A Focus on Botanical Products in Diabetes." *Diabetes Spectrum* 2001;14:199–208.

[250] Ibid.

[251] Olin, B. R., ed. "Gymnema." *The Lawrence Review of Natural Products*. St. Louis, MO: Facts and Comparisons, 1993.

[252] Trejo-Gonzalez, A., et al. "A Purified Extract from Prickly Pear Cactus (*Opuntia fuliginosa*) Controls Experimentally Induced Diabetes in Rats." *J. Ethnopharmacol.* 1996;55:27–33.

[253] Laurenz, J. C., et al. "Hypoglycaemic Effect of *Opuntia lindheimeri Englem.* in a Diabetic Pig Model." *Phytother. Res.* 2003;17:26–29.

[254] Frati-Munari, A. C., et al. "Hypoglycemic Effect of *Opuntia streptacantha Lemaire* in NIDDM." *Diabetes Care* 1988;11:63–66.

[255] Curi, R., et al. "Effect of *Stevia rebaudiana* on Glucose Tolerance in Normal Adult Humans." *Braz. J. Med. Biol. Res.* 1986;19:771–774.

[256] Surwit, R. S., and Schneider, M. S. "Role of Stress in the Etiology and Treatment of Diabetes Mellitus." *Psychosom. Med.* 1993;55:380–393.

[257] Jaber, L. A., et al. "The Effect of Stress on Glycemic Control in Patients with Type II Diabetes during Glyburide and Glipizide Therapy." *J. Clin. Pharmacol.* 1993;33:239–245.

[258] Surwit, R. S., et al. "Stress Management Improves Long-Term Glycemic Control in Type 2 Diabetes." *Diabetes Care* 2002;25:30–34.

[259] Luftman, P. J., et al. "Effects of Alprazolam on Glucose Regulation in Diabetes: Results of Double-Blind, Placebo-Controlled Trial." *Diabetes Care* 1995;18:1133–1139.

[260] Katon, W. J., et al. "The Association of Comorbid Depression with Mortality in Patients with Type 2 Diabetes." *Diabetes Care* 2005;28:2668–2672.

[261] Karter, A. J., et al. "Achieving Good Glycemic Control: Initiation of New Antihyperglycemic Therapies in Patients with Type 2 Diabetes from the Kaiser Permanente Northern California Diabetes Registry." *Am. J. Managed Care* 2005;11:262–270.

[262] Ibid.

[263] Saenz, A., et al. "Metformin Monotherapy for Type 2 Diabetes Mellitus." *The Cochrane Library* 2005.

[264] Khan, M., et al. "Pioglitazone and Reductions in Post-Challenge Glucose Levels in Patients with Type 2 Diabetes." *Diabetes Obes. Metab.* 2006;8:31–38.

[265] Betteridge, D.J., and Verges, B. "Long-Term Effects on Lipids and Lipoproteins of Pioglitazone versus Metformin Addition to Sulphonylurea in the Treatment of Type 2 Diabetes." *Diabetologia* 2005;48: 2477–2481.

[266] Nishio, K., et al. "A Randomized Comparison of Pioglitazone to Inhibit Restenosis after Coronary Stenting in Patients with Type 2 Diabetes." *Diabetes Care* 2006;29:101–106.

[267] Goldberg, R. B., et al. "A Comparison of Lipid and Glycemic Effects of Pioglitazone and Rosiglitazone in Patients with Type 2 Diabetes and Dyslipidemia." *Diabetes Care* 2005;28:1547–1554.

[268] Whitelaw, D. C., et al. "Effects of the New Oral Hypoglycaemic Agent Nateglinide on Insulin Secretion in Type 2 Diabetes Mellitus." *Diabetic Medicine* 2000;17:225–229.

[269] Rosenstock, J., et al. "Repaglinide versus Nateglinide Monotherapy: A Randomized, Multicenter Study." *Diabetes Care* 2004;27:1265–1270.

[270] Reboussin, D. M., et al. "The Combination Oral and Nutritional Treatment of Late-Onset Diabetes Mellitus (Control DM) Trial Results." *Diabet. Med.* 2004;21:1082–1089.

[271] Horton, E. S., et al. "Nateglinide Alone and in Combination with Metformin Improves Glycemic Control by Reducing Mealtime Glucose Levels in Type 2 Diabetes." *Diabetes Care* 2000;23:1660–1665.

[272] Moses, R., et al. "Effect of Repaglinide Addition to Metformin Monotherapy on Glycemic Control in Patients with Type 2 Diabetes." *Diabetes Care* 1999;22:119–124.

[273] "Byetta Exenatide Injection" Web site (http://www.byetta.com), 02-05-1136-A; EX-35924, 2005.

Eczema

[274] Williams, H. C. "Atopic Dermatitis." *N. Engl. J. Med.* 2005;352:2314–2324.

[275] British Academy of Dermatology patient brochure online: www.bad.org.uk/patients/disease/atopic.

[276] Choi, M. J., and Maibach, H. I. "Role of Ceramides in Barrier Function of Healthy and Diseased Skin." *Am. J. Clin. Dermatol.* 2005;6:215–223.

[277] Hon, K. L., et al. "A Survey of Bathing and Showering Practices in Children with Atopic Eczema." *Clin. Exp. Dermatol.* 2005;30:351–354.

[278] Williams, op. cit., p. 2317.

[279] Gutgesell, C., et al. "Double-Blind Placebo-Controlled House Dust Mite Control Measures in Adult Patients with Atopic Dermatitis." *Br. J. Dermatol.* 2001;145:70–74.

[280] Williams, op. cit., p. 2321.

[281] Weston, S., et al. "Effects of Probiotics on Atopic Dermatitis: A Randomised Controlled Trial." *Arch. Dis. Child.* 2005;90:892–897.

[282] Viljanen, M., et al. "Probiotics in the Treatment of Atopic Eczema/Dermatitis Syndrome in Infants: A Double-Blind Placebo-Controlled Trial." *Allergy* 2005;60:494–500.

[283] Rosenfeldt, V., et al. "Effect of Probiotic *Lactobacillus* Strains in Children with Atopic Dermatitis." *J. Allergy Clin. Immunol.* 2003;111:389–395.

[284] Viljanen, M., et al. "Induction of Inflammation as a Possible Mechanism of Probiotic Effect in Atopic Eczema-Dermatitis Syndrome." *J. Allergy. Clin. Immunol.* 2005;115:1254–1259.

[285] Senok, A. C., et al. "Probiotics—Facts and Myths." *Clin. Microbiol. Infect.* 2005;11:958–966.

[286] Henriksson, A., et al. "Probiotics Under the Regulatory Microscope." *Expert Opin. Drug Saf.* 2005;4:1135–1143.

[287] Laitinen, K., et al. "Evaluation of Diet and Growth in Children with and without Atopic Eczema: Follow-Up Study from Birth to 4 Years." *Br. J. Nutr.* 2005;94:565–574.

[288] Kirjavainen, P. V., et al. "Probiotic Bacteria in the Management of Atopic Disease: Underscoring the Importance of Viability." *J. Ped. Gastroent. Nutr.* 2003;36:223–227.

[289] Van Gool, C. J. A. W., et al. "Oral Essential Fatty Acid Supplementation in Atopic Dermatitis—A Meta-Analysis of Placebo-Controlled Trials." *Br. J. Dermatol.* 2004;150:728–740.

[290] Takwale, A., et al. "Efficacy and Tolerability of Borage Oil in Adults and Children with Atopic Eczema: Randomised, Double Blind, Placebo Controlled, Parallel Group Trial." *BMJ* 2003;327:1385–1390.

[291] Callaway, J., et al. "Efficacy of Dietary Hempseed Oil in Patients with Atopic Dermatitis." *J. Dermatolog. Treat.* 2005;16:87–94.

[292] Ehlers, I., et al. "Sugar Is Not an Aggravating Factor in Atopic Dermatitis." *Acta Derm. Venereol.* 2001; 81:282–284.

[293] Olivry, T., et al. "Evidence-Based Veterinary Dermatology: A Systematic Review of the Pharmaco-therapy of Canine Atopic Dermatitis." *Vet. Dermatol.* 2003;14:121–146.

[294] Uehara, M., et al. "A Trial of Oolong Tea in the Management of Recalcitrant Atopic Dermatitis." *Arch. Dermatol.* 2001;137:42–43.

[295] Tsoureli-Nikita, E., et al. "Evaluation of Dietary Intake of Vitamin E in the Treatment of Atopic Dermatitis: A Study of the Clinical Course and Evaluation of the Immunoglobulin E Serum Levels." *Int. J. Dermatol.* 2002;41:146–150.

[296] Ross, S. M. "An Integrative Approach to Eczema (Atopic Dermatitis)." *Holist. Nurs. Pract.* 2003;17:56–62.

[297] Al-Waili, N. S. "Topical Application of Natural Honey, Beeswax and Olive Oil Mixture for Atopic Dermatitis or Psoriasis: Partially Controlled, Single-Blinded Study." *Complement. Ther. Med.* 2003;11: 226–234.

[298] Williams, op. cit.

[299] Saeedi, M., et al. "The Treatment of Atopic Dermatitis with Licorice Gel." *J. Dermatolog. Treat.* 2003;14: 153–157.

[300] Autio, P., et al. "Heliotherapy in Atopic Dermatitis: A Prospective Study on Climatotherapy Using the SCORAD Index." *Acta Derm. Venereol.* 2002;82:436–440.

[301] Van Coevorden, A. M., et al. "Comparison of Oral Psoralen–UV-A with a Portable Tanning Unit at Home vs Hospital-Administered Bath Psoralen–UV-A in Patients with Chronic Hand Eczema." *Arch. Dermatol.* 2004;140:1463–1466.

[302] Schiffner, R., et al. "Dead Sea Treatment-Principle for Outpatient Use in Atopic Dermatitis: Safety and Efficacy of Synchronous Balneophototherapy Using Narrowband UVB and Bathing in Dead Sea Salt Solution." *Eur. J. Dermatol.* 2002;12:543–548.

[303] Proksch, E., et al. "Bathing in a Magnesium-Rich Dead Sea Salt Solution Improves Skin Barrier Function, Enhances Skin Hydration, and Reduces Inflammation in Atopic Dry Skin." *Int. J. Dermatol.* 2005;44:151–157.

[304] Ernst, E., et al. "Complementary/Alternative Medicine in Dermatology: Evidence-Assessed Efficacy of Two Diseases and Two Treatments." *Am. J. Clin. Dermatol.* 2002;3:341–348.

[305] Kimata, H. "Listening to Mozart Reduces Allergic Skin Wheal Responses and In Vitro Allergen-Specific IgE Production in Atopic Dermatitis Patients with Latex Allergy." *Behav. Med.* 2003;29:15–19.

Foot Odor

[306] Jonski, G., et al. "Insoluble Zinc, Cupric and Tin Pyrophosphates Inhibit the Formation of Volatile Sulphur Compounds." *Eur. J. Oral Sci.* 2004;112:429–432.

[307] Giffard, C. J., et al. "Administration of Charcoal, *Yucca schidigera*, and Zinc Acetate to Reduce Malodorous Flatulence in Dogs." *J. Am. Vet. Med. Assoc.* 2001;218:892–896.

[308] Sugiura, T., et al. "Chronic zinc toxicity in an infant who received zinc therapy for atopic dermatitis." *Acta Paediatr.* 2005;94:1333–1335.

Gas (Flatulence)

[309] Watson, W. C. "Speaking the Unspeakable." *N. Engl. J. Med.* 1978;299:494.

[310] Serra, J., et al. "Mechanisms of Intestinal Gas Retention in Humans: Impaired Propulsion Versus Obstructed Evacuation." *Am. J. Physiol. Gastrointel. Liver Physiol.* 2001;282:G138–G143.

[311] Quigley, E. M. M. "From Comic Relief to Real Understanding; How Intestinal Gas Causes Symptoms." *Gut* 2003;52:1659–1661.

[312] Kurbel, S., et al. "Intestinal Gases and Flatulence: Possible Causes of Occurrence." *Med. Hypotheses* 2006;March 27 [Epub ahead of print].

[313] Azpiroz, F. "Intesttinal Gas Dynamics: Mechanisms and Clinical Relevance." *Gut* 2005;54:893–895.

[314] Van Ness, M. M., and Cattau, Jr., E.L. "Flatulence: Pathophysiology and Treatment." *Am. Fam. Physician.* 1985;31:198–208.

[315] Suarez, F. L. and Levitt, M. D. "An Undestanding of Excessive Intestinal Gas." *Curr. Gastroenterol. Rep.* 2000;2:413–419.

[316] Levitt, M. D., et al. "Studies of a Flatulent Patient." *N. Engl. J. Med.* 1976;295:260–262.

[317] Green, Peter H. R., and Jones, R. *Celiac Disease: A Hidden Epidemic.* New York: Collins, 2006.

[318] Rabkin, E. S. and Silverman, E. J. "Passing Gas." *Human Nature* 1979;2:50–55.

[319] Ganiats, T. G., et al. "Does Beano Prevent Gas?: A Double-Blind Crossover Study of Oral Alpha-Galactosidase to Treat Dietary Oligosaccharide Intolerance." *J. Fam. Pract.* 1994;39:441–445.

[320] Lettieri, J. T. and Dain, B. "Effects of Beano on the Tolerability and Pharmacodynamics of Acarbose." *Clin. Ther.* 1998;20:497–504.

[321] Ohge, H., et al. "Effectiveness of Devices Purported to Reduce Flatus Odor." *Am. J. Gastroenterol.* 2005;100:397–400.

[322] Hall, R. G., et al. "Effects of Orally Administered Activated Charcoal on Intestinal Gas." *Am. J. Gastroenterol.* 1981;75:192–196.

[323] Suarez, F. L., et al. "Failure of Activated Charcoal to Reduce the Release of Gases Produced by the Colonic Flora." *Am. J. Gastroenterol.* 1999;94:208–212.

[324] Suarez, op. cit.

[325] Suarez, F. L., et al. "Bismuth Subsalicylate Markedly Decreases Hydrogen Sulfide Release in the Human Colon." *Gastroenterol.* 1998;114:923–929.

[326] Di Stefano, M., et al. "Probiotics and Functional Abdominal Bloating." *J. Clin. Gastroenterol.* 2004;38: S102–S103.

[327] Nobaek, S., et al. "Alterations of Intestinal Microflora is Associated with Reduction in Abdominal Bloating and Pain in Patients with Irritable Bowel Syndrome." *Am. J. Gastroenterol.* 2000;95:1231–1238.

Headaches and Migraines

[328] Edmeads, J. "Analgesic-Induced Headache: An Unrecognized Epidemic." *Headache* 1990;30:614–617.

[329] Larsson, B., et al. "Relaxation Treatment of Adolescent Headache Sufferers: Results from a School-Based Replication Series." *Headache* 2005;45:692–704.

[330] Bren, L. "Managing Migraines." *FDA Consumer* 2006;40:30–36.

[331] Holzhammer, J., and Wober, C. "Alimentary Trigger Factors that Provoke Migraine and Tension-Type Headache." *Schmerz* 2006;20:151–159.

[332] Marcus, D. A., et al. "A Double-Blind Provocative Study of Chocolate as a Trigger of Headache." *Cephalalgia* 1997;17:855–862.

[333] Boehnke, C., et al. "High-Dose Riboflavin Treatment Is Efficacious in Migraine Prophylaxis: An Open Study in a Tertiary Care Center." *Eur. J. Neurol.* 2004;11:475–477.

[334] Maizels, M., et al. "A Combination of Riboflavin, Magnesium, and Feverfew for Migraine Prophylaxis: a Randomized Trial." *Headache* 2004;44:885–890.

[335] Tassorelli, C., et al. "Parthenolide Is the Component of *Tanacetum parthenium* That Inhibits Nitroglycerin-Induced Fos Activation: Studies in an Animal Model of Migraine." *Cephalalgia* 2005;25:612–621.

[336] Pittler, M. H., and Ernst, E. "Feverfew for Preventing Migraine." *Cochrane Database Syst. Rev.* 2004;(1): CD002286.

[337] Diener, H. C., et al. "Efficacy and Safety of 6.25 mg t.i.d. Feverfew CO_2-extract (MIG-99) in Migraine Prevention—A Randomized, Double-Blind, Multicentre, Placebo-Controlled Study." *Cephalalgia* 2005;25:1031–1041.

[338] Cady, R. K., et al. "GelStat Migraine (Sublingually Administered Feverfew and Ginger Compound) for Acute Treatment of Migraine When Administered During the Mild Pain Phase." *Med. Sci. Monit.* 2005;11:P165–P169.

[339] Diener, H. C., et al. "The First Placebo-Controlled Trial of a Special Butterbur Root Extract for the Prevention of Migraine: Reanalysis of Efficacy Criteria." *Eur. Neurol.* 2004;51:89–97.

[340] Lipton, R. B., et al. "*Petasites hybridus* Root (Butterbur) Is an Effective Preventive Treatment for Migraine." *Neurology* 2004;63:2240–2244.

[341] Pothmann, R., and Danesch, U. "Migraine Prevention in Children and Adolescents: Results of an Open Study with a Special Butterbur Root Extract." *Headache* 2005;45:196–203.

[342] Danesch, U., and Rittinghausen, R. "Safety of a Patented Special Butterbur Root Extract for Migraine Prevention." *Headache* 2003;43:76–78.

[343] Kroll, D. Personal communication, April 26, 2006.

[344] Allais, G., et al. "Acupuncture in the Prophylactic Treatment of Migraine Without Aura: A Comparison with Flunarizine." *Headache* 2002;42:855–861.

[345] Vickers, A. J., et al. "Acupuncture for Chronic Headache in Primary Care: Large, Pragmatic, Randomised Trial." *BMJ* 2004;328:744.

[346] Ernst, E. "Acupuncture—A Critical Analysis." *J. Intern. Med.* 2006;259:125–137.

[347] MacPherson, H., and Thomas, K. "Short Term Reactions to Acupuncture—A Cross-Sectional Survey of Patient Reports." *Acupunct. Med.* 2005;23:112–120.

[348] Linde, K., et al. "Acupuncture for Patients with Migraine: A Randomized Controlled Trial." *JAMA* 2005;293:2118–2125.

[349] Diener, H. C., et al. "Efficacy of Acupuncture for the Prophylaxis of Migraine: A Multicentre Randomised Controlled Clinical Trial." *Lancet Neurol.* 2006;5:310–316.

[350] Melchart, D., et al. "Acupuncture Versus Placebo Versus Sumatriptan for Early Treatment of Migraine Attacks: A Randomized Controlled Trial." *J. Intern. Med.* 2003;253:181–183.

[351] Peres, M. F., et al. "Melatonin, 3 mg, Is Effective for Migraine Prevention." *Neurology* 2004;63:757.

[352] Sandor, P. S., et al. "Efficacy of Coenzyme Q_{10} in Migraine Prophylaxis: A Randomized Controlled Trial." *Neurology* 2005;64:713–715.

[353] Scharff, L., et al. "A Controlled Study of Minimal-Contact Thermal Biofeedback Treatment in Children with Migraine." *J. Pediatr. Psychol.* 2002;27:109–119.

[354] Rios, J., and Passe, M. M. "Evidence-Based Use of Botanicals, Minerals, and Vitamins in the Prophylactic Treatment of Migraines." *J. Am. Acad. Nurse Pract.* 2004;16:251–256.

[355] Codispoti, J. R., et al. "Efficacy of Nonprescription Doses of Ibuprofen for Treating Migraine Headache: A Randomized Controlled Trial." *Headache* 2001;41:665–679.

[356] Kellstein, D. E., et al. "Evaluation of a Novel Solubilized Formulation of Ibuprofen in the Treatment of Migraine Headache: A Randomized, Double-Blind, Placebo-Controlled, Dose-Ranging Study." *Cephalalgia* 2000;20:233–243.

[357] Goldstein, J., et al. "Acetaminophen, Aspirin, and Caffeine in Combination Versus Ibuprofen for Acute Migraine: Results From a Multicenter, Double-Blind, Randomized, Parallel-Group, Single-Dose, Placebo-Controlled Study." *Headache* 2006;46:444–453.

[358] Goldstein, J., et al. "Acetaminophen, Aspirin, and Caffeine Versus Sumatriptan Succinate in the Early Treatment of Migraine: Results from the ASSET Trial." *Headache* 2005;45:973–982.

[359] Diener, H. C., et al. "Efficacy, Tolerability and Safety of Oral Eletriptan and Ergotamine plus Cafeine (Cafergot) in the Acute Treatment of Migraine: A Multicentre, Randomised, Double-Blind, Placebo-Controlled Comparison." *Eur. Neurol.* 2002;47:99–107.

[360] Christie, S., et al. "Crossover Comparison of Efficacy and Preference for Rizatriptan 10 mg Versus Ergotamine/Caffeiine in Migraine." *Eur. Neurol.* 2003;49:20–29.

[361] Freedom of Information Act request File Number F95-00866, From Bernice Carter, Freedom of Information Officer, Center for Drug Evaluation and Research, January 23, 1995: Memorandum N20-070, December 28, 1992 from Paul Leber, M.D., Director Division of Neuropharmacological Drug Products to Robert Temple, M.D., Director, Office of Drug Evaluation I.

[362] Saper, J. Personal communication, January 7, 2006.

[363] Winner, P., et al. "Topiramate for Migraine Prevention in Children: A Randomized, Double-Blind, Placebo-Controlled Trial." *Headache* 2005;45:1304–1312.

[364] Wenzel, R. G., et al. "Topiramate for Migraine Prevention." *Pharmacotherapy* 2006;26:375–387.

[365] Bussone, G., et al. "Topiramate 100 mg/Day in Migraine Prevention: A Pooled Analysis of Double-Blind Randomised Controlled Trials." *Int. J. Clin. Pract.* 2005;59:961–968.

[366] Wenzel, op. cit.

[367] Charles, J. A., et al. "Prevention of Migraine with Olmesartan in Patients with Hypertension/Prehypertension." *Headache* 2006;46:503.

[368] Silberstein, S. D., et al. "Botulinum Toxin Type A for the Prophylactic Treatment of Chronic Daily Headache: A Randomized, Double-Blind, Placebo-Controlled Trial." *Mayo Clin. Proc.* 2005;80:1126–1137.

[369] Dodick, D. W., et al. "Botulinum Toxin Type A for the Prophylaxis of Chronic Daily Headache: Subgroup Analysis of Patients Not Receiving Other Prophylactic Medications: A Randomized, Double-Blind, Placebo-Controlled Study." *Headache* 2005;45:315–324.

[370] Mathew, N. T., et al. "Botulinum Toxin Type A (BOTOX) for the Prophylactic Treatment of Chronic Daily Headache: A Randomized, Double-Blind, Placebo-Controlled Trial." *Headache* 2005;45:293–307.

[371] Martin, V., and Behbehani, M. "Ovarian Hormones and Migraine Headache: Understanding Mechanisms and Pathogenesis—Part 2." *Headache* 2006;46:365–386.

[372] Ibid.

[373] Al-Waili, N. S. "Treatment of Menstrual Migraine with Prostaglandin Synthesis Inhibitor Mefenamic Acid: Double-Blind Study with Placebo." *Eur. J. Med. Res.* 2000;5:176–182.

[374] Facchinetti, F., et al. "Magnesium Prophylaxis of Menstrual Migraine: Effects on Intracellular Magnesium." *Headache* 1991;31:298–301.

[375] Burke, B. E., et al. "Randomized, Controlled Trial of Phytoestrogen in the Prophylactic Treatment of Menstrual Migraine." *Biomed. Pharmacother.* 2002;56:283–288.

[376] Ferrante, F., et al. "Phyto-oestrogens in the Prophylaxis of Menstrual Migraine." *Clin. Neuropharmacol.* 2004;27:137–140.

[377] Allais, G., et al. "Advanced Strategies of Short-Term Prophylaxis of Menstrual Migraine: State of the Art and Prospects." *Neurol. Sci.* 2005;26:S125–S129.

[378] Ibid.

[379] Cutrer, F. M., and Boes, C. J. "Cough, Exertional, and Sex Headaches." *Neurol. Clin.* 2004;22:133–149.

Heartburn

[380] Hippocrates. *On Regimen in Acute Diseases.* 400 BCE, Appendix Part 18. Adams, F., translator. Williams and Wilkins, 1946.

[381] Koelz, H. R. "Gastric Acid in Vertebrates." *Scand. J. Gastroenterol.* 1992;27(Suppl. 193):2–6.

[382] Penagini, R., et al. "Effect of Increasing the Fat Content but Not the Energy Load of a Meal on Gastro-Oesophageal Reflux and Lower Oesaphageal Sphincter Motor Function." *Gut* 1998;42:330–333.

[383] Ibid.

[384] Kaltenbach, T., et al. "Are Lifestyle Measures Effective in Patients with Gastroesophageal Reflux Disease? An Evidence-Based Approach." *Arch. Intern. Med.* 2006;166:965–971.

[385] Yudkin, J., and Evans, E. "The Low-Carbohydrate Diet in the Treatment of Chronic Dyspepsia." *Proc. Nutr. Soc.* 1972;31:12A.

[386] Yancey, W. S., et al. "Improvement of Gastroesophageal Reflux Disease After Initiation of a Low-Carbohydrate Diet: Five Brief Case Reports." *Altern. Ther. Health Med.* 2001;7:116–119.

[387] Austin G. L., et al. "A Very Low Carbohydrate Diet Improves Gastroesophageal Reflux and Its Symptoms." *Digestive Diseases and Sciences.* 2006; July 27 [Epub ahead of print].

[388] Richter, J. "Do We Know the Cause of Reflux Disease?" *Eur. J. Gastroenterol. Hepatol.* 1999;11(Suppl. 1): S3–S9.

[389] Vakevainen, S., et al. "Hypochlorhydria Induced by a Proton Pump Inhibitor Leads to Intragastric Microbial Production of Acetaldehyde from Ethanol." *Aliment. Pharmacol. Ther.* 2000;14:1511–1518.

[390] Holtmann, G., et al. "A Placebo-Controlled Trial of Itopride in Functional Dyspepsia." *N. Engl. J. Med.* 2006;354:832–840.

[391] Kim, Y. S., et al. "Effect of Itopride, a New Prokinetic, in Patients with Mild GERD: A Pilot Study." *World J. Gastroenterol.* 2005;11:4210–4214.

[392] Helf, J. F., et al. "Effect of Esophageal Emptying and Saliva on Clearance of Acid from the Esophagus." *N. Engl. J. Med.* 1984;310:284–288.

[393] Smoak, B. R., and Koufman, J. A. "Effects of Gum Chewing on Pharyngeal and Esophageal pH." *Ann. Otol. Rhinol. Laryngol.* 2001;110:1117–1119.

[394] Polland, K. E., et al. "Salivary Flow Rate and pH During Prolonged Gum Chewing in Humans." *J. Oral. Rehabil.* 2003;30:861–865.

[395] von Schonfeld, J., et al. "Oesophageal Acid and Salivary Secretion: Is Chewing Gum a Treatment Option for Gastro-Oesophageal Reflux?" *Digestion* 1997;58:111–114.

[396] Moazzez, R., et al. "The Effect of Chewing Sugar-Free Gum on Gastro-Esophageal Reflux." *J. Dent. Res.* 2005;84:1062–1065.

[397] Avidan, B., et al. "Walking and Chewing Reduce Postprandial Acid Reflux." *Aliment. Pharmacol. Ther.* 2001;15:151–155.

[398] Szolcsanyi, J., and Bartho, L. "Capsaicin-Sensitive Afferents and Their Role in Gastroprotection: An Update." *J. Physiol. Paris* 2001;95:181–188.

[399] Bortolotti, M., et al. "Red Pepper and Functional Dyspepsia." *N. Engl. J. Med.* 2002; 346:947–948.

[400] Ibid.

[401] Holzer, P., et al. "Intragastric Capsaicin Protects Against Aspirin-Induced Lesion Formation and Bleeding in the Rat Gastric Mucosa." *Gastroenterology* 1989;96:1425–1433.

[402] Lazebnik, N., et al. "Spontaneous Rupture of the Normal Stomach After Sodium Bicarbonate Ingestion." *J. Clin. Gastroenterol.* 1986;8:454–456.

[403] Baraona, E., et al. "Bioavailability of Alcohol: Role of Gastric Metabolism and Its Interactions with Other Drugs." *Dig. Dis.* 1994;12:351–367.

[404] Arora, S., et al. "Alcohol Levels are Increased in Social Drinkers Receiving Ranitidine." *Am. J. Gastroenterol.* 2000;95:208–213.

[405] Calculated from Vaczek, D. "Top 200 Prescription Drugs of 2004." *Pharmacy Times*, May 2004, p. 41 (data courtesy of IMS Health) and *Drug Topics*, February 21, 2005, and March 7, 2005 (data courtesy of Verispan).

[406] Laheij, R. J., et al. "Risk of Community-Acquired Pneumonia and Use of Gastric Acid-Suppressive Drugs." *JAMA* 2004;292:1955–1960.

[407] Dial, S., et al. "Use of Gastric Acid-Suppressive Agents and the Risk of Community-Acquired *Clostridium difficile*-Associated Disease." *JAMA* 2005;294:2989–2995.

[408] Graedon, J., and Graedon, T. *Joe Graedon's The New People's Pharmacy: Drug Breakthroughs of the '80s.* New York: Bantam Books, 1985, p. 147.

[409] Schell, T. G. "Acid Suppression and Adenocarcinoma of the Esophagus: Cause or Cure?" *Am. J. Gastroenterol.* 2004;99:1884–1886.

[410] Ibid.

[411] Waldum, H. L., and Brenna, E. "Personal Review: Is Profound Acid Inhibition Safe? *Aliment. Pharmacol. Ther.* 2000;14:15–22.

[412] Jensen, R. T. "Consequences of Long-Term Proton Pump Blockade: Insights from Studies of Patients with Gastrinomas." *Basic Clin. Pharmacol. Toxicol.* 2006;98:4–19.

[413] Ibid.

[414] Waldum, op. cit.

[415] Gillen, D., and McColl, K. E. L. "Problems Associated with the Clinical Use of Proton Pump Inhibitors." *Pharmacol. Toxicol.* 2001;89:281–296.

[416] Fossmark, R., et al. "Rebound Acid Hypersecretion After Long-Term Inhibition of Gastric Acid Secretion." *Aliment. Pharmacol. Ther.* 2005;21:149–154.

[417] Sandvik, A. K., et al. "Review Article: The Pharmacological Inhibition of Gastric Acid Secretion— Tolerance and Rebound." *Aliment. Pharmacol. Ther.* 1997;11:1013–1018.

[418] Gillen, op. cit.

Heart Disease and High Cholesterol

[419] American Heart Association Statistics Committee and Stroke Statistics Subcommittee. "Heart Disease and Stroke Statistics—2006 Update. A Report From the American Heart Association Statistics Committee and Stroke Statistics Subcommittee." *Circulation* 2006;113:e85–e151.

[420] Ibid.

[421] Jemal, A., et al. "Trends in the Leading Causes of Death in the United States, 1970–2002." *JAMA* 2005; 294:1255–1259.

[422] American Heart Association Statistics Committee, op. cit.

[423] Fernandez, M. L. "Dietary Cholesterol Provided by Eggs and Plasma Lipoproteins in Healthy Populations." *Curr. Opin. Clin. Nutr. Metab. Care* 2006;9:8–12.

[424] Ibid.

[425] Greene, C. M., et al. "Plasma LDL and HDL Characteristics and Carotenoid Content Are Positively Influenced by Egg Consumption in an Elderly Population." *Nutr. Metab.* 2006;3:6.

[426] Yancy, W. S., et al. "A Low-Carbohydrate, Ketogenic Diet Versus a Low-Fat Diet to Treat Obesity and Hyperlipidemia." *Ann. Int. Med.* 2004;140:769–777.

[427] Ibid.

[428] Westman, E. C., et al. "Effect of a Low-Carbohydrate, Ketogenic Diet Program Compared to a Low-Fat Diet on Fasting Lipoprotein Subclasses." *Int. J. Cardiol.* 2005;November 15 [Epub, ahead of print].

[429] Wood, R. J., et al. "Carbohydrate Restriction Alters Lipoprotein Metabolism by Modifying VLDL, LDL and HDL Subfraction Distribution and Size in Overweight Men." *J. Nutr.* 2006;136:384–389.

[430] Foster, G. D., et al. "A Randomized Trial of a Low-Carbohydrate Diet for Obesity." *N. Engl. J. Med.* 2003;348:2082–2090.

[431] Fernandez, op. cit.

[432] Hays, J. H., et al. "Effect of a High Saturated Fat and No-Starch Diet on Serum Lipid Subfractions in Patients with Documented Atherosclerotic Cardiovascular Disease." *Mayo Clin. Proc.* 2003;78:1331–1336.

[433] Dansinger, M. L., et al. "Comparison of the Atkins, Ornish, Weight Watchers, and Zone Diets for Weight Loss and Heart Disease Risk Reduction: A Randomized Trial." *JAMA* 2005;293:43–53.

[434] Howard, B. V., et al. "Low-Fat Dietary Pattern and Risk of Cardiovascular Disease: The Women's Health Initiative Randomized Controlled Dietary Modification Trial." *JAMA* 2006;295:655–666.

[435] Bogani, P., et al. "Postprandial Anti-Inflammatory and Antioxidant Effects of Extra Virgin Olive Oil." *Atherosclerosis* 2006;February 17 [Epub ahead of print].

[436] Perona, J. S., et al. "The Role of Virgin Olive Oil Components in the Modulation of Endothelial Function." *J. Nutr. Biochem.* 2005;December 12 (Epub ahead of print].

[437] Wahle, K. W., et al. "Olive Oil and Modulation of Cell Signaling in Disease Prevention." *Lipids* 2004; 39:1223–1231.

[438] Konishi, M., et al. "Association of Serum Total Cholesterol, Different Types of Stroke, and Stenosis Distribution of Cerebral Arteries. The Akita Pathology Study." *Stroke* 1993;24:954–964.

[439] Schatz, I. J., et al. "Cholesterol and All-Cause Mortality in Elderly People from the Honolulu Heart Program: A Cohort Study." *Lancet* 2001;358:351–355.

[440] Ibid.

[441] Ibid.

[442] Fackelmann, K. A. "Japanese Stroke Clues: Are There Risks to Low Cholesterol?" *Science News* 1989; 135:250–253.

[443] Iso, H., et al. "Prospective Study of Fat and Protein Intake and Risk of Intraparenchymal Hemorrhage in Women." *Circulation* 2001;103:856–863.

[444] Willett, W. Personal Communication, August 5, 2000.

[445] Winslow, R. "New Prescription for Zocor Users." *Wall Street Journal*, June 17, 2006; p. A2.

[446] Topol, E. J. "Intensive Statin Therapy—A Sea Change in Cardiovascular Prevention." *N. Engl. J. Med.* 2004;350:1562–1564.

[447] Nissen, S. Communication on *The People's Pharmacy* radio show.

[448] Mosca, L. "C-Reactive Protein—To Screen or Not to Screen." *N. Engl. J. Med.* 2002;347:1615–1617.

[449] Sirois, B. C., and Burg, M. M. "Negative Emotion and Coronary Heart Disease: A Review." *Behav. Modif.* 2003;27:83–102.

[450] Ramachandruni, S., et al. "Mental Stress Provokes Ischemia in Coronary Artery Disease Subjects Without Exercise- or Adenosine-Induced Ischemia." *J. Am. Coll. Cardiol.* 2006;47:987–991.

[451] Hamilton, C. "Marital Strife a Heartbreak in More Ways than One." *The Salt Lake Tribune*, March 5, 2006.

[452] Boyle, S. H., et al. "Hostility, Age, and Mortality in a Sample of Cardiac Patients." *Am. J. Cardiol.* 2005; 96:64–66.

[453] Boyle, S. H., et al. "Hostility as a Predictor of Survival with Coronary Artery Disease." *Psychosom. Med.* 2004;66:629–632.

[454] Smith, T., et al. "Hearts Hurt When Spouses Spat." *Newswise* report about key findings presented at the American Psychosomatic Society meetings, March 3, 2006, Denver, Colorado.

[455] Cromie, W. J. "Better Way to Predict Heart Attacks Is Discovered." *The Harvard University Gazette*, March 23, 2000.

[456] Verma, S., et al. "C-Reactive Protein Comes of Age." *Nat. Clin. Pract. Cardiovasc. Med.* 2005;2:29–36.

[457] Kerr, M. "Mediterranean Diet Has Anti-Inflammatory Effects." *Reuters Health*, March 8, 2006, a report from the American Heart Association's 46th Annual Conference on Cardiovascular Disease Epidemiology.

[458] Wannamethee, S. G., et al. "Associations of Vitamin C Status, Fruit and Vegetable Intakes, and Markers of Inflammation and Hemostasis." *Am. J. Clin. Nutr.* 2006;83:567–574.

[459] Liepa, G. U., and Basu, H. "C-Reactive Proteins and Chronic Disease: What Role Does Nutrition Play?" *Nutr. Clin. Pract.* 2003;18:227–233.

[460] De Bacquer, D., et al. "Epidemiological Evidence for an Association Between Habitual Tea Consumption and Markers of Chronic Inflammation." *Atherosclerosis* 2006; Jan. 25 [Epub ahead of print].

[461] Dalen, J. E. "Aspirin to Prevent Heart Attack and Stroke: What's the Right Dose?" *Am. J. Med.* 2006;119:198–202.

[462] Bhatt, D. L., et al. "Clopidogrel and Aspirin Versus Aspirin Alone for the Prevention of Atherothrombotic Events." *N. Engl. J. Med.* 2006;354 [Epub March 12, ahead of print].

[463] Craven, L. L. "Acetylsalicylic Acid, Possible Preventive of Coronary Thrombosis." *Ann. Western Med.* 1950;4:95–99.

[464] Craven, L. L. "Prevention of Coronary and Cerebral Thrombosis." *Mississippi Medical Valley J.* 1953; 75:38–44.

[465] Antithrombotic Trialists' Collaboration. "Collaborative Meta-Analysis of Randomised Trials of Antiplatelet Therapy for Prevention of Death, Myocardial Infarction, and Stroke in High Risk Patients." *BMJ* 2002;324:71–86.

[466] Hayden, M., et al. "Aspirin for the Primary Prevention of Cardiovascular Events: A Summary of the Evidence for the U.S. Preventive Services Task Force." *Ann. Intern. Med.* 2002;136:161–172.

[467] de Lorgeril, M., and Salen, P. "The Mediterranean-Style Diet for the Prevention of Cardiovascular Diseases." *Public Health Nutr.* 2006;9:118–123.

[468] Mori, T. A., and Woodman, R. J. "The Independent Effects of Eicosapentaenoic Acid and Docosahexaenoic Acid on Cardiovascular Risk Factors in Humans." *Curr. Opin. Clin. Nutr. Metab. Care* 2006; 9:95–104.

[469] Hu, F. B., and Stampfer, M. J. "Nut Consumption and Risk of Coronary Heart Disease: A Review of the Epidemiologic Evidence." *Curr. Atheroscler. Rep.* 1999;1:205–210.

[470] Albert, C. M., et al. "Nut Consumption and Decreased Risk of Sudden Cardiac Death in the Physicians' Health Study." *Arch. Intern. Med.* 2002;162:1382–1387.

[471] Feldman, E. B. "The Scientific Evidence for a Beneficial Health Relationship Between Walnuts and Coronary Heart Disease." *J. Nutr.* 2002;132:1062S–1101S.

[472] Mukuddem-Petersen, J., et al. "A Systematic Review of the Effects of Nuts on Blood Lipid Profies in Humans." *J. Nutr.* 2005;135:2082–2089.

[473] Zibaeenezhad, M. J., et al. "Walnut Consumption in Hyperlipidemic Patients." *Angiology* 2005;56: 581–583.

[474] Koren, J., et al. "Walnut Polyphenolics Inhibit in Vitro Human Plasma and LDL Oxidation." *J. Nutr.* 2001;131:2837–2842.

[475] Ros, E., et al. "A Walnut Diet Improves Endothelial Function in Hypercholesterolemic Subjects: A Randomized Crossover Trial." *Circulation* 2004;109:1609–1614.

[476] Kris-Etherton, P. M., et al. "The Effect of Nuts on Coronary Heart Disease Risk." *Nutr. Rev.* 2001; 59:103–111.

[477] Feldman, op. cit.

[478] Jenkins, D. J. A., et al. "Direct Comparison of a Dietary Portfolio of Cholesterol-Lowering Foods with a Statin in Hypercholesterolemic Participants." *Am. J. Clin. Nutr.* 2005;81:380–387.

[479] Klatsky, A. L. et al. "Moderate Drinking and Reduced Risk of Heart Disease." *Alcohol Res. Health.* 1999; 23:15–23.

[480] Maclure, M. "Demonstration of Deductive Meta-Analysis: Ethanol Intake and Risk of Myocardial Infarction. *Epidemiol. Rev.* 1993;15:328–351.

[481] Mukamal, K. J., et al. "Roles of Drinking Pattern and Type of Alcohol Consumers in Coronary Heart Disease in Men." *N. Engl. J. Med.* 2003;348:109–118.

[482] Elkind, M. S., et al. "Moderate Alcohol Consumption Reduces Risk of Ischemic Stroke: The Northern Manhattan Study." *Stroke* 2006;37:1–2.

[483] Mukamal, K. J., et al. "Alcohol and Risk for Ischemic Stroke in Men: The Role of Drinking Patterns and Usual Beverage." *Ann. Intern. Med.* 2005;142:11–19.

[484] Howard, A. A., et al. "Effect of Alcohol Consumption on Diabetes Mellitus: A Systematic Review." *Ann. Intern. Med.* 2004;140:211–219.

[485] Mukamal, K. J., et al. "Prospective Study of Alcohol Consumption and Risk of Dementia in Older Adults." *JAMA* 2003;289:1405–1413.

[486] Stein, J. H., et al. "Purple Grape Juice Improves Endothelial Function and Reduces the Susceptibility of LDL Cholesterol to Oxidation in Patients with Coronary Artery Disease." *Circulation* 1999;100:1050–1055.

[487] Folts, J. D. "Potential Health Benefits from the Flavonoids in Grape Products on Vascular Disease." *Adv. Exp. Med. Biol.* 2002;505:95–111.

[488] Albers, A. R., et al. "The Antiinflammatory Effects of Purple Grape Juice Consumption in Subjects with Stable Coronary Artery Disease." *Arterioscler. Thromb. Vasc. Biol.* 2004;24:e179–e180.

[489] Aviram, M., et al. "Pomegranate Juice Consumption Reduces Oxidative Stress, Atherogenic Modifications to LDL, and Platelet Aggregations: Studies in Humans and in Atherosclerotic Apolipoprotein E-Deficient Mice." *Am. J. Clin. Nutr.* 2000;71:1062–1076.

[490] Fuhrman, B., et al. "Pomegranate Juice Inhibits Oxidized LDL Update and Cholesterol Biosynthesis in Macrophages." *J. Nutr. Biochem.* 2005;16:570–576.

[491] Aviram, M., et al. "Pomegranate Juice Consumption for 3 Years by Patients with Carotid Artery Stenosis Reduces Common Carotid Intima-Media Thickness, Blood Pressure and LDL Oxidation." *Clin. Nutr.* 2004;23:423–433.

[492] Aviram, M., and Dornfeld, L. "Pomegranate Juice Consumption Inhibits Serum Angiotensin Converting Enzyme Activity and Reduces Systolic Blood Pressure." *Atherosclerosis* 2001;158:195–198.

[493] Esmaillzaden, A., et al. "Concentrated Pomegranate Juice Improves Lipid Profiles in Diabetic Patients with Hypelipidemia." *J. Med. Food* 2004;7:305–308.

[494] Sumner, M. D., et al. "Effects of Pomegranate Juice Consumption on Myocardial Perfusion in Patients with Coronary Heart Disease." *Am. J. Cardiol.* 2005;96:810–814.

[495] Azadzoi, K. M., et al. "Oxidative Stress in Arteriogenic Erectile Dysfunction: Prophylactic Role of Antioxidants." *J. Urol.* 2005;174:386–393.

[496] Malik, A., et al. "Pomegranate Fruit Juice for Chemoprevention and Chemotherapy of Prostate Cancer." *Proc. Natl. Acad. Sci. USA* 2005;102:14813–14818.

[497] Malic, A., and Mukhtar, H. "Prostate Cancer Prevention Through Pomegranate Fruit." *Cell Cycle* 2006;February 15;5(4) [Epub ahead of print].

[498] Ahmed, S., et al. "*Punica granatum L.* Extract Inhibits IL-1 Beta-Induced Expression of Matrix Metalloproteinases by Inhibiting the Activation of MAP Kinases and NF-KabbaB in Human Chondrocytes In Vitro." *J. Nutr.* 2005;135:2096–2102.

[499] Hidaka, M., et al. "Effects of Pomegranate Juice on Human Cytochrome P450 3A (CYP3A) and Carbamazepine Pharmacokinetics in Rats." *Drug Metab. Dispos.* 2005;33:644–648.

[500] Gorinstein, S., et al. "Red Grapefruit Positively Influences Serum Triglyceride Level in Patients Suffering from Coronary Atherosclerosis: Studies in Vitro and in Humans." *J. Agric. Food Chem.* 2006;54:1887–1892.

[501] Grassi, D., et al. "Short-Term Administration of Dark Chocolate Is Followed by a Significant Increase in Insulin Activity and a Decrease in Blood Pressure in Healthy Persons." *Am. J. Clin. Nutr.* 2005;81:611–614.

[502] Hermann, F., et al. "Dark Chocolate Improves Endothelial and Platelet Function." *Heart* 2006;92:119–120.

[503] Keen, C. L., et al. "Cocoa Antioxidants and Cardiovascular Health." *Am. J. Clin. Nutr.* 2005;81:298S–303S.

[504] Schroeter, H., et al. "(-)-Epicatechin Mediates Beneficial Effects of Flavanol-Rich Cocoa on Vascular Function in Humans." *Proc. Natl. Acad. Sci. USA* 2006;103:1024–1029.

[505] Pearson, D. A., et al. "Flavanols and Platelet Reactivity." *Clin. Dev. Immunol.* 2005;12:1–9.

[506] Innes, A. J., et al. "Dark Chocolate Inhibits Platelet Aggregation in Healthy Volunteers." *Platelets* 2003;14:325–327.

[507] Mursu, J., et al. "Dark Chocolate Consumption Increases HDL Cholesterol Concentration and Chocolate Fatty Acids May Inhibit Lipid Peroxidation in Healthy Humans." *Free Radic. Biol. Med.* 2004;37:1351–1359.

[508] Buijsse, B., et al. "Cocoa Intake, Blood Pressure, and Cardiovascular Mortality: The Zutphen Elderly Study." *Arch. Int. Med.* 2006;166:411–417.

[509] Grassi, D., et al. "Cocoa Reduces Blood Pressure and Insulin Resistance and Improves Endothelium-Dependent Vasodilation in Hypertensives." *Hypertension* 2005;46:e17.

[510] Imparl-Radosevich, J., et al. "Regulation of PTP-1 and Insulin Kinase by Fractions from Cinnamon: Implications for Cinnamon Regulation of Insulin Signalling." *Horm. Res.* 1998;50:177–182.

[511] Broadhurst, C. L., et al. "Insulin-Like Biological Activity of Culinary and Medicinal Plant Aqueous Extracts in Vitro." *J. Agric. Food Chem.* 2000;48:849–852.

[512] Lee, J. S., et al. "Cinnamate Supplementation Enhances Hepatic Lipid Metabolism and Antioxidant Defense Systems in High Cholesterol-Fed Rats." *J. Med. Food* 2003;6:183–191.

[513] Khan, A., et al. "Cinnamon Improves Glucose and Lipids of People with Type 2 Diabetes." *Diabetes Care* 2003;26:3215–3218.

[514] The Heart Outcomes Prevention (HOPE) 2 Investigators. "Homocysteine Lowering with Folic Acid and B Vitamins in Vascular Disease." *N. Engl. J. Med.* 2006:354:1567–1577.

[515] Bonaa, K. H., et al. "Homocysteine Lowering and Cardiovascular Events After Acute Myocardial Infarction." *N. Engl. J. Med.* 2006;354:1578–1588.

[516] Conner, P. L., et al. "Fifteen Year Mortality in Coronary Drug Project Patients: Long-Term Benefit with Niacin." *J. Am. Coll. Cardiol.* 1986; 8:1245–1255.

[517] Abbott, R. D., et al. "Dietary Magnesium Intake and the Future Risk of Coronary Heart Disease (the Honolulu Heart Program)." *Am. J. Cardiol.* 2003;92:665–669.

[518] Anderson, J. W., et al. "Cholesterol-Lowering Effects of Psyllium Hydrophilic Mucilloid for Hypercholesterolemic Men." *Arch. Intern. Med.* 1988;148:292–296.

[519] Bell, L. P., et al. "Cholesterol-Lowering Effects of Psyllium Hydrophilic Mucilloid." *JAMA* 1989;261:3419–3423.

[520] Anderson, J. W., et al. "Long-Term Cholesterol-Lowering Effects of Psyllium as an Adjunct to Diet Therapy in the Treatment of Hypercholesterolemia." *Am. J. Clin. Nutr.* 2000;71:1433–1438.

[521] Anderson, J. W., et al. "Cholesterol-Lowering Effects of Psyllium Intake Adjunctive to Diet Therapy in Men and Women with Hypercholesterolemia: Meta-Analysis of 8 Controlled Trials." *Am. J. Clin. Nutr.* 2000;71:472–479.

[522] Anderson, J. W. "Diet First, Then Medication for Hypercholesterolemia." *JAMA* 2003;290:531–533.

[523] Jenkins, D. J. A., et al. "Effects of a Dietary Portfolio of Cholesterol-Lowering Foods vs. Lovastatin on Serum Lipids and C-Reactive Protein." *JAMA* 2003;290:502–510.

[524] Jenkins, D. J. A., et al. "Assessment of the Longer-Term Effects of a Dietary Portfolio of Cholesterol-Lowering Foods in Hypercholesterolemia." *Am. J. Clin. Nutr.* 2006;83:582–591.

[525] Moreyra, A. E., et al. "Effect of Combining Psyllium Fiber with Simvastatin in Lowering Cholesterol." *Arch. Intern. Med.* 2005;165:1161–1166.

[526] Chen, J. T., et al. "Meta-Analysis of Natural Therapies for Hyperlipidemia: Plant Sterols and Stanols Versus Policosanol." *Pharmacotherapy* 2005;25:171–183.

[527] Varady, K. A., et al. "Role of Policosanols in the Prevention and Treatment of Cardiovascular Disease." *Nutr. Rev.* 2003;61:376–383.

[528] Monograph. "Policosanol." *Altern. Med. Rev.* 2004;9:312–317.

[529] Ibid.

[530] Castano, F., et al. "Effects of Addition of Policosanol to Omega-3 Fatty Acid Therapy on the Lipid Profile of Patients with Type II Hypercholesterolaemia." *Drugs R. D.* 2005;6:207–219.

[531] Berthold, H. K., et al. "Effect of Policosanol on Lipid Levels among Patients with Hypercholesterolemia or Combined Hyperlipidemia: A Randomized Controlled Trial." *JAMA* 2006; 295:2262–2269.

[532] Heber, D., et al. "Cholesterol-Lowering Effects of a Proprietary Chinese Red-Yeast Rice Dietary Supplement." *Am. J. Clin. Nutr.* 1999;69:231–236.

[533] Heber, D., et al. "An Analysis of Nine Proprietary Chinese Red Yeast Rice Dietary Supplements: Implications of Variability in Chemical Profile and Contents." *J. Altern. Complement. Med.* 2001;7: 133–139.

[534] Zhaoping, L., et al. "Plasma Clearance of Lovastatin Versus Chinese Red Yeast Rice in Healthy Volunteers." *J. Altern. Complement. Med.* 2005;11:1031–1038.

[535] Winslow, op. cit.

[536] Nissen, S. E., et al. "Effect of Very High-Intensity Statin Therapy on Regression of Coronary Atherosclerosis." *JAMA* 2006;295 [Published online March 13].

[537] Pignone, M., et al. "Aspirin, Statins, or Both Drugs for the Primary Prevention of Coronary Heart Disease Events in Men: A Cost-Utility Analysis." *Ann. Intern. Med.* 2006;144:326–336.

[538] Mata, P., et al. "Benefits and Risks of Simvastatin in Patients with Familial Hypercholesterolaemia." *Drug Saf.* 2003;26:769–786.

[539] Elrod, J. W., and Lefer, D. J. "The Effects of Statins on Endothelium, Inflammation and Cardio-protection." *Drug News Perspect.* 2005;18:229–236.

[540] Hansson, G. K. "Inflammation, Atherosclerosis, and Coronary Artery Disease." *N. Engl. J. Med.* 2005;352:1685–1695.

[541] Chan, K. Y., et al. "HMG-CoA Reductase Inhibitors for Lowering Elevated Levels of C-Reactive Protein." *Am. J. Health Syst. Pharm.* 2004;61:1676–1681.

[542] Pignone, M., et al. "Aspirin, Statins, or Both Drugs for the Primary Prevention of Coronary Heart Disease Events in Men: A Cost-Utility Analysis." *Ann. Intern. Med.* 2006;144:326–336.

[543] Katan, M. B. Book Reviews: "Nutrition in the Prevention and Treatment of Disease." N. *Engl. J. Med.* 2002;346:1754.

[544] Law, M., and Rudnicka, A. R. "Statin Safety: A Systematic Review." *Am. J. Cardiol.* 2006;97(8A):52C–60C.

[545] Laino, C. "Discontinuing Statins Can Lead to Rapid Rise in Cholesterol and C-Reactive Protein." *WebMD Medical News*, March 15, 2006, based on data presented at the annual meeting of the American College of Cardiology, March 11–14, 2006.

[546] Sinatra, Stephen T. *The Sinatra Solution: Metabolic Cardiology.* North Bergen, NJ: Basic Health, 2005; p. 68.

[547] Sinatra, op cit, p. 75.

[548] UCSD Statin Study Group. "Answers to Most Commonly Asked Questions About Statins." Personal Communication.

High Blood Pressure

[549] Mancia, G., et al. "Ambulatory Blood Pressure Monitoring Use in Hypertension Research and Clinical Practice." *Hypertension* 1993;21:510–523.

[550] Turjanmaa, V., et al. "Diurnal Blood Pressure Profiles and Variability in Normotensive Ambulant Subjects." *Clin. Physiol.* 1987;7:389–401.

[551] Robertson, D., et al. "Effects of Caffeine on Plasma Renin Activity, Catecholamines and Blood Pressure." *N. Engl. J. Med.* 1978;298:181–186.

[552] Turjanmaa, V., et al. "Blood Pressure and Heart Rate Variability and Reactivity as Related to Daily Activities in Normotensive Men Measured with 24-H Intra-Arterial Recording." *J. Hypertens.* 1992;10:665–673.

[553] Kassabeh, E., et al. "Inflammatory Aspects of Sleep Apnea and Their Cardiovascular Consequences." *South. Med. J.* 2006;99:58–67.

[554] Tuomisto, M. T., et al. "Diurnal and Weekly Rhythms of Health-Related Variables in Home Recording for Two Months." *Physiol. Behav.* 2006; Feb. 23 [Epub ahead of print].

[555] Mancia, G., et al. "Effects of Blood-Pressure Measurement by the Doctor on Patient's Blood Pressure and Heart Rate." *Lancet* 1983;2:695–698.

[556] Houweling, S. T., et al. "Pitfalls in Blood Pressure Measurement in Daily Practice." *Fam. Pract.* 2006; 23:20–27.

[557] Pickering, T. G., et al. "Recommendations for Blood Pressure Measurement in Humans and Experimental Animals: A Statement for Professionals from the Subcommittee of Professional and Public Education of the American Heart Association Council on High Blood Pressure Research." *Circulation* 2005;111:697–716.

[558] "Blood Pressure Monitors" and "Ratings Blood Pressure Monitors: The Tests Behind the Ratings." *ConsumerReports.org.* June 2003.

[559] Le Pailleur, C., et al. "Talking Effect and White Coat Phenomenon in Hypertensive Patients." *Behav. Med.* 1996;22:114–122.

[560] Saunders, E. "Building on the Specialist's Antihypertensive Treatment Recommendation: It's Just the Beginning." *J. Clin. Hypertens. (Greenwich)* 2006;81(Suppl. 1):31–39.

[561] Prospective Studies Collaboration. "Age-Specific Relevance of Usual Blood Pressure to Vascular Mortality: A Meta-Analysis of Individual Data for One Million Adults in 61 Prospective Studies." *Lancet* 2002;360:1903–1913.

[562] Qiu, C., et al. "Decline in Blood Pressure Over Time and Risk of Dementia: A Longitudinal Study from the Kungsholmen Project." *Stroke* 2004;35:1810–1815.

[563] Psaty, B. M., and Furberg, C. D. "British Guidelines on Managing Hypertension." *BMJ* 1999;319: 589–590.

[564] Volpe, M, et al. "Beyond Hypertension: Toward Guidelines for Cardiovascular Risk Reduction." *Am. J. Hypertens.* 2004;17:1068–1074.

[565] Matthews, K. A., et al. "Blood Pressure Reactivity to Psychological Stress and Coronary Artery Calcification in the Coronary Artery Risk Development in Young Adults Study." *Hypertension* 2006;47:391–395.

[566] Tuomisto, op. cit.

[567] Lynch, J. J., et al. "The Effects of Talking on the Blood Pressure of Hypertensive and Normotensive Individuals." *Psychosom. Med.* 1981;43:25–33.

[568] Le Pailleur, op. cit.

[569] Le Pailleur, C., et al. "Talking Effect and 'White Coat' Effect in Hypertensive Patients: Physical Effort or Emotional Content?" *Behav. Med.* 2001;26:149–157.

[570] Freed, C. D., et al. "Blood Pressure, Heart Rate, and Heart Rhythm Changes in Patients with Heart Disease During Talking." *Heart Lung* 1989;18:17–22.

[571] Yucha, C. B., et al. "Biofeedback-Assisted Relaxation Training for Essential Hypertension: WhoIis Most Likely to Benefit." *J. Cardiovasc. Nurs.* 2005;20:198–205.

[572] Nakao, M., et al. "Blood Pressure-Lowering Effects of Biofeedback Treatment in Hypertension: A Meta-Analysis of Randomized Controlled Trials." *Hypertens. Res.* 2003;26:37–46.

573 Yucha, op cit.

574 Joseph, C. N., et al. "Slow Breathing Improves Arterial Baroreflex Sensitivity and Decreases Blood Pressure." *Hypertension* 2005;46:714–718.

575 Viskoper, R., et al. "Nonpharmacologic Treatment of Resistant Hypertensives by Device-Guided Slow Breathing Exercises." *Am. J. Hypertens.* 2003;16:484–487.

576 Meles, E., et al. "Nonpharmacologic Treatment of Hypertension by Respiratory Exercise in the Home Setting." *Am. J. Hypertens.* 2004;17:370–374.

577 Eliott, W. J., et al. "Graded Blood Pressure Reduction in Hypertensive Outpatients Associated with Use of a Device to Assist with Slow Breathing." *J. Clin. Hypertens. (Greenwich)* 2004;6:553–559.

578 Hawkley, L. C., et al. "Loneliness is a Unique Predictor of Age-Related Differences in Systolic Blood Pressure." *Psychol. Aging* 2006;21:152–164.

579 Craddick, S. R., et al. "The DASH Diet and Blood Pressure." *Curr. Atheroscler. Rep.* 2003;5:484–491.

580 Bacon, S. L., et al. "Effects of Exercise, Diet and Weight Loss on High Blood Pressure." *Sports Med.* 2004;34:307–316.

581 Ard, J. D., et al. "One-Year Follow-Up Study of Blood Pressure and Dietary Patterns in Dietary Approaches to Stop Hypertension (DASH)-Sodium Participants." *Am. J. Hypertens.* 2004;17:1156–1162.

582 Champagne, C. M. "Dietary Interventions on Blood Pressure: The Dietary Approaches to Stop Hypertension (DASH) Trials." *Nutr. Rev.* 2006;64:S53–S56.

583 Appel, L. J., et al. "Effects of Protein, Monunsaturated Fat, and Carbohydrate Intake on Blood Pressure and Serum Lipids: Results of the OmniHeart Randomized Trial." *JAMA* 2005;294: 2455–2464.

584 Neter, J. E., et al. "Influence of Weight Reduction on Blood Pressure: A Meta-Analysis of Randomized Controlled Trials." *Hypertension* 2003;42:878–884.

585 Graudal, N. A., et al. "Effects of Sodium Restriction on Blood Pressure, Renin, Aldosterone, Catecholamines, Cholesterols, and Triglyceride: A Meta-Analysis." *JAMA* 1998;279:1383–1391.

586 Cohen, H. W., et al. "Sodium Intake and Mortality in the NHANES II Follow-up Study." *Am. J. Med.* 2006;119:275.e7–275.e14.

587 Aviv, A. "Salt and Hypertension: The Debate that Begs the Bigger Question." *Arch. Int. Med.* 2001;161:507–510.

588 Weinberger, M. H., et al. "Salt Sensitivity, Pulse Pressure and Death in Normal and Hypertensive Humans." *Hypertension* 2001;37:429–432.

589 Aviv, op. cit.

590 Robertson, D., et al. "Effects of Caffeine on Plasma Renin Activity, Catecholamines and Blood Pressure." *N. Engl. J. Med.* 1978;298:181–186.

591 Noordzij, M., et al. "Blood Pressure Response to Chronic Intake of Coffee and Caffeine: A Meta-Analysis of Randomized Controlled Trials." *J. Hypertens.* 2005;23:921–928.

592 Klag, M. J., et al. "Coffee Intake and Risk of Hypertension." *Arch. Intern. Med.* 2002;162:657–662.

593 Cornelis, M. C., et al. "Coffee, CYP1A2 Genotype, and Risk of Myocardial Infarction." *JAMA* 2006;295:1135–1141.

594 Yang, Y. C., et al. "The Protective Effect of Habitual Tea Consumption on Hypertension." *Arch. Intern. Med.* 2004;164:1534–1540.

595 Aviram, M., and Dornfeld, L. "Pomegranate Juice Consumption Inhibits Serum Angiotensin Converting Enzyme Activity and Reduces Systolic Blood Pressure." *Atherosclerosis* 2001;158:195–198.

596 Aviram, M., and Dornfeld, L. "Pomegranate Juice Consumption Inhibits Serum Angiotensin Converting Enzyme Activity and Reduces Systolic Blood Pressure." *Atherosclerosis* 2001;158:195–198.

597 Sumner, M. D., et al. "Effects of Pomegranate Juice Consumption on Myocardial Perfusion in Patients with Coronary Heart Disease." *Am. J. Cardiol.* 2005;96:810–814.

598 Honsho, S., et al. "A Red Wine Vinegar Beverage Can Inhibit the Renin-Angiotensin System: Experimental Evidence In Vivo." *Biol. Pharm. Bull.* 2005;28:1208–1210.

599 Takahara, A., et al. "The Endothelium-Dependent Vasodilator Action of a New Beverage Made of Red Wine Vinegar and Grape Juice." *Biol. Pharm. Bull.* 2005;28:754–756.

600 Stein, J. H., et al. "Purple Grape Juice Improves Endothelial Function and Reduces the Susceptibility of LDL Cholesterol to Oxidation in Patients with Coronary Artery Disease." *Circulation* 1999; 100:1050–1055.

601 Folts, J. D. "Potential Health Benefits from the Flavonoids in Grape Products on Vascular Disease." *Adv. Exp. Med. Biol.* 2002;505:95–111.

602 Park, Y. K., et al. "Concord Grape Juice Supplementation Reduces Blood Pressure in Korean Hypertensive Men: Double-Blind, Placebo Controlled Intervention Trial." *Biofactors* 2004;22:145–147.

603 Vlachopoulos, C., et al. "Effect of Dark Chocolate on Arterial Function in Healthy Individuals." *Am. J. Hypertens.* 2005;18:785–791.

604 Buijsse, B., et al. "Cocoa Intake, Blood Pressure, and Cardiovascular Mortality: The Zutphen Elderly Study." *Arch. Int. Med.* 2006;166:411–417.

605 Grassi, D., et al. "Cocoa Reduces Blood Pressure and Insulin Resistance and Improves Endothelium-Dependent Vasodilation in Hypertensives." *Hypertension* 2005;46:e17.

606 Buijsse, op. cit.

607 Jee, S. H., et al. "The Effect of Magnesium Supplementation on Blood Pressure: A Meta-Analysis of Randomized Clinical Trials." *Am. J. Hypertens.* 2002;15:691–696.

608 Welton, P. K., et al. "Effects of Oral Potassium on Blood Pressure: A Meta-Analysis of Randomized Controlled Clinical Trials." *JAMA* 1997;277:1624–1632.

609 Griffith, L. E., et al. "The Influence of Dietary and Nondietary Calcium Supplementation on Blood Pressure: An Updated Metaanalysis of Randomized Controlled Trials." *Am. J. Hypertens.* 1997;12: 84–92.

610 Shechter, M., et al. "Effects of Oral Magnesium Therapy on Exercise Tolerance, Exercise-Induced Chest Pain, and Quality of Life in Patients with Coronary Artery Disease." *Am. J. Cardiol.* 2003;91: 517–521.

611 Fujioka, Y., and Yokoyama, M. "Magnesium, Cardiovascular Risk Factors and Atherosclerosis." *Clin. Calcium* 2005;15:221–225.

612 Maier, J. A., et al. "Low Magnesium Promotes Endothelial Cell Dysfunction: Implications for Atherosclerosis, Inflammation and Thrombosis." *Biochem. Biophys. Acta* 2004;1689:13–21.

613 Atabek, M. E., et al. "Serum Magnesium Concentrations in Type 1 Diabetic Patients: Relation to Early Atherosclerosis." *Diabetes Res. Clin. Pract.* 2006;72:42–47.

614 King, D. E., et al. "Dietary Magnesium and C-Reactive Protein." *J. Am. Coll. Nutr.* 2005;24:166–171.

615 Maier, J. A. "Low Magnesium and Atherosclerosis: An Evidence-Based Link." *Mol. Aspects Med.* 2003;24:137–146.

616 He, K., et al. "Magnesium Intake and Incidence of Metabolic Syndrome Among Young Adults." *Circulation* 2006;March 27 [Epub ahead of print].

617 Shechter, M., et al. "Oral Magnesium Therapy Improves Endothelial Function in Patients with Coronary Artery Disease." *Circulation* 2000;102:2353–2358.

618 Singh, R. B., et al. "Magnesium Metabolism in Essential Hypertension." *Acta Cardiol.* 1989;44:313–322.

619 Rahman, K., and Lowe, G. M. "Garlic and Cardiovascular Disease: A Critical Review." *J. Nutr.* 2006;136:736S–740S.

620 Ackerman, R. T., et al. "Garlic Shows Promise for Improving Some Cardiovascular Risk Factors." *Arch. Int. Med.* 2001;161:813–824.

621 Wilburn, A. J., et al. "The Natural Treatment of Hypertension." *J. Clin. Hypertens.* 2004;6:242–248.

[622] Hitti, M. "Grape Seed Extract for Blood Pressure?" *WebMD*, March 27, 2006, based on a presentation by Tissa Kappagoda, MD, PhD, to the American Chemical Society National Meeting, Atlanta, March 26–30, 2006.

[623] Messerli, op. cit.

[624] Williams, F., and The CAFE Investigators, et al. "Differential Impact of Blood Pressure-Lowering Drugs on Central Aortic Pressure and Clinical Outcomes: Principal Results of the Conduit Artery Function Evaluation (CAFE) Study." *Circulation* 2006;113:1213–1225.

[625] Lindholm, L. H., et al. "Should Beta-Blockers Remain First Choice in the Treatment of Primary Hypertension? A Meta-Analysis." *Lancet* 2005;366:1545–1553.

[626] Kaplan, N. M., and Opie, L. H. "Controversies in Hypertension." *Lancet* 2006;367:168–176.

[627] Messerli, F. H., et al. "Beta-Blockers in Hypertension—The Emperor Has No Clothes: An Open Letter to Present and Prospective Drafters of New Guidelines for the Treatment of Hypertension." *Am. J. Hypertens.* 2003;16:870–873.

[628] Beevers, D. G. "The End of Beta-Blockers for Uncomplicated Hypertension?" *Lancet* 2005;366:1510–1512.

[629] Carlberg, B., et al. "Atenolol in Hypertension: Is It a Wise Choice?" *Lancet* 2004;364:1684–1689.

[630] Sharma, A. M., et al. "Beta-Adrenergic Receptor Blockers and Weight Gain: A Systematic Analysis." *Hypertension* 2001;37:250–254.

[631] ALLHAT Collaborative Research Group. "Major Outcomes in High-Risk Hypertensive Patients Randomized to Angiotensin-Converting Enzyme Inhibitor or Calcium Channel Blocker vs. Diuretic: The Antihypertensive and Lipid-Lowering Treatment to Prevent Heart Attack Trial (ALLHAT)." *JAMA* 2002;288:2981–2987.

[632] Ernst, M. E., et al. "Comparative Antihypertensive Effects of Hydrochlorothiazide and Chlorthalidone on Ambulatory and Office Blood Pressure." *Hypertension* 2006;47:352–358.

[633] Sica, D. A. "Chlorthalidone: Has It Always Been the Best Thiazide-Type Diuretic?" *Hypertension* 2006;47:321–322.

[634] Grimm, R. H. Jr., et al. "Long-Term Effects on Sexual Function of Five Antihypertensive Drugs and Nutritional Hygienic Treatment in Hypertensive Men and Women: Treatment of Mild Hypertension (TOMHS)." *Hypertension* 1997;29:8–14.

[635] Furberg, C. Personal communication, December 19, 2002.

[636] Gillespie, E. L., et al. "The Impact of ACE Inhibitors or Angiotensin II Type 1 Receptor Blockers on the Development of New-Onset Type 2 Diabetes." *Diabetes Care* 2005;28:2261–2266.

[637] Furberg, C. Personal communication, April 4, 2006.

[638] Verma, S., and Strauss, M. "Angiotensin Receptor Blockers and Myocardial Infarction: These Drugs May Increase Myocardial Infarction—and Patients May Need to Be Told." *BMJ* 2004;329: 1248–1249.

[639] Volpe, M., et al. "Angiotensin II Receptor Blockers and Myocardial Infarction: Deeds and Misdeeds." *J. Hypertens.* 2005:23:2113–2118.

[640] Schunkert, H. "Pharmacotherapy for Prehypertension—Mission Accomplished? *N. Engl. J. Med.* 2006; March 14 [Epub ahead of print].

Hyperhydrosis

[641] "Don't Sweat It: Epidemiology, Pathophysiology, and Treatment of Hyperhidrosis." *Pharmacy Times* 2006; ACPE Program ID Number: 290-000-06-001-H01.

[642] Ibid.

[643] Hornberger, J., et al. "Recognition, Diagnosis, and Treatment of Primary Focal Hyperhidrosis." *J. Am. Acad. Dermatol.* 2004;51:274.

644 Gupta, V. B., et al. "Aluminum in Alzheimer's Disease: Are We Still at a Crossroad?" *Cell Mol. Life Sci.* 2005;62:143–158.

645 Darbre, P. D. "Aluminum, Antiperspirants and Breast Cancer." *J. Inorg. Biochem.* 2005;99:1912–1919.

646 Darbre, P. D. "Metalloestrogens: An Emerging Class of Inorganic Xenoestrogens with Potential to Add to the Oestrogenic Burden of the Human Breast." *J. Appl. Toxicol.* 2006; [http://dx.doi.org/10.1002/jat.1135].

647 *Pharmacy Times*, op. cit.

648 Benohanian, A., et al. "Localized Hyperhidrosis Treated with Aluminum Chloride in a Salicylic Acid Gel Base." *Int. J. Dermatol.* 1998;37:701.

649 Heckmann, M., et al. "Low-Dose Efficacy of Botulinum Toxin A for Axillary Hyperhidrosis: A Randomized, Side-by-Side, Open Label Study." *Arch. Dermatol.* 2005;141:1255–1259.

Hypothyroidism

650 Shomon, M. *Living Well with Hypothyroidism.* New York: HarperResource, 2005. p. 470.

651 Crane, H. M., et al. "Effects of Ammonium Perchlorate on Thyroid Function in Developing Fathead Minnows, *Pimephales promelas.*" *Environ. Health Perspect.* 2005;113:396–401.

652 Porterfield, S. P. "Thyroidal Dysfunction and Environmental Chemicals—Potential Impact on Brain Development." *Environ. Health Perspect.* 2000;108 (Suppl. 3):433–438.

653 Wang, S.-L., et al. "In Utero Exposure to Dioxins and Polychlorinated Biphenyls and Its Relations to Thyroid Function and Growth Hormone in Newborns." *Environ. Health Perspect.* 2005;113:1645–1650.

654 http://www.ecy.wa.gov/news/2006news/2006-012.html.

655 White, G. H., and Walmsley, R. N. "Can the Initial Clinical Assessment of Thyroid Function Be Improved?" *Lancet* 1978;ii:933–935. Cited in *Bandolier*, 1997;46–45.

656 Dickey, R. A., et al. "Optimal Thyrotropin Level: Normal Ranges and Reference Intervals Are Not Equivalent." *Thyroid* 2005;15:1035–1039.

657 Meier, C., et al. "Restoration of Euthyroidism Accelerates Bone Turnover in Patients with Subclinical Hypothyroidism: A Randomized Controlled Trial." *Osteoporos. Int.* 2004;15:209–216.

658 Arem, R. *The Thyroid Solution.* New York: Ballantine Books, 1999. p. 284.

659 Bunevicius, R., et al. "Effects of Thyroxine as Compared with Thyroxine Plus Triiodothyronine in Patients with Hypothyroidism." *N. Engl. J. Med.* 1999;340:424–429.

660 Escobar-Morreale, H. F., et al. "Treatment of Hypothyroidism with Combinations of Levothyroxine plus Liothyronine." *J. Clin. Endocrinol. Metab.* 2005;90:4946–4954. [

661 Escobar-Morreale, H. F., et al. "Thyroid Hormone Replacement Therapy in Primary Hypothyroidism: A Randomized Trial Comparing L-Thyroxine plus Liothyronine with L-Thyroxine Alone." *Ann. Int. Med.* 2005;142:412–424.

662 Arem, op. cit.

663 Blanchard, K. "Dosage Recommendations for Combination Regimen of Thyroxine and 3,5,3'-Triiodothyronine." *J. Clin. Endocrinol. Metab.* 2004;89:1486–1487.

664 Ditkoff, B. A., and Lo Gerfo, P. *The Thyroid Guide.* New York: HarperCollins, 2000.

665 Chong, W., et al. "Multivariate Analysis of Relationships between Iodine Biological Exposure and Subclinical Thyroid Dysfunctions." *Chin. Med. Sci. J.* 2005;20:202–205.

666 Doerge, D. R., and Chang, H. C. "Inactivation of Thyroid Peroxidase by Soy Isoflavones, In Vitro and In Vivo." *J. Chromatogr. B Analyt. Technol. Biomed. Life Sci.* 2002;777:269–279.

667 Doerge, D. R., and Sheehan, D. M. "Goitrogenic and Estrogenic Activity of Soy Isoflavones." *Environ. Health Perspect.* 2002;110:349–353.

[668] Arem, op. cit., p. 298.

[669] Arem, op. cit., p. 302.

[670] Shomon, M. J. *The Thyroid Diet: Manage Your Metabolism for Lasting Weight Loss.* New York: HarperResource, 2004. p. 53.

Insomnia

[671] Kamel, N. S., and Gammack, J. K. "Insomnia in the Elderly: Cause, Approach, and Treatment." *Am. J. Med.* 2006;119:463–469.

[672] Baron-Faust, R. *Sleep Disorders: Common Problems and Treatments.* Norwalk, CT: Belvoir Media Group, 2006.

[673] Buscemi, N., et al. *Manifestations and Management of Chronic Insomnia in Adults.* Evidence Report/Technology Assessment Number 125. Rockville, MD: Agency for Healthcare Research and Quality, June 2005.

[674] Schernhammer, E. S., et al. "Night Work and Risk of Breast Cancer." *Epidemiology* 2006;17:108–111.

[675] Mills, E., et al. "Melatonin in the Treatment of Cancer: A Systematic Review of Randomized Controlled Trials and Meta-Analysis." *J. Pineal Res.* 2005;39:360–366.

[676] Harder, B. "Bright Lights, Big Cancer." *Science News* 2006;169:8–10.

[677] Baron-Faust, op. cit., pp. 19–20.

[678] Leppamaki, S., et al. "Drop-Out and Mood Improvement: A Randomized Controlled Trial with Light Exposure and Physical Exercise." *BMC Psychiatry* 2004;4:22.

[679] Knight, J. A., et al. "Light and Exercise and Melatonin Production in Women." *Am. J. Epidemiol.* 2005;162:1114–1122.

[680] Li, F., et al. "Tai Chi and Self-Rated Quality of Sleep and Daytime Sleepiness in Older Adults: A Randomized Controlled Trial." *J. Am. Geriatr. Soc.* 2004;52:892–900.

[681] Tworoger, S. S., et al. "Effects of a Yearlong Moderate-Intensity Exercise and a Stretching Intervention on Sleep Quality in Postmenopausal Women." *Sleep* 2003;26:830–836.

[682] Baron-Faust, op. cit., pp. 64–65.

[683] "TV in the Bedroom Halves Your Sex Life." Reuters Health Information, January 16, 2006.

[684] Lai, H.-L., and Good, M. "Music Improves Sleep Quality in Older Adults." *J. Adv. Nursing* 2005;49:234–244.

[685] Viens, M., et al. "Trait Anxiety and Sleep-Onset Insomnia: Evaluation of Treatment Using Anxiety Management Training." *J. Psychosom. Res.* 2003;54:31–37.

[686] Sivertsen, B., et al. "Cognitive Behavioral Therapy vs Zopiclone for Treatment of Chronic Primary Insomnia in Older Adults: A Randomized Controlled Trial." *JAMA* 2006;295:2851–2858.

[687] Wurtman, J., and Suffes, S. *The Serotonin Solution.* New York: Fawcett, 1996, p. 186.

[688] Durlach, J., et al. "Chronopathological Forms of Magnesium Depletion with Hypofunction or with Hyperfunction of the Biological Clock." *Magnes. Res.* 2002;15:263–268.

[689] Hornyak, M., et al. "Magnesium Therapy for Periodic Leg Movements-Related Insomnia and Restless Legs Syndrome: An Open Pilot Study." *Sleep* 1998;21:501–505.

[690] Lewith, G. T., et al. "A Single-Blinded, Randomized Pilot Study Evaluating the Aroma of *Lavandula augustifolia* as a Treatment for Mild Insomnia." *J. Alt. Complement. Med.* 2005;11:631–637.

[691] Goel, N., et al. "An Olfactory Stimulus Modifies Nighttime Sleep in Young Men and Women." *Chronobiol. Int.* 2005;22:889–904.

[692] Koon, J., et al. "Odorant Administration on Sleep Quality, Mood, and Cognitive Performance." Student Research Symposium, Wheeling Jesuit University, April 15, 2003 [(1:15)(P 5)].

[693] Kuroda, K., et al. "Sedative Effects of the Jasmine Tea Odor and (R)-(-)-Linalool, One of Its Major Odor Components, on Autonomic Nerve Activity and Mood States." *Eur. J. Appl. Physiol.* 2005;95:107–114.

[694] Buscemi, N., et al. "The Efficacy and Safety of Exogenous Melatonin for Primary Sleep Disorders: A Meta-Analysis." *J. Gen. Intern. Med.* 2005;20:1151–1158.

[695] Brzezinski, A., et al. "Effects of Exogenous Melatonin on Sleep: A Meta-Analysis." *Sleep Med. Rev.* 2005;9:41–50.

[696] Kayumov, L., et al. "A Randomized, Double-Blind, Placebo-Controlled Crossover Study of the Effect of Exogenous Melatonin on Delayed Sleep Phase Syndrome." *Psychosom. Med.* 2001;63:40–48.

[697] Sok, S., and Kim, K. B. "Effects of Auricular Acupuncture on Insomnia in Korean Elderly." *Taehan. Kanho. Hakhoe. Chi.* 2005;35:1014–1024.

[698] Chen, M. L., et al. "The Effectiveness of Acupressure in Improving the Quality of Sleep of Institutionalized Residents." *J. Gerontol. A Biol. Sci. Med. Sci.* 1999;54:M389–M394.

[699] Hadley, S., and Petry, J. J. "Valerian." *Am. Fam. Physician* 2003;67:1755–1758.

[700] Glass, J. R., et al. "Acute Pharmacological Effects of Temazepam, Diphenhydramine, and Valerian in Healthy Elderly Subjects." *J. Clin. Psychopharmacol.* 2003;23:260–268.

[701] Wheatley, D. "Medicinal Plants for Insomnia: A Review of their Pharmacology, Efficacy, and Tolerability." *J. Psychopharmacol.* 2005;19:414–421.

[702] Glass, J., et al. "Sedative Hypnotics in Older People with Insomnia: Meta-Analysis of Risks and Benefits." *BMJ* 2005;331:1169–1176.

[703] Ibid.

[704] Ibid.

[705] Dundar, Y., et al. "Comparative Efficacy of Newer Hypnotic Drugs for the Short-Term Management of Insomnia: A Systematic Review and Meta-Analysis." *Human Hum. Psychopharmacol. Clin. Exp.* 2004; 19:305–322.

[706] Abramowicz, M., ed. "Ambien CR for Insomnia." *Med. Lett. Drugs Ther.* 2005;47:97–98.

[707] Abramowicz, M., ed. "Remelteon (Rozerem) for Insomnia." *Med. Lett. Drugs Ther.* 2005;47:89–91.

[708] Campbell, S. S., et al. "Light Treatment for Sleep Disorders; Consensus Report." *J. Biol. Rhythms* 1995;10:151–154.

[709] Cole, R. J., et al. "Bright-Light Mask Treatment of Delayed Sleep Phase Syndrome." *J. Biol. Rhythms* 2002;17:89–101.

[710] Abramowicz, M., ed. "Treatment of Insomnia." *Treatment Guidelines from The Medical Letter* 2006;4:5–10.

[711] Silver, M. H. "Chronic Insomnia." *N. Engl. J. Med.* 2005;353:803–810.

Leg Cramps

[712] Panel on Dietary Reference Intakes for Electrolytes and Water. *Dietary Reference Intakes for Water, Potassium, Sodium Chloride, and Sulfate.* Washington, DC: The National Academies Press, 2004.

[713] Roffe, C., et al. "Randomised, Cross-Over, Placebo-Controlled Trial of Magnesium Citrate in the Treatment of Chronic Persistent Leg Cramps." *Med. Sci. Monit.* 2002;8:CR326–CR330.

[714] Dahle, L. O., et al. "The Effect of Oral Magnesium Substitution on Pregnancy-Induced Leg Cramps." *Am. J. Obstet. Gynecol.* 1995;173:175–180.

[715] Hammar, M., et al. "Calcium and Magnesium Status in Pregnant Women. A Comparison between Treatment with Calcium and Vitamin C in Pregnant Women with Leg Cramps." *Int. J. Vitam. Nutr. Res.* 1987; 57:179–183.

[716] Young, G. L., and Jewell, D. "Interventions for Leg Cramps in Pregnancy." *Cochrane Database Syst. Rev.* 2002;(1):CD000121.

[717] Chan, P., et al. "Randomized, Double-Blind, Placebo-Controlled Study of the Safety and Efficacy of Vitamin B Complex in the Treatment of Nocturnal Leg Cramps in Elderly Patients with Hypertension." *J. Clin. Pharmacol.* 1998;38:1151–1154.

[718] "More on Nighttime Leg Cramps." *Harvard Health Letter*, April 2005, p. 7.

[719] Butler, J. V., et al. "Nocturnal Leg Cramps in Older People." *Postgrad. Med. J.* 2002;78:596–598.

[720] Diener, H. C., et al. "Effectiveness of Quinine in Treating Muscle Cramps: A Double-Blind, Placebo-Controlled, Parallel-Group, Multicentre Trial." *Int. J. Clin. Pract.* 2002;56:243–246.

Menopause

[721] *Menopause: A Clinician's Guide*, Section A. Cleveland, OH: North American Menopause Society, October 2004.

[722] *Menopause: A Clinician's Guide*, Section A. op. cit. p. 9.

[723] Colditz, G. A., et al. "The Use of Estrogens and Progestins and the Risk of Breast Cancer in Postmenopausal Women." *N. Engl. J. Med.* 1995;332:1589–1593.

[724] Colditz, G. A. "Estrogen, Estrogen Plus Progestin Therapy, and Risk of Breast Cancer." *Clin. Cancer Res.* 2005;11:909s–917s.

[725] Chlebowski, R. T., et al. "Influence of Estrogen Plus Progestin on Breast Cancer and Mammography in Healthy Postmenopausal Women: The Women's Health Initiative Randomized Trial." *JAMA* 2003; 289:3243–3253.

[726] Love, S. M., and Lindsey, K. *Dr. Susan Love's Hormone Book*. New York: Random House, 1997. p. 160.

[727] MacLennan, A. H., et al. "Oral Oestrogen and Combined Oestrogen/Progestogen Therapy Versus Placebo for Hot Flushes (Review)." *The Cochrane Database of Systematic Reviews* 2004; 4: Art. No: CD002978.pub2. DOI:10.1002/14651858.CD002978.pub2.

[728] Ibid.

[729] Writing Group for the Women's Health Initiative Investigators. "Risks and Benefits of Estrogen Plus Progestin in Healthy Postmenopausal Women: Principal Results from the Women's Health Initiative Randomized Controlled Trial." *JAMA* 2002;288:321–333.

[730] Ibid.

[731] Hsia, J., et al. "Conjugated Equine Estrogens and Coronary Heart Disease: The Women's Health Initiative." *Arch. Intern. Med.* 2006;166:357–365.

[732] Ibid.

[733] Lemaitre, R., et al. "Esterified Estrogen and Conjugated Equine Estrogen and the Risk of Incident Myocardial Infarction and Stroke." *Arch. Intern. Med.* 2006;166:399–404.

[734] Beasley, D. "Use of 'Bioidentical' Female Hormones Questioned." *Reuters Health* October 31, 2005.

[735] Ibid.

[736] Komesaroff, P. A., et al. "Effects of Wild Yam Extract on Menopausal Symptoms, Lipids, and Sex Hormones in Healthy Menopausal Women." *Climacteric* 2001;4:144–150.

[737] Hermann, A. C., et al. "Over-the-Counter Progesterone Cream Produces Significant Drug Exposure Compared to a Food and Drug Administration-Approved Oral Progesterone Product." *J. Clin. Pharmacol.* 2005;45:614–619.

[738] North American Menopause Society. "Treatment of Menopause-Associated Vasomotor Symptoms: Position Statement of the North American Menopause Society." *Menopause* 2004;11:11–33.

[739] Osmers, R., et al. "Efficacy and Safetey of Isopropanolic Black Cohosh Extract for Climacteric Symptoms." *Obstet. Gynecol.* 2005;105:1074–1083.

[740] Nappi, R. E., et al. "Efficacy of *Cimicifuga racemosa* on Climacteric Complaints: A Randomized Study Versus Low-Dose Transdermal Estradiol." *Gynecol. Endocrinol.* 2005;20:30–35.

[741] Ibid.

[742] Kligler, B. "Black Cohosh." *Am. Fam. Physician* 2003;68:114–116.

[743] Osmers, et al. op. cit. p. 1081.

[744] Huntley, A., and Ernst, E. "A Systematic Review of the Safety of Black Cohosh." *Menopause* 2003;10:58–64.

745 Haimov-Kochman, R., and Hochner-Celnikier, D. "Hot Flashes Revisited: Pharmacological and Herbal Options for Hot Flashes Management. What Does the Evidence Tell Us?" *Acta Obstet. Gynecol. Scand.* 2005; 84:972–979.

746 Ibid.

747 Verhoeven, M. O., et al. "Effect of a Combination of Isoflavones and *Actaea racemosa Linnaeus* on Climacteric Symptoms in Healthy Symptomatic Perimenopausal Women: A 12-Week Randomized, Placebo-Controlled, Double-Blind Study." *Menopause* 2005;12:412–420.

748 Messina, M., and Hughes, C. "Efficacy of Soyfoods and Soybean Isoflavone Supplements for Alleviating Menopausal Symptoms Is Positively Related to Initial Hot Flush Frequency." *J. Med. Food* 2003;6:1–11.

749 Huntley, A. L., and Ernst, E. "Soy for the Treatment of Perimenopausal Symptoms—A Systematic Review." *Maturitas* 2004;47:1–9.

750 Faure, E. D., et al. "Effects of a Standardized Soy Extract on Hot Flushes: A Multicenter, Double-Blind, Randomized, Placebo-Controlled Study." *Menopause* 2002;9:329–334.

751 van de Weijer, P. H. M., and Barentsen, R. "Isoflavones from Red Clover (Promensil) Significantly Reduce Menopausal Hot Flush Symptoms Compared with Placebo." *Maturitas* 2002;42:187–193.

752 Tice, J. A., et al. "Phytoestrogen Supplements for the Treatment of Hot Flashes: The Isoflavone Clover Extract (ICE) Study." *JAMA* 2003;290:207–214.

753 Haimov-Kochman, R., and Hochner-Celnikier, D, op. cit. pp. 976–977.

754 Giardinelli, M. "[Effect of Alpha-Tocopherol in Some Disorders of the Menopause and in Atrophy of the Vaginal Mucosa.]" *Minerva Ginecol.* 1952;4579–4587.

755 Stearns, V., et al. "Paroxetine Is an Effective Treatment for Hot Flashes: Results from a Prospective Randomized Clinical Trial." *J. Clin. Oncol.* 2005;23:6919–6930.

756 Loprinzi, C. L., et al. "Venlafaxine in Management of Hot Flashes in Survivors of Breast Cancer: A Randomised Controlled Trial." *Lancet* 2000;356:2059–2063.

757 Boekhout, A. H., et al. "Symptoms and Treatment in Cancer Therapy-Induced Early Menopause." *Oncologist* 2006;11:641–654.

758 Kendall, A., et al. "Caution: Vaginal Estradiol Appears to Be Contraindicated in Postmenopausal Women on Adjuvant Aromatase Inhibitors." *Ann. Oncol.* 2006;17:584–587

Nail Fungus

759 "Vicks VapoRub Might Help Fight Toenail Fungus." *Consumer Reports* 2006;71:49.

760 Ibid.

761 Farber, E. M., and South, D. A. "Urea Ointment in the Nonsurgical Avulsion of Nail Dystrophies." *Cutis* 1978;22:689–692.

762 Sigurgeirsson, B., et al. "Long-Term Effectiveness of Treatment with Terbinafine vs Itraconazole in Onychomycosis." *Arch. Dermatol.* 2002;138:353–357.

763 Warshaw, E. M. "Evaluating Costs for Onychomycosis Treatments: A Practitioner's Perspective." *J. Am. Podiatr. Med. Assoc.* 2006;96:38–52.

764 Gupta, A. K., et al. "The Use of Terbinafine in the Treatment of Onychomycosis in Adults and Special Populations: A Review of the Evidence." *J. Drugs Dermatol.* 2005;4:302–308.

765 Novartis prescribing information T2005-37.

Osteoporosis

766 National Institutes of Health, Osteoporosis and Related Bone Diseases, National Resource Center Web site (http://www.osteo.org).

767 Ibid.

[768] Moynihan, R., and Cassels, A. *Selling Sickness: How the World's Biggest Pharmaceutical Companies Are Turning Us All into Patients.* New York: Nation Books, 2005.

[769] Moynihan, R., and Henry, D. "The Fight against Disease Mongering: Generating Knowledge for Action." *PLoS Med.* 2006;3:e191.

[770] Neuner, J. M., et al. "Bone Density Testing in Older Women and Its Association with Patient Age." *J. Am. Geriatr. Soc.* 2006;54:485–489.

[771] Abramowicz, M., ed. *Treatment Guidelines from The Medical Letter: Drugs for Prevention and Treatment of Postmenopausal Osteoporosis.* 2005;3:69–74.

[772] Moynihan and Cassels, *op. cit.*, p. 142.

[773] Notelovitz, M., et al. *Stand Tall! Every Woman's Guide to Preventing and Treating Osteoporosis.* Gainesville, FL: Triad Publishing Company, 1998. pp. 114–115.

[774] Boonen, S., et al. "Fracture Risk with Calcium and Vitamin D: A Review of the Evidence." *Calcif. Tissue Int.* 2006 [April 21—Epub ahead of print].

[775] Dawson-Hughes, B. "Interaction of Dietary Calcium and Protein in Bone Health in Humans." *J. Nutr.* 2003;133:852S–854S.

[776] Dawson-Hughes, B., et al. "Effect of Calcium and Vitamin D Supplementation on Bone Density in Men and Women 65 Years of Age or Older." *N. Engl. J. Med.* 1997;337:670–676.

[777] Chapuy, M. C., et al. "Combined Calcium and Vitamin D_3 Supplementation in Elderly Women: Confirmation of Reversal of Secondary Hyperparathyroidism and Hip Fracture Risk: The Decalyos II Study." *Osteoporos. Int.* 2002;13:257--64.

[778] Lilliu, H., et al. "Calcium-Vitamin D_3 Supplementation Is Cost-Effective in Hip Fractures Prevention." *Maturitas* 2003;44:299–305.

[779] Jackson, R. D., et al. "Calcium Plus Vitamin D Supplementation and the Risk of Fractures." *N. Engl. J. Med.* 2006;354:750–752.

[780] Holick, M. F., and Jenkins, M. *The UV Advantage.* New York: ibooks, 2003. p. 153.

[781] Bischoff-Ferrari, H. A., et al. "Fracture Prevention with Vitamin D Supplementation: A Meta-Analysis of Randomized Controlled Trials." *JAMA* 2005;293:2257–2264.

[782] Abramowicz, et al., op. cit., p.71.

[783] Abramowicz, et al., op. cit., p. 69.

[784] Atkinson, H. G., ed. "Calcium + Vitamin D Offers Small Bone Improvements." *HealthNews* 2006;12:6–7.

[785] Writing Group for the Women's Health Initiative Randomized Controlled Trial. "Risks and Benefits of Estrogen Plus Progestin in Healthy Postmenopausal Women." *JAMA* 2002;288:321–333.

[786] "Menostar—A Low-Dose Estrogen Patch for Osteoporosis." *Med. Lett. Drugs Ther.* 2004;46:69–70.

[787] Johnson, S. R., et al. "Uterine and Vaginal Effects of Unopposed Ultralow-Dose Transdermal Estradiol." *Obstet. Gynecol.* 2005;105:779–787.

[788] Ettinger, B., et al. "Effects of Ultralow-Dose Transdermal Estradiol on Bone Mineral Density: A Randomized Clinical Trial." *Obstet. Gynecol.* 2004;104:443–451.

[789] Ettinger, B., et al. "Reduction of Vertebral Fracture Risk in Postmenopausal Women with Osteoporosis Treated with Raloxifene: Results from a 3-Year Randomized Clinical Trial." Multiple Outcomes of Raloxifene Evaluation (MORE) Investigators. *JAMA* 1999;282:637–645.

[790] Martino, S., et al. "Safety Assessment of Raloxifene over Eight Years in a Clinical Trial Setting." *Curr. Med. Res. Opin.* 2005;21:1441–1452.

[791] Barrett-Connor, E., et al. "Effects of Raloxifene on Cardiovascular Events and Breast Cancer in Postmenopausal Women." *N. Engl. J. Med.* 2006;355:125–137.

[792] Black, D. M., et al. "Randomised Trial of Effect of Alendronate on Risk of Fracture in Women with Existing Vertebral Fractures. Fracture Intervention Trial Research Group." *Lancet* 1996;348:1535–1541.

[793] Bonnick, S., et al. "Comparison of Weekly Treatment of Postmenopausal Osteoporosis with Alendronate versus Risedronate Over Two Years." *J. Clin. Endocrinol. Metab.* 2006 [April 24—Epub ahead of print].

[794] McClung, M. R., et al. "Effect of Risedronate on the Risk of Hip Fracture in Elderly Women. Hip Intervention Program Study Group." *N. Engl. J. Med.* 2001;344:333–340.

[795] "Alendronate (Fosamax) and Risedronate (Actonel) Revisited." *Med. Lett. Drugs Ther.* 2005;47:33–34.

[796] "Ibandronate (Boniva): A New Oral Bisphosphonate." *Med. Lett. Drugs Ther.* 2005;47:35–36.

[797] Fraunfelder, F. W., and Fraunfelder, F. T. "Bisphosphonates and Ocular Inflammation." *N. Engl. J. Med.* 2003;348:1187.

[798] Wysowski, D. K., and Chang, J. T. "Alendronate and Risedronate: Reports of Severe Bone, Joint, and Muscle Pain." *Arch. Intern. Med.* 2005;165:346.

[799] "Teriparatide (Forteo) for Osteoporosis." *Med. Lett. Drugs Ther.* 2003;45:9–11.

[800] Body, J. J., et al. "A Randomized Double-Blind Trial to Compare the Efficacy of Teriparatide [Recombinant Human Parathyroid Hormone (1-34)] with Alendronate in Postmenopausal Women with Osteoporosis." *J. Clin. Endocrinol. Metab.* 2002;87:4528–4535.

[801] Abramowicz, op. cit., p. 74.

[802] Ofluoglu, D., et al. "The Effect of Calcitonin on Beta-Endorphin Levels in Postmenopausal Osteoporotic Patients with Back Pain." *Clin. Rheumatol.* 2006 [March 31—Epub ahead of print].

[803] Papadokostakis, G., et al. "The Effectiveness of Calcitonin on Chronic Back Pain and Daily Activities in Postmenopausal Women with Osteoporosis." *Eur. Spine J.* 2006;15:356–362.

[804] Fadanelli, M. E., and Bone, H. G. "Combining Bisphosphonates with Hormone Therapy for Postmenopausal Osteoporosis." *Treat. Endocrinol.* 2004;3:361–369.

[805] Gaspard, U., and Van den Brule, F. "Medication of the Month. Angeliq: New Hormonal Therapy of Menopause, with Antialdosterone and Antiandrogenic Properties." *Rev. Med. Liege.* 2004;59:162–166.

[806] Abramowicz, op. cit., p. 73.

Tinnitus

[807] Noell, C. A., and Meyerhoff, W. L. "Tinnitus: Diagnosis and Treatment of this Elusive Symptom." *Geriatrics* 2003;58:28–34.

[808] Lockwood, A. H., et al. "Tinnitus." *N. Engl. J. Med.* 2002;347:904–910.

[809] Ibid.

[810] Rossiter, S., et al. "Tinnitus and Its Effect on Working Memory and Attention." *J. Speech Lang. Hear. Res.* 2006;49:150–160.

[811] Lockwood, op. cit.

[812] Dobie, R. A. "A Review of Randomized Clinical Trials in Tinnitus." *Laryngoscope* 1999;109:1202–1211.

[813] Dobie, R. A., et al. "Antidepressant Treatment of Tinnitus Patients: Report of a Randomized Clinical Trial and Clinical Prediction of Benefit." *Am. J. Otol.* 1993;14:18–23.

[814] Noell, op. cit.

[815] Sierpina, V. S., et al. "Ginkgo Biloba." *Am. Fam. Physician* 2003;68:923–926.

[816] Ernst, E., and Stevinson, C. "Ginkgo Biloba for Tinnitus: A Review." *Clin. Otolaryngol.* 1999;24: 164–167.

[817] Drew, S., and Davies, E. "Effectiveness of Ginkgo Biloba in Treating Tinnitus: Double Blind, Placebo Controlled Trial." *BMJ* 2001;322:73–78.

[818] Rejali, D., et al. "Ginkgo Biloba Does Not Benefit Patients with Tinnitus: A Randomized Placebo-Controlled Double-Blind Trial and Meta-Analysis of Randomized Trials." *Clin. Otolaryngol. Allied Sci.* 2004;29:226–231.

[819] Arda, H. N., et al. "The Role of Zinc in the Treatment of Tinnitus." *Otol. Neurol.* 2003;24:86–89.

[820] Herxheimer, A., and Petrie, K. J. "Melatonin for the Prevention and Treatment of Jet Lag." *Cochrane Database Syst. Rev.* 2002;(2):CD001520.

[821] Buscemi, N., et al. "The Efficacy and Safety of Exogenous Melatonin for Primary Sleep Disorders: A Meta-Analysis." *J. Gen. Intern. Med.* 2005;20:1151–1158.

[822] Buscemi, N., et al. "Efficacy and Safety of Exogenous Melatonin for Secondary Sleep Disorders and Sleep Disorders Accompanying Sleep Restriction: Meta-Analysis." *BMJ* 2006;332:385–393.

[823] Rosenberg, S. I., et al. "Effect of Melatonin on Tinnitus." *Laryngoscope* 1998;108:305–310.

[824] Megwalu, U. C., et al. "The Effects of Melatonin on Tinnitus and Sleep." *Otolaryngol. Head Neck Surg.* 2006;134:210–213.

[825] Yilmaz, I., et al. "Misoprostol in the Treatment of Tinnitus: A Double-Blind Study." *Otolaryngol. Head Neck Surg.* 2004;130:604–620.

[826] Briner, W., et al. "Synthetic Prostaglandin E1 Misoprostol as a Treatment for Tinnitus." *Arch. Otolaryngol. Head Neck Surg.* 1993;119:652–654.

[827] Ibid.

[828] Akkuzu, B., et al. "Efficacy of Misoprostol in the Treatment of Tinnitus in Patients with Diabetes and/or Hypertension." *Auris Nasus Larynx* 2003;31:226–232.

[829] Yilmaz, I., op. cit.

Weight Loss

[830] Dansinger, M. L., et al. "Comparison of the Atkins, Ornish, Weight Watchers, and Zone Diets for Weight Loss and Heart Disease Risk Reduction: A Randomized Trial." *JAMA* 2005;293:43–53.

[831] Nordmann, A. J., et al. "Effects of Low-Carbohydrate vs Low-Fat Diets on Weight Loss and Cardiovascular Risk Factors: A Meta-analysis of Randomized Controlled Trials." *Arch. Intern. Med.* 2006; 166:285–293.

[832] Katzen, M., and Willett, W. C. *Eat, Drink, and Weigh Less: A Flexible and Delicious Way to Shrink Your Waist Without Going Hungry.* New York: Hyperion, 2006. pp. 96-101.

[833] Popkin, B. M., et al. "A New Proposed Guidance System for Beverage Consumption in the United States." *Am. J. Clin. Nutr.* 2006;83:529–542.

[834] Wyatt, H. R., et al. "Long-Term Weight Loss and Breakfast in Subjects in the National Weight Control Registry." *Obes. Res.* 2002;10:78–82.

[835] Wolfram, S., et al. "Anti-Obesity Effects of Green Tea: From Bedside to Bench." *Mol. Nutr. Food Res.* 2006;50;176–187.

[836] Pittler, M. H., et al. "Adverse Events of Herbal Food Supplements for Body Weight Reduction: Systematic Review." *Obes. Rev.* 2005;6:93–111.

[837] Heymsfield, S. B., et al. "*Garcinia cambogia* (Hydroxycitric Acid) as a Potential Antiobesity Agent: A Randomized Controlled Trial." *JAMA* 1998;80:1596–1600.

[838] Kernan, W. N., et al. "Phenylpropanolamine and the Risk of Hemorrhagic Stroke." *N. Engl. J. Med.* 2000;243:1826–1832.

[839] Hertzman, P. "The Cost Effectiveness of Orlistat in a 1-Year Weight-Management Programme for Treating Overweight and Obese Patients in Sweden: A Treatment Responder Approach." *Pharmacoeconomics* 2005;23:1007–1020.

[840] Despres, J.-P., et al. "Effects of Rimonabant on Metabolic Risk Factors in Overweight Patients with Dyslipidemia." *N. Engl. J. Med.* 2005;353:2121–2134.

[841] Van Gaal, L. F., et al. "Effects of the Cannabinoid-1 Receptor Blocker Rimonabant on Weight Reduction and Cardiovascular Risk Factors in Overweight Patients: 1-Year Experience from the RIO-Europe Study." *Lancet* 2005;365:1389–1397.

[842] Pi-Sunyer, F. X., et al. "Effect of Rimonabant, a Cannabinoid-1 Receptor Blocker, on Weight and Cardiometabolic Risk Factors in Overweight or Obese Patients: RIO-North America: A Randomized Controlled Trial." *JAMA* 2006;295:761–775.

[843] Marx, J. "Drugs Inspired by a Drug." *Science* 2006;311:322–325.

THE PEOPLE'S PHARMACY
FAVORITE PICKS

Over the last 30 years we have heard from a lot of our newspaper column readers and radio show listeners about their favorite remedies for a variety of conditions. Suffering is the mother of creativity, so people have come up with ingenious ways to relieve their discomfort. Some of these are astonishingly inexpensive, and others are just plain astonishing.

People reach for what they have on hand, which might account for why common household products show up so frequently in strange home remedies. Perhaps that is why some folks have tried rinsing their itchy scalp with Listerine for flaky dandruff. How did someone come up with the idea of applying Vicks VapoRub to fungus-infected toenails or of sloshing a laxative (milk of magnesia) on armpits as a deodorant? We may never know what prompted these experiments, but readers tell us they are effective.

There are few, if any, double-blind, placebo-controlled trials of home remedies. Such studies generally cost millions of dollars and involve randomizing subjects to either an active treatment, such as a drug or dietary supplement, or a placebo. The dummy pills are identical in appearance to the active agent, and neither the investigators nor the human guinea pigs know which is which. The goal of this type of protocol is to eliminate bias and suggestibility. Such studies are the gold standard of scientific research, but who would spend good money to test the effectiveness of vinegar soaks against nail fungus? And how would you create a placebo vinegar solution?

Many of the simple approaches detailed in this book won't work for everyone. But then again, prescription drugs don't work for everyone, either. We have heard from so many people about their successes with particular treatments that we wanted to share them with you. The cost of trying them, in most cases, is minimal—certainly far less than that of most prescription medications.

We have collected some of our favorite treatments below. They should never be substituted for proper medical diagnosis and care. But you may find that some of these approaches are practical, affordable, and effective. Any condition that does not respond promptly to self-care or that continues to get worse should be reviewed with a health-care professional.

BLACK PEPPER FOR BLEEDING

Physicians often look down their noses at home remedies. In an era of "evidence-based medicine," such treatments are considered quaint at best and harmful at worst. The fear is that people will try something dangerous or delay seeking appropriate treatment for a severe problem. We understand and share these concerns. We would never advocate using a home remedy for a serious condition that would be better treated with a prescription medicine. But sometimes people need to make do with what they have at hand.

Although double-blind, placebo-controlled trials are the standard for assessing any therapy, common sense and personal experience are also worthwhile. As far as we can tell, there has never been a well-controlled study of using black pepper to stop bleeding. Nevertheless, our own experience tells us that this one works. It is one of the most astonishing home remedies we have ever heard about.

Nell Heard and her family were camping in Yellowstone National Park, far from any medical facility. A mug fell out of their RV's cupboard and hit Nell's brother-in-law Wendall on the head. The long, shallow gash started to bleed profusely, but Wendall, a wood-carver, suggested sprinkling ground black pepper on it. This worked very well to stop the bleeding.

We shared this report with readers of our newspaper column. Since then, we have heard from many folks who used black pepper successfully, but the most dramatic story came from Stephen Scott:

“*Once I was working alone in wintertime in a church. I was pushing a duct together and my hand slipped. The raw edge of the metal cut my hand open. Picture the cut you would need if you were removing a thumb—about 3 inches long and right to the bone at the joint. Pressure wasn't working, there was no telephone, and it was about 10 degrees outside. I had been dropped off there and had no idea where I was.*

I remembered my mother telling me that either black pepper or cobwebs would stop bleeding. I found some pepper in the church kitchen, and after applying great pressure, I opened my hand and the wound, and I dumped about a half shaker of pepper directly into the gaping cut. I pushed it shut again, put a pot-holder over it, and secured it with some electrical tape. The bleeding stopped immediately, and in a matter of minutes there was no pain. After about 20 minutes I got bored and went back to work. I finished out the day, but when I got home, my wife started screaming for me to rush to the hospital.

When I got to the emergency room there was more screaming. The doctor and nurses thought I was an idiot for putting pepper in the cut and insisted that every bit be washed out. Of course, as they fiddled with it, large amounts of blood began pouring out and it hurt like hell again. Finally, my patience ran out and I held some gauze over the cut and left. I immediately went down to the cafeteria, opened a bunch of those little pepper packages, poured the wound full again, and drove myself home. My wife complained that I was stupid and unreasonable, but the entire unstitched, un-doctored, bone-deep wound healed without a scar. I have used black pepper to heal cuts ever since. "

We would never suggest that anyone consider using black pepper to treat such a serious wound. This sort of injury needs immediate medical attention and stitches, which were not initially available to Stephen. We were astonished and delighted to learn of his success, however. For minor cuts, then, we think black pepper has something to offer. Here's an example that makes sense to us: "Soon after reading about black pepper I cut myself while opening a letter. I immediately plunged the finger into my small tin of black pepper and in an instant the bleeding stopped. It didn't burn or hurt." We, too, have had similar success with black pepper. Others tell us that cayenne pepper also works.

CINNAMON FOR BLOOD SUGAR AND CHOLESTEROL

There is growing evidence that spices that we take for granted may have powerful pharmacological effects. Cinnamon is our favorite example. Research suggests that ¼ to ½ teaspoon of cinnamon can lower blood sugar, apparently by increasing insulin sensitivity.[1] Diabetic mice given a cinnamon extract had lower blood sugar, higher HDL cholesterol, and lower triglyceride levels.[2] Some of the research in humans corroborates the blood sugar–lowering effects of cinnamon.[3]

Cinnamon off the spice rack may be contaminated with coumarin, which can damage the liver. Water-extracted capsules are not. If you take cinnamon, you must be under medical supervision and constantly monitor blood glucose to keep it at the right level. Alternative approaches should never be substituted for medically supervised diabetes management!

> *I'm a type 2 diabetic. I read that cinnamon can reduce blood sugar levels, but it doesn't work for me. I've been having two cinnamon buns for breakfast every day and my blood sugar has gone up. (Just kidding!)*
>
> *Actually, I've been adding half a teaspoon of cinnamon to my lunchtime sugar-free shake four or five times a week and there's been a noticeable reduction in my readings the next morning.*

No one should ever use cinnamon or any other home remedy to substitute for careful diabetes management by a physician. Nevertheless, we have heard from lots of folks who have improved control over the condition with these remedies. Some of these people have combined two different approaches, such as cinnamon and mustard. As crazy as it may seem to expect mustard to lower the blood glucose level, several animal studies have shown that curcumin, the active ingredient in the yellow spice turmeric, does just that. Turmeric gives mustard its yellow color.

> *I have been using cinnamon to help control my blood sugar for the last 4 years. Using ¼ teaspoon in boiling water to make a cinnamon tea lowers my blood sugar readings from about 185 to 135 in 1 hour.*

> *Yellow mustard works even more effectively. I take about ½ teaspoon per meal, depending on the amount of carbohydrates in the food. Both cinnamon and yellow mustard can be overdone and make blood sugar go too low, so you have to be cautious.*

Some readers report that they have also been able to improve their cholesterol and other lipid blood levels with cinnamon. One downside: Some people complain of heartburn. Please check with your physician before considering long-term use of cinnamon. It might also interact with some prescription medicines.

> *I've been trying to improve my cholesterol levels with exercise and healthy diet. For 10 years, my typical LDL was 135 while my HDL was 35.*
>
> *This year's numbers were 114 and 43. My total cholesterol dropped from 192 to 170 and my triglycerides went from 98 to 65. The only change I've made was to have ¼ teaspoon cinnamon on my breakfast cereal every morning. I am pleasantly surprised.*

COCONUT FOR DIARRHEA

In 1998 Donald Agar wrote to tell us that eating two Archway coconut macaroon cookies daily could overcome chronic diarrhea. Donald stumbled upon this remedy by accident. He had suffered with Crohn's disease (an inflammatory bowel disorder marked by severe diarrhea) for 40 years. After eating the cookies, though, his problem virtually disappeared.

Over the last several years we have heard from dozens of people who have found that coconut is helpful in controlling diarrhea. Some suffer from irritable bowel syndrome (IBS), while others found coconut useful against diarrhea triggered by chemotherapy drugs. One young man even reported that coconut-containing candy bars (such as Mounds) helped his antibiotic-induced diarrhea. Not everyone will benefit from this treatment, but those who do are extremely pleased.

❝ *I want to thank you for the remedy that has changed my life! I have severe ulcerative colitis. For 14 years, I had 30 loose, bloody bowel movements a day along with unbearable cramps. Six months ago I started eating two Archway coconut macaroon cookies with breakfast. I now have just three bowel movements a day. The stools are solid with no bleeding and I have virtually no cramps at all.*

As a 43-year-old fitness nut engaged in weight training, I am in great shape and feel better than I did 20 years ago. I still take maintenance medicine to be safe, but the cookies made all the difference. ❞

We don't think there is anything special about Archway brand coconut macaroons. You could make your own macaroon cookies or just try plain shredded coconut. We've heard from people who got no benefit from cookies but found that 2 or 3 teaspoons of shredded coconut sprinkled on their breakfast cereal did the trick. Dog owners have given shredded coconut to their pets when nothing the vet prescribed worked well for doggie diarrhea. We urge caution, however. Too much coconut can be constipating, as this letter shows.

❝ *I saw a mention of macaroons curing diarrhea, but 4 years ago I knew nothing of this. My husband brought home some delicious macaroons and I pigged out on them.*

The next day I was in so much pain I passed out and had to be taken to the emergency room. My bowels were bound. They pumped my stomach, starved me, put an IV in me, threatened surgery, and kept me for 5 days. I escaped surgery, but what an experience! Now when I tell people macaroons can have a constipating effect, I know firsthand. ❞

DUCT TAPE FOR WARTS

Who says home remedies don't work? When it comes to warts, even dermatologists sometimes use unorthodox approaches. Over the years, these specialists have occasionally shared the tricks of their trade. Some have claimed that they can "buy" a wart from a child by rubbing a shiny new penny on it. Others have used a magnifying glass to focus the rays of the sun on the base of the wart.

> *I had a small wart on the back of my hand that the dermatologist treated with liquid nitrogen. Two applications did not work.*
>
> *Next I tried taping a small piece of banana peel, wet side to skin, over the wart. With diligent use of the banana peel, the wart has gone and not returned.*

We have collected dozens of other wart remedies over the decades. They include soaking the wart in vinegar or hot water; applying castor oil, nail polish, instant (cyanoacrylate) glue, or potato peel; and taking oral cimetidine (Tagamet). None has any real scientific basis, but people swear that they work. It's possible that vinegar creates an inhospitable environment for the virus that causes warts. Hot water may somehow stimulate the immune system to defeat the virus. But we have no clinical data to support the effectiveness of these remedies or understand why they work.

That's why we were so excited to see a dermatological study on using duct tape to treat children's warts. Researchers divided the children into two groups, and half received the standard liquid nitrogen therapy to freeze their warts. The remaining children had a tiny piece of duct tape applied to the wart for 6 days. After this time, parents were instructed to remove the duct tape, soak the wart in water, and then sand it down with an emery board. The duct tape was left off overnight and then reapplied for another 6 days. This procedure was repeated for up to 2 months or until the wart disappeared.

The treatment was successful in 60 percent of the children treated with liquid nitrogen and in 85 percent of those treated with duct tape. The investigators speculated that the duct tape had somehow stimulated the children's immune system because some untreated warts also disappeared. The researchers concluded that "the use of duct tape appears promising as a safe and nonthreatening treatment modality for children."[4]

These results are all the more impressive in light of an overview of standard wart treatments published in the *British Medical Journal*.[5] The researchers reviewed the effectiveness of wart remedies containing salicylic acid (such as Wart-Off, Compound W, and Clear Away) as well as cryotherapy, laser surgery, and other expensive high-tech treatments. Salicylic acid was the only method with data to support its efficacy.

> *As a doctor, I don't embrace all home remedies, but I like the duct tape idea with warts. It really works. In fact, I had one teenager with warts all over his finger and around the fingernail—which is very difficult to treat. He tried athletic tape, which looks a little better than duct tape, and the warts disappeared within a month. We think the tape causes some local inflammatory reaction that induces the immune system to kill the wart virus.*

KEYS FOR NOSEBLEEDS

Nosebleeds are common, messy, and embarrassing. No one likes to drip blood all over everything. Children are especially prone to nosebleeds, perhaps because they are also more likely to pick their noses. Other causes include dry air, a blow to the nose, frequent sneezing, and high blood pressure.

Some doctors recommend blowing the nose to clear out the clots and then applying pressure by pinching the nose shut for 10 to 15 minutes. Others suggest placing an ice pack over the bridge of the nose. Although this conventional medical wisdom may work for some, it doesn't always solve the problem.

A reader shared one of the most unusual home remedies we have ever received: "A few years ago, a co-worker developed a major nosebleed. I tried ice and pressure to no avail. The bleeding had me worried. A co-worker stopped by and asked, 'Where are your car keys?' The person with the nosebleed handed her his huge key ring and she loosened his shirt and dropped the keys down his back. Within 30 seconds the bleeding stopped! Her grandmother had used this method for years."

We had never encountered this approach before. In fact, we thought it was so ridiculous we almost did not share it. But since then we have heard that it works from so many people that we can no longer ignore this simple trick. We've even tried it ourselves, with immediate results.

Some sleuthing has revealed that this folk remedy was known in colonial America and seems to have come from the British Isles. The Maharani of Jaipur, Gayatri Devi, reported in her memoir, *A Princess Remembers*, that when she got a nosebleed at age 11, the actor Douglas Fairbanks Sr. "put a key down my back to stop the bleeding." Nuns and teachers seem particularly fond of this remedy.

> *I was teaching in a rural school in south Georgia in a four-pod classroom with 120 first-graders and four teachers. Kids played hard in the heat and humidity and many children came in with nosebleeds. I used the old methods of squeezing their nostrils and having them hold their heads back or putting ice on the backs of their necks to try to stop the bleeding.*
>
> *One day an elderly custodian who had lived in the South all her life took out her car keys, asked for some string to tie through the key ring, placed the string around the neck of the child with the nosebleed and dropped the keys down the child's back under her shirt. That nosebleed was no longer a frightening problem!*
>
> *I treated nosebleeds this way and never had a problem again. That's 120 first-graders a year for 15 years, which sounds like a pretty big number to me!*

If such an old-fashioned home remedy doesn't work or if you just prefer drugstore solutions, consider Nosebleed QR. It contains hydrophilic polymer powder and potassium salt. In one study, it stopped a nosebleed in less than a minute for most patients. You can buy Nosebleed QR in the pharmacy without a prescription. More information is available at 800-722-7559 or on the Web at www.biolife.com.

When folk treatments or over-the-counter

(OTC) medicines don't work promptly, medical attention is essential. Prolonged nosebleeds (15 to 20 minutes) require a trip to the emergency room.

LISTERINE FOR ATHLETE'S FOOT, DANDRUFF, AND JOCK ITCH

The smell and taste of original Listerine are so distinctive that they can never be forgotten. Gargling with this mouthwash can't be described as pleasant. The taste is bitter. It puckers the mouth and makes the tongue tingle. The aftertaste lingers.

It is astonishing that a product that has been described as tasting terrible has remained so popular for so long. Listerine was originally developed in 1879 not for use as a mouthwash, but as an antiseptic for use prior to surgery. Its inventor, Jordan Lambert, named it in honor of Dr. Joseph Lister, the pioneer of antiseptic surgery.

In 1895 the product was marketed to dentists to kill bacteria in the mouth. By 1914, Lambert and his son Gerald began offering Listerine to the public as a mouthwash, and one of America's most enduring personal-care products was launched. Listerine has maintained its popularity in part because of its distinctive taste. Although the company has new flavors and colors, the old-fashioned amber liquid still has devotees. And we keep hearing from readers about new uses for this old patent medicine.

One of those "new" uses is actually a rediscovered old use. Back in the early 20th century, Listerine was advertised as a cure for infectious dandruff. The original formulation contains a number of herbal oils—including thymol, eucalyptol, menthol, and methyl salicylate—that seem to have antifungal activity. We've heard that these various herbs may work better together than any of them can alone, but it seems that doing research to substantiate bizarre uses is not on the manufacturer's agenda, so we have no clinical data to support that claim.

> *I have suffered from severe dandruff all of my life, and nothing helped. I tried washing my hair with Listerine and have been dandruff free since. It's nothing short of a miracle cure.*

Some years back, a man called our public radio show to say that his vet had recommended Listerine mixed with baby oil for treating hot spots on his Doberman dogs and his horses. It worked so well on the animals that he decided to try it on his own dandruff, and he reported to us that it worked within a few days. We have since heard from many readers who have had success with this approach. Because dandruff is often triggered by a yeast called *Malassezia* that is susceptible to antifungal treatments, we no longer think that it is surprising.

If Listerine (the original formula) does indeed fight fungal infection, it's easy to imagine that it might work against conditions like athlete's foot and jock itch, which are also caused by fungi. That is also what we hear from readers who want us to know that this treatment can be inexpensive and effective, although it may sting when first applied to the skin.

> *Forty-plus years ago when I was a glue chemist, we kept a crystal of thymol in our pH buffers to prevent the growth of organisms like fungi and bacteria.*
>
> *So I tried sloshing Listerine on a paper towel and applying it to my scalp. It worked against dandruff. I reasoned that since Listerine is okay in the mouth, it should be safe for regular skin. Listerine also turns out to be wonderful for treating jock itch and smelly feet.*

In addition to seborrheic dermatitis (severe dandruff caused by *Malassezia* that may appear on the face as well as the scalp), fungal infections of the nails may respond to this treatment. One reader told us that painting his toenails morning and night with a solution of half Listerine and half white vinegar got rid of his nail fungus within several months. Others are enthusiastic about using Listerine as a way to avoid lice infestation. Some readers have also tried using Listerine on the painful rash caused by shingles. Most report that it relieves the pain rapidly.

> *I called my aunt in Virginia and told her to try Listerine on the shingles. She is at the point she would try anything at all. Last night she took a shower and coated the affected areas with Listerine mouthwash. She had her first pain-free night in years.*

> *This morning, she took another shower and applied Listerine and again, she had no pain today. This may be an off-the-wall solution, but it is working for my aunt.*

MUSTARD FOR BURNS, HEARTBURN, AND LEG CRAMPS

When a gentleman from South Carolina called our syndicated radio show to tell us that plain old yellow mustard helps minor skin burns heal faster, we tried to talk him out of it. We suggested that rapid application of ice water was preferable. He insisted, though, that mustard really will do the trick.

Then we heard from a person who had seen this remedy work up close and personal. At the age of 7, he and his twin brother were tearing around his grandmother's kitchen in the mountains of North Carolina. His brother tripped and stuck out his hands to catch himself. One hand landed on the red-hot eye of the woodstove. His dad scooped the kid up and plunged the burned hand into a gallon jar of yellow mustard that was in the fridge. The only area that was red the next day was where the boy had peeled away the dried mustard "glove." We think the cold mustard must have stopped the tissue injury instantly. In addition, the turmeric in yellow mustard may have healing properties.

We have also heard that swallowing a teaspoonful of yellow mustard can stop heartburn quickly. That may seem counterintuitive, but we have heard from enough people that we think there is some merit to this remedy.

> *My husband and I use a teaspoon of yellow mustard to relieve heartburn. I was in a chat room a while ago when one of the chatters complained about her heartburn. Another said, "Try mustard." We all thought this was ludicrous, but she did try it and it helped.*
>
> *The next time my husband had one of his terrible roll-on-the-floor-in-agony bouts of heartburn, I suggested mustard. I figured it couldn't hurt any more than what he already had. Amazingly, it worked, faster than Tums or DiGel. Our friends have had good results also.*

Another popular use for this cheap kitchen staple is for stopping leg cramps. It does not work for everyone, but many readers have had surprising success with this unorthodox approach to easing a muscle spasm.

> *My husband had severe leg cramps for years. While he was at the eye doctor, the receptionist excused herself, saying, "I've got leg cramps. I've gotta grab the dill pickle juice!"*
>
> *When my husband got leg cramps a few nights later, he grabbed the dill pickle jar and poured himself a swig of juice. Almost instantly, the cramps were gone!*
>
> *Once we were out of pickle juice and he took a tablespoon of mustard. Voilà! He got the same result! Now he keeps little packets of mustard in the car and the truck just in case.*

OLIVE OIL FOR HEMORRHOIDS

Hemorrhoids can be quite painful. Physicians frequently recommend a warm sitz bath to help ease the discomfort. That basically boils down to sitting in the bathtub a few times a day. The problem is that this common practice has no scientific evidence to support it.[6] Nevertheless, if it helps you, don't worry about the lack of research. If it doesn't, here are some other options.

Witch hazel is a time-honored topical treatment for hemorrhoids. Buy a generic brand and saturate some toilet paper. Gently wiping or patting it on the hemorrhoid is all you need to do.

Some people insist that Vicks VapoRub can relieve the discomfort of hemorrhoids, but we generally advise against this application. Another option is warm rutabaga. A reader suggested this root vegetable could do wonders for hemorrhoids. Peel and boil a rutabaga, then drain the fiber well to make a poultice. Spread it on gauze and put it on the hemorrhoids while the rutabaga mush is still warm. She learned this approach from her Scottish mother.

Olive oil is another option. It has anti-inflammatory properties in the diet. One reader reports that it can soothe irritated hemorrhoids when used topically.

> *Hemorrhoids are a real pain in the rump! When I ran out of Preparation H for an attack, I read the ingredients to see what I could substitute. I was astonished to see shark liver oil. Good grief!*

I made a little pad out of toilet paper and put some olive oil on it. As soon as I applied it, my pain was soothed. The hemorrhoids also disappeared. I don't know if I am imagining things, but olive oil worked for me. People who are allergic to olive oil obviously shouldn't try it.

TURMERIC FOR PSORIASIS

Americans are gradually rediscovering some natural medicines that have long been popular in other parts of the world. One of these is turmeric, the spice that makes curry yellow. It's also found in yellow mustard.

Turmeric comes from the rhizome of a plant, *Curcuma longa*, that is related to ginger and native to India. It has long been used in that country in the traditional practice of Ayurvedic medicine and in traditional Chinese medicine as well. The most active component of turmeric, curcumin, has powerful antioxidant activity. Scientists have been testing turmeric and curcumin for treating a variety of serious health problems, including Alzheimer's disease, arthritis, cancer, Crohn's disease, cardiovascular diseases, diabetes, osteoporosis, and psoriasis.[7]

Readers started reporting that taking turmeric could alleviate their hard-to-treat skin problems around the same time that some researchers were identifying its potential usefulness for psoriasis.[8] We received this amazing message in August 2003:

A few months ago you wrote about turmeric being used for boils and also being studied for treating arthritis and cancer. This bit of information has changed my life. I've suffered with psoriasis for 25 years, having it over nearly half of my body. I've seen many physicians and tried every medication and ultraviolet treatment. The cost has been enormous, matched only by my disappointment with the failures.

When I read that turmeric might have anti-inflammatory action, I wondered if it could help me. I immediately bought some and sprinkled a rounded teaspoonful on my cereal. I continued the regimen daily and the results are unbelievable! After 10 days, the awful itching and bleeding had ceased. My scalp, which had been heavily flaked and itchy, was returning to normal. The skin problems on my legs and thighs cleared up after 8 weeks. Now, 5 months later, I have no psoriasis, just a few reddened areas where it was bad. I am grateful to you for the information that made a huge difference for me.

Physicians frequently find such stories hard to believe. They are clearly anecdotal and not scientific. We have heard from others, however, that turmeric has helped clear their psoriasis. One mother reported that nothing else had worked well for her daughter's psoriasis, but after 3 weeks of turmeric treatment, the girl's arms had no more red, itchy patches. Doctors usually chalk up such positive results to the placebo effect.

We find it harder to explain how animals could be responding to a placebo. In addition to psoriasis, turmeric has been used for arthritis or joint pain. Since it has anti-inflammatory properties, there is some scientific basis for this use, though few clinical trials exist.

> ❝ My pet potbellied pig (Bradford) was down for 6 weeks with a disc problem in his back. We tried everything to help him, including prednisone. What finally saved him, just before the vet was set to euthanize him, was turmeric!
>
> A friend recommended giving him curcumin pills. They had worked wonders for her son after surgery. Once Brad ate them, his recovery was almost a miracle. For the first time in 6 weeks he got up and made himself a bed, he ate without being spoon-fed and drank from a dish rather than a syringe. I believe it saved his life. We cancelled the vet appointment and he's been a happy, pain-free pig ever since (about 2 years).
>
> In addition, I have another pig, Snippet, with arthritic front feet who is getting turmeric daily and shows improvement. Snip gets ½ teaspoon of turmeric twice a day right from the spice can with a meal. He seems to like the taste. ❞

Another reader discovered an odd side effect when she started taking turmeric for knee pain. Her desire to gamble disappeared. This has not shown up anywhere in the medical literature. One might even dismiss it as totally ludicrous, except the opposite effect has also been reported. Some patients on a drug to treat Parkinson's disease have experienced a compulsion to gamble.[9]

> ❝ All my life my knees have ached at night. I would use Aleve, arthritis-strength aspirin, or Tylenol and usually woke up and had to take more about 3 a.m. I read in your column about using turmeric for arthritis pain and I bought some turmeric capsules. I took one with milk and a cookie at bedtime and slept pain-free all night and every night since then. It is almost miraculous.
>
> There is another interesting effect. I used to enjoy playing the slot machines. With video slot machines in bars and restaurants here in Oregon, I was playing the slots once or twice a week. I felt I was a little too interested in the slots but I'd still find myself spending more on them than I intended. Since that first capsule of turmeric, I have had no interest whatsoever in gambling. It was like flipping off a switch.
>
> I'd think this was simply an odd coincidence, but I recall reading about a prescription drug with the opposite effect. It triggered a gambling compulsion that went away when the drug was discontinued. Gambling is hard to kick, so I thought you might be interested in my experience. Turmeric has been a godsend to me on two fronts. ❞

Other readers have discovered some hazards not yet reported in the medical literature. Susceptible people may suffer allergic reactions (such as rash) to turmeric. We also caution patients on warfarin (Coumadin) that one reader experienced a significant increase in that drug's anticoagulant effect when she added turmeric to her regimen. Fortunately, it was discovered before it caused a dangerous hemorrhage.

VICKS VAPORUB FOR JUST ABOUT EVERYTHING

The never-ending story of "off-label" uses for Vicks VapoRub got its start many years ago when foot-care nurse Jane Kelley, RN, contacted us to report that vinegar soaks could be helpful for nail fungus. She added, almost as an afterthought, that some people were coating infected nails with Vicks ointment twice a day and getting good results.

Almost as a lark, we wrote about this unique use for Vicks in our newspaper column. Then the letters started pouring in. People shared amazing stories about using the ointment to clear up difficult-to-treat cases of nail fungus. Michigan State University researchers finally verified what we had been talking about for almost a decade. They found that daily applications of Vicks cleared fungal infection in 32 of 85 patients. Patience is necessary, though, since it took anywhere from 5 to 16 months to achieve results.[10] We can't tell you why some folks see fabulous results and others get no benefit. But then again, the same thing happens with pricey prescription products.

> *I'd like to add to your library of success stories with Vicks VapoRub. My husband had a toenail he called his 'eagle claw.'*
> *I told him what I had read about Vicks Vapo-Rub for nails. He used it religiously, once a day, for about 3 months. He was then able to clip this 'eagle claw' toenail away. That very hard nail softened and grew out normal with the use of Vicks.*

UNIQUE USES FOR VAPORUB

- Ant repellant
- Calluses
- Chest congestion
- Chigger bites
- Coughs
- Cracked fingertips
- Dandruff
- Fire ant bites
- Fungus on skin or nails
- Headaches
- Hemorrhoids (external)
- Kitten scratches
- Leg cramps
- Mosquito bites
- Paper cuts
- Poison ivy
- Scaly skin
- Seborrheic dermatitis
- Sore heels
- Squirrel repellant
- Tennis elbow

We heard from another nurse that smearing Vicks on the soles of the feet could help a child with a cough sleep through the night.

People wrote about using Vicks on paper cuts, mosquito and fire ant bites, and seborrheic dermatitis.

> *My son continues to have problems with ear infections, although he had tubes put in them at 8 months old. He is now 30 months old and has an ear infection with nasal and chest congestion.*
>
> *I was looking for home remedies for coughs when I found your Web site. I read the idea of putting Vicks VapoRub on the soles of the feet. Within 10 minutes he was asleep without a cough.*

Cat lovers have used Vicks to keep frisky kittens from scratching their legs. Scientists have used it to keep polar bears from rejecting foster cubs. Horse trainers have used it under stallions' nostrils when they are being trained as racehorses to keep them from being distracted by nearby fillies. And quite a few birdwatchers have come up with the idea of smearing it on the birdfeeder pole to repel squirrels; this is occasionally successful. It needs to be kept away from places where birds might perch on or accidentally ingest it.

> *My elbows were very scaly and getting uncomfortable to lean on. Since scaly skin could be a sign of fungus and I had Vicks VapoRub on hand, I tried it.*
>
> *My elbows are now about 85 percent better,*

> *but here is the really cool thing. I am an artist. Since I turned 50, my fingertips would split and bleed whenever I handled paper, worked in the garden, or washed too often. It was almost impossible to put any kind of pressure on my fingers. I was wearing bandages on my fingertips and feeling debilitated.*
>
> *Since treating my elbows for fungus, my hands have stopped splitting and bleeding. They had been so sore I had trouble doing any fine finger work. I conclude my fingers must also have had a fungal infection and the oils in the VapoRub have helped my skin stay whole.*

Some individuals have found the ointment useful for softening calluses on their feet or scaly skin on elbows. A few brave souls insist that it can relieve the discomfort of hemorrhoids, but we generally advise against this application. John Welter, an essayist who tried it, reported: "The active ingredients in Vicks—which I think are menthol, camphor, and napalm—instantly engulfed my hemorrhoidal locality in spontaneous combustion."

There is another place one should probably not put Vicks. We recently received this message from a reader: "I was experimenting with Vicks VapoRub to see if it would help my jock itch. I inadvertently got some where I shouldn't. I believe I have found a poor man's Viagra!"

This is not the first time we'd heard of this effect. Pharmacist Anna Barrigan told us of her experience in Alaska in the 1950s, when most of the jobs were in construction, gold dredging, bars, and the military. With a ratio of 50 to 60 men for every woman, there were long lines outside the houses of prostitution every payday. The "ladies of the evening" all got paid the same, so if they wanted to make more they had to work quicker. Apparently some of them sped things along with a tiny dab of Vicks in a critical location. According to Ms. Barrigan, "It would get the blood flowing to that organ in very little time. I guess this was an early form of Viagra." We urge readers *not* to try this at home! Vicks VapoRub is intended for external use only and is not to be applied to delicate tissues.

VINEGAR FOR DANDRUFF, DRY SKIN, AND WARTS

Vinegar might just be one of the most versatile home remedies there is. Perhaps because everyone has vinegar in the kitchen cupboard, it has been put to use for an astounding range of common ailments. As for most home remedies, there is little, if any, scientific research to back up the claims. Then again, vinegar is inexpensive, and the likelihood of side effects is low. After all, if we use it in salads, how dangerous can it be?

One of the ways we think vinegar works against the fungus among us is by changing the pH of the skin and scalp. Although it is a temporary effect, fungi (including yeast, which is a type of fungus) have a hard time surviving in an acidic environment. Vinegar is, after all, acetic acid.

Since fungal infections are the cause of everything from athlete's foot and dandruff to jock itch and nail infections, it does not surprise us that our readers report that vinegar works for all these conditions. Doctors sometimes recommend flushing the ear with a mixture of one part white vinegar to five parts tepid water to discourage a type of fungus that causes itching in the ear. Athlete's foot often responds well to being soaked in a vinegar solution (half vinegar, half water) or swabbing with straight vinegar. Don't put it on broken

---

UNIQUE USES FOR VINEGAR

- Arthritis
- Athlete's foot
- Bee stings
- Cholesterol
- Constipation
- Dandruff
- Dry skin
- Fire ant bites
- Fungus in ears or on nails
- Granuloma annulare
- Heartburn
- High blood sugar
- Jock itch
- Nits
- Smelly armpits
- Warts

skin, though, because it will sting and be uncomfortable.

> *All my life I have used dilute vinegar to rinse my hair after shampooing. It works well against dandruff and you can also use it on your feet to stop odor. Best of all, it's cheap!*

There are so many dandruff shampoos readily available that it seems unlikely that many people would use vinegar to treat dandruff. But every year we hear from readers who find this inexpensive approach works better on their dandruff than the fancy medicated shampoos do. As we mentioned, dandruff is partly triggered by a yeast called *Malassezia* that lives on the scalp. Presumably, vinegar clears up dandruff by making the environment unfriendly to yeast.

> *My wife reads your column and told me about using a vinegar rinse to control my dry scalp. I have suffered from this problem for years. I have used a huge variety of shampoos, including expensive prescription ones. Sometimes my scalp would itch so badly it was difficult to sleep.*
>
> *The vinegar mixed with an equal amount of water has made a huge difference. Thank you for helping me to control my dry scalp.*
>
> *I have even started rinsing my dog's coat with this solution after bathing him. He had some areas where the hair was very thin and it has grown back. We spent hundreds on vet bills*

for him, and I am pleased to have solved this problem so inexpensively.

Another use for vinegar on the hair, this one endorsed by the medical establishment, is to loosen the glue that holds nits to hair. This makes combing out nits after treating the lice much easier, though it will never be pleasant. Vinegar alone does not kill the lice, but it can help get rid of the nits so the infestation does not continue.

> *Last year it seemed every kid in the state contracted lice, and I caught them from my granddaughter. She and I tried every possible shampoo, rinse, and remedy and combed our hair with special combs, all to no avail. It was awful!*
>
> *What finally worked was white vinegar. Wet the hair and towel it partly dry. Pour the white vinegar all over the hair and let it set there awhile. That's all we had to do to end the nightmare.*

Jock itch is closely related to athlete's foot, with a similar fungus being implicated in both. Over-the-counter medicines as well as prescription creams will fight this fungus, but many men find that vinegar is at least as effective and far less expensive.

> *The constant itch in my groin continues all year-round though summer is worse. Lotrimin antifungal spray is effective but expensive.*
>
> *A lady told me that her husband suffers from the same trouble. She advised rubbing the area*

with vinegar. This smells strong, but it makes the itch go away for a longer time. It's much easier to get this remedy from the kitchen than to pay high prices for medicine."

Until the early 1990s doctors rarely treated nail fungus except in diabetics, for whom foot problems are a serious concern. The prescription drugs that they used worked slowly and were inconvenient. They also had side effects. With the introduction of newer, more effective nail fungus treatments, physicians are quicker to prescribe medications for infected nails. But even the new pills work slowly and have some worrisome side effects. Treating the fungus with vinegar requires a lot of patience, but many readers have found that it can banish nail fungus at a very low cost and with minimal risk.

"*I have fought toenail fungus for years, even having several toenails removed from each foot.* No fun! *Then I read somewhere that fungus can't live in an acidic environment.*

Two years ago I began putting white vinegar on each toenail with a cotton swab twice a day. I do this in the morning as I have a cup of coffee and read my e-mail, then again each evening after supper. After about 6 weeks, all evidence of toenail fungus disappeared.

I noticed an extra benefit. I am an avid hunter, but wearing hunting boots all day makes my feet sweat profusely. In the fall I've always had smelly feet and athlete's foot. I tried all the pow-

ders and creams and even a prescription from my doc. The vinegar cured it all. I will swear to my grave: vinegar cures foot fungus and prevents its recurrence."

Other skin conditions not caused by fungus or yeast also seem to respond to treatment with vinegar. We have heard that vinegar can considerably ease dry skin. One reader uses a solution of two-thirds vinegar and one-third water to spray on her hands and feet in the shower. Vinegar is also a very popular way to treat warts.

"*I have had a wart on my finger for more than 2 years. I tried Compound W for 2 months or so with no noticeable effect.*

After reading your column, I tried wrapping it with banana peel, dousing it with iodine, and then with castor oil. After 2 months of each, nothing!

Then, based on your latest advice, I began swabbing it with vinegar. After 2 months it is decreasing in size and no longer stands above the surface of the skin. This appears to be working on a second wart, too."

Some folks find that vinegar is an inexpensive way to deal with underarm odor rather than using aluminum salts or other potentially irritating chemicals. One woman wrote, "I had chemo treatment for breast cancer in 2002 and found that all antiperspirants caused redness and irritation. My doctor advised me not to use any deodorant, but that did not suit me.

I tried plain white vinegar, and it worked so well I've kept it up ever since."

A mixture of vinegar and baking soda makes an impressive bubbling poultice for bee or wasp stings and even for fire ant bites. It seems to help alleviate the pain immediately and decrease the subsequent inflammation. Besides, the fizzing looks cool, and that alone may be enough to charm a child into smiling. Of course, no such home remedy is appropriate for someone having a serious allergic reaction to a sting with swelling or wheezing. Emergency medical care is called for in such situations.

> *The tip on using vinegar and baking soda for fire ant bites worked well the day my toddler was playing hide-and-seek and chose to hide in an ant bed. There were marks for a few days, but none of the usual blistering. The bites did not seem to bother her.*

The internal uses for vinegar cover an even wider range. Some people claim that a vinegar concoction (1 teaspoon vinegar, 2 teaspoons honey, and 4 ounces of hot water), taken daily, is great for preventing constipation. Others are enthusiastic about the benefits of vinegar as first aid for heartburn. It seems like the last thing anyone with heartburn would want to swallow, yet some people swear that it helps.

> *A doctor advised a family friend to take a tablespoon of vinegar for heartburn relief. I tried 2 teaspoons of apple cider vinegar and it worked.*

> *It tastes strong for a few minutes and I thought the heartburn was worse. Then the pain went away for good.*

One of the most fascinating uses of vinegar is in a cholesterol-lowering mixture. We haven't seen any research that suggests vinegar will actually have an impact on blood lipids, though it is a persistent and widespread belief. We have received many testimonials claiming that a combination of juice and vinegar has had a beneficial effect on cholesterol.

> *I have a friend who has a cholesterol problem but can't take medication for it because of elevated liver enzymes. Her doctor told her to mix 4 cups of apple juice with 3 cups of white grape juice and half a cup of apple cider vinegar. She is supposed to drink 6 ounces of this mixture every morning. She's been following this regimen for approximately 6 months and her cholesterol is going down.*

Another intriguing use for vinegar is to keep blood sugar under control after a high-carbohydrate meal. Unlike other vinegar remedies, this one is actually supported by some scientific research. Investigators in Sweden report that vinegar given with white bread reduces blood sugar and insulin. It also helps people feel fuller for up to 2 hours later.[11] Swedish nutrition scientists have also found that potato salad prepared with a vinegar dressing does not have the same dramatic effect on blood sugar as regular potatoes do.[12]

Japanese researchers have found that vinegar can counteract the effect of white rice on blood sugar.[13] And investigators at Arizona State University report that 2 tablespoons of vinegar taken before a starchy meal can significantly reduce the rise in blood glucose.[14]

> ❝ *I suffer with type 2 diabetes. My doctor prescribed Glucotrol for my blood sugar. It has helped to a degree, but I have found that by also adding apple cider vinegar and cinnamon to a careful diet, I can control my blood sugar even better.* ❞

YOGURT FOR HANGNAILS

Hangnails are one of life's little miseries. It's hard to understand how such a small sliver of skin can catch on so many things. And if you bite, tear, or clip it off, there is always the possibility of inflammation and infection. You can soak the finger in a variety of solutions, from Epsom salts or kosher salt to 4 capfuls of bath oil (such as Alpha Keri) in 2 cups of warm water. Another option, according to a reader, is to stick the finger in an active culture of yogurt.

> ❝ *I had a hangnail that had gotten very inflamed. A friend of mine from Iran told me to buy plain yogurt that had active culture and soak my finger in it. She said Iranians use plain yogurt for numerous things.*
>
> *I tried the yogurt and my hangnail cleared up very quickly. Maybe the probiotics in yogurt have anti-inflammatory properties.* ❞

REFERENCES

[1] Broadhurst, C. L., et al. "Insulin-Like Biological Activity of Culinary and Medicinal Plant Aqueous Extracts in Vitro." *J. Agric. Food Chem.* 2000;48:849–852.

[2] Kim, S. H., et al. "Antidiabetic Effect of Cinnamon Extract on Blood Glucose in db/db Mice." *J. Ethnopharmacol.* 2005;Oct 3 [Epub ahead of print].

[3] Khan, A., et al. "Cinnamon Improves Glucose and Lipids of People with Type 2 Diabetes." *Diabetes Care* 2003;26:3215–3218.

[4] Focht, D. R., et al. "The Efficacy of Duct Tape vs Cryotherapy in the Treatment of Verruca Vulgaris (the Common Wart)." *Arch. Pediatr. Adolesc. Med.* 2002;156:971–974.

[5] Gibbs, S., et al. "Local Treatments for Cutaneous Warts: Systematic Review." *BMJ* 2002;325:461–469.

[6] Tejirian, T. and Abbas, M. A. "Sitz Bath: Where Is the Evidence? Scientific Basis of a Common Practice." *Dis. Colon Rectum* 2005;48:2336–2340.

[7] Shishodia, S., et al. "Curcumin: Getting Back to the Roots." *Ann. N.Y. Acad. Sci.* 2005;1056:206–217.

[8] Pol, A., et al. "Comparison of Antiproliferative Effects of Experimental and Established Antipsoriatic Drugs on Human Keratinocytes, Using a Simple 96-Well-Plate Assay." *In Vitro Cell Dev. Biol. Anim.* 2003;39:36–42.

[9] Dodd, M. L., et al. "Pathological Gambling Caused by Drugs Used to Treat Parkinson Disease." *Arch. Neurol.* 2005;62:1377–1381.

[10] "Vicks VapoRub Might Help Fight Toenail Fungus." *Consum. Rep.* 2006;71:49.

[11] Ostman, E., et al. "Vinegar Supplementation Lowers Glucose and Insulin Responses and Increases Satiety After a Bread Meal in Healthy Subjects." *Eur. J. Clin. Nutr.* 2005;59:983–988.

[12] Leeman, M., et al. "Vinegar Dressing and Cold Storage of Potatoes Lowers Postprandial Glycaemic and Insulinaemic Responses in Healthy Subjects." *Eur. J. Clin. Nutr.* 2005;59:1266–1271.

[13] Sugiyama, M., et al. "Glycemic Index of Single and Mixed Meal Foods among Common Japanese Foods with White Rice as a Reference Food." *Eur. J. Clin. Nutr.* 2003;57:743–752.

[14] Johnston, C. S., et al. "Vinegar Improves Insulin Sensitivity to a High-Carbohydrate Meal in Subjects with Insulin Resistance or Type 2 Diabetes." *Diabetes Care* 2004;27:281–282.

APPENDIX

HOW I LOWERED MY LDL CHOLESTEROL 44 POINTS IN 5 WEEKS WITHOUT DRUGS*

by Laura Effel

Authors' note: A listener of our radio show contacted us about her success with diet and cholesterol control. She wrote to tell us how she had lowered her cholesterol without drugs. We were so impressed with her story that we wanted to share it. Not everyone can achieve such dramatic results with diet alone, but Laura's story demonstrates that diet can make a difference. And lest you think this was a flash in the pan, we heard that three months later Laura had maintained her success and even managed to achieve greater improvement by lowering her LDL cholesterol to 70.

*Reprinted with permission from Laura Effel.

At the age of 60 I got my first bad news about cholesterol in the mail from my doctor: LDL cholesterol of 155—near alarming—accompanied by a prescription for Zocor (simvastatin) and a recommendation that I take it. Since I took no regular prescriptions and had heard of the many problems caused by statin drugs, such as muscle weakness, I wanted to try reducing my bad cholesterol without drugs.

Undoubtedly, the unexpected increase in my LDL cholesterol was caused by the drop in estrogen after I stopped hormone replacement therapy, which I had started after having a complete hysterectomy. I never thought that hot flashes were a reason to take medicine, but I knew my hot flashes were telling me something about changes in my body.[*] Now I knew what the message was: Your LDL cholesterol is up!

With the help of a food scientist and the skeptical cooperation of my physician, I set about changing my diet to make a difference. Five weeks later, from changes in diet alone, my LDL cholesterol was down 44 points. I had a new way of eating, a permanent change, and I knew my cholesterol would continue to improve.

My old way of eating had not been disastrous, especially not before the loss of estro-gen. After all, at the age of 60, I weighed little more than I had the day I graduated from high school at 18. But I made changes that made a difference.

Here is what I did:

- Avoided spikes in blood sugar
- Eliminated refined carbohydrates
- Ate a high-protein breakfast
- Substituted olive oil for other fats
- Added soluble fiber to meals other than breakfast
- Focused on fish
- Drank green tea
- Consumed other antioxidants
- Stopped eating before bed

The experiment worked. My LDL cholesterol not only went down 44 points in 5 weeks, it also continued on its downward course.

1. Avoided Spikes in Blood Sugar

Most people know that eating saturated fat causes their bodies to make cholesterol, but relatively few have gotten the message that excess blood sugar does the same. When my body takes in more energy than it needs for current use, it stores the energy and thus needs cholesterol to carry it around in the bloodstream. Avoiding spikes in blood sugar reduces the body's need to produce cholesterol. This is the same diet principle that keeps blood sugar in check for a diabetic. If everyone ate like a diabetic, Lipitor (atorvastatin) might not be the top-selling prescription drug that it is.

---

[*]My doctor's comment was that postmenopausal women have predictable changes that lead to higher risk of development of coronary disease: substantially higher LDL cholesterol, total cholesterol, and triglycerides and a concomitant decrease in HDL (good) cholesterol.

2. Eliminated Refined Carbohydrates

The carbohydrates to avoid are the ones that are quickly turned into blood sugar: white sugar, white flour, white potatoes, and any other food with a high glycemic index, a notion that has gained publicity recently. I did not give up all carbohydrates, but I included primarily whole foods or whole-grain foods to the extent possible. I gave up juice, choosing whole fruit instead. Oranges were on my list of acceptable foods; orange juice was out. I had never consumed sodas anyway.

I used a glycemic index list from a published source since not all the categorizations are obvious. For example, raisins are high glycemic foods, but dried figs and prunes are low glycemic foods.

3. Ate a High-Protein Breakfast

I started my day with a high-protein breakfast, with added fat from olive oil, and fruit. Since I have an intolerance for eggs, one obvious source of breakfast protein was not available to me. I frequently eat nonfat cottage cheese, with black pepper and extra virgin olive oil, perhaps with sliced tomato if ripe tomatoes are available.

When I first started my new regimen, I ate fish for breakfast most days, with either olive oil or additional omega-3 fish oil on it, and a piece of fruit, but that was austere even for a determined fanatic like me. Rarely do I include any carbohydrate-rich foods at breakfast. The protein is transformed into energy slowly and sustains me through the morning if I eat enough of it.

4. Substituted Olive Oil for Other Fats

I not only put extra-virgin olive oil on my cottage cheese for breakfast and on salads of all kinds, I also use olive oil (but not extra-virgin) for cooking.

In fact, garlic sautéed in olive oil makes almost everything taste better. Even my picky 17-year-old son will devour spinach cooked this way.

5. Added Soluble Fiber to Meals Other Than Breakfast

Due to a cereal producer's promotional campaign, most people have heard that oatmeal can reduce cholesterol. But if they eat sweetened instant oatmeal for breakfast, they may accomplish nothing.* Soluble fiber works best if it is consumed, unsweetened, before a meal to slow the absorption of energy and thus slow the rise in blood sugar occasioned by eating a meal's worth of food. Consuming it during or right after the meal works pretty well, too. This was probably the most effective step I took toward reducing my LDL cholesterol.

The usefulness of soluble fiber in reducing cholesterol is not well publicized, even

*By the time the oatmeal is processed to death, sweetened, and loaded with nonnutritive additives, it is worthless.

though it is well known in the food industry. A glimmer of this mysterious dichotomy between industry and public knowledge can be seen on the label of the house brand of psyllium capsules sold at Wal-Mart under the name Equate Fiber Therapy. In small red letters at the bottom of the label, highlighted in yellow, are the words, "Peel here for more information." Then, under the label that describes the product's use as a bulk-forming laxative is a second label, this one describing its use to reduce cholesterol!

My soluble fiber choice is usually psyllium seed husk, also called *psyllium*. If I am eating out, as I frequently do at lunch, I take six capsules of psyllium with water before the meal. The capsules are available in any drugstore. I avoid the sweetened varieties of psyllium and brand names in favor of store-brand capsules with no added ingredients.

At home, I use bulk psyllium, purchased at a health-food store, and mix about 3 heaping tablespoons with skim milk to consume before lunch or dinner. It sets up thickly and sometimes has to be eaten with a spoon. The taste is a bit like shredded wheat.

Later, I began adding other ingredients to the psyllium that I take before dinner: 2 heaping tablespoons of ground flaxseed (a source of omega-3 oil) and 1 level teaspoon of cinnamon. I mix the dry items together before stirring in the skim milk. The cinnamon was recommended on *The People's Pharmacy* radio show on public radio. Taking this mixture before dinner isn't quite like having dessert first, but it comes close now that I am no longer eating pastries.

Another soluble fiber that I sometimes use is called konjac. Konjac is difficult to find in powdered or capsule form, though 4 capsules of konjac instead of 6 capsules of psyllium before lunch are much to be desired. However, noodles made from konjac are available in the refrigerated case of some Asian stores. Including them in a meal instead of regular pasta or noodles satisfies the need for soluble fiber.

6. Focused on Fish

I have tried to make my primary source of protein fish instead of meat or poultry. Due to concerns about mercury, I prefer to eat fish that is not farm-raised. Fatty fish, like salmon (the wild Pacific Ocean kind), mackerel, and bluefish have the added advantage of omega-3 fish oil. Almost any fish is good, and I see no need to limit its consumption to once or twice a week if I am careful to avoid mercury poisoning.

7. Drank Green Tea

Unsweetened green tea, brewed and drunk hot, suppresses my appetite and reduces my craving for sweets and snacks outside of meals. Since it also contains antioxidants, it may contribute to lowering my LDL cholesterol. The Japanese drink copious amounts of it and rarely have elevated LDL cholesterol. Because it has caffeine (but less than coffee has), I have to let up on drinking it late in the day. Occasionally I consider giving up coffee and just drinking green tea, but I love my morning coffee too much to become a complete convert to green tea.

8. Consumed Other Antioxidants

I took recommendations from a selection of sources for healthy foods to add to my diet or to eat more of.

Eating cruciferous vegetables was a recommendation that appeared in many sources. The list of cruciferous vegetables I used was this: cabbage, broccoli, cauliflower, kale, watercress, brussels sprouts, bok choy, collards, turnips and turnip greens, and rutabaga. One of my favorite new items is shredded raw brussels sprouts dressed with vinegar and olive oil.

Other "super" foods appearing on many health-oriented lists include berries, nuts and seeds (like sunflower seeds), winter squash, beans, tomatoes, and kiwifruit.

9. Stopped Eating before Bed

Late-evening snacks just before bedtime seem inherently dangerous to cholesterol levels. If I eat just before going to bed, then surely I am taking in energy that I won't need while sleeping. Excess intake of energy requires my body to manufacture cholesterol to carry it to its storage site.

Sometimes I need that late-night snack anyway. I make it light but high in protein and hope I have done enough other good things to carry me through.

INDEX

<u>Underscored</u> page references indicate boxed text. **Boldface** references indicate main discussion of medical conditions.

A

CRP. *See* C-reactive protein
Cruciferous vegetables, for cholesterol reduction, 471
Culturelle, for gas, 195
Curcumin, 11, 92–93, 94, 450, 457, 458
Cymbalta, 132, 135
Cytomel, 321, 322, 326
Cytotec, for tinnitus, 401–2, <u>401</u>

D

Dalmane, 336
Dandruff, **121–29**, 454, 455, 462
DASH diet, for blood pressure reduction, 286, <u>286</u>, 287, 306
Daypro, 296
Decongestants
   for allergies, 63–64
   prostate enlargement and, 56, 64
   sleep problems from, 328
Dehumidification, for reducing allergens, 53, 64
Dehydration, leg cramps from, 342
Dementia, 141, 253, 282
Denorex, 126
Depo-Provera, 359
Depression, **129–43**
   causes of
      beta-blockers, 299
      progesterone, 358, 360
      reserpine, 282, 300
      tinnitus, 396, 402
      Zocor, 269
   diabetes and, 161
   signs of, 129, <u>130</u>
   treatments for
      drug, 131–38, 142–43
      nondrug, 138–42, 143
      old-time, 130–31
Dermatitis
   atopic (*see* Eczema)
   seborrheic, 122, 126, 128, 455
Desipramine, 131, 138
Desloratadine, 60
Dexatrim, 408
Dexfenfluramine, 410
Dextromethorphan, 115, 118, 120
Diabetes, **143–65**
   complications from, 143, 144
   controlling, with
      drugs, 161–65
      nondrug approaches, 152–53, 155–61, 165
   curcumin and, 93

description of, 143, 144
drug-induced, 153, <u>154</u>, 155
incidence of, 144
nail fungus and, 372, 373, 382
possible causes of, 144–45
preventing, 39, 145–52, 165, 249
risk factors for, 145
Diarrhea, coconut for, 450–51
Diazepam, 12, 160, 219, 333
Diclofenac
   acupuncture and, 99
   side effects of, 7–8, 68, 75, 296
   topical, 76, 77, <u>78</u>
Diet. *See also* Low-carb diet; Low-fat diet
   heartburn and, 219–20
   for prevention of
      diabetes, 39, 145–49, 165
      heart disease, 39
   for treatment of
      acne, 38–40, 49
      arthritis, 79, 83
      constipation, 103, 105–8, 111, 112, 113
      diabetes, 155
      eczema, 167–72
      high blood pressure, 286–87
      high cholesterol, 238–41, <u>262</u>, 263–64, <u>263</u>, 277, 467–71
   for weight loss, 403, 404–5, 411
Dietary diary
   for heartburn sufferers, 220
   for weight loss, 405–6, <u>405</u>, 411
Diet pills, 407–11
Dilantin, vs. generic phenytoin, 12–13, 25
Diltiazem, 305
Dimetane, 60
Dimetapp, 60
Diovan, 348
Diphenhydramine
   for allergies, 60, 61
   in cough medicine, 120
   for insomnia, 335, 340
Disprin, 73
Diuretics
   blood sugar increased by, 153
   for high blood pressure, 4–5, 300–303, <u>300</u>, 306
   mineral depletion from, 261, 292, 302, <u>302</u>, 348
Divalproex, for migraines, 213
Docusate calcium, 110
Docusate sodium, 110, <u>110</u>, 113
Doxazosin, 5, 300, 301
Doxepin, 131
Doxycycline, 44

Relaxation techniques
    for headaches, 203, 217
    for insomnia, 329–30, 341
ReliOn blood pressure monitor, 280
Remifemin, for hot flashes, 360, 360, 364, 371
Repaglinide, 161, 164, 165
Replens, for vaginal dryness, 367
Reserpine, 282, 300
Resorcinol, 43
RESPeRATE, for blood pressure control, 285, 285
Restless leg syndrome, 331
Restoril, 333, 335, 336
Retin-A, 44, 44, 49
Revlimid, 16
Rheumatrex, 76
Riboflavin, for migraines, 205–6, 217
Richardson, Lunsford, 376
Rimonabant, 287, 410–11, 411
Risedronate, 189, 328, 390
Ritalin, 19
Rofecoxib, 7
Rolaids Extra Strength, 229
Rosemary, for dandruff, 125–26, 125, 128
Rosiglitazone, 164
Rosuvastatin, 10, 189, 238, 267
Rozerem, 337, 338–39, 339
Rutabaga, for hemorrhoids, 456

S

SAD, 139
Sage, for dandruff, 125–26, 125, 128
Salicylic acid, 43
Saline, for nose cleaning, 54–55, 64
Saliva, for heartburn relief, 222–23, 222, 236
Salmeterol, 8–9
Salsa, for eczema, 170–71, 171, 179
Salsalate, for arthritis, 74, 74
Salt, for foot odor, 182, 186
Salt restriction, blood pressure and, 287–88
SAM-e, for arthritis, 98
Sears Kenmore vacuum cleaner, 54
Seasonal affective disorder (SAD), 139
Seborrheic dermatitis, 122, 126, 128, 455
Sebulex, 126
Selective serotonin reuptake inhibitors (SSRIs)
    efficacy rate of, 6, 6
    homicidal ideation from, 133, 134
    for hot flashes, 363, 371
    STAR*D trial on, 134–35

suicide and, 8, 132–34, 142
    vs. tricyclic antidepressants, 131–32
Selegiline patch, 141–42, 143
Selenium
    for arthritis, 79–80, 80, 326
    for thyroid function, 324, 325
Selsun Blue, 126
Serax, 335
Serevent, 8
Serostim, 28
Sertraline, 21, 132, 135, 189, 328
Serutan, 109
Serzone, 132, 136
Sex headaches, 215–16, 217
Shampoos, dandruff, 122, 127–128, 129
Shingles, Listerine for, 455
Shoes, for reducing foot odor, 181, 186
Side effects, xviii, 7, 10–11, 31. See also specific drugs
Sildenafil, 26
Simethicone, for gas, 193
Simvastatin, 10, 21, 189, 238, 257, 264, 267, 269
Sinequan, 131
Singulair, 57, 62–63
Sinus cleaning, neti pot for, 54–55, 64
Sitz bath, for hemorrhoids, 456
Skin cleansers, for acne, 41, 49
Sleeping pills, 333, 336–40, 341
Sleep problems. See Insomnia
Smart Balance, 242
Soap under sheets, for leg cramps, 342–43, 342, 351
Social interaction, for blood pressure control, 286, 306
Socks, for foot odor, 181, 186
Soda, high blood pressure and, 288–89, 306
Sodium bicarbonate. See Baking soda
Sodium restriction, blood pressure and, 287–88
Somatropin, 28
Sonata, 337, 339–40, 339
Sotalol, 20
Sotret, 47, 49
Soup
    chicken, for cough, 114, 116–17, 120, 121
    spicy, for migraines, 209, 210, 217
Soy isoflavones, for preventing menstrual migraines, 214–15
Soy products
    for hot flashes, 360–61, 361, 371
    thyroid function and, 323–24, 326
Spicy soup, for migraines, 209, 210, 217
Spironolactone
    for acne, 46, 49
    for high blood pressure, 302, 305–6, 348

ABOUT THE AUTHORS

JOE GRAEDON, MS

Joe Graedon received his BS from Pennsylvania State University in 1967 and went on to do research on mental illness, sleep, and basic brain physiology at the New Jersey Neuropsychiatric Institute in Princeton. In 1971 he received his MS in pharmacology from the University of Michigan. Joe was conferred the degree of Doctor of Humane Letters *honoris causa* from Long Island University in 2006 as one of the country's leading drug experts for the consumer.

Joe has lectured at the Duke University School of Nursing, the University of California, San Francisco (UCSF) School of Pharmacy, and the University of North Carolina School of Pharmacy. He taught pharmacology at the School of Medicine of the Universidad Autonoma "Benito Juarez" of Oaxaca, Mexico, from 1971 to 1974. He served as a consultant to the Federal Trade Commission on over-the-counter drug issues from 1978 to 1983 and was on the Advisory Board for the Drug Studies Unit at UCSF from 1983 to

1989. He has been an adjunct assistant professor, Division of Pharmacotherapy and Experimental Therapeutics, School of Pharmacy, University of North Carolina (UNC) at Chapel Hill since 1986 and was a member of the National Policy Advisory Board for the UNC Center for Education and Research on Therapeutics (CERTS). He is a member of the American Association for the Advancement of Science (AAAS), the Society for Neuroscience, and the New York Academy of Science.

Joe has served as an editorial advisor to *Men's Health Newsletter*. He was elected to the rank of AAAS Fellow for "exceptional contribution to the communication of the rational use of pharmaceutical products and an understanding of health issues to the public" in 2005. Joe is an advisory board member of the American Botanical Council (Herbalgram) and he has served as a member of the Board of Visitors, University of North Carolina at Chapel Hill School of Pharmacy, since 1989.

Joe's features on health and pharmaceuticals have been syndicated nationally to public television stations via Intraregional Program Service member exchange. A TV pledge special was underwritten by PBS in 1998. He is considered one of the country's leading drug experts for consumers and speaks frequently on issues of pharmaceuticals, nutrition, herbs, home remedies, and self-care. He has appeared as a guest on many major US national television shows, including *Dateline, 20/20*, the *Geraldo Rivera Show*, the *Oprah Winfrey Show, Live with Regis and Kathie Lee, Today, Good Morning America, CBS Morning News, NBC Nightly News with Tom Brokaw, Extra*, the *Phil Donahue Show*, and the *Tonight Show with Johnny Carson*.

TERESA GRAEDON, PhD

Medical anthropologist Teresa Graedon is a best-selling author, syndicated newspaper columnist, and award-winning internationally syndicated radio talk-show host. Teresa Graedon received her AB from Bryn Mawr College in 1969, graduating magna cum laude with a major in anthropology. She attended graduate school at the University of Michigan, receiving her AM in 1971. She received a fellowship from the Institute for Environmental Quality (1972–1975), which enabled her to pursue doctoral research on health and nutritional status in a migrant community in Oaxaca, Mexico. Her doctorate was awarded in 1976.

Teresa taught at the Duke University School of Nursing with an adjunct appointment in the Department of Anthropology from 1975 to 1979. Since that time she has periodically taught courses in medical anthropology and international health at Duke University. From 1982 to 1983 she pursued postdoctoral training in medical anthropology at the University of California, San Francisco.

Teresa is a member of the Society for Applied Anthropology, the American Anthropological Association, and the Society for Medical Anthropology. She has served on the Foundation Board of the University of North Carolina School of Nursing.

JOE AND TERRY

For over a decade Joe and Terry contributed a regular column on self-medication for Tom Ferguson, MD's magazine, *Medical Self-Care*. Their thrice-weekly newspaper column, *The People's Pharmacy*, has been syndicated nationally by King Features Syndicate since 1978. Circulation of client papers exceeds 6 million. The *People's Pharmacy* radio show won a Silver Award from the Corporation for Public Broadcasting in 1992. It is syndicated to hundreds of radio stations in the United States and around the world on public radio and the In Touch Radio Reading Service. In 2003 Joe and Teresa received the Alvarez Award at the 63rd annual conference of the American Medical Writers Association for "excellence in medical communications."

Joe and Terry were charter members of the North Carolina Consortium of Natural Medicine and Public Health and served on the Consortium Executive Committee in 2003. They are members of the Patient Safety and Quality Assurance Committee of the Duke University Health System Board of Directors. Joe and Terry serve on the Patient Advocacy Council of Duke University Health System.

The Graedons have coauthored the following books: *The People's Pharmacy-2* (Avon, 1980), *Joe Graedon's The New People's Pharmacy: Drug Breakthroughs for the '80s* (Bantam, 1985), *The People's Pharmacy, Totally New and Revised* (St. Martin's Press, 1985), *50+: The Graedons' People's Pharmacy for Older Adults* (Bantam, 1988), *Graedons' Best Medicine: From Herbal Remedies to High-Tech Rx Breakthroughs* (Bantam, 1991), *The Aspirin Handbook: A User's Guide to the Breakthrough Drug of the '90s* (Bantam, 1993), *The People's Guide to Deadly Drug Interactions* (St. Martin's Press, 1995; 1997), *The People's Pharmacy, Completely New and Revised* (1996, 1998) and *The People's Pharmacy Guide to Home and Herbal Remedies* (St. Martin's Press, 1999). Total books in print exceed 2 million. Terry and Joe contributed a chapter on over-the-counter medications to *The Merck Manual of Medical Information Home Edition* (1997) and to *Health Care Choices for Today's Consumer: Guide to Quality and Cost* (1997).

Terry and Joe were presented with the America Talks Health "Health Headliner of 1998" award for "superior contribution to the advancement of medicine and public health education." Together they have been designated Ambassadors Plenipotentiary by the City of Medicine, Durham, North Carolina, where they live. You can communicate with the Graedons through their Web site, www.peoplespharmacy.com.

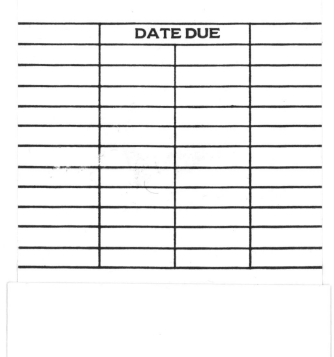

DATE DUE

WITHDRAWN